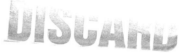

SEAFOOD CHOICES
BALANCING BENEFITS AND RISKS

Committee on Nutrient Relationships in Seafood:
Selections to Balance Benefits and Risks
Food and Nutrition Board

Maldon C. Nesheim and Ann L. Yaktine, *Editors*

INSTITUTE OF MEDICINE
OF THE NATIONAL ACADEMIES

THE NATIONAL ACADEMIES PRESS
Washington, D.C.
www.nap.edu

THE NATIONAL ACADEMIES PRESS   500 Fifth Street, N.W.   Washington, DC 20001

NOTICE: The project that is the subject of this report was approved by the Governing Board of the National Research Council, whose members are drawn from the councils of the National Academy of Sciences, the National Academy of Engineering, and the Institute of Medicine. The members of the committee responsible for the report were chosen for their special competences and with regard for appropriate balance.

The study was supported by Contract No. DG133R04CQ0009 TO #8 between the National Academy of Sciences and the Department of Commerce, and Contract No. 223-01-2460 TO #29 between the National Academy of Sciences and the U.S. Food and Drug Administration. Any opinions, findings, conclusions, or recommendations expressed in this publication are those of the authors and do not necessarily reflect the views of the organizations or agencies that provided support for the project.

Library of Congress Cataloging-in-Publication Data

Seafood choices : balancing benefits and risks/Committee on Nutrient Relationships in Seafood: Selections to Balance Benefits and Risks, Food and Nutrition Board ; Malden C. Nesheim, and Ann L. Yaktine, editors.
    p. ; cm.
  Includes bibliographical references and index.
  The study was supported by Contract No. DG133R04CQ0009 TO #8 between the National Academy of Sciences and the Department of Commerce, and Contract No. 223-01-2460 TO #29 between the National Academy of Sciences and the U.S. Food and Drug Administration.
  ISBN-13: 978-0-309-10218-6 (hardback)
  ISBN-10: 0-309-10218-9 (hardback)
  1. Seafood—Health aspects. 2. Seafood poisoning. I. Nesheim, Malden C. II. Yaktine, Ann L. III. Institute of Medicine (U.S.). Committee on Nutrient Relationships in Seafood: Selections to Balance Benefits and Risk.
  [DNLM: 1. Seafood—standards. 2. Consumer Participation. 3. Food Contamination. 4. Nutritive Value. 5. Risk Assessment. WB 426 S438 2007]
  RA602.F5.S428 2007
  363.19'29—dc22
                                                                    2006035748

Additional copies of this report are available from the National Academies Press, 500 Fifth Street, N.W., Lockbox 285, Washington, DC 20055; (800) 624-6242 or (202) 334-3313 (in the Washington metropolitan area); Internet, http://www.nap.edu.

For more information about the Institute of Medicine, visit the IOM home page at: **www. iom.edu.**

The serpent has been a symbol of long life, healing, and knowledge among almost all cultures and religions since the beginning of recorded history. The serpent adopted as a logotype by the Institute of Medicine is a relief carving from ancient Greece, now held by the Staatliche Museen in Berlin.

"Knowing is not enough; we must apply.
Willing is not enough; we must do."
—Goethe

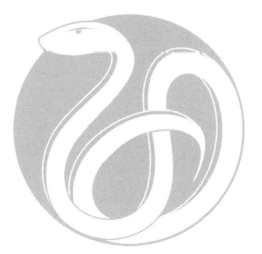

INSTITUTE OF MEDICINE
OF THE NATIONAL ACADEMIES

Advising the Nation. Improving Health.

THE NATIONAL ACADEMIES
Advisers to the Nation on Science, Engineering, and Medicine

The **National Academy of Sciences** is a private, nonprofit, self-perpetuating society of distinguished scholars engaged in scientific and engineering research, dedicated to the furtherance of science and technology and to their use for the general welfare. Upon the authority of the charter granted to it by the Congress in 1863, the Academy has a mandate that requires it to advise the federal government on scientific and technical matters. Dr. Ralph J. Cicerone is president of the National Academy of Sciences.

The **National Academy of Engineering** was established in 1964, under the charter of the National Academy of Sciences, as a parallel organization of outstanding engineers. It is autonomous in its administration and in the selection of its members, sharing with the National Academy of Sciences the responsibility for advising the federal government. The National Academy of Engineering also sponsors engineering programs aimed at meeting national needs, encourages education and research, and recognizes the superior achievements of engineers. Dr. Wm. A. Wulf is president of the National Academy of Engineering.

The **Institute of Medicine** was established in 1970 by the National Academy of Sciences to secure the services of eminent members of appropriate professions in the examination of policy matters pertaining to the health of the public. The Institute acts under the responsibility given to the National Academy of Sciences by its congressional charter to be an adviser to the federal government and, upon its own initiative, to identify issues of medical care, research, and education. Dr. Harvey V. Fineberg is president of the Institute of Medicine.

The **National Research Council** was organized by the National Academy of Sciences in 1916 to associate the broad community of science and technology with the Academy's purposes of furthering knowledge and advising the federal government. Functioning in accordance with general policies determined by the Academy, the Council has become the principal operating agency of both the National Academy of Sciences and the National Academy of Engineering in providing services to the government, the public, and the scientific and engineering communities. The Council is administered jointly by both Academies and the Institute of Medicine. Dr. Ralph J. Cicerone and Dr. Wm. A. Wulf are chair and vice chair, respectively, of the National Research Council.

www.national-academies.org

Independent Report Reviewers

This report has been reviewed in draft form by individuals chosen for their diverse perspectives and technical expertise, in accordance with procedures approved by the National Research Council's Report Review Committee. The purpose of this independent review is to provide candid and critical comments that will assist the institution in making its published report as sound as possible and to ensure that the report meets institutional standards for objectivity, evidence, and responsiveness to the study charge. The review comments and draft manuscript remain confidential to protect the integrity of the deliberative process. We wish to thank the following individuals for their review of this report:

Henry B. Chin, The Coca-Cola Company, Atlanta, GA

Rebecca Goldburg, Environmental Defense, New York

Scott M. Grundy, The University of Texas Southwestern Medical Center at Dallas, TX

Sheila M. Innis, University of British Columbia, Vancouver, Canada

Lester Lave, Graduate School of Industrial Administration, Carnegie Mellon University, Pittsburgh, PA

Robert S. Lawrence, Johns Hopkins Bloomberg School of Public Health, Baltimore, MD

Alice Lichtenstein, Jean Mayer USDA Human Nutrition Research Center on Aging, Tufts University, Boston, MA

Barbara J. Petersen, Exponent, Inc., Washington, DC

Hildegard Przyrembel, Federal Institute for Risk Assessment, Berlin, Germany

Nadine R. Sahyoun, Center on Aging, University of Maryland, College Park, MD

Sally E. Shaywitz, Yale University School of Medicine, New Haven, CT

Alan Stern, Bureau of Risk Analysis, Division of Science and Research and Technology, New Jersey Department of Environmental Protection, Trenton

Michael R. Taylor, University of Maryland School of Medicine, Baltimore, MD

Although the reviewers listed above have provided many constructive comments and suggestions, they were not asked to endorse the conclusions or recommendations nor did they see the final draft of the report before its release. The review of this report was overseen by **Johanna T. Dwyer,** Tufts University School of Medicine and Friedman School of Nutrition Science & Policy and Tufts–New England Medical Center and **Catherine E. Woteki,** Mars, Inc. Appointed by the National Research Council and Institute of Medicine, they were responsible for making certain that an independent examination of this report was carried out in accordance with institutional procedures and that all review comments were carefully considered. Responsibility for the final content of this report rests entirely with the authoring committee and the institution.

Preface

When I was growing up, fish were considered "brain food." I was told that eating fish was good for you and would make you smart. Amazingly, there now is some evidence that this old food lore may have some scientific basis, as mothers who consume seafood may provide benefits to the developing fetal nervous system from fatty acids in the seafood. It is not clear, however, whether this will make you smarter as an adult.

Seafood is a good source of high-quality protein, is low in saturated fat, and is rich in many micronutrients. Seafood is also a major source of the long-chain polyunsaturated omega-3 fatty acids eicosapentaenoic acid (EPA) and docosahexaenoic acid (DHA), which are synthesized in limited amounts by the human body from alpha-linolenic acid (ALA), an omega-3 fatty acid found in several vegetable, nut, and seed oils. Though these fatty acids are found in other foods, some seafood is an unusually rich source. In the past several years, research has implicated seafood and/or EPA and DHA in an array of health benefits for the developing fetus, infants, and also for adults, especially those prone to heart disease. This has led to recommendations by several health authorities to include seafood in a healthy diet.

Seafood is the only animal protein food that is still provided in significant amounts to human diets through capture of wild species. Though our oceans are being depleted of some wild species, and aquaculture has become an important source of seafood, wild capture still provides a significant portion of the seafood we consume. The pollution of our oceans both through natural processes and practices of an increasingly industrialized world raise concern about the contaminants found in our seafood supply. As aquaculture of some species also uses fish meal and fish oil produced from captured wild sources, farmed seafood is not free from potential risks of further reducing ocean stocks or from potential contaminants. As consumption of seafood rises, there has been an increasing awareness of the potential risks from seafood consumption due to the presence of microbial contaminants; persistent organic pollutants; and heavy metals, especially mercury, in our oceans and inland waters.

Consumers are therefore confronted with a dilemma: they are told that seafood is good for them and should be consumed in larger amounts than current consumption, while at the same time the federal government and virtually all the state governments have issued advisories urging caution in consumption of fish of certain species or from specific waters. Clearly, it should be an environmental priority to eliminate the sources of contamination of this important component of our food supply so that such a contradiction is avoided.

The National Oceanic and Atmospheric Administration (NOAA) provides federal leadership in marine science and conservation. The seafood industry contributes a large part of the nation's economic health, and as an agency of the US Department of Commerce, NOAA works to advance fisheries management policies and programs to ensure that fishery resources are healthy and sustainable so that they will remain a safe, nutritious, and affordable component of the US food supply. In light of these considerations, NOAA recognized the need for an independent group to examine the scientific evidence on the nutritional benefits obtained from seafood balanced against potential risks from exposure to contaminants, and ways to guide US consumers to make selections appropriate to their needs. Thus, NOAA asked the Institute of Medicine (IOM) to convene a committee with a diverse background and a broad scope of expertise to address the task put before them.

The committee was charged to identify and prioritize adverse health effects from both naturally occurring and introduced toxicants in seafood; assess evidence on availability of specific nutrients in seafood compared to other food sources; determine the impact of modifying food choices to reduce intake of naturally occurring and introduced toxicants on nutrient intake and nutritional status within the US population; develop a decision path for US consumers to balance their seafood choices to obtain nutritional benefits while minimizing exposure risks; and identify data gaps and recommend future research. The committee's report recommends approaches to decision-making for selecting seafood to obtain the greatest nutritional benefits balanced against exposure to potential toxicants, and identifies data gaps and research needs. The committee concentrated on issues affecting marine species and has not dealt in detail with freshwater fisheries.

The task has not been an easy one. The committee reviewed the existing literature on benefits of seafood consumption and has attempted to make judgments as to the strength of the evidence. In many cases, we have deemed the evidence for benefit insufficient or too preliminary. Similarly, the committee reviewed the data on contaminants and risks they imply. We were surprised at the lack of good data on the distribution of some contaminants in the seafood supply. There is likewise little available evidence as to how beneficial effects of seafood may counteract some of the risks from contaminants.

The committee also considered how consumers make decisions as to what they eat and tried to advise on how to approach the task of communicating benefits and risks to consumers. We have not regarded it the committee's task to set specific dietary standards for seafood or EPA/DHA consumption and we have considered our findings in the light of the dietary recommendations of the Dietary Guidelines Advisory Committee as well as other authoritative groups.

The Committee on Nutrient Relationships in Seafood was made up of committed members with widely varied expertise who volunteered countless hours to the research, deliberations, and preparation of the report. Many other individuals volunteered significant time and effort to address and educate our committee members during the first open session, workshop, and through consultations, and we are grateful for their contributions.

The report could not have been produced without the dedicated guidance and expertise of the study director, Ann Yaktine, and her colleagues; Cara James, research associate; and Sandra Amamoo-Kakra, senior program assistant. We also thank Geraldine Kennedo for administrative support, Greg Fulco for graphic design, and Hilary Ray for technical and copy editing. This project benefited from the support and wisdom of Linda Meyers, director of the Food and Nutrition Board.

Malden C. Nesheim, *Chair*
Committee on Nutrient Relationships in Seafood

Contents

APPENDIXES

Summary

Seafood (referring in this report to all commercially obtained fish, shellfish, and mollusks, both marine and freshwater) is a nutrient-rich food source that is widely available to most Americans. It is a good source of high-quality protein, is low in saturated fat, and is rich in many micronutrients. Seafood is often also a rich source of the preformed long-chain polyunsaturated omega-3 fatty acids eicosapentaenoic acid (EPA) and docosahexaenoic acid (DHA), which are synthesized in limited amounts by the human body from alpha-linolenic acid (ALA), a fatty acid found in several vegetable, nut, and seed oils (e.g., walnut and flaxseed oils). In the past several years, research has implicated seafood, particularly its contribution of EPA and DHA, in various health benefits identified for the developing fetus and infants, and also for adults, including those at risk for cardiovascular disease. Contamination of aquatic food sources, however, whether by naturally-occurring or introduced toxicants, is a concern for US consumers because of adverse health effects that have been associated with exposure to such compounds. Methylmercury can accumulate in the lean tissue of seafood, particularly large, predatory species such as swordfish, certain shark, tilefish, and king mackerel. Lipophilic compounds such as dioxins and polychlorinated biphenyls (PCBs) can be found in the fatty tissue of some fish. High levels of particular microbial pathogens may be present during certain seasons in various geographic areas, which can compromise the safety of products commonly eaten raw, such as oysters. Additionally, some population groups have been identified as being at greater risk from exposure to certain contaminants in seafood.

In consideration of these issues, the US Department of Commerce,

1

National Oceanic and Atmospheric Administration (NOAA) asked the Institute of Medicine (IOM) of the National Academies to examine relationships between benefits and risks associated with seafood consumption to help consumers make informed choices. The expert committee was asked to prioritize the potential for adverse health effects from both naturally occurring and introduced toxicants in seafood, assess evidence on availability of specific nutrients in seafood compared to other food sources, determine the impact of modifying food choices to reduce intake of naturally occurring and introduced toxicants on nutrient intake and nutritional status within the US population, develop a decision path for US consumers to weigh their seafood choices to obtain nutritional benefits balanced against exposure risks, and identify data gaps and recommend future research.

The committee concentrated primarily on seafood derived from marine (saltwater) sources and included freshwater fisheries when appropriate to the discussion. Further, the committee recognized that these sources vary greatly in their level of contamination depending on local conditions, and that individual states have issued a large number of advisories based on assessment of local conditions. Although the committee was not asked to consider questions or make recommendations about environmental concerns related to seafood, it recognizes that the impact of changes in seafood production, harvesting, and processing have important environmental consequences.

To address the task of assessing benefit-risk trade-offs, the committee took a three-step approach. The steps that framed this analytical approach were: (1) analysis and balancing of the benefits and risks (including attention to characteristics that distinguish target populations as well as substitution predictions); (2) analysis of consumer perceptions and decision-making (understanding decision contexts and their variability, and assessing consumers' behavior regarding how they perceive and make choices); and (3) design and evaluation of the decision support program itself (including format and structure of information, media, and combination of communication products and processes). The aim of the analysis in step 1 is to assess the overall effect of seafood selections rather than the assessment of reduction in a specific risk or enhancement of a specific benefit.

ANALYSIS OF THE BALANCING OF BENEFITS AND RISKS OF SEAFOOD CONSUMPTION

The scientific assessment and balancing of the benefits and risks associated with seafood consumption is a complex task. Diverse evidence, of varying levels of completeness and uncertainty, on different types of benefits and risks must be combined to carry out the assessment required as a first step in designing consumer guidance. In light of the uncertainty in the available scientific information associated with both nutrient intake and contaminant exposure from seafood, no summary metric adequately captures the complexity of seafood benefit/risk trade-offs. Thus, the committee developed a four-part qualitative protocol adapted from previous work (IOM, 2003) to evaluate and balance benefits and risks. Following the protocol, the committee considered consumption patterns of seafood; the scope of the benefits and risks associated with different patterns of consumption for the population as a whole and, if appropriate, for specific target populations; and changes in benefits and risks associated with changes in consumption patterns. It then balanced the benefits and risks to come to specific guidance for healthy consumption for the population as a whole, and, as appropriate, for specific target populations.

Consumption of Seafood in the United States

Seafood consumption has increased over the past century, reaching a level of more than 16 pounds per person per year in 2003. The ten types of seafood consumed in the greatest quantities among the US general population (from highest to lowest) are shrimp, canned tuna, salmon, pollock, catfish, tilapia, crab, cod, clams, and flatfish (e.g., flounder and sole). The nation's seafood supply is changing, however, and this may have a significant impact on seafood choices in the future. The preference among consumers for marine types of seafood is leading to supply deficits, and seafood produced by aquaculture is replacing captured supplies for several of these types.

While seafood is recognized as a primary source of the omega-3 long-chain polyunsaturated fatty acids EPA and DHA, not all seafood is rich in these fatty acids. Among types of seafood, shrimp and canned light tuna are the two most commonly consumed, and they are not especially high in EPA and DHA. Eggs and chicken, although not particularly rich sources,[1] may contribute to the EPA and DHA content of the US diet because of their frequent consumption. Relative to other foods in the meat, poultry, fish, and eggs group, however, seafood is generally lower in saturated fatty acids and higher in EPA, DHA, and selenium, all of which have been associated with health benefits.

Primary Findings

1. Average quantities of seafood consumed by the general US population, and by several specific population groups, are below levels suggested by

---

[1]Because of changes in feed composition the current levels of EPA/DHA in chicken and eggs may be less than that reported in food databases.

many authoritative groups, including levels recommended by the American Heart Association for cardiovascular disease prevention; and

2. For many ethnic and geographic subgroups, there are insufficient data to characterize the intake levels of seafood, EPA, DHA, and other dietary constituents, and to assess the variability of those intakes.

Benefits Associated with Nutrients from Seafood

The high nutritional quality of seafood makes it an important component of a healthy diet. While protein is an important macronutrient in the diet, most Americans already consume enough and do not need to increase their intake. Fats and oils are also part of a healthful diet, but the type and amount of fat can be important—for example, with regard to cardiovascular disease. Many Americans consume greater than recommended amounts of saturated fat as well as cholesterol from high-fat protein foods such as beef and pork. Many seafood selections are lower in total and saturated fats and cholesterol than some more frequently selected animal protein foods such as fatty cuts of beef, pork, and poultry, and are equivalent in amount of fat to some leaner cuts of meat. Since it is lower in saturated fats, however, by substituting seafood more often for other animal foods, consumers can decrease their overall intake of both total and saturated fats while retaining the nutritional quality of other protein food choices.

Seafood is also a primary source of EPA and DHA in the American diet. The contribution of these nutrients to improving health and reducing risk for certain chronic diseases in adults has not been completely elucidated. There is evidence, however, to suggest there are benefits to the developing infant, such as increasing length of gestation, improved visual acuity, and improved cognitive development. In addition, there is evidence to support an overall benefit to the general population for reduced risk of heart disease among those who eat seafood compared to those who do not, and there may be benefits from consuming EPA and DHA for adults at risk for coronary heart disease.

Primary Findings

1. Seafood is a nutrient-rich food that makes a positive contribution to a healthful diet. It is a good source of protein, and relative to other protein foods, e.g., meat, poultry, and eggs, is generally lower in saturated fatty acids and higher in the omega-3 fatty acids EPA and DHA as well as selenium;

2. The evidence to support benefits to pregnancy outcome in females who consume seafood or fish-oil supplements as part of their diet during pregnancy is derived largely from observational studies. Clinical trials and epidemiological studies have also shown an association between increased

duration of gestation and intake of seafood or fish-oil supplements. Evidence that the infants and children of mothers who consume seafood or EPA/DHA supplements during pregnancy and/or lactation may have improved developmental outcomes is also supported largely by observational studies;

3. Observational evidence suggests that increased seafood consumption is associated with a decreased risk of cardiovascular deaths and cardiovascular events in the general population. Evidence is insufficient to assess if this association is mediated through an increase in EPA and DHA consumption and/or a decrease in saturated fat consumption and/or other correlates of seafood consumption;

4. Evidence is inconsistent for protection against further cardiovascular events in individuals with a history of myocardial infarction from consumption of EPA/DHA-containing seafood or fish-oil supplements. The protection evidenced by population (observational) studies has not been consistently observed in randomized clinical trials; and

5. Evidence for a benefit associated with seafood consumption or fish-oil supplements on blood pressure, stroke, cancer, asthma, type II diabetes, or Alzheimer's disease is inconclusive. Whereas observational studies have suggested a protective role of EPA/DHA for each of these diseases, supportive evidence from randomized clinical trials is either nonexistent or inconclusive.

Risks Associated with Seafood

The safety of seafood in the US has increased in recent decades, although there are still a number of chemical and microbial hazards that are present in seafood. Whether a contaminant poses a health risk to consumers depends on the amount present in the food and the potential outcome from exposure. Consumers are exposed to a complex mixture of dietary and non-dietary contaminants. However, most studies of the risks associated with seafood focus on one contaminant at a time rather than a mixture. The extent to which such coexposures might affect the toxicity of seafoodborne contaminants is largely unknown. Similarly, few data are available on the extent to which beneficial components of seafood, such as selenium, might mitigate the risks associated with seafoodborne contaminants. The evidence reviewed indicates that the levels of different contaminants in seafood depend on several factors such as species, size, location, age, and feed source. Levels of some contaminants in seafood vary substantially due to their geographic localization; areas of highest variation tend to be mostly freshwater.

Consumption of aquatic foods is the major route of human exposure to methylmercury (MeHg). The seafood choices a consumer makes and the frequency with which different species are consumed are thus important determinants of methylmercury intake. Exposure to MeHg among US consumers in general is a concern because there is uncertainty about the potential for subtle adverse health outcomes. Since the most sensitive sub-group of the population to MeHg exposure is the developing fetus, intake recommendations are developed for and directed to the pregnant woman rather than to the general population.

Persistent organic pollutants (POPs), including dioxins and PCBs, can be found in the fatty tissue of all animal-derived foods, including seafood. Exposure to these compounds among the general population has been de-creasing in recent decades. The greatest concern is for population groups exposed to POPs in seafood obtained through cultural, subsistence, or recreational fishing, because of reliance on fish from locations that may pose a greater risk.

In contrast to heavy metal contaminants and POPs, the number of re-ported illnesses from seafoodborne microbial contaminants has remained steady over the past several decades. Exposure to *vibrio* and *norovirus* infec-tions is still a concern, however, because they continue to be associated with consumption of raw molluscan shellfish. Strategies for minimizing the risk of seafoodborne illnesses are, to some extent, hazard-specific, but overall include avoiding types of seafood identified as being more likely to contain certain contaminants, and following general food safety guidelines, which include proper cooking.

Primary Findings

1. Levels of contaminants in seafood depend on several factors, includ-ing species, size, harvest location, age, and composition of feed. MeHg is the seafoodborne contaminant for which the most exposure and toxicity data are available; levels of MeHg in seafood have not changed substantially in recent decades. Exposure to dioxins and PCBs varies by location and vulnerable subgroups (e.g., some American Indian/Alaskan Native groups living near contaminated waters) may be at increased risk. Microbial illness from seafood is acute, persistent, and a potentially serious risk, although incidence of illness has not increased in recent decades.

2. Considerable uncertainties are associated with estimates of the health risks to the general population from exposures to methylmercury and persis-tent organic pollutants at levels present in commercially obtained seafood. The available evidence to assess risks to the US population is incomplete and useful to only a limited extent.

3. Consumers are exposed to a complex mixture of dietary and non-dietary contaminants whereas most studies of risks associated with seafood focus on a single contaminant.

Balancing Benefits and Risks

From its review of consumption, benefits, and risks, the committee recommends that:

Recommendation 1: Dietary advice to the general population from federal agencies should emphasize that seafood is a component of a healthy diet, particularly as it can displace other protein sources higher in saturated fat. Seafood can favorably substitute for other high biologic value protein sources while often improving the overall nutrient profile of the diet.

Recommendation 2: Although advice from federal agencies should also support inclusion of seafood in the diets of pregnant females or those who may become pregnant, any consumption advice should stay within federal advisories for specific seafood types and state advisories for locally caught fish.

Recommendation 3: Appropriate federal agencies (the National Oceanic and Atmospheric Administration [NOAA], the US Environmental Protection Agency [USEPA], and the Food and Drug Administration of the US Department of Health and Human Services [FDA]) **should increase monitoring of methylmercury and persistent organic pollutants in seafood and make the resulting information readily available to the general public.** Along with this information, these agencies should develop better recommendations to the public about levels of pollutants that may present a risk to specific population subgroups.

Recommendation 4: Changes in the seafood supply (source and type of seafood) must be accounted for—there is inconsistency in sampling and analysis methodology used for nutrients and contaminant data that are published by state and federal agencies. Analytical data is not consistently revised, with separate data values presented for wild-caught, domestic, and imported products.

Drawing on these recommendations and its benefit-risk assessment protocol, the committee identified four population groups for which the data support subgroup-specific conclusions. In the committee's judgement, the variables that distinguish between these populations facing different benefit-risk balances based on existing evidence are (1) age, (2) gender, (3) pregnancy or possibility of becoming pregnant, or breastfeeding, and (4) risk of coronary heart disease, although the evidence for a benefit to adult males and females who are at risk for coronary heart disease is not sufficient to warrant inclusion as a separate group within the decision-making framework. The groups and appropriate guidance are listed in Box S-1 below.

To balance the benefits and risks, the recommendations, as they apply to the target population groups 1–3, are arrayed in a decision pathway (shown in Figure S-1) that illustrates the committee's resulting analysis of the balance between benefits and risks associated with seafood consumption.

BOX S-1
Population Groups and Appropriate Guidance

1. *Females who are or may become pregnant or who are breastfeeding:*
    a. May benefit from consuming seafood, especially those with relatively higher concentrations of EPA and DHA;
    b. A reasonable intake would be two 3-ounce (cooked) servings but can safely consume 12 ounces per week;
    c. Can consume up to 6 ounces of white (albacore) tuna per week;
    d. Should avoid large predatory fish such as shark, swordfish, tilefish, or king mackerel.
2. *Children up to age 12:*
    a. May benefit from consuming seafood, especially those with relatively higher concentrations of EPA and DHA;
    b. A reasonable intake would be two 3-ounce (cooked), or age-appropriate, servings but can safely consume 12 ounces per week;
    c. Can consume up to 6 ounces (or age-appropriate) of white (albacore) tuna per week;
    d. Should avoid large predatory fish such as shark, swordfish, tilefish, or king mackerel.
3. *Adolescent males, adult males, and females who will not become pregnant:*
    a. May reduce their risk for cardiovascular disease by consuming seafood regularly, e.g., two 3-ounce servings per week;
    b. Who consume more than two servings a week should choose a variety of types of seafood to reduce the risk for exposure to contaminants from a single source.
4. *Adult males and females who are at risk of cardiovascular disease:*
    a. May reduce their risk of cardiovascular disease by consuming seafood regularly, e.g., two 3-ounce servings per week;
    b. Although supporting evidence is limited, there may be additional benefits from including high EPA/DHA seafood selections;
    c. Who consume more than two servings a week should choose a variety of types of seafood to reduce the risk for exposure to contaminants from a single source.

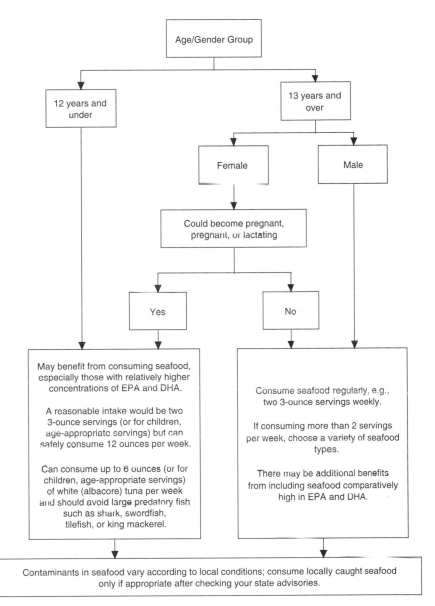

FIGURE S-1 The committee's decision pathway derived from the balance between benefits and risks associated with seafood consumption. The diagram highlights the variables that group consumers into target populations that face different benefits and risks and should receive tailored advice.

NOTE: The wording in this figure has not been tested among consumers. Designers will need to test the effects of presenting information on seafood choices in alternative formats.

UNDERSTANDING CONSUMER DECISION MAKING AS THE BASIS FOR THE DESIGN OF CONSUMER GUIDANCE

The second step in the approach to balancing benefits and risks associated with seafood consumption is developing an understanding of the context within which consumers make seafood choices. Receiving new information, such as dietary guidance, does not automatically lead consumers to change their food consumption patterns. Food choice is influenced by a complex information environment that includes taste, availability, and price, as well as guidance, point-of-purchase information, labeling, and advice from health care providers. In the context of this environment, specific pieces of guidance may have limited impact, although evidence suggests that this impact varies significantly and in many instances is not well measured or understood. There are several factors that mitigate against current advice having the intended consequences in terms of consumer choice. Increased understanding of the individual, socio-cultural, and environmental factors that influence consumer choice is necessary for the design of consumer guidance, especially where the intent is to communicate balancing of benefits and risks associated with seafood consumption.

Seafood choices, like all consumption choices, entail value trade-offs; some individuals will choose high risks to achieve what they value as high benefits (e.g., consume raw seafood because of its pleasurable taste), while others may prefer to "play it safe." Individual differences in tastes, preferences, beliefs and attitudes, and situations complicate the task of informing and supporting benefit-risk trade-off decisions. Audience segmentation and targeting, therefore, is essential for effective communication, because decision objectives, risk attitudes, and people's knowledge about and interest in decision-making vary. Guidance in making seafood choices should allow consumers to access information in a clear and easy-to-understand format. It should also be structured to support decision-making, and allow consumers to access additional layers of information when they want them.

BALANCING CHOICES: SUPPORTING CONSUMER SEAFOOD CONSUMPTION DECISIONS

The third design step for developing specific support for seafood consumption decisions is production and evaluation of the information itself, including ways to integrate the benefit and risk considerations in mock-up examples of how such information might be provided. It is apparent in any discussion of seafood consumption that "one size does not fit all" and that messages about consumption often have to be individualized for different groups, such as subsistence fishers, pregnant women, children, and native populations, to mention a few. The committee's balancing of the benefits and risks of different patterns of seafood consumption for different subpopulations is illustrated in Figure S-1. Different subpopulations could be used by federal agencies as the basis for targeting advice to consumers on seafood consumption. Resulting communication products should be tested empirically. Through a brief set of questions, a decision pathway can segment and channel consumers into relevant benefit-risk subpopulations in order to provide benefit and risk information that is tailored to each group. The inclusion of alternative presentations of benefit-risk advice and information in the design of consumer advice recognizes that while some consumers prefer to follow the advice given to them by experts, others want to decide on the benefit-risk trade-offs for themselves.

One of the challenges in supporting informed consumer choice is how governmental agencies communicate health benefits and risks to both the general population and to specific subgroups or particularly vulnerable populations. Developing effective tools to disseminate current and emerging information to the public requires formal evaluation, as well as an iterative approach to design. The use of tailored messages and community-level involvement on an ongoing basis is likely to improve the effectiveness of communication between federal agencies and target populations.

Primary Findings

1. Advice to consumers from the federal government and private organizations on seafood choices to promote human health has been fragmented. Benefits have been addressed separately from risks; portion sizes differ from one piece of advice to another. Some benefits and some risks have been addressed separately from others for different physiological systems and age groups. As a result, multiple pieces of guidance—sometimes conflicting—simultaneously exist for seafood.

2. Given the uncertainties present in underlying exposure data and health impact analysis, there is no single summary metric that adequately captures the complexity of balancing benefits and risks associated with seafood for purposes of providing guidance to consumers. An expert judgement technique can be used to consider benefits and risks together, to yield specific suggested consumption guidance.

Recommendations

Recommendation 5: Appropriate federal agencies should develop tools for consumers, such as computer-based, interactive decision support and visual representations of benefits and risks that are easy to use and to interpret. An example of this kind of tool is the health risk appraisal (HRA), which allows individuals to enter their own specific information and returns appropriate recommendations to guide their health actions. The model developed here provides this kind of evidence-based recommendations regarding seafood consumption. Agencies should also develop alternative tools for populations with limited access to computer-based information.

Recommendation 6: New tools apart from traditional safety assessments should be developed, such as consumer-based benefit-risk analyses. A better way is needed to characterize the risks combined with benefit analysis.

Recommendation 7: A consumer-directed decision path needs to be properly designed, tested, and evaluated. The resulting product must undergo methodological review and update on a continuing basis. Responsible agencies will need to work with specialists in risk communication and evaluation, and tailor advice to specific groups as appropriate.

Recommendation 8: Consolidated advice is needed that brings together different benefit and risk considerations, and is tailored to individual circumstances, to better inform consumer choices. Effort should be made to improve coordination of federal guidance with that provided through partnerships at the state and local level.

Recommendation 9: Consumer messages should be tested to determine if there are spillover effects for segments of the population not targeted by the message. There is suggestive evidence that risk-avoidance advice for sensitive subpopulations may be construed by other groups or the general population as appropriate precautionary action for themselves. While emphasizing trade-offs may reduce the risk of spillover effects, consumer testing of messages should address the potential for spillover effects explicitly.

Recommendation 10: The decision pathway the committee recommends, which illustrates its analysis of the current balance between benefits and risks associated with seafood consumption, should be used as a basis for developing consumer guidance tools for selecting seafood to obtain nutritional benefits balanced against exposure risks. Real-time, interactive decision tools, easily available to the public, could increase informed actions for a significant portion of the population, and help to inform important intermediaries, such as physicians.

Recommendation 11: The sponsor should work together with appropriate federal and state agencies concerned with public health to develop an interagency task force to coordinate data and communications on seafood consumption benefits, risks, and related issues such as fish stocks and seafood sources, and begin development of a communication program to help consumers make informed seafood consumption decisions. Empirical evaluation of consumers' needs and the effectiveness of communications should be an integral part of the program.

Recommendation 12: Partnerships should be formed between federal agencies and community organizations. This effort should include targeting and involvement of intermediaries, such as physicians, and use of interactive

Internet communications, which have the potential to increase the usefulness and accuracy of seafood consumption communications.

RESEARCH GAPS AND RECOMMENDATIONS

Seafood Consumption

Recommendation 1: Research is needed on systematic surveillance studies of targeted subpopulations. Such studies should be carried out using state-of-the-art assessment methods to determine the intake levels of seafood, EPA/DHA and other dietary constituents, and the variability of those intake levels among population groups.

Recommendation 2: Sufficiently large analytic samples of the most common seafood types need to be obtained and examined. These samples should be used to determine the levels of nutrients, toxicants, and contaminants in each species and the variability between them, which should be reported transparently.

Recommendation 3: Additional data is needed to assess benefits and risks associated with seafood consumption within the same population or population subgroup.

Pregnant and Lactating Women

Recommendation 4: Better data are needed to determine if outcomes of increasing consumption of seafood or increasing EPA/DHA intake levels in US women would be comparable to outcomes of populations in other countries. Such studies should be encouraged to include populations of high fish-consumers outside the United States to determine if there are differences in risks for these populations compared to US populations.

Recommendation 5: Dose-response studies of EPA/DHA in pregnant and lactating women are needed. This information will help determine if higher intakes can further increase gestation duration, reduce premature births, and benefit infant development. Other studies should include assessing whether DHA alone can act independently of EPA to increase duration of gestation.

Infants and Toddlers

Recommendation 6: Research is needed to determine if cognitive and developmental outcomes in infants are correlated with performance later in childhood. This should include:

- Evaluating preschool and school-age children exposed to EPA/DHA in utero and postnatally, at ages beginning around 4 years when executive function is more developed; and
- Evaluating development of school-age children exposed to variable EPA/DHA levels in utero and postnatally with measures of distractibility, disruptive behavior, and oppositional defiant behavior, as well as more commonly assessed cognitive outcomes and more sophisticated tests of visual function.

Recommendation 7: Additional data are needed to better define optimum intake levels of EPA/DHA for infants and toddlers.

Children

Recommendation 8: Better-designed studies about EPA/DHA supplementation in children with behavioral disorders are needed.

Adults at Risk for Chronic Disease

Recommendation 9: In the absence of meta-analyses that systematically combine quantitative data from multiple studies, further meta-analyses and larger randomized trials are needed to assess outcomes other than cardiovascular, in particular total mortality, in order to explore possible adverse effects of EPA/DHA supplementation.

Recommendation 10: Additional clinical research is needed to assess a potential effect of seafood consumption and/or EPA/DHA supplementation on stroke, cancer, Alzheimer's disease, and depression.

Recommendation 11: Future epidemiological studies should assess intake of specific species of seafood and/or biomarkers, in order to differentiate the health effects of EPA/DHA from the health effects of contaminants such as methylmercury.

Health Risks Associated with Seafood Consumption

Recommendation 12: More complete data are needed on the distribution of contaminant levels among types of fish. This information should be made available in order to reduce uncertainties associated with the estimation of health risks for specific seafoodborne contaminant exposures.

Recommendation 13: More quantitative characterization is needed of the dose-response relationships between chemical contaminants and adverse health effects, in the ranges of exposure represented in the general US population. Such information will reduce uncertainties associated with recommendations for acceptable ranges of intake.

Recommendation 14: In addition, the committee recommends more research on useful biomarkers of contaminant exposures and more precise quantitative characterization of the dose-response relationships between chemical contaminants and adverse health effects, in the ranges of exposure represented in the general US population, in order to reduce uncertainties associated with recommendations for acceptable ranges of intake.

Designing Consumer Guidance

Recommendation 15: Research is needed to develop and evaluate more effective communication tools for use when conveying the health benefits and risks of seafood consumption as well as current and emerging information to the public. These tools should be tested among different communities and subgroups within the population and evaluated with pre- and post-test activities.

Recommendation 16: Among federal agencies there is a need to design and distribute better consumer advice to understand and acknowledge the context in which the information will be used by consumers. Understanding consumer decision-making is a prerequisite. The information provided to consumers should be developed with recognition of the individual, environmental, social, and economic consequences of the advice. In addition, it is important that consistency between agencies be maintained, particularly with regard to communication information using serving sizes.

CONCLUSION

For most of the general population, balancing benefits and risks associated with seafood consumption to obtain nutritional and health benefits can be achieved by selecting seafood from available options in quantities that fall within accepted dietary guidelines. For the specific subgroups identified by the committee, making such selections requires that consumers are aware of both nutrients and contaminants in the seafood available and are provided useful information on both benefits and risks to inform their choices. The committee has put forward its interpretation of the evidence for benefits and risks associated with seafood and considered the balance between them. Recommendations are made to facilitate development of appropriate consumer guidance for making seafood selections, based on the committee's findings, and research opportunities are identified that will contribute to filling knowledge gaps.

1

Introduction

Federal agencies and private organizations have recommended including seafood as part of a healthy diet because of the variety of nutrients it provides. However, contamination of seafood, whether by naturally occurring or introduced contaminants, remains a concern for US consumers because of the potential for adverse health effects. The extent to which a contaminant in a food may be considered a risk to health depends upon the nature and level of the compound present, and the sensitivity of individuals or groups in a population to potentially toxic compounds. Specific population groups have been identified as being at particular risk from exposure to contaminants in seafood. Paradoxically, these population groups may especially benefit from the nutrients in seafood. For most of the general population, optimal benefits from seafood can be obtained by making choices to maximize intake of desirable nutrients balanced against exposure to contaminants that may pose a health risk. Making such selections, however, requires that consumers are aware of the variety of seafood available and are provided information on both benefits and risks to inform their choices.

For the purposes of this report, the term seafood refers to all commercially obtained fish, shellfish, and mollusks, both marine and freshwater. When marine mammals are pertinent to the discussion, they will be identified separately. The impact of seafood obtained by subsistence and recreational harvesting is considered as far as the more limited data allow.

RECOMMENDATIONS TO ENCOURAGE SEAFOOD CONSUMPTION

Seafood contributes a variety of nutrients to the American diet, including protein and important micronutrients, and its eicosapentaenoic acid (EPA) and docosahexaenoic acid (DHA) content distinguishes it as providing a unique nutritional benefit. EPA and DHA are abundant in some seafood types and the conversion from alpha-linolenic acid (ALA) is inefficient in humans (Burdge, 2004). Seafood is not a primary source for ALA. EPA and DHA are believed to be important in reducing the risk of cardiovascular disease, lengthening gestation, and possibly promoting fetal and infant neurological development. For these reasons, several groups have recommended inclusion of seafood, particularly those choices high in EPA/DHA, in the American diet (see Appendix Table B-3). These recommendations frequently refer to servings per week; throughout this report, unless otherwise stated, a serving of seafood is defined as 4 ounces raw, which yields 3 ounces cooked. As noted later in this chapter and throughout the report, some federal and state agencies and nonfederal organizations include larger (8 ounce) serving sizes in their recommendations and advisories. This committee has adopted the convention of the Dietary Guidelines Advisory Committee (see below) in considering a serving size from the meat, poultry, fish, and egg food group to be 4 ounces raw, or 3 ounces cooked.

Dietary Guidelines Advisory Committee

Every 5 years, an expert Dietary Guidelines Advisory Committee (DGAC) is appointed to make recommendations to the Secretaries of the Department of Health and Human Services (HHS) and the Department of Agriculture (USDA) concerning revision of the *Dietary Guidelines for Americans* (DGA). In 2005, the DGAC issued its own report, separate from the Dietary Guidelines, which reviewed the preponderance of scientific and medical knowledge and suggested a set of key messages (DGAC, 2005).

One of these messages, in the section on dietary fats, was "the consumption of two servings (approximately 6–8 ounces) per week of fish high in EPA and DHA is associated with reduced risk of both sudden death and death from coronary heart disease in adults. To benefit from the potential cardioprotective effects of EPA and DHA, the weekly consumption of two servings of fish, particularly fish rich in EPA and DHA, is suggested. Other sources of EPA and DHA may provide similar benefits; however, further research is warranted." The strength of this message was tempered somewhat by the section on food safety, which warned of the potential danger of methylmercury in fish.

Dietary Guidelines for Americans

The *Dietary Guidelines for Americans* provide science-based advice to promote health and reduce risk for major chronic diseases through diet and physical activity. The DGA are a statement of federal nutrition policy and, as such, form the basis of all federal food assistance as well as nutrition education and information programs. For example, the DGA are used in menu planning in the National School Lunch Program; in educational materials used by the Special Supplemental Nutrition Program for Women, Infants, and Children (WIC); and in setting the Healthy People objectives for the nation. In addition, the Secretaries of HHS and USDA review all federal publications related to dietary guidance to ensure consistency with the DGA.

Developed for policy makers, nutrition professionals, and educators, the DGA were initially published in 1980 by HHS and USDA, and have been updated every 5 years. The most recent edition was drafted in 2005 by a committee of scientists after reviewing the recommendations of the DGAC (see above) and the associated public comments. Because of the competing benefits and risks associated with seafood consumption pointed out in the DGAC report, drafters of the DGA stopped short of making a quantified key recommendation for fish or seafood. Instead, they recommended that individuals "Keep total fat intake between 20 to 35 percent of calories, with most fats coming from sources of polyunsaturated and monounsaturated fatty acids, such as fish, nuts, and vegetable oils" (DGA, 2005). The accompanying text cites evidence for a reduced risk of cardiovascular disease among the general population associated with the consumption of certain fatty acids from seafood.

MyPyramid

After the release of the DGA, the USDA released the MyPyramid food guidance system along with the new MyPyramid symbol (USDA, 2005). This food guidance system was developed to help Americans make healthy food choices, given their sex, age, and activity level. Recommended quantities are provided for each food group (grains, fruits, vegetables, milk, meat and beans, oils, and discretionary calories), with fish represented in the meat and beans group. While no specific quantity of fish is recommended, "selection tips" suggest that Americans "select fish rich in omega-3 fatty acids, such as salmon, trout, and herring, more often" (Source: http://www.mypyramid.gov).

American Heart Association Guidelines

The American Heart Association (AHA) Dietary Guidelines are based on the findings of the nutrition committee of the AHA and were last revised

TABLE 1-1 Summary of American Heart Association Recommendations for Omega-3 Fatty Acid Intake[a]

Population	Recommendation
Patients without documented coronary heart disease (CHD)	Eat a variety of (preferably fatty) fish at least twice a week. Include oils and foods rich in alpha-linolenic acid (flaxseed, canola, and soybean oils; flaxseed and walnuts).
Patients with documented CHD	Consume about 1 g of EPA+DHA per day, preferably from fatty fish. EPA+DHA supplements could be considered in consultation with the physician.
Patients who need to lower triglycerides	2 to 4 g of EPA+DHA per day provided as capsules under a physician's care.

[a]Patients taking more than 3 g of omega-3 fatty acids from supplements should do so only under a physician's care. High intakes could cause excessive bleeding in some people.

SOURCE: AHA, 2005.

in 2000 (Krauss et al., 2000). The AHA recommendations are aimed at reducing risk for cardiovascular disease by altering dietary and lifestyle factors among the general population, although there are individualized approaches for specific subgroups with medical concerns such as lipid disorders and diabetes. The AHA dietary guidelines include a recommendation that healthy adults eat fish at least twice a week. Altogether, the AHA has three recommended intake levels for EPA and DHA, corresponding to research findings on associations between EPA/DHA intake and cardiac risk reduction. The AHA (2005) recommendations, posted on its website (Source: http://www.americanheart.org/presenter.jhtml?identifier=851), are shown in Table 1-1.

The basis for the AHA recommendations is research suggesting that adopting healthy food habits that include eating two 3-ounce servings of seafood per week can help reduce three major risk factors for heart attack—high blood cholesterol, high blood pressure, and excess body weight (see Chapter 3 for discussion). Reducing blood pressure may also help reduce the major risk factors for stroke. Recognizing the importance of primary prevention, i.e., preventing the development of cardiovascular risk factors before symptoms arise, the American Heart Association also endorses the recommendation that children aged 2 years and above increase consumption of "oily" fish prepared by broiling or baking (Gidding et al., 2005).

The American Dietetic Association

The American Dietetic Association and the Dietitians of Canada (ADA, 2003) published a position paper on vegetarian diets that addressed inclusion of omega-3 fatty acids. Vegetarian diets, which are rich in omega-6 but poor in omega-3 fatty acids, may contribute to decreased production of EPA and DHA in vegetarians. Apart from fish and eggs, omega-3 fatty acids can be obtained from microalgae, which is now available as a dietary supplement.

The Dietary Reference Intake (IOM, 2002/2005) recommendation for an adequate intake (AI) of 1.6 and 1.1 grams of ALA per day for men and women, respectively, assumes some intake of EPA and DHA to meet targeted omega-3 levels. However, since vegetarians may not consume adequate levels of preformed EPA and DHA from seafood, and ALA is not efficiently converted to EPA/DHA, this recommendation may not be adequate for their needs. The joint World Health Organization/Food and Agriculture Organization *Consultation on Diet, Nutrition and the Prevention of Chronic Disease* (WHO/FAO, 2003) recommendation of an intake of 5–8 percent of daily calories from omega-6 and 1–2 percent from all omega-3 (EPA, DHA, and ALA) sources also falls short of vegetarians' needs if an algal source is not included in the diet.

The position of the American Dietetic Association is that vegetarians should include good sources of ALA, such as flaxseed, flaxseed oil, soy, or walnut oil in their diets. In addition, for those with increased requirements, including pregnant and lactating females, direct sources of EPA and DHA such as microalgae should be included in the diet.

ADVISORIES AND WARNINGS ABOUT SEAFOOD CONSUMPTION

The levels of different toxic compounds in seafood vary within and among species due to the chemical properties of the contaminant and the characteristics of the seafood. For example, compounds such as dioxins and polychlorinated biphenyls (PCBs) accumulate in fat tissue and are found predominantly in fatty fish and fish that live in fresh or coastal waters, including striped bass, bluefish, American eel, lake trout, and farmed Atlantic salmon. Heavy metals such as methylmercury accumulate in lean tissue and are found in the muscle tissue of older, predatory fish such as shark, swordfish, king mackerel, and tilefish.

Federal Advisories

The Food and Drug Administration (FDA) of the US Department of Health and Human Services announced in 2001 its advice to pregnant females and those of childbearing age who may become pregnant on the hazard of consuming fish that may contain high levels of methylmercury. In 2004, the advice was jointly reissued by FDA and the US Environmental Protection Agency (US EPA), and was updated to include the message that seafood makes an important contribution to the diet (US EPA/FDA, 2004).

The FDA advice states that women should select a variety of seafood including shellfish, canned fish, smaller ocean fish or farm-raised fish, and that they could safely consume 12 ounces per week of cooked fish (four 3-ounce servings). The US EPA/FDA joint advisory also includes information on specific types of fish that are low or high in methylmercury and advice to consumers to check their local advisories about the safety of locally caught fish. The advisory further cautions pregnant women and women of child-bearing age who may become pregnant, as well as women who are nursing and young children, to avoid consuming shark, swordfish, king mackerel, and tilefish. This recommendation applies to commercially obtained as well as consumer-caught fish. The US EPA national fishing advisory states that, for consumer-caught fish, consumers should first consult their local advisories, or in the case where no advisory exists, to restrict consumption of consumer-caught fish to one "8-ounce (raw; 6 ounces cooked) meal per week" (US EPA, 2004a) for an adult with a body weight of 70 kilograms (kg) (154 pounds) (see Table 1-2).

State Advisories

The five primary bioaccumulative pollutants for which fishing advisories have been established are mercury, PCBs, chlordane, dioxins, and DDT and its metabolites, although approximately 76 percent of all advisories issued addressed mercury contamination. States establish their own advisory criteria, which may be based on established federal advisories, and determine which water bodies to monitor; these may include coastal waters, rivers, and lakes. Across the states and territories of the United States, the number of waterbodies under advisory represents 35 percent of total lake acres (approximately 101,818 lakes), 24 percent of total river miles (approximately 846,310 river miles), and 71 percent of the contiguous coastal waters (US EPA, 2004b).

The National Listing of Fish Advisories database (Source: http://www. epa.gov/waterscience/fish/advisories/index.html) listed 3,089 advisories in 48 states, the District of Columbia, and the US Territory of American Samoa in 2003 (US EPA, 2005b).

In 2003, 31 states had statewide advisories in effect, including new statewide advisories for all rivers and lakes in Montana and Washington, and an advisory for marine fish in Hawaii. In addition to advisories in place in 2003, 16 states across the United States had Safe Eating Guidelines, either for specific waterbodies or inclusive of all rivers and lakes statewide. The guidelines are issued to inform and reassure the public that certain species of fish taken from these waterbodies have been tested and shown to contain very low levels of contaminants. The only state within the continental United States that did not have an advisory of any type in 2003 was Wyoming

TABLE 1-2 Federal Fish Advisories in the United States

Organization	Audience	Reasons for Advisories/Restrictions	Fish Advisories/Restrictions[a]		
			Type of Fish/Seafood	Serving Size	Number of Servings
Environmental Protection Agency	Not specified	Inform the public from which specific bodies of water or which species of fish it is safe to eat	Noncommercial fish (where there is no local advisory)	8 ounces raw (6 ounces cooked)[b]	Once per week
Food and Drug Administration	Pregnant women and women of childbearing age	Receive the benefits of eating fish and shellfish and be confident of reductions in exposure to the harmful effects of methylmercury	A variety of fish includes shellfish, canned fish, smaller ocean fish, or farm-raised fish	6 ounces cooked	Twice per week
Environmental Protection Agency and Food and Drug Administration	Pregnant women, women of childbearing age, nursing women, and children	These fish contain high levels of methylmercury	Shark, swordfish, king mackerel, tilefish	Any	Avoid
Environmental Protection Agency and Food and Drug Administration	Pregnant women, women of childbearing age, nursing women, and children	Albacore ("white") tuna has more methylmercury than canned light tuna	Albacore ("white") tuna and locally caught fish	6 ounces	Once per week[c]

[a]When consuming noncommercial fish, always check for local fishing advisories.
[b]For an adult with an average body weight of 70 kilograms (154 pounds), based on a reference dose for methylmercury of 1×10^{-4} mg/kg/day.
[c]If consuming locally caught fish, do not consume any other fish that week.

SOURCES: US EPA, 2004a; FDA, 2001; US EPA/FDA, 2004.

(Source: http://www.epa.gov/waterscience/fish/advisories/fs2004.html). The number of total state and territory advisories increased to 3,221 in 2004; however, the number of Safe Eating Guidelines issued by states increased as well to 1,213 in 2004.

ADVICE ON SEAFOOD CONSUMPTION OUTSIDE THE US

The United Kingdom's Scientific Advisory Committee on Nutrition

In the United Kingdom (UK), the Food Standards Agency (FSA) and the Department of Health sought advice from the Scientific Advisory Committee on Nutrition (SACN) and the Committee on Toxicity of Chemicals in Food, Consumer Products and the Environment (COT) on the benefits and risks of fish consumption, with particular reference to "oily" fish (fish high in EPA/DHA). A joint SACN/COT subgroup was convened to deliberate and produce a report. The report (SACN, 2004) assessed the risks associated with consumption of seafood, weighed the nutritional benefits against possible risks, and developed coherent dietary advice for the public on the consumption of seafood.

A summary of the benefits and risks associated with seafood consumption was reviewed in the report. Among the conclusions reached by the SACN/COT regarding those benefits and risks associated with increased consumption of seafood and fish oils were that:

1. SACN endorsed the general population recommendation to eat at least two servings of fish per week, of which one should be oily, and agreed that this recommendation should also apply to pregnant women;

2. An increase in oily fish consumption to one serving a week, from the current levels of about a third of a serving a week, would probably confer significant public health benefits in terms of reduced risk of cardiovascular disease;

3. There is further evidence that increased seafood consumption might have beneficial effects on fetal development;

4. The evidence to support benefits at higher levels of consumption is insufficient to enable accurate quantification; and

5. Exceeding designated intake guideline ranges over the short-term would not be deleterious, but long-term exceedances could have deleterious effects in sensitive individuals. In the case of pregnant and lactating women, for example, a woman who had not consistently exceeded the guideline range previously, could increase her oily fish consumption throughout pregnancy and lactation above the guideline range (e.g., to two to three servings of oily fish a week) without detrimental effects from exposure to persistent organic pollutants such as dioxins and PCBs.

The European Food Safety Authority

Recognizing that fish is a source of nutritional benefit but also of contaminants of concern, particularly methylmercury, dioxins, and dioxin-like compounds (DLCs), the European Food Safety Authority (EFSA) was asked by the European Parliament to assess health risks associated with consumption of farmed and wild-caught fish, including an assessment of the safety of consuming Baltic herring (EFSA, 2005a). EFSA reviewed evidence on the benefits of nutrients, especially omega-3 fatty acids, in fish; sources of contaminants of concern in seafood; and risks to health from consuming fish and generated exposure scenarios from data on consumption of and contaminants in fish. The conclusions and recommendations of EFSA were published as an opinion on the health risks related to consumption of wild and farmed fish (Source: http://www.efsa. eu.int/science/contam/contam_opinions/1007_en.html).

The report pointed out that fish obtained from the Baltic Sea are likely to contain higher levels of contaminants, particularly dioxins and PCBs, than comparable fish obtained from other sources. For some EU member countries, i.e., Sweden and Finland, there is specific national advice for consumers, particularly girls (due to childbearing potential), about consuming Baltic fish that may be contaminated with dioxins and PCBs. Apart from fish obtained from the Baltic Sea, the EFSA opinion states that there are no consistent differences between wild and farmed fish regarding either safety or nutritional value, and that consumption of fish, especially fish high in EPA/DHA, is beneficial to cardiovascular health and to fetal development.

The report noted that fish is a valuable source of many nutrients, including protein, iodine, selenium, and vitamins A and D. The EFSA statement was further qualified, however, with the advice that vulnerable population groups, such as pregnant women and women of childbearing age, should consider the nutritional benefits of fish weighed against potential risks from contaminants in certain types of fish. The EFSA panel also stated that advice regarding fish consumption should take into account other comparable sources of contaminants, particularly dioxin-like compounds and PCBs, that are present in the fatty components of other animal foods. Pregnant women were advised to consume up to two servings of fish per week as long as certain types of fish, e.g., long-lived predatory fish such as swordfish and tuna, were avoided (for additional information see Cossa et al., 1989; Claisse et al., 2001). Lastly, the EFSA panel recommended development of a consistent and agreed-upon methodology for carrying out quantitative assessments of benefits and risks related to food consumption.

World Health Organization

A Joint WHO/FAO Expert Consultation on Diet, Nutrition and the Prevention of Chronic Diseases met in Geneva in 2002 to evaluate evidence for the role of diet in the prevention of nutritional deficiency and chronic disease. The Joint WHO/FAO committee's report *Diet, Nutrition and the Prevention of Chronic Diseases* recommends a shift in the conceptual framework for developing health care strategies that would place nutrition, together with the other principal risk factors for chronic disease, at the forefront of public health policies and programs (WHO/FAO, 2003).

The report examined the role of omega-6 and omega-3 fatty acids in the prevention of chronic disease, including cancer and cardiovascular disease. Recommendations included that diets should provide a total intake of omega-6 and omega-3 fatty acids in the range of 6–10 percent of daily energy (caloric) intake, but an optimal balance would include 5–8 percent of those percent as n-6 and 1–2 percent as n-3 fatty acids. Omega-3 fatty acids include α-linolenic (ALA), eicosapentaenoic (EPA), and docosahexaenoic (DHA). Whereas certain fish are the primary source of EPA and DHA, ALA is derived primarily from plant sources, e.g., soybean, flaxseed, and walnut oils. The WHO/FAO (2003) recommendation on the consumption of fish is that "Regular fish consumption (1–2 servings per week) is protective against coronary heart disease and ischaemic stroke and is recommended. The serving should provide an equivalent of 200–500 mg of eicosapentaenoic and docosahexaenoic acid. People who are vegetarians are recommended to ensure adequate intake of plant sources of α-linolenic acid."

THE CHARGE TO THE COMMITTEE

Considering the recommendations and suggestions to increase seafood intake to promote cardiovascular health, and the somewhat conflicting messages to avoid certain fish, consumers and health professionals may feel confused regarding the healthfulness of consuming seafood. For this reason, the National Marine Fisheries Service (NMFS) of the Department of Commerce, National Oceanic and Atmospheric Administration (NOAA), in particular the National Marine Fisheries Science Board, asked the Institute of Medicine to convene an ad hoc committee to (1) identify and prioritize the potential for adverse health effects from both naturally occurring and introduced toxicants in seafood, (2) assess evidence on availability of specific nutrients in seafood compared to other food sources, (3) determine the impact of modifying food choices to reduce intake of naturally occurring and introduced toxicants on nutrient intake and nutritional status within the US population, (4) develop a decision path, appropriate to the needs of US consumers, for selecting seafood to balance their choices to obtain nutritional benefits against exposure risks, and (5) identify data gaps and recommend future research.

Many of the contaminants that are present in seafood and have a role in influencing selections to balance benefits and risks are introduced, and thus may be controlled. For this reason, an examination of the sources of toxicants and the pathways by which they enter and bioaccumulate in the seafood supply is important. However, the committee was not asked to make recommendations to mitigate contaminant sources in seafood.

Approach to the Task

Following a request by NOAA to the National Academies, an expert committee was appointed to review evidence on ways for the US consumer to balance the benefits of seafood consumption against potential risks from exposure to contaminants they may contain, and to recommend ways to guide US consumers in making selections appropriate to their needs. The committee approached its task by gathering information from existing literature and from workshop presentations by recognized experts (see Appendix D for workshop agendas), consulting with experts in relevant fields, performing analyses on data collected in the most recent National Health and Nutrition Examination Survey (NHANES), deliberating on issues relevant to the task, and formulating an approach to address the scope of work

ORGANIZATION OF THE REPORT

This report is organized into seven chapters that describe what is known about the benefits associated with nutrients in seafood, particularly omega-3 fatty acids; risks associated with contaminants found in seafood; and ways to balance benefits and risks and guide consumers in making selections appropriate to their needs. Chapter 2 provides information on seafood consumption patterns, and nutrients and contaminants in seafood. Chapter 3 provides in-depth evaluation of the literature on benefits of consuming seafood, particularly omega-3 fatty acids, and the impact of seafood consumption on health outcomes. Chapter 4 reviews risks associated with introduced and naturally occurring contaminants in seafood and potential health outcomes from exposure. Chapter 5 discusses the scientific assessment and analysis of risks and benefits from seafood consumption and ways that benefits and risks could vary depending on the type of fish consumed. Chapter 6 discusses consumer decision-making and the current consumer information environment and Chapter 7 discusses approaches to designing consumer information and supporting seafood consumption decisions.

REFERENCES

ADA (American Dietetic Association). 2003. Position of the American Dietetic Association and Dietitians of Canada: Vegetarian diets. *Journal of the American Dietetic Association* 103(6):748–765.

AHA (American Heart Association). 2005. *Fish and Omega-3 Fatty Acids: AHA Recommendation.* [Online]. Available: http://www.americanheart.org/presenter.jhtml?identifier=4632 [accessed December 9, 2005].

AHA. 2006. *Our 2006 Diet and Lifestyle Recommendations.* [Online]. Available: http://www.americanheart.org/presenter.jhtml?identifier=851 [accessed September 6, 2006].

Burdge G. 2004. Alpha-linolenic acid metabolism in men and women: Nutritional and biological implications. *Current Opinion in Clinical Nutrition and Metabolic Care* 7(2):137–144.

Claisse D, Cossa D, Bretaudeau-Sanjuan J, Touchard G, Bombled B. 2001. Methylmercury in molluscs along the French coast. *Marine Pollution Bulletin* 42(4):329–332.

Cossa D, Auger D, Averty B, Lucon M, Masselin P, Noel J, SanJuan J. 1989. *Atlas Des Niveaux de Concentration en Metaux Metalloides et Composes Organochlores dans les Produits de la Peche Cotiere Francaise. Technical Report.* Nantes, France: IFREMER.

DGA (Dietary Guidelines for Americans). 2005. Washington, DC: Department of Health and Human Services and the Department of Agriculture. [Online]. Available: http://www.health.gov/dietaryguidelines/dga2005/document/ [accessed November 29, 2005].

DGAC (Dietary Guidelines Advisory Committee). 2005. *Dietary Guidelines Advisory Committee Report.* Washington, DC: Department of Health and Human Services and the Department of Agriculture. [Online]. Available: http://www.health.gov/dietaryguidelines/dga2005/report/ [accessed November 29, 2005].

EFSA (European Food Safety Authority). 2005a. *Opinion of the CONTAM Panel Related to the Safety Assessment of Wild and Farmed Fish.* [Online]. Available: http://www.efsa.eu.int/science/contam/contam_opinions/1007_en.html [accessed December 4, 2006].

EFSA. 2005b. Opinion of the scientific panel on contaminants in the food chain on a request from the European Parliament related to the safety assessment of wild and farmed fish. *The EFSA Journal* 236:1–118. [Online]. Available: http://www.efsa.eu.int/press_room/press_release/258_en.html [accessed October 6, 2005].

FDA (Food and Drug Administration). 2001. *FDA Announces Advisory on Methyl Mercury in Fish.* [Online]. Available: http://www.fda.gov/bbs/topics/ANSWERS/2001/ANS01065.html [accessed May 9, 2006].

Gidding SS, Dennison BA, Birch LL, Daniels SR, Gilman MW, Lichtenstein AH, Rattay KT, Steinberger J, Stettler N, Van Horn L. 2005. Dietary recommendations for children and adolescents: A guide for practitioners. Consensus statement from the American Heart Association. *Circulation* 112(13):2061–2075.

IOM (Institute of Medicine). 2002/2005. Dietary Reference Intakes for Energy, Carbohydrates, Fiber, Fat, Fatty Acids, Cholesterol, Protein, and Amino Acids. Washington, DC: The National Academies Press.

Krauss RM, Eckel RH, Howard B, Appel LJ, Daniels SR, Deckelbaum RJ, Erdman JW, Kris-Etherton P, Goldberg IJ, Kotchen, TA, Lichtenstein AH, Mitch WE, Mullis R, Robinson K, Wylie-Rosett J, St. Jeor S, Suttie J, Tribble DL, Bazzarre TL. 2000. AHA Dietary Guidelines Revision 2000: A statement for healthcare professionals from the Nutrition Committee of the American Heart Association. *Circulation* 102:2284–2299.

SACN (Scientific Advisory Committee on Nutrition). 2004. *Advice on Fish Consumption: Benefits & Risks.* London, UK: TSO (The Stationery Office). [Online]. Available: http://www.sacn.gov.uk/reports/#/ [accessed September 8, 2005].

US EPA (US Environmental Protection Agency). 2004a (March 11). *Origin of 1 Meal/Week Noncommerical Fish Consumption Rate in National Advisory for Mercury. Technical Memorandum.* [Online]. Available: http://www.epa.gov/waterscience/fishadvice/1-meal-per-week.pdf [accessed September 8, 2005].

US EPA. 2004b. *National Listing of Fish Advisories: Fact Sheet.* EPA-823-F-04-016. [Online]. Available: http://www.epa.gov/waterscience/fish/advisories/factsheet.pdf [accessed September 8, 2005].

US EPA. 2005a. *2004 National Listing of Fish Advisories: Fact Sheet (September 2005).* [Online]. Available: http://www.epa.gov/waterscience/fish/advisories/fs2004.html [accessed September 13, 2005].

US EPA. 2005b. *The National Listing of Fish Advisories (NLFA).* [Online]. Available: http://www.epa.gov/waterscience/fish/advisories/index.html [accessed September 13, 2005].

US EPA/FDA (US Environmental Protection Agency and the Food and Drug Administration). 2004. *What You Need to Know About Mercury in Fish and Shellfish.* EPA-823-R-04-005. [Online]. Available: http://www.epa.gov/waterscience/fishadvice/advice/html or http://www.cfsan.fda.gov/~dms/admehg3.html [accessed September 8, 2005].

USDA. 2005. *My Pyramid: Steps to a Healthier You.* [Online]. Available: http://www.mypyramid.gov [accessed September 27, 2005].

WHO/FAO (World Health Organization/Food and Agriculture Organization) Expert Consultation on Diet, Nutrition and the Prevention of Chronic Diseases. 2003. *Diet, Nutrition and the Prevention of Chronic Diseases.* Geneva, Switzerland: World Health Organization. [Online]. Available: http://www.who.int/dietphysicalactivity/publications/trs916/kit/en/ [accessed October 27, 2005].

2

Consumption Patterns and Composition of Seafood

This chapter provides a discussion of seafood consumption in terms of trends over time, major types of seafood, and current intake among the general population and various subgroups. This is followed by a discussion of future trends in seafood supplies that may have an impact on seafood selections. The discussion then reviews information on the consumption and sources of nutrients, particularly the omega-3 fatty acids eicosapentaenoic acid (EPA) and docosahexaenoic acid (DHA), because seafood is their primary source in the US diet. Finally, the overall nutrient profiles of seafood are compared to those of other foods in the diet.

SEAFOOD CONSUMPTION

Trends over Time

Trends in seafood consumption can be tracked using national food supply data. These data are especially useful because the methodology for collecting and analyzing them has remained consistent for nearly 100 years. Per capita seafood consumption is calculated by the National Marine Fisheries Service (NMFS) of the Department of Commerce using a disappearance model. This model estimates, on an annual basis, the total US supply of imported and landed seafood converted to raw edible weight, minus exports and other decreases in supply. The edible supply determined by this method is then divided by the total population to estimate per capita consumption (Source: http://www.nmfs.noaa.gov). The estimate can be considered an upper bound of seafood consumption, because some amount

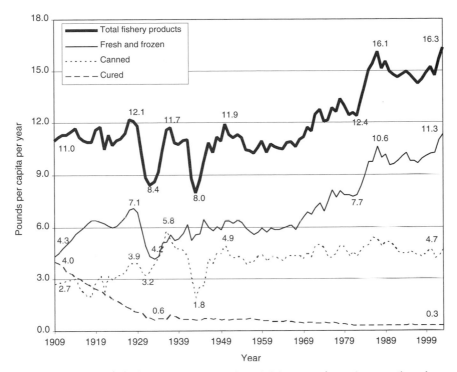

FIGURE 2-1 Trends in US consumption of total fishery products, by type (boneless, trimmed [edible] weight), in pounds per capita per year, 1909–2003. Figures are calculated on the basis of edible raw meat. Excludes edible offal, bones, and viscera for fishery products. Excludes game consumption for fishery product. Calculated from data not rounded.
SOURCE: ERS, 2004.

of the product is wasted at the household level. As shown in Figure 2-1, seafood consumption has increased since 1909, with notable exceptions during the Depression and the Second World War. In 2003, per capita seafood consumption was 16.3 pounds per person (Source: http://www.ers.usda.gov/data/foodconsumption/spreadsheet.mtfish.xls). As can be seen from Figure 2-1, the increase in seafood consumption results from an increase in consumption of fresh and frozen forms rather than canned and cured seafood.

Major Types of Seafood

There are several ways to consider the major types of seafood consumed, as shown in Tables 2-1 through 2-3. NMFS data are useful for

TABLE 2-1 NMFS Disappearance Data Ranked by Seafood Type for 2004 and 1994

	2004		1994	
Rank	Fish	Estimated Per Capita Consumption (pounds)	Fish	Estimated Per Capita Consumption (pounds)
1	Shrimp	4.2	Canned tuna	3.3
2	Canned tuna	3.3	Shrimp	2.5
3	Salmon	2.2	Pollock	1.5
4	Pollock	1.3	Salmon	1.1
5	Catfish	1.1	Cod	0.9
6	Tilapia	0.7	Catfish	0.9
7	Crab	0.6	Clams	0.5
8	Cod	0.6	Flatfish	0.4
9	Clams	0.5	Crab	0.3
10	Flatfish[a]	0.3	Scallops	0.3

NOTES: The figures are calculated on the basis of raw, edible meat, that is, excluding such offals as bones, viscera, and shells. Excludes game fish consumption.

   [a]Includes flounder and sole.

SOURCE: NFI, 2005.

examining the top species entering retail distribution channels in a given year. Table 2-1 shows estimated US per capita consumption calculated from disappearance data by type of seafood for 1994 and 2004. Over this decade, shrimp and tuna remained the most frequently consumed seafood; the top

TABLE 2-2 Percentage of Persons (Aged 2 and Older) Reporting Having Eaten Different Types of Seafood in Last 30 Days, 1999–2000

Rank	Seafood Type	Percent Consuming
1	Shrimp	84.6
2	Tuna	49.1
3	Crab	25.3
4	Breaded fish[a]	23.6
5	Salmon	20.2
6	Clams	15.2
7	Catfish	14.9
8	Scallops	13.2
9	Lobster	12.3
10	Oysters	10.1

   [a]Breaded fish, although not identified by type, is commonly pollock, which explains its high ranking among the top 10 seafoods consumed.

SOURCE: CDC/NCHS, 1999/2000.

TABLE 2-3 Proportion of Total Seafood Consumed on a Given Day, for Various Types of Seafood, 1999–2000

Rank	Seafood Type	Percent Consumed
1	Tuna	22.1
2	Shrimp	16.1
3	Salmon	8.9
4	Mix of fish	8.1
5	Crab	7.5
6	Cod	5.1
7	Flounder	4.5
8	Catfish	4.2
9	Don't know type	3.4
10	Clams	2.4

SOURCE: DGAC, 2005.

ten seafood types were consistent, except that tilapia replaced scallops. The data represented in Table 2-1 docs not take into account possible regional differences in seafood consumption. Rupp et al. (1980) reported that most regional differences in seafood consumption were attributable to freshwater and shellfish. Generally, consumption of freshwater species was greater in inland compared to coastal regions. Miller and Nash (1971) reported that overall shellfish consumption was greater in coastal regions, but the species consumed varied between northern and southern coastal areas, e.g., consumption of clams was greater in New England whereas consumption of oysters was greater in South Atlantic and Pacific states.

Another way of considering the top seafood is to compare the percentage of the population having eaten different types of seafood. In 1999–2000, the National Health and Nutrition Examination Survey (NHANES) queried respondents about their frequency of consumption of various seafood types in the previous 30 days. Table 2-2 provides a ranking of these by the percentage reporting consumption at least once. Consistent with the NMFS data, shrimp and tuna are the types consumed by the largest percentage of respondents, and crab, salmon, clams, catfish, scallops, and cod are included among the top choices. "Breaded fish" is not identified by type, and could represent some double-counting with other types, but is of interest for its relatively high use and caloric density.

Finally, another indication of the top types of seafood can be gleaned from the 1999–2000 NHANES 24-hour recalls of dietary intake. While respondents report seafood consumption in various ways—consumed with or without other ingredients added—the seafood portion alone can be examined by disaggregating all the ingredients using the US Department of Agriculture's (USDA) FoodLink database. Table 2-3 provides the major types of seafood consumed in the United States, using food intake data from all respondents aged 2 years and over. The types of seafood accounting for the greatest proportion consumed on a given day were tuna, about 22 percent; shrimp, about 16 percent; salmon, about 9 percent; mixed fish, about 8 percent; and crab, about 7 percent (DGAC, 2005).

The congruence of disappearance and consumption data on the types of seafood consumed in the diet of the US population provides a solid basis from which to make recommendations for consumer choices. Notably, the four fish (shark, swordfish, king mackerel, and tilefish) identified in federal advisories (US EPA/FDA, 2004) as those which pregnant women should avoid eating are not among those that are widely consumed by the general population.

It should also be noted that tuna consumption shown on Tables 2-1 to 2-3 represents an aggregate of both "light" and "white" tuna. According to the USDA, approximately 75 percent of tuna consumed is light and 25 percent is white (DGAC, 2005). Substantial differences exist between light and white tuna, in both fatty acid composition and potential toxicants (see Box 2-1). The significance of this aggregation will become evident in the following discussions.

Current Seafood Intake by the General Population

Food intake data obtained using 24-hour recalls from a representative sample are generally considered the best source of point estimate consumption data for a population. As shown in Table 2-4, about 16 percent of individuals consume some seafood on a given day, with the average quantity consumed being 89 grams (g) or approximately 3 ounces. These are quantities reported as eaten, so they generally represent cooked weights. Adult males and pregnant/lactating women whose intake was at or above the 95th percentile of quantities consumed reported intakes exceeding 280 g or about 10 ounces for days they consumed seafood.

The percentage of individuals consuming seafood varies among age groups, with children and adolescents being least, and those aged 40 to 59 years most, likely to consume seafood on a given day. Within each age category, there is little difference between the percentage of males and females consuming seafood. If the entire population consumed two 3-ounce servings (4 ounces raw) per week, the average quantity consumed per person per day would be expected to be 24 g per day (28 g per ounce × 6 ounces per week/7 days per week). Table 2-4 shows that no groups averaged this level of intake, and few groups even came close. These data suggest that seafood consumption for most individuals in the population is below targeted intake levels. Further, the committee recognizes that because of limitations in the supply of available seafood along with reported seafood consumption pat-

BOX 2-1
Tuna: White vs. Light

Tuna is the most popular fish used for canning and is the second most consumed type of seafood in the United States. Japan and the United States consume 36 and 31 percent, respectively, of the global tuna catch.

Tuna is a predatory fish that, if consumed in large quantities, may contain levels of methylmercury that exceed recommended safe levels. Although many different tuna species are fished, the most popular commercial varieties are described below.

White Tuna
Albacore—high in fat and rich in EPA/DHA; it has the whitest flesh and is typically referred to as white tuna; it is eaten both canned and fresh. Albacore generally contains more methylmercury than other types of tuna and may also contain more lipophilic compounds.
Northern Bluefin—high in fat and EPA/DHA; it is a slow-growing and thus rarer species than albacore and has a very high-quality meat; its major market is Japan, where it is used for sashimi.
Southern Bluefin—stocks are in decline and thus it is harder to obtain than other tunas. It is the most expensive fresh tuna.

Light Tuna
Skipjack—leaner than albacore tuna; it is the most commonly used tuna for canning.
Yellowfin—larger and leaner than albacore; it has pale pink flesh and is the second most popular species of tuna used in canning.
Bigeye—similar to yellowfin; it has a milder flavor than skipjack or yellowfin and is frequently used in canning.

Most canned tuna sold in the United States is available as "solid," also called "fancy" (a solid piece of loin, cut to fit the can); or "chunk" (a mixture of cut pieces). Canned tuna comes packed in either oil or water and is labeled either "white" or "light." Chunk light tuna packed in water is the most popular form of canned tuna sold in the United States. The source for most of this tuna is skipjack, although individual cans may contain more than one species of tuna. Albacore or "white" tuna is almost always packed in water in solid form.

NOTES: A standard of identity is used to define the species of fish that may be canned under the name "tuna" (21 CFR 161.190[a]). There is also a standard for fill-of-container of canned tuna (21 CFR 161.190[c]). These standards provide for various styles of pack, including solid pack, chunk or chunk style, flakes, and grated tuna. Provision is also made for type of packing media (water or oil), certain specified seasonings and flavorings, color designations, and methods for determining fill-of-containers (Source: http://www.cfsan.fda.gov/~dms/qa-ind4g.html).

SOURCE: Derived from US Tuna Foundation (http://www.tunafacts.org/abouttuna/index.html).

TABLE 2-4 Total Seafood: Percentage of Persons Using Food and Quantities Consumed in a Day

| Statistic | All Individuals Aged 2 and Over | Age (years) and Sex | | | |
		2–5 Males and Females	6–11 Males and Females	12–19 Males	Females
Number in sample	17,107	1521	2098	2244	2261
Percent of persons using in 1 day	15.9	10.2	9.9	7.9	11.2
Quantity consumed in 1 day, by users (1 ounce = 28 g)					
Mean	89.2	49.6	58.5	77.4	62.2
SEM	2.6	4.7	4.4	7.2	6.2
5th percentile	0.2	5.4	0.1	0.4	0.1
10th percentile	7.0	7.0	6.1	12.3	0.1
25th percentile	27.9	14.8	23.7	24.7	13.8
50th percentile	60.8	37.3	47.4	56.2	39.4
75th percentile	114.2	65.4	84.4	102.3	89.8
90th percentile	192.7	108.1	111.6	170.7	151.8
95th percentile	267.1	149.9	153.5	227.5	201.2
Average quantity consumed per person per day					
Mean	14.2	5.0	5.8	6.1	6.9
SEM	0.7	0.7	0.8	0.8	0.8

[a]Indicates a statistic that is potentially unreliable because of small sample size or large coefficient of variation (CVs have yet to be determined).

[b]Indicates a percentage that is greater than 0 but less than 0.05 or a mean, SEM, or percentile that is greater than 0 but less that 0.5.

SOURCE: CDC/NCHS, 1999–2002.

terns for most Americans, it is unlikely that targeted intake levels will be achieved on a population-wide scale.

Figure 2-2 provides an indication of where people are most likely to consume seafood. According to data from the 1999–2000 NHANES, about 58 percent of seafood is consumed at home or in someone else's home, 25 percent is consumed in a restaurant, and 8 percent at work or school. Only about 4 percent is consumed at a fast-food restaurant, though some at-home consumption could include seafood brought into the house from a fast-food outlet.

20–39		40–59		60 and older		Pregnant/ Lactating Women	Females, Age 15 to 45
Males	Females	Males	Females	Males	Females		
1372	1844	1345	1361	1512	1549	709	3658
16.6	17.2	19.3	19.4	17.8	18.2	19.3	16.4
110.7	83.3	112.3	82.1	101.8	76.7	97.7	81.9
7.4	6.4	7.8	6.4	7.5	5.2	15.7	5.8
3.1	0.1	4.6	0.1	2.8	3.6	0.1	0.1
8.5	4.9	16.8	1.5	16.8	11.3	0.1	3.6
29.6	26.9	49.4	27.9	41.9	25.6	37.3	24.5
72.8	58.5	90.0	55.8	83.4	56.2	60.8	55.8
151.1	95.6	137.3	118.7	118.2	105.2	119.7	98.6
257.7	172.5	237.2	178.5	220.6	166.0	268.6	174.2
292.6	268.6	294.9	252.8	352.9	192.2	306.9	262.5
18.4	14.3	21.6	15.9	18.1	14.0	18.8	13.4
1.6	1.6	1.7	1.9	1.8	0.9	3.4	1.4

Current Seafood Intake by Population Subgroups

Results from several studies indicate differences in seafood consumption among specific ethnic groups (Burger et al., 1999; Burger, 2002; Sechena et al., 2003; Sharma et al., 2003, 2004; Arnold and Middaugh, 2004; Ballew et al., 2004). Some of these population groups may have higher exposure to contaminants as a result of their seafood consumption practices. For example, they may consume more fish, compared to the general population, from waters in locations known to be contaminated. While data from studies of consumption practices are not directly comparable because of

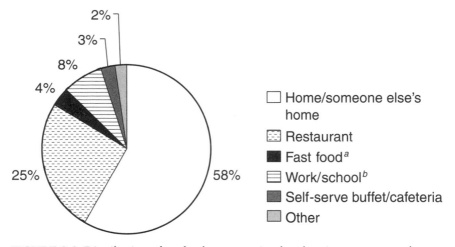

FIGURE 2-2 Distribution of seafood consumption by place it was consumed.
[a]Includes food eaten at takeout restaurant, in store, and in car.
[b]Includes food eaten by children in day care.
SOURCE: CDC/NCHS, 1999/2000.

methodological and reporting differences, they are useful for gleaning some insights into differences in consumption among different groups.

Multiethnic Cohort Study

The Multiethnic Cohort (MEC) Study is a large, population-based study designed to assess variations in specific rates of cancer occurrence among various ethnic groups and to characterize both environmental and genetic factors contributing to cancer incidence. Conducted between 1993 and 1996, the study collected comprehensive lifestyle and dietary data on the cohort (Sharma et al., 2003, 2004). The cohort reflected a range of educational levels, although cohort members were more educated than the general population.

Study participants in Hawaii and Los Angeles, California, included population samples from five self-identified ethnic groups—African Americans, Latinos, Japanese Americans, Native Hawaiians, and Whites—aged 45 to 75 years, who completed a mailed self-administered quantitative Food Frequency Questionnaire (FFQ) that was developed specifically for the study population (Sharma et al., 2004). The study objectives included providing prospective data on exposures and biomarkers thought to alter cancer risk; data collected from the questionnaires included information on dietary and other lifestyle and health practices (Kolonel et al., 2004). Table 2-5 shows

TABLE 2-5 Mean Seafood Intake Consumed Per Week Among Various Ethnic Groups, in the Multiethnic Cohort Study (1993–1996)

Ethnic Group	Mean + SD[a], Amount Consumed Per Week (ounces)
African Americans	
Men (n=11,772)	4.9±4.9
Women (n=20,130)	4.2±4.2
Latinos, born in Mexico, South or Central America	
Men (n=10,180)	4.9±5.6
Women (n=10,903)	3.5±4.9
Latinos, born in United States	
Men (n=10,613)	3.5±4.2
Women (n=11,255)	2.8±3.5
Japanese Americans	
Men (n=25,893)	7.0±6.3
Women (n=28,355)	5.6±4.9
Native Hawaiians	
Men (n=5979)	9.1±9.1
Women (n=7650)	7.7±7.7
Whites	
Men (n=21,933)	4.9±4.9
Women (n=25,303)	3.5±3.5

NOTE: The daily amounts reported in the study were converted to weekly amounts for this table.

[a]SD = Standard Deviation.

SOURCES: Derived from Sharma et al., 2003, 2004.

information collected from the MEC study on consumption of seafood by specific ethnic groups. The study reported food intakes in terms of ounces of lean meat equivalents, which for seafood can generally be thought of as ounces of cooked seafood consumed. The daily amounts reported in the study were converted to weekly amounts for Table 2-5. While these data are not representative of every ethnic group in the United States, and there is large variation in intakes among all groups; the means suggest there may be higher intakes among Native Hawaiians and Japanese Americans than among African Americans, Latinos, and Whites.

Asian American Populations

Among Asian American and Pacific Island members of the population in the contiguous United States, seafood consumption is an important aspect of cultural behavior. Self-harvesting and consuming seafood are seen as healthy activities that echo a culturally familiar lifestyle, but may also be an economic necessity. Asian American and Pacific Island groups consume greater amounts, different types, and different parts of seafood than the general population (Sechena et al., 2003).

A large population of Laotian immigrants (Hmong) who settled in Wisconsin have been studied to determine how their fishing and seafood consumption habits differ from those of the general US population. Hutchison and Kraft (1994) found that individuals in Hmong households in Green Bay, Wisconsin, consumed an average of 30 fish meals per year compared to 18 fish meals per year consumed by Wisconsin anglers in the general population. About one-third of the fish caught were reported to come from lakes where fishing advisories warned against eating locally caught fish, suggesting that this group is at greater risk from exposure to contaminants in fish than the general population.

Some members of the Asian American population have undergone acculturation resulting in food choices that are more similar to those of the general US population than population groups from their country of origin (Kudo et al., 2000; Kim and Chan, 2004). Kudo et al. (2000) studied the eating patterns of Japanese immigrants and their US-born descendants. Their findings show dietary changes among succeeding generations of Japanese American females, and suggest that acculturation-related changes may contribute to decreased intake of many traditional foods, including fish.

American Indian/Alaskan Native and First Nations Populations

Many indigenous peoples, particularly those who live in Alaska and northern Canada, maintain a subsistence life-style and diet. The dietary practices of these populations are an important part of their self-definition, culture, health, and well-being, as well as a part of the socioeconomic structure of their communities.

A survey of coastal First Nations communities in British Columbia indicated that, although traditional dietary patterns have changed considerably since the introduction of Europeans to the Americas, seafood and other marine food sources remain an important part of the culture and nutritional resources of this population group (Mos et al., 2004). The survey showed that fishing and gathering of seafood was practiced regularly among 46 percent of respondents and that traditional methods were used 94 percent of the time. Among the types of seafood consumed by First Nations communities, salmon was the most popular; 95 percent of respondents reported consuming salmon each year and an average of 42 percent of all seafood meals consisted of salmon.

Availability of data on seafood consumption practices among Alaskan Natives and other Northern Dwellers is limited. Further, traditional foods that are consumed in Alaska vary by region, local preference, and seasonal availability. The range of traditional foods available includes fish, marine mammals, shellfish, ascidians (sea squirts), sea cucumbers, and seaweed. Also included are nonmarine game meats, berries, and edible plants (Kuhnlein et al., 2000). Specific examples of wild-caught foods commonly consumed by Northern Dwellers include caribou meat, arctic char, Beluga (whale), muktuk, geese, whitefish, and trout (see Glossary for definitions) (Kuhnlein et al., 2000).

Muckle et al. (2001) reported that among Inuit women of childbearing age, about 80 percent consumed fish at least once per week and the average frequency of consumption of fish meals was 3.3 times per week. This population also consumed traditional products including beluga whale fat, muktuk, and seal fat, meat, and liver; their consumption of these foods increased during pregnancy.

Kuhnlein et al. (2004) report that since the introduction of nonnative foods to the Canadian Arctic at the turn of the 20th century, the use of native (traditional) foods has declined such that, among adults, only 10–36 percent of dietary energy is derived from traditional foods. Additionally, Receveur et al. (1997) found that traditional food consumption among Dene/Métis communities was associated with greater intake of iron, zinc, and potassium, and lower intake of sodium, fat, saturated fat, and sugar. Considered in conjunction with the cultural integration and importance of dietary traditions, advice to indigenous peoples to change their long-standing dietary patterns in order to reduce exposure to contaminants may not only not be beneficial, but could have deleterious health effects (Marien and Patrick, 2001).

Sport and Subsistence Fishers

The number of subsistence fishers in the United States and the amount of seafood they consume is difficult to estimate due to the challenge of identifying members of this population and a lack of data collected on them. By and large, individuals who engage in sport and subsistence fishing tend to consume more fish than the general population (Burger, 2002). Among anglers (those who crab and/or fish) in the Newark Bay Complex area of New Jersey, Blacks and Hispanics ate more fish than Whites or Asians (Burger, 2002). Similarly, Burger et al. (1999) noted that Blacks living along the Savannah River in South Carolina consumed both larger portions of seafood as well as higher total amounts compared to Whites. In that study, levels of intake were also related to education: those who did not graduate from high school ate seafood more often, consumed more total seafood, and consumed more intact fish than those with at least a high school degree.

While Alaskan Natives fish for sustenance (Ballew et al., 2004), others, e.g., the Newark Bay Complex group (Burger, 2002), angled primarily for recreation, relaxation, and communing with nature, and more than 30 percent did not eat the crab or fish they caught. Thus, quantities obtained from fishing do not provide an accurate indicator of consumption.

FUTURE SEAFOOD SUPPLIES

Changes in Supply and Demand

The nation's seafood supply is changing in ways that are likely to have a significant impact on consumer choice in the future. Changes in amounts, types, sources, and cost of seafood are predicted to continue in the next decades due largely to increasing demand. Over the past two decades the US population has grown by about 20 percent, and consumer demand for seafood fluctuated between about 14.5 and 16.5 pounds per person (see Figure 2-1). As mentioned previously, per capita seafood consumption was 16.6 pounds in 2004 (NMFS, 2005a), which represents almost 4.7 billion pounds of seafood.

The demand for seafood in the United States now exceeds domestic supplies, and fulfilling that demand requires more dependence on international sources. Seafood on the international market currently accounts for over 75 percent of the world marine fisheries' catch, and a trend of increasing consumption is expected to continue (Watson and Pauly, 2001). The world production of edible fishery products, defined as both captured and farmed fish, reached a total of 103 million metric tons in 2003, which provided an estimated annual per capita supply of 16.3 kilograms or 35.9 pounds (live-weight equivalents) (FAO, 2004). Predictions about future world seafood supplies suggest that, at current rates of consumption, the world seafood supply will not keep pace with demand. The deficit is forecast to be 9.4 million metric tons by 2010, increasing to 10.9 million tons by 2015 (FAO, 2004). Although a recommendation to consume two 3-ounce servings of seafood per week may be beneficial to consumers (discussed in Chapter 3), if the entire population increased current consumption to meet this proposed consumption level, the supply of seafood would likely not be able to support the increased demand.

Impact of Aquaculture on Seafood Supplies

Aquaculture is one alternative that may contribute to closing the gap between diminishing seafood supplies and increasing demand. World production of seafood from farms or aquaculture operations is growing more rapidly than production of all other food-producing animals in the world (FAO, 2004). Between 1970 and 2002, the percentage of total seafood product weight provided by aquaculture production increased from 3.9 to almost

30 percent (FAO, 2004). This represents an increase of approximately one percent per year; however, that rate cannot keep pace with anticipated increases in seafood demand. Furthermore, the total aquaculture production figures can be deceiving in that the major portion of world aquaculture production involves freshwater species, e.g., carp (FAO, 2004). This fish is not a common consumer selection in most developed nations, particularly the United States.

The top ten seafood types consumed in the United States (shown in Table 2-1) are marine (or saltwater) species, although not all are wild-caught. Current seafood consumption patterns are beginning to lead to reductions in supply for some species that will influence future availability and price. For example, flatfish (e.g., flounder, sole, and halibut), among the top ten types of seafood consumed in 1990, are less prevalent today.

Aquacultured seafood (e.g., salmon, catfish, and shrimp) is now supplementing the supply for some of these seafood choices of long-standing popularity. The recent increase in per capita consumption of shrimp over tuna was in part due to the increasing supply and lower price resulting from aquaculture. Aquaculture has also contributed to the 100-fold increase in salmon consumption and introduced a new selection, tilapia, to the top ten per capita seafood consumed in 2004.

An emerging concern about aquaculture is that it is largely used for production of carnivorous species such as salmon, and the feed used is based on fish meal. The source of fish meal is considered an industrial product (wild-caught fish that is not used for human consumption) obtained from capture fisheries (FAO, 2002). Pound for pound, however, the amount of wild-caught fish needed to produce fish meal exceeds by more than two times the amount of fish produced by aquaculture for human consumption (Naylor et al., 2000).

Future Trends

Future trends in availability for the most popular seafood consumed in the United States can be estimated from comparisons of annual production over the past 10 years (Table 2-6). These estimates are based on total reported catch from 1995 through predictions for 2005.

While the NMFS and the eight regional Fishery Management Councils report that 2004 assessments of domestic stocks indicated that fishery management strategies have resulted in increases in some stocks to a sustainable yield, most of the top ten seafood choices were not among them (NMFS, 2005b). Limited availability of these popular seafood types may translate into more resource competition and higher prices.

The additional competition of recreational fishing has a further impact on seafood supplies. Coleman et al. (2004) concluded that the less-regulated

TABLE 2-6 General Trends and Predictions for the Supply and Sources of Popular Fish Consumed in the United States from 1995 through 2005

Seafood Type	Supply Trend	Domestic Supply		Imported Supply	
		Catch	Farmed	Catch	Farmed
Salmon	Increasing[e]	Limited	Limited	Increasing	Increasing
Tilapia	Increasing	Limited	Increasing	Limited	Increasing
Catfish[a]	Increasing	Limited	Limited	Increasing	Increasing
Cod	Limited[f]	Limited	N/A	Limited	Increasing
Flatfish/Soles[b]	Limited	Limited	N/A	Limited	Increasing
Tuna[c]	Limited	Limited	N/A	Limited	N/A
Haddock	Limited	Limited	N/A	N/A	N/A
Halibut	Limited	Limited	N/A	N/A	N/A
O. perch	Limited	Limited	N/A	Limited	N/A
Pollock	Limited	Limited	N/A	Limited	N/A
O. roughy	Declining[f]	N/A[g]	N/A	Limited	N/A
Rockfishes	Declining	Declining	N/A	N/A	N/A
K. mackerel[d]	Limited	Limited	N/A	N/A	N/A
Swordfish[d]	Limited	Limited	N/A	Limited	N/A
Tilefish[d]	Declining	Declining	N/A	N/A	N/A
Sharks[d]	Limited	Limited	N/A	Declining	N/A

NOTE: The listings include some of, but are not limited to, the most popular fish relative to consumption totals based on annual fishery reports and other sources.

[a]Catfish can include domestic cultured varieties as well as imported varieties.

[b]Flatfish can include flounders and sole.

[c]Tuna includes all major commercial species; tuna is also "farmed" in some countries through the capture of smaller fish, which are fed in pens.

[d]The four fish targeted by the FDA/US EPA advisory on methylmercury (FDA/US EPA, 2004).

[e]Increasing = More annual supply can be available than is currently produced either from underfished resources and/or aquaculture (existing or emerging).

[f]Supply is described as either limited or declining due to overfishing (the domestic resources are near or exceed steady state annual yield as estimated by NMFS [2005]).

[g]N/A = The resource is not available in the respective situation or data is not available per the listing.

SOURCES: FAO, 2004; NMFS, 2005a,b; SAFMC, 2005; Personal communication, W. Swingle, Gulf of Mexico Fishery Management Council, January 2006; Personal communication, G. Waugh, Deputy Executive Director, South Atlantic Fishery Management Council, January 10, 2006.

recreational fishery is exerting a large impact on certain popular seafood selections. They reported that in 2002, the recreational catch of fish "populations of concern" (i.e., popular types that were at risk for overfishing) accounted for 64, 38, 59, and 12 percent of the catch in the Gulf of Mexico, South Atlantic, Pacific, and Northeastern coastal waters, respectively. Some of these recreationally caught and consumed types, e.g., king mackerel, have been identified in advisories as fish that pregnant women should not consume. In the Gulf of Mexico, the regional fishery management plans allocate 68 percent of the king mackerel harvest to recreational fishermen (GMFMC, 2006).

Table 2-6 shows that several popular species are overfished and supplies are declining. Among capture fisheries worldwide, 28 percent of fish stocks have been estimated to be depleted or overexploited (FAO, 2002). In the United States, over 18 percent of the 236 fish stocks or stock complexes with known overfishing status have a mortality rate that exceeds the overfishing threshold (i.e., subject to overfishing) (NMFS, 2005b). Supply predictions for shark (Baum et al., 2003), tilefish, king mackerel, and swordfish (identified in the joint FDA/US EPA methylmercury advisory) suggest that they will likely decrease. In addition, changes in the supply of other wild-caught seafood will also influence seafood selections for all segments of the population in the future.

NUTRIENT PROFILES OF SEAFOOD COMPARED TO OTHER FOODS IN THE DIET

Foods with similar nutrient profiles are often grouped together for the purpose of making dietary recommendations. Seafood is grouped with meats, poultry, eggs, nuts, legumes, and seeds as major contributors (supplying >50 percent) of protein, niacin, zinc, and vitamin B6 to the diet. These foods are also substantial contributors (supplying >10 percent) of vitamins E and B12, thiamin, riboflavin, phosphorus, magnesium, iron, copper, potassium, and linoleic acid. Among these foods, however, higher levels of selenium and the omega-3 fatty acids EPA and DHA and generally lower levels of saturated fats are unique to seafood. Although EPA and DHA are found in other protein-rich foods (i.e., poultry and eggs), fish that are high in EPA/DHA (e.g., salmon, lake trout, and white [albacore] tuna) have the highest concentration per serving among food sources. Table 2-7 provides a comparison of the availability of some macro- and micronutrients, including the omega-3 fatty acids EPA (20:5 n-3) and DHA (22:6 n-3) in three types of seafood, as well as chicken, beef, and eggs, and the alpha-linolenic acid (ALA; 18:3 n-3) in walnuts.

EPA and DHA

An important reason for choosing seafood over other protein food sources is that it is a primary source of the omega-3 fatty acids EPA and DHA. The benefits of these two fatty acids are described in detail in Chapter 3. The following discussion provides information about sources and consumption patterns of EPA/DHA.

TABLE 2-7 Nutrients in Selected Seafoods and Other Comparable Foods

Food	Content per 100 g		
	Energy (kcal)	Protein (g)	Total Fat (g)
FISH			
Tuna, canned, light, packed in water	116	25.51	0.82
Tuna, canned, white, packed in water	128	23.62	2.97
Shrimp, mixed species, cooked, moist heat	99	20.91	1.08
Salmon, Atlantic, farmed, cooked, dry heat	206	22.10	12.35
Pollock, Atlantic, cooked, dry heat	118	24.92	1.26
Catfish, channel, farmed, cooked, dry heat	152	18.72	8.02
Cod, Atlantic, cooked, dry heat	105	22.83	0.86
Crab, blue, cooked, moist heat	102	20.20	1.77
Halibut, Atlantic and Pacific, cooked, dry heat	140	26.69	2.94
BEEF			
Ground beef, 80% lean, patty, cooked, broiled	271	25.75	17.82
Eye of round roast, all grades, trimmed to 1/8" fat, cooked	208	28.31	9.65
Top sirloin, all grades, trimmed to 1/8" fat, cooked, broiled	243	26.96	14.23
PORK			
Cured ham, boneless, regular, roasted	178	22.62	9.02
Pork loin, center rib, boneless, cooked, roasted	252	26.99	15.15
Ground fresh pork, cooked	297	25.69	20.77
POULTRY			
Chicken breast, meat and skin, cooked, roasted[b]	197	29.80	7.78
Chicken breast, meat only, cooked, roasted[b]	165	31.02	3.57
Turkey, meat and skin, cooked, roasted	208	28.10	9.73
Turkey, ground, cooked	235	27.36	13.15
SAUSAGES AND LUNCHEON MEATS			
Frankfurter, meat	290	10.26	25.76
Frankfurter, beef	330	11.24	29.57
Turkey roll, light meat	147	18.70	7.22
Bologna, beef and pork	308	15.20	24.59
OTHER			
Egg, poached[b]	147	12.53	9.90
Egg, omega[c]	125	10.00	10.00
Walnuts, English	654	15.23	65.21
Seeds, flaxseed	534	18.29	42.16

[a]Total 18:3 fatty acid.

[b]EPA/DHA levels in chicken and egg are based on existing published data; changes in the use of fishmeal in feed sources may impact levels detected in the future.

[c]Derived from Sindelar et al., 2004.

—No data available.

SOURCE: USDA National Nutrient Database for Standard Reference, Release 18 (unless otherwise specified).

SFA (g)	EPA (g)	DHA (g)	ALA (g)	Ca (mg)	Fe (mg)	Zn (mg)	Se (µg)	B-6 (mg)
0.234	0.047	0.223	0.002[a]	11	1.53	0.77	80.4	0.350
0.792	0.233	0.629	0.071[a]	14	0.97	0.48	65.7	0.217
0.289	0.171	0.144	0.012[a]	39	3.09	1.56	39.6	0.127
2.504	0.690	1.457	0.113[a]	15	0.34	0.43	41.4	0.647
0.170	0.091	0.451	—	77	0.59	0.60	46.8	0.331
1.789	0.049	0.128	0.082[a]	9	0.82	1.05	14.5	0.163
0.168	0.004	0.154	0.001[a]	14	0.49	0.58	37.6	0.283
0.228	0.243	0.231	0.021[a]	104	0.91	4.22	40.2	0.180
0.417	0.091	0.374	0.083[a]	60	1.07	0.53	46.8	0.397
6.766	—	—	0.050	24	2.48	6.25	21.5	0.367
3.664	—	—	0.093[a]	7	2.29	4.70	28.7	0.372
5.603	—	—	0.127[a]	20	1.73	4.87	29.2	0.564
3.120	—	—	0.240[a]	8	1.34	2.47	19.8	0.310
5.350	—	—	0.030[a]	6	0.93	2.64	40.3	0.363
7.720	—	—	0.070[a]	22	1.29	3.21	35.4	0.391
2.190	0.010	0.030	0.060[a]	14	1.07	1.02	24.7	0.560
1.010	0.010	0.020	0.030[a]	15	1.04	1.00	27.6	0.600
2.840	—	0.040	0.110[a]	26	1.79	2.96	32.9	0.410
3.390	—	0.030	0.150[a]	25	1.93	2.86	37.2	0.390
7.667	—	—	0.146[a]	99	1.09	1.20	12.5	0.166
11.688	—	—	0.176[a]	14	1.51	2.46	8.2	0.089
2.020	—	0.020	0.090[a]	40	1.28	1.56	22.3	0.320
9.301	—	—	0.055[a]	85	1.21	2.30	24.6	0.297
3.087	0.004	0.037	0.033[a]	53	1.83	1.10	31.6	0.142
2.500	—	0.170	0.420	—	—	—	—	—
6.126	—	—	9.080[a]	98	2.91	3.09	4.9	0.537
3.663	—	—	22.813[a]	255	5.73	4.34	25.4	0.473

Sources of EPA and DHA

Seafood is the primary source for EPA and DHA in human diets. Estimated amounts of EPA and DHA in the top seafood types consumed are shown in Table 2-8. The figures suggest that, other than salmon, the most frequently consumed types of fish are not particularly rich sources of these fatty acids.

The fatty acid concentration of farmed fish reflects the composition of the diets they are fed (Bell et al., 2003). Fish, like mammals, have a limited ability to deposit EPA and DHA in their tissues even when they are fed diets high in ALA (Tocher et al., 2003). Thus, farmed salmon need to be fed a source of EPA and DHA (e.g., fish oil) to have a fatty acid profile similar to that of wild salmon. Feeding diets that are high in fish oil for a period prior to harvest elevates levels of EPA and DHA in farmed salmon previously fed vegetable oils during part of their growing period (Bell et al., 2003).

TABLE 2-8 Mean Levels of EPA and DHA in the Top 10 Seafood Types Consumed in the United States

Seafood (type)[a]	# Data Points	Standard Error	EPA Content (g/100 g)	DHA Content (g/100 g)	Total n-3 Content (g/100 g)
Shrimp	11	N/A[b]	0.17	0.14	0.31
Light tuna	5	N/A	0.05	0.22	0.27
Salmon	2	N/A	0.69	1.46	2.15
Pollock	0[c]	N/A	0.09	0.45	0.54
Catfish	3	N/A	0.05	0.13	0.18
Tilapia	2	N/A	0.00	0.11	0.11
Crab	12 (EPA) 10 (DHA)	0.021 (EPA) 0.008 (DHA)	0.30	0.12	0.42
Cod	0[c]	N/A	0.00	0.15	0.15
Clams	0[c]	N/A	0.14	0.15	0.29
Flatfish	11	32.5 (EPA) 22.3 (DHA)	0.24	0.26	0.50

[a]Shrimp = Mixed, cooked, moist heat; Light tuna = light, canned in water, drained; Salmon = Atlantic, farmed, cooked; Pollock = Atlantic, cooked, dry heat; Catfish = Channel, farmed, cooked, dry heat; Tilapia = Cooked, dry heat; Crab = Alaska king, cooked, moist heat; Cod = Atlantic, cooked, dry heat; Clams = Mixed, cooked, moist heat; Flatfish = Flounder and sole species, cooked, dry heat.

[b]N/A means that the values are not available.

[c]As reported in USDA Nutrient Database Release 18 (http://www.nal.usda.gov/fnic/foodcomp/Data/SR18/sr18.html). Zeroes indicate that value was not derived analytically but was either calculated by difference or imputed from the value for some other similar food(s).

SOURCES: National Fisheries Institute (http://www.aboutseafood.com/media/top_10.cfm) and USDA Nutrient Database Release 18 (http://www.nal.usda.gov/fnic/foodcomp/Data/SR18/sr18.html).

As discussed in Chapter 1, the *Dietary Guidelines Advisory Committee Report* (DGAC, 2005) recommends that adults consume two portions (each 4 ounces raw/3 ounces cooked) of seafood per week. Following this recommendation would provide the consumer with a range of intake levels from 60 mg to 700 mg of EPA and DHA combined per day, depending on the type of seafood consumed.

Table 2-9 shows mean dietary intake levels of EPA, DHA, and EPA and DHA combined, for several sex/age groups from the 1999–2002 NHANES. Mean intake levels for the total population are estimated to be 35 mg of EPA and 68 mg of DHA per day. Although adults had greater intakes than children, and men greater intakes than women, none of the sex/age groups shown had average intakes of even 200 mg per day of EPA and DHA combined.

Consumption of High Compared to Low EPA/DHA Content Seafood

An analysis of NHANES data classified all seafood types as either high (> 500 milligrams per 3-ounce serving) or low (< 500 milligrams per 3-ounce serving) in EPA and DHA combined (DGAC, 2005). High EPA/DHA seafood includes anchovy, mackerel, pompano, salmon, sardines, sea bass, swordfish, and trout. Low EPA/DHA types include carp, catfish, clams, conches, cod, crabs, croaker, flounder, frogs, haddock, halibut, lobster, mullet, octopuses/squid, oysters, perch, pike, pollock, porgy, scallops, shrimp, snapper, and whiting.

In the NHANES survey, tuna was considered separately, because although there are both high- and low-EPA/DHA varieties of tuna, respondents usually cannot distinguish between them. Therefore, 75 percent of the tuna consumed was assigned to the low EPA/DHA group and the remainder to the high EPA/DHA group in accordance with USDA figures (DGAC, 2005). Figure 2-3 shows that the greatest percentage of seafood consumed is low in EPA/DHA, and that salmon, white tuna, sea bass, and trout are the most commonly consumed types of seafood high in EPA/DHA.

Another way to consider sources of EPA/DHA is to examine which foods contribute the most to the population's intake, a method that takes into account not only each food's fatty acid content but also in what quantities it is consumed. Tables 2-10 and 2-11 show the foods contributing the most to EPA and DHA intakes, respectively, according to data from the NHANES 1999–2002. Not surprisingly, various seafood types are among the major contributors of both fatty acids. What might not be expected, however, is that chicken and eggs contributed measurable amounts to EPA intake over this time period. Soups, while only contributing 1.8 percent of the EPA, are a curious addition to the table. These include not only fish chowders, but soups made from chickens that have been fed fishmeal. Whether chicken

TABLE 2-9 Dietary Intake of Linolenic Fatty Acid, Eicosapentaenoic Fatty Acid (EPA), Docosahexaenoic Fatty Acid (DHA), and EPA and DHA Combined

Statistic	All Individuals Aged 2 and Over	Age (years) and Sex			
		2–5 Males and Females	6–11 Males and Females	12–19 Males	Females
Number in sample	17,107	1521	2098	2244	2261
	g				
Linolenic fatty acid					
Mean	1.41	0.90	1.16	1.49	1.23
SEM	0.01	0.02	0.03	0.04	0.03
	mg				
Eicosapentaenoic fatty acid (EPA)					
Mean	35.26	11.94	14.16	16.91	16.78
SEM	1.99	2.10	1.74	1.91	1.68
Docosahexaenoic fatty acid (DHA)					
Mean	67.98	27.99	37.72	43.75	39.89
SEM	2.66	3.18	4.09	3.12	3.23
EPA and DHA combined					
Mean	103.25	39.93	51.87	60.67	56.66
SEM	4.53	5.21	5.59	4.64	4.68

SOURCE: CDC/NCHS, 1999–2002.

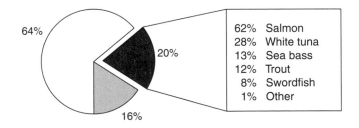

■ High Omega-3 Fish   ▨ Light Tuna (Low Omega-3)   ☐ Other Low Omega-3 Fish

FIGURE 2-3 Consumption estimates, as a percentage of total seafood consumed, by EPA/DHA content classification. High-EPA/DHA seafood is further delineated by type; white (albacore) tuna is high in EPA/DHA but light (e.g., skipjack) tuna is not.
SOURCE: DGAC, 2005.

20–39		40–59		60 and older		Pregnant/ Lactating Women	Females, Aged 15 to 45 Years
Males	Females	Males	Females	Males	Females		
1372	1844	1345	1361	1512	1549	709	3658
1.74	1.33	1.75	1.33	1.45	1.18	1.47	1.32
0.04	0.04	0.04	0.04	0.03	0.02	0.06	0.03
42.83	32.66	56.42	42.99	43.17	36.43	40.13	34.09
4.23	2.73	5.14	7.56	4.60	3.19	8.80	4.69
82.43	63.01	108.92	72.55	78.14	64.88	73.19	62.11
6.22	5.15	7.83	7.82	5.89	4.01	10.54	4.93
125.26	95.67	165.33	115.54	121.31	101.31	113.32	96.19
10.19	7.66	12.59	14.96	10.27	7.11	18.72	9.33

and egg products will continue to contribute significant amounts of DHA is uncertain because of changes in feed composition aimed at reducing amount of fishmeal used in animal feeds (Barlow, 2001).

As with farmed fish, feeding practices used in the poultry and egg industries may affect the content of EPA/DHA in these foods. Poultry feeds are predominantly vegetable- and grain-based, supplemented with animal and grain by-products (IOM, 2003), with cost driving the feed formulation. Fat sources used in poultry feed formulations can include animal fat, vegetable fat or oil, or feed-grade fat products (Hulan et al., 1989; Ratnayake and Ackman, 1989; Cantor, 1999; Gonzalez-Esquerra and Leeson, 2000). The feed ingredients most frequently used to increase the long-chain polyunsaturated fatty acid (LCPUFA) content of poultry meat include fish oil, flaxseed oil, and rapeseed (canola) oil (Komprda et al., 2005). The amount of fish meal used in a formulation has typically been about 1 percent of the total ingredients (IOM, 2003). Recent changes in fat sources used in poultry feed resulting in a lower fish meal content (Barlow, 2001) suggest a probable

TABLE 2-10 Food Sources of EPA Among the US
Population, Aged 2 Years and Older, 1999–2002

Food Group[a]	Percent of EPA	Cumulative Percent of EPA
Salmon	19.8	19.8
Shrimp	18.8	38.6
Chicken[b]	8.9	47.5
Crab	5.6	53.1
Trout	3.6	56.7
Tuna	3.2	59.9
Sardines	2.1	62.0
Catfish	2.0	64.0
Soups	1.8	65.8
Cod	1.6	67.4
Eggs	1.5	68.9
Fish, mixed types	1.5	70.4
Flounder	1.2	71.6
Other fish[c]	20.9	92.5

NOTE: Species not shown contributed <1 percent each.

[a]Includes mixed dishes composed mainly of this item.

[b]New data forthcoming show most nutrient levels comparable to earlier sample, but EPA/DHA levels as undetectable.

[c]Includes types not specified by respondent and types other than those listed elsewhere in table.

SOURCE: CDC/NCHS, 1999–2002.

decrease in detectable EPA/DHA levels in poultry and egg products. New forthcoming data on chicken and eggs show levels of most nutrients are comparable to earlier samples, but EPA/DHA levels as undetectable.

When egg-producing hens are fed diets enriched with EPA and DHA, their egg lipid content reflects their diet composition (Scheideler and Froning, 1996; Van Elswyk, 1997; Cantor, 1999; Bean and Leeson, 2003). Scheideler and Froening (1996) showed that the DHA content of eggs could be increased by about 3.5 times over that of unmodified eggs by feeding hens diets containing 5 percent whole flaxseed (2.8 times for a diet containing 5 percent ground flaxseed) compared to unmodified diets for control hens, indicating that some conversion of ALA to DHA occurs in the hen. The ALA content of the eggs increased nearly eightfold under the same conditions. Similarly, hens fed a diet with 2.5 percent dried algae meal high in DHA produced eggs with about 150 mg DHA per egg (Herber and Van Elswyk, 1996), similar to the level produced by feeding 1.5 percent fish oil.

Non-Animal Sources of Omega-3 Fatty Acids It is important for consumers to understand that there are different sources of omega-3 fatty acids. EPA and DHA are not endogenously synthesized from saturated, monounsatu-

TABLE 2-11 Food Sources of DHA Among the US Population, Aged 2 and Older, 1999–2002.

Food Group[a]	Percent of DHA	Cumulative Percent of DHA
Chicken[b]	15.6	15.6
Salmon	14.3	30.0
Eggs	9.4	39.4
Shrimp	8.6	48.0
Tuna	7.6	55.6
Trout	4.9	60.5
Catfish	3.1	63.6
Crab	2.9	66.5
Cod	1.6	68.1
Poultry, cold cuts/ground	1.3	69.4
Sardines	1.3	70.7
Fish, mixed types[c]	1.1	71.8
Turkey	1.0	72.8
Other fish	16.9	89.7

NOTE: Species not shown contributed < 1 percent each.

[a]Includes mixed dishes composed mainly of this item.

[b]New data forthcoming show most nutrient levels comparable to earlier sample, but EPA/DHA levels as undetectable.

[c]Includes types not specified by respondent and types other than those listed elsewhere in table.

SOURCE: CDC/NCHS, 1999–2002.

rated, or omega-6 fatty acids; they can only be made from the precursor omega-3 fatty acid ALA. Some current recommendations include the use of plant sources, such as walnuts and flaxseed oil, to obtain sufficient amounts of EPA and DHA in the diet (ADA, 2003). This suggestion is based on the observation that some vegetable oils contain significant amounts of ALA, and thus could be used as an alternative to direct consumption of EPA and DHA (refer to Supplemental Information, Appendix A for detailed information). However, as mentioned previously, humans do not convert EPA or DHA from ALA at rates high enough to reach recommended intake levels (Pawlosky et al., 2001). Furthermore, based on in vivo isotope studies, the rates of conversion differ between young men and women (Burdge et al., 2002; Burdge and Wootton, 2002), and between nonpregnant, pregnant, lactating and nonpregnant, and nonmenopausal women (Burdge and Wootton, 2002). Additionally, the extent to which ALA is utilized for energy rather than converted into EPA and DHA is likely driven by both the physiologic requirements for these fatty acids and by the quantity available in the diet (Burdge et al., 2002). For example, if the physiologic requirement for EPA is high, e.g., during pregnancy and lactation, and other energy needs are being met, there is likely to be more efficient utilization of ALA as a precursor source for EPA in women. On the other hand, an adult male who is not at risk for heart disease and whose energy needs are greater than his intake of calories from other sources would preferentially utilize ALA as an energy source rather than as a source of omega-3 fatty acids.

Production of long-chain polyunsaturated fatty acids from microorganisms, including lower fungi, bacteria, and marine microalgae, appears to be a promising source of omega-3 fatty acids, especially DHA (Cohen et al., 1995). The organisms *Schizochytrium* sp. and *Crypthecodinium cohnii* are currently used in commercial production of DHA. Sijtsma and de Swaaf (2004) have estimated that 50 large bioreactors could produce up to 10 percent of the quantity of DHA currently obtained from global production of fish oil.

The production of EPA and DHA in mustard seed has recently been achieved by application of genetic engineering techniques by Wu et al. (2005). The oil in the engineered mustard seeds contained 15 percent EPA and 1.5 percent DHA. The investigators were optimistic that a higher content of DHA could be achieved in further work. Therefore, although fish are presently the principal source of EPA and DHA available for human diets, there are several alternative sources available and more in development.

Dietary Supplements as Sources of EPA and DHA

The use of fish-oil supplements has increased over the past three decades, presumably as a result of publicity regarding the many studies showing a relationship between fish-oil supplementation and reduced risk for heart disease (e.g., Blonk et al., 1990; Reis et al., 1990; Bairati et al., 1992; Bucher et al., 2002; Marchioli et al., 2002; Vanschoonbeek et al., 2003). In 1998, Nutrition Business International (1998) forecast a market growth of 14–16 percent annually for fish-oil supplements compared to the industry's supplement average of 13 percent.

Fish oils used as food ingredients and dietary supplements are derived from a variety of different fish and are processed in different ways; consequently, their fatty acid profiles differ, especially in their content of the principal omega-3 fatty acids, EPA and DHA. The EPA and DHA content of some typical fish-oil supplements is shown in Table 2-12. The first five entries in this table are fish oils that have been determined to be generally recognized as safe (GRAS) for addition to foods and for which notices were submitted to the Food and Drug Administration (FDA).[1] Some fish oils are specially processed to increase the concentration of EPA and DHA, but unmodified fish oils contain from about 10 to 30 percent of these fatty acids, respectively.

---

[1]Information on sample number and variability not available.

TABLE 2-12 EPA and DHA Content of Fish-Oil Supplements

Fish Oil	Manufacturer	EPA Content (g/100 g)	DHA Content (g/100 g)	Data Source[a]
Small Planktivorous Pelagic Fish Body Oil (SPPFBO)	Jedwards	18.0	12.0	GRAS Notice #102, 2002
Fish Oil Concentrate	Unilever	20.0	18.0	GRAS Notice #105, 2002
Tuna Oil	Clover	6.0	26.5	GRAS Notice #109, 2002
18/12 Triglycerides	Ocean Nutrition Canada (ONC)	18.5	11.8	GRAS Notice #138, 2003
Salmon Oil	Jedwards	8.0	12.0	GRAS Notice #146, 2004
Menhaden Oil	Unspecified	13.1	6.7	FDA, 1997 (Federal Register 62, No. 108, Rules and Regulations)
Herring Oil	Unspecified	6.3	4.2	USDA Nutrient Database for Standard Reference, Release 18
Salmon Oil	Unspecified	13.0	18.2	USDA Nutrient Database for Standard Reference, Release 18
Sardine Oil	Unspecified	10.1	10.7	USDA Nutrient Database for Standard Reference, Release 18

[a]Information on sample number and variability not available.

A variety of fatty acids other than EPA and DHA are also found in fish oils. While these oils are generally lower in saturated fatty acids than other animal-derived fats and oils, they do contain about 20–25 percent saturated fatty acids by weight, as well as from about 20 to about 55 percent mono-unsaturated fatty acids (Table 2-12).

CONTAMINANTS OF CONCERN IN SEAFOOD

Methylmercury

Methylmercury is an environmental contaminant found in nearly all seafood. It is a potent neurotoxin (ATSDR, 1999; NRC, 2000; Satoh, 2003). Its origin and metabolism are discussed in a recent NRC report (NRC, 2000). Table 2-13 presents the average mercury concentrations in

TABLE 2-13 Methylmercury Concentrations in Seafood

Seafood Type	Mercury Concentration (ppm)[a] Mean	Median	Min	Max	*n*	Source[b]	Market[c] (%)
Anchovies	0.04	NA	ND	0.34	40	NMFS 1978	0.5
Bass (saltwater)[d]	0.27	0.15	0.06	0.96	35	FDA 1990–03	0.6
Bluefish	0.31	0.30	0.14	0.63	22	FDA 2002–03	0.1
Buffalo fish	0.19	0.14	0.05	0.43	4	FDA 1990–02	0.0
Butterfish	0.06	NA	ND	0.36	89	NMFS 1978	0.1
Carp	0.14	0.14	0.01	0.27	2	FDA 1990–02	0.0
Catfish	0.05	ND	ND	0.31	22	FDA 1990–02	4.8
Clams	ND	ND	ND	ND	6	FDA 1990–02	1.7
Cod	0.11	0.10	ND	0.42	20	FDA 1990–03	4.7
Crab[e]	0.06	ND	ND	0.61	59	FDA 1990–02	4.7
Crawfish	0.03	0.03	ND	0.05	21	FDA 2002–03	0.6
Croaker (Atlantic)	0.05	0.05	0.01	0.10	21	FDA 1990–03	0.3
Croaker white (Pacific)	0.29	0.28	0.18	0.41	15	FDA 1990–03	0.0
Flatfish[f]	0.05	0.04	ND	0.18	22	FDA 1990–02	3.6
Grouper	0.55	0.44	0.07	1.21	22	FDA 2002–03	0.2
Haddock	0.03	0.04	ND	0.04	4	FDA 1990–02	0.6
Hake	0.01	ND	ND	0.05	9	FDA 1990–02	0.3
Halibut	0.26	0.20	ND	1.52	32	FDA 1990–02	0.9
Herring	0.04	NA	ND	0.14	38	NMFS 1978	2.5
Jacksmelt	0.11	0.06	0.04	0.50	16	FDA 1990–02	0.0
Lobster (Northern/American)	0.31	NA	0.05	1.31	88	NMFS 1978	1.3
Lobster (spiny)	0.09	0.14	ND	0.27	9	FDA 1990–02	0.8
Mackerel, Atlantic (N. Atlantic)	0.05	NA	0.02	0.16	80	NMFS 1978	0.3
Mackerel, chub (Pacific)	0.09	NA	0.03	0.19	30	NMFS 1978	0.2
Mackerel, king	0.73	NA	0.23	1.67	213	Gulf 2000	0.1
Mackerel, Spanish (Gulf of Mexico)	0.45	NA	0.07	1.56	66	NMFS 1978	0.0
Mackerel, Spanish (S. Atlantic)	0.18	NA	0.05	0.73	43	NMFS 1978	0.0
Marlin	0.49	0.39	0.10	0.92	16	FDA 1990–02	0.0
Monkfish	0.18	NA	0.02	1.02	81	NMFS 1978	0.4
Mullet	0.05	NA	ND	0.13	191	NMFS 1978	0.2
Orange roughy	0.54	0.56	0.30	0.80	26	FDA 1990–03	0.2
Oysters	ND	ND	ND	0.25	34	FDA 1990–02	0.8
Perch (freshwater)	0.14	0.15	ND	0.31	5	FDA 1990–02	0.0
Perch ocean	ND	ND	ND	0.03	6	FDA 1990–02	0.5
Pickerel	ND	ND	ND	0.06	4	FDA 1990–02	0.1
Pollock	0.06	ND	ND	0.78	37	FDA 1990–02	11.1
Sablefish	0.22	NA	ND	0.7	102	NMFS 1978	0.3
Salmon (canned)	ND	ND	ND	ND	23	FDA 1990–02	0.9
Salmon (fresh/frozen)	0.01	ND	ND	0.19	34	FDA 1990–02	7.9
Sardine	0.02	0.01	ND	0.04	22	FDA 2002–03	1.2
Scallops	0.05	NA	ND	0.22	66	NMFS 1978	0.8
Scorpion fish	0.29	NA	0.02	1.35	78	NMFS 1978	0.9

TABLE 2-13 Continued

Seafood Type	Mercury Concentration (ppm)[a]				n	Source[b]	Market[c] (%)
	Mean	Median	Min	Max			
Shad (American)	0.07	NA	ND	0.22	59	NMFS 1978	0.0
Shark[g]	0.99	0.83	ND	4.54	351	FDA 1990–02	0.1
Sheepshead	0.13	NA	0.02	0.63	59	NMFS 1978	0.0
Shrimp	ND	ND	ND	0.05	24	FDA 1990–02	15.1
Skate	0.14	NA	0.04	0.36	56	NMFS 1978	0.3
Snapper	0.19	0.12	ND	1.37	25	FDA 2002–03	0.5
Squid	0.07	NA	ND	0.40	200	NMFS 1978	1.0
Swordfish	0.97	0.86	0.10	3.22	605	FDA 1990–02	0.4
Tilapia	0.01	ND	ND	0.07	9	FDA 1990–02	1.9
Tilefish (Atlantic)	0.15	0.10	0.06	0.53	17	FDA 2002–03	0.0
Tilefish (Gulf of Mexico)	1.45	NA	0.65	3.73	60	NMFS 1978	0.0
Trout (freshwater)	0.03	0.02	ND	0.13	17	FDA 2002–03	0.7
Tuna (canned, albacore)	0.35	0.34	ND	0.85	179	FDA 1990–03	5.3
Tuna (canned, light)	0.12	0.08	ND	0.85	131	FDA 1990–03	13.4
Tuna (fresh/frozen)	0.38	0.30	ND	1.30	131	FDA 1990–02	1.8
Weakfish (sea trout)	0.25	0.16	ND	0.74	27	FDA 1990–03	0.1
Whitefish	0.07	0.05	ND	0.31	25	FDA 1990–03	0.2
Whiting	ND	ND	ND	ND	2	FDA 1990–02	4.1

[a]Mercury was measured as total mercury and/or methylmercury. ND—mercury concentration below the level of detection (LOD = 0.01 ppm). NA—data not available.

[b]Source of data: FDA Surveys 1990–2003 (FDA, 2004), *National Marine Fisheries Service Survey of Trace Elements in the Fishery Resource* (Hall et al., 1978), *A Survey of the Occurrence of Mercury in the Fishery Resources of the Gulf of Mexico* (Ache et al., 2000).

[c]Market share calculation based on 2001 National Marine Fisheries Service published landings data (NMFS, 2002).

[d]Includes sea bass/striped bass/rockfish.

[e]Includes blue, king, and snow crab.

[f]Includes flounder, plaice, sole.

[g]Includes multiple species of shark.

SOURCE: Derived from *Regulatory Toxicology and Pharmacology* 40(3), Carrington CD, Montwill B, Bolger PM. An intervention analysis for the reduction of exposure to methylmercury from the consumption of seafood by women of child-bearing age, 274–280, 2004, with permission from Elsevier.

species of fish and shellfish reported consumed by women in the 1999–2000 NHANES (Carrington et al., 2004). Mercury levels in fish do not appear to have changed appreciably over recent decades, although the data are limited (US EPA, 1997).

Persistent Organic Pollutants

Persistent organic pollutants (POPs) are lipophilic contaminant compounds and tend to bioaccumulate up the food chain. They include such substances as dioxins, dioxin-like compounds (DLCs), and polychlorinated biphenyls (PCBs), including those with dioxin-like activity. Dioxins, dioxin-like compounds (including PCBs with dioxin-like activity) (DLCs) and PCBs are the most frequently occuring POPs in seafood. A variety of lipophilic pesticide contaminants have been found in fish from the Great Lakes (Giesy et al., 1994; Anderson et al., 1998; Chernyak et al., 2005) and both farmed and wild-caught salmon from European waters (Food Safety Authority of Ireland, 2002; Foran et al., 2004; Hites et al., 2004b; Hamilton et al., 2005). Among these contaminants, aldrin and dieldrin have been found in amounts exceeding 1 µg/kg body weight in the Great Lakes (Anderson et al., 1998; Cole et al., 2002; Schmitt et al., 1999). The Salton Sea, a large manmade lake in California, was reported to have high levels of some organochlorine compounds (OCs) in 2001 (Sapozhnikova et al., 2004). The toxicity of these compounds varies widely, and the implications for human health remain controversial.

Several investigators have found that levels of many POPs are higher in commercially available farmed fish than in wild-caught fish (Easton et al., 2002; Hites et al., 2004a,b; Foran et al., 2005). Van Leeuwen and de Boer (2004) tabulated contaminant data for PCBs, OCs, polychlorinated dibenzo-*p*-dioxins (PCDDs), polychlorinated dibenzofurans (PCDFs), dioxin-like PCBs, polybrominated diphenyl ethers (PBDEs), and others. Table 2-14 shows estimated DLC levels in seafood from the FDA Total Diet Study Market Basket Survey. The reported values differ from 2001 through 2004, in part because of changes in analytical detection techniques.

Impact of Toxicants on Selenium Status

Several environmental organic toxicants have a direct or indirect impact on antioxidant status or oxidative stress of various organisms (Halliwell and Gutteridge, 1999). Therefore, studies have examined what influences such compounds may have on selenoproteins involved in modulation of oxidative stress.

Dioxin

2,3,7,8-Tetrachlorodibenzo-*p*-dioxin (TCDD) inhibits hepatic selenium-dependent but not selenium-independent glutathione peroxidase in hamsters (Hassan et al., 1983). Supplemental dietary selenium will partially protect against TCDD toxicity in rats (Hassan et al., 1985).

Polychlorinated Biphenyls

PCB exposure causes significant increases in hepatic levels of lipid

TABLE 2-14 Total Diet Study Analyses of Dioxin-like Compounds in Seafood, 2001–2004

Seafood Type	PCDD[a] TEQ[b], Pg/g[c], ND = LOD/2[d] (by year reported)			
	2001	2002	2003	2004
Tuna, canned in oil	0.0057	0.0050	N/A	N/A
Tuna, canned in water	N/A	N/A	0.0110	0.0182
Tuna noodle casserole	0.0334	0.0318	0.0826	0.0159
Fish sticks, frozen	0.0335	0.0667	0.0126	0.0053
Shrimp, boiled	0.0597	0.0834	0.0032	0.0151
Salmon, fillets	0.3257	0.1504	0.2585	0.0795
Fish sandwich, fast-food	0.0138	0.0059	0.0152	0.0078
Clam chowder, canned	0.0054	0.0169	0.0096	0.0154
Catfish, cooked in oil	N/A	N/A	0.2971	0.2055

[a]PCDD = Polychlorinated dibenzo-*p*-dioxin.

[b]TEQ = Toxicity Equivalents (see Chapter 4 for explanation).

[c]Pg/g = Picograms of contaminant per gram of food (see Chapter 4 for explanation).

[d]ND = LOD/2 refers to the non-detect limit expressed as the limit of detection×0.5.

SOURCE: USDA Total Diet Study (http://www.cfsan.fda.gov/~lrd/dioxdata. html).

peroxidation, glutathione, glutathione reductase, glucose-6-phosphate dehydrogenase, and glutathione S-transferase in rats fed diets low in selenium but not in rats fed adequate selenium (Chow and Gairola, 1981; Chow et al., 1981). Thus, dietary selenium deprivation renders rats more sensitive to PCB effects.

FINDINGS

1. Seafood is a primary source of the omega-3 long-chain polyunsaturated fatty acids (LCPUFA) eicosapentaenoic acid (EPA) and docosahexaenoic acid (DHA), but not all seafood is rich in these fatty acids.

2. Relative to other foods in the meat, poultry, fish, and egg group, fish is generally lower in saturated fatty acids and higher in EPA, DHA, and selenium than most other choices.

3. Seafood may also contain chemical contaminants (e.g., methylmercury, POPs). While there are data on the methylmercury content of many types of seafood, there are virtually no data on other contaminants and pollutants.

4. Average quantities of seafood consumed by the general US population, and by several specific population groups, are below levels suggested by

many authoritative groups including levels recommended by the American Heart Association for cardiovascular disease prevention.

5. Average quantities of EPA and DHA consumed by the general US population, and by several specific population groups, are also below levels recommended by many authoritative groups.

6. For many ethnic and geographic subgroups, there are insufficient data to characterize the intake levels of seafood, EPA, DHA, and other dietary constituents, and to assess the variability of those intakes.

7. Chicken and eggs, although not particularly rich sources, have contributed over 10 percent of the EPA and about 25 percent of the DHA in the US diet in recent years because of their frequent consumption. However, changes in feeding practices may be making these contributions negligible. New forthcoming data on chicken and eggs show most nutrient levels comparable to earlier samples, but EPA/DHA levels as undetectable.

8. Shrimp and tuna are the two most commonly consumed types of seafood in the United States. Shrimp and canned/packaged light tuna—the major type of tuna consumed—are not especially rich in EPA and DHA; nor are they especially high in mercury. However, albacore (white) tuna, a good source of EPA/DHA, can be higher in mercury than other tuna.

9. Shark, swordfish, king mackerel, and tilefish—the four types of seafood identified in the FDA/US EPA joint advisory as being most highly contaminated with mercury—are not among the types of seafood most frequently consumed in the United States, and supply trends suggest their future availability will be increasingly limited.

10. Forces such as consumer trends, increasing dependence on aquaculture, and increased imports are influencing the availability of many popular seafood selections.

RESEARCH RECOMMENDATIONS

Recommendation 1: Research is needed on systematic surveillance studies of targeted subpopulations. Such studies should be carried out using state-of-the-art assessment methods to determine the intake levels of seafood, EPA/DHA and other dietary constituents, and the variability of those intake levels among population groups.

Recommendation 2: Sufficiently large analytic samples of the most common seafood types need to be obtained and examined. These samples should be used to determine the levels of nutrients, toxicants, and contaminants in each species and the variability between them, which should be reported transparently.

Recommendation 3: Additional data is needed to assess benefits and risks associated with seafood consumption within the same population or population subgroup.

REFERENCES

Ache BW, Boyle JD, Morse CE. 2000. *A Survey of the Occurrence of Mercury in the Fishery Resources of the Gulf of Mexico*. Stennis Space Center, MS: Battelle.

ADA (American Dietetic Association). 2003. Position of the American Dietetic Association and Dietitians of Canada: Vegetarian diets. *Journal of the American Dietetic Association* 103(6):748–765.

Anderson HA, Falk C, Hanrahan L, Olson J, Burse VW, Needham L, Paschal D, Patterson D Jr, Hill RH Jr, and The Great Lakes Consortium. 1998. Profiles of Great Lakes critical pollutants: A sentinel analysis of human blood and urine. *Environmental Health Perspectives* 106(5):279–289.

Arnold SM, Middaugh JP. 2004 (December 2). Use of traditional foods in a healthy diet in Alaska: Risks in perspective (Mercury). *State of Alaska Epidemiology Bulletin* 8(11):1–48.

ATSDR (Agency for Toxic Substances and Disease Registry). 1999. *Toxicological Profile for Mercury*. Atlanta, GA: US Department of Health and Human Services, Public Health Service.

Bairati I, Roy L, Meyer F. 1992. Double-blind, randomized, controlled trial of fish oil supplements in prevention of recurrence of stenosis after coronary angioplasty. *Circulation* 85(3):950–956.

Ballew C, Ross A, Wells RS, Hiratsuka V, Hamrick KJ, Nobmann ED, Bartell S. 2004. *Final Report on the Alaska Traditional Diet Survey*. Anchorage, AK: Alaska Native Health Board, Alaska Native Epidemiology Center.

Barlow S. 2001 (October). *Fishmeal and Oil—Supplies and Markets*. A presentation to Group Fish Forum, St. Albans, UK, International Fishmeal and Fish Oil Organization. [Online]. Available: http://www.iffo.org.uk/Supplies.pdf#search=%22Fishmeal%20and%20oil%3A%20resources%20and%20markets%22 [accessed August 24, 2006].

Baum JK, Myers RA, Kehler DG, Worm B, Harley SJ, Doherty PA. 2003. Collapse and conservation of shark populations in the Northwest Atlantic. *Science* 299(5605):389–392.

Bean LD, Leeson S. 2003. Long-term effects of feeding flaxseed on performance and egg fatty acid composition of brown and white hens. *Poultry Science* 82(3):388–394.

Bell JG, Tocher DR, Henderson RJ, Dick JR, Crampton VO. 2003. Altered fatty acid compositions in atlantic salmon (*Salmo salar*) fed diets containing linseed and rapeseed oils can be partially restored by a subsequent fish oil finishing diet. *Journal of Nutrition* 133(9):2793–2801.

Blonk MC, Bilo HJ, Nauta JJ, Popp-Snijders C, Mulder C, Donker AJ. 1990. Dose-response effects of fish oil supplementation in healthy volunteers. *American Journal of Clinical Nutrition* 52(1):120–127.

Bucher HC, Hengstler P, Schindler C, Meier G. 2002. N-3 polyunsaturated fatty acids in coronary heart disease: A meta-analysis of randomized controlled trials. *American Journal of Medicine* 112(4):298–304.

Burdge GC, Wootton SA. 2002. Conversion of alpha-linolenic acid to eicosapentaenoic, docosapentaenoic and docosahexaenoic acids in young women. *British Journal of Nutrition*. 88(4):411–420.

Burdge GC, Jones AE, Wootton SA. 2002. Eicosapentaenoic and docosapentaenoic acids are the principal products of alpha-linolenic acid metabolism in young men. *British Journal of Nutrition* 88(4):355–363.

Burger J. 2002. Consumption patterns and why people fish. *Environmental Research* 90(2): 125–135.

Burger J, Stephens WL Jr, Boring CS, Kuklinski M, Gibbons JW, Gochfeld M. 1999. Factors in exposure assessment: Ethnic and socioeconomic differences in fishing and consumption of fish caught along the Savannah River. *Risk Analysis* 19(3):427–438.

Cantor AH, Decker EA, Collins VP. 1999. Chapter 7: Fatty acids in poultry and egg products. In: Chow CK, ed. *Fatty Acids in Foods and Their Health Implications.* New York: Marcel Dekker, Inc. Pp. 125–151.

Carrington CD, Montwill B, Bolger PM. 2004. An intervention analysis for the reduction of exposure to methylmercury from the consumption of seafood by women of child-bearing age. *Regulatory Toxicology and Pharmacology* 40(3):272–280.

CDC/NCHS (Centers for Disease Control and Prevention/National Center for Health Statistics). 1999–2000. *National Health and Nutrition Examination Survey.* Hyattsville, MD: US Department of Health and Human Services, Centers for Disease Control and Prevention.

Chernyak SM, Rice CP, Quintal RT, Begnoche LJ, Hickey JP, Vinyard BT. 2005. Time trends (1983–1999) for organochlorines and polybrominated diphenyl ethers in rainbow smelt (*Osmerus mordax*) from Lakes Michigan, Huron, and Superior, USA. *Environmental Toxicology and Chemistry* 24(7):1632–1641.

Chow CK, Gairola CC. 1981. Influence of dietary selenium on the hepatic and pulmonary enzymes in polychlorobiphenyls-treated rats. *Cancer Detection and Prevention* 4(1–4):135–139.

Chow CK, Thacker R, Gairola C. 1981. Dietary selenium and levels of L-ascorbic acid in the plasma, livers and lungs of polychlorinated biphenyls-treated rats. *International Journal of Vitamin and Nutrition Research* 51(3):279–283.

Cohen Z, Norman HA, Heimer YM. 1995. Microalgae as a source of omega 3 fatty acids. *World Review of Nutrition and Dietetics* 77:1–31.

Cole DC, Sheeshka J, Murkin EJ, Kearney J, Scott F, Ferron LA, Weber JP. 2002. Dietary intakes and plasma organochlorine contaminant levels among Great Lakes fish eaters. *Archives of Environmental Health* 57(5):496–509.

Coleman FC, Figueira WF, Ueland JS, Crowder LB. 2004. The impact of United States recreational fisheries on marine fish populations. *Science* 305(5692):1958–1960.

DGAC (Dietary Guidelines Advisory Committee). 2005. *Dietary Guidelines Advisory Committee Report.* Washington, DC: Department of Health and Human Services and the Department of Agriculture. [Online]. Available: http://www.health.gov/dietaryguidelines/dga2005/report/ [accessed November 29, 2005].

Easton MD, Luszniak D, Von der Geest E. 2002. Preliminary examination of contaminant loadings in farmed salmon, wild salmon and commercial salmon feed. *Chemosphere* 46(7):1053–1074.

ERS (Economic Research Service). 2004 (December 21). *Data: Food Availability: Spreadsheets. Fish and Shellfish.* [Online]. Available: http://www.ers.usda.gov/data/foodconsumption/spreadsheets/mtfish.xls [accessed December 22, 2005].

FAO (Food and Agriculture Organization). 2002. Part I: World review of fisheries and aquaculture. In: *The State of World Fisheries and Aquaculture.* FAO Information Division Rome, Italy: Food and Agriculture Organization. [Online]. Available: http://www.fao.org/docrep/005/y7300e/y7300e04.htm#P0_0 [accessed August 24, 2006].

FAO. 2004. Part I: World review of fisheries and aquaculture. In: *The State of World Fisheries and Aquaculture.* Rome, Italy: FAO Information Division. [Online]. Available: http://www.fao.org/documents/show_cdr.asp?url_file=/docrep/007/y5600e/y5600e04.htm [accessed October 10, 2005].

FDA (Food and Drug Administration). 2004. *Mercury Levels in Commercial Fish and Shellfish.* [Online]. Available: http://www.cfsan.fda.gov/~frf/sea-mehg.html [accessed December 5, 2006].

Food Safety Authority of Ireland. 2002. *Investigation on PCDDs/PCDFs and Several PCBs in Fish Liver Oil Capsules.* Hamburg, Germany: ERGO Forschungsgesellschaft mbH, Germany.

Foran JA, Hites RA, Carpenter DO, Hamilton MC, Mathews-Amos A, Schwager SJ. 2004. A survey of metals in tissues of farmed Atlantic and wild Pacific salmon. *Environmental Toxicology and Chemistry* 23(9):2108–2110.

Foran JA, Carpenter DO, Hamilton MC, Knuth BA, Schwager SJ. 2005. Risk-based consumption advice for farmed Atlantic and wild Pacific salmon contaminated with dioxins and dioxin-like compounds. *Environmental Health Perspectives* 113(5):552–556.

Giesy JP, Vergrugge DA, Othout RA, Bowerman WW, Mora MA, Jones PD, Newsted JL, Vandervoort C, Heaton SN, Auerlich RJ, Bursian SJ, Ludwig JP, Ludwig M, Dawson GA, Kubiak TJ, Best DA, Tillitt DE. 1994. Contaminants in fishes from Great Lakes–influenced sections and above dams on three Michigan rivers. I: Concentrations of organo-chlorine insecticides, polychlorinated biphenyls, dioxin equivalents, and mercury. *Archives of Environmental Contamination and Toxicology* 27(2):202–212.

GMFMC (Gulf of Mexico Fishery Management Council). 2006. *Coastal Migratory Pelagics Fishery Management Plan*. [Online]. Available: http://www.gulfcouncil.org/Beta/GMFM-CWeb/FMPs/migratory_pelagics_amendments.htm [accessed May 9, 2006].

Gonzalez-Esquerra R, Leeson S. 2000. Effects of menhaden oil and flaxseed in broiler diets on sensory quality and lipid composition of poultry meat. *British Poultry Science* 41(4):481–488.

Hall RA, Zook EG, Meaburn GM. 1978. *National Marine Fisheries Service Survey of Trace Elements in the Fishery Resource*. Seattle, WA: US Department of Commerce, National Oceanic and Atmospheric Administration, National Marine Fisheries Service.

Halliwell B, Gutteridge JMC. 1999. Free radicals, "reactive species" and toxicology. In: *Free Radicals in Biology and Medicine*. Oxford, UK: Oxford University Press. Pp. 544–616.

Hamilton MC, Hites RA, Schwager SJ, Foran JA, Knuth BA, Carpenter DO. 2005. Lipid composition and contaminants in farmed and wild salmon. *Environmental Science and Technology* 39(22):8622–8629.

Hassan MQ, Stohs SJ, Murray WJ. 1983. Comparative ability of TCDD to induce lipid peroxidation in rats, guinea pigs, and Syrian golden hamsters. *Bulletin of Environmental Contamination and Toxicology* 31(6):649–657.

Hassan MQ, Stohs SJ, Murray WJ, Birt DF. 1985. Dietary selenium, glutathione peroxidase activity, and toxicity of 2,3,7,8-tetrachloro-dibenzo-p-dioxin. *Journal of Toxicology and Environmental Health* 15(3-4):405–415.

Herber SM, Van Elswyk ME. 1996. Dietary marine algae promotes efficient deposition of n-3 fatty acids for the production of enriched shell eggs. *Poultry Science* 75(12):1501–1507.

Hites RA, Foran JA, Carpenter DO, Hamilton MC, Knuth BA, Schwager SJ. 2004a. Global assessment of organic contaminants in farmed salmon. *Science* 303(5655):226–229.

Hites RA, Foran JA, Schwager SJ, Knuth BA, Hamilton MC, Carpenter DO. 2004b. Global assessment of polybrominated diphenyl ethers in farmed and wild salmon. *Environmental Science and Technology* 38(19):4945–4949.

Hulan HW, Ackman RG, Ratnayake WM, Proudfoot FG. 1989. Omega-3 fatty acid levels and general performance of commercial broilers fed practical levels of redfish meal. *Poultry Science* 68(1):153–162.

Hutchison R, Kraft CE. 1994. Hmong fishing activity and fish consumption. *Journal of Great Lakes Research* 20(2):471–478.

IOM (Institute of Medicine). 2003. *Dioxins and Dioxin-like Compounds in the Food Supply: Strategies to Decrease Exposure*. Washington, DC: The National Academies Press.

Kim J, Chan MM. 2004. Acculturation and dietary habits of Korean Americans. *British Journal of Nutrition* 91(3):469–478.

Kolonel LN, Altshuler D, Henderson BE. 2004. The Multiethnic Cohort Study: Exploring genes, lifestyle and cancer risk. *Nature Reviews Cancer* 4(7):519–527.

Komprda T, Zelenka J, Fajmonova E, Fialova M, Kladroba D. 2005. Arachidonic acid and long-chain n-3 polyunsaturated fatty acid contents in meat of selected poultry and fish species in relation to dietary fat sources. *Journal of Agricultural and Food Chemistry* 53(17):6804–6812.

Kudo Y, Falciglia GA, Couch SC. 2000. Evolution of meal patterns and food choices of Japanese-American females born in the United States. *European Journal of Clinical Nutrition* 54(8):665–670.

Kuhnlein HV, Receveur O, Chan HM, Loring E. 2000. *Assessment of Dietary Benefit: Risk in Inuit Communities*. Ste-Anne-de-Bellevue, Québec: Centre for Indigenous Peoples' Nutrition and Environment (CINE) and Inuit Tapirisat of Canada.

Kuhnlein HV, Receveur O, Soueida R, Egeland GM. 2004. Arctic indigenous peoples experience the nutrition transition with changing dietary patterns and obesity. *Journal of Nutrition* 134(6):1447–1453.

Marchioli R, Barzi F, Bomba E, Chieffo C, Di Gregorio D, Di Mascio R, Franzosi MG, Geraci E, Levantesi G, Maggioni AP, Mantini L, Marfisi RM, Mastrogiuseppe G, Mininni N, Nicolosi GL, Santini M, Schweiger C, Tavazzi L, Tognoni G, Tucci C, Valagussa F, GISSI-Prevenzione Investigators. 2002. Early protection against sudden death by n-3 polyunsaturated fatty acids after myocardial infarction: Time-course analysis of the results of the Gruppo Italiano per lo Studio della Sopravvivenza nell'Infarto Miocardico (GISSI)-Prevenzione. *Circulation* 105(16):1897–1903.

Marien K, Patrick GM. 2001. Exposure analysis of five fish-consuming populations for overexposure to methylmercury. *Journal of Exposure Analysis and Environmental Epidemiology* 11(3):193–206.

Miller MM, Nash DA. 1971. *Regional and Other Related Aspects of Shellfish Consumption, Circular 361*. Seattle, WA: National Marine Fisheries Service.

Mos L, Jack J, Cullon D, Montour L, Alleyne C, Ross PS. 2004. The importance of marine foods to a near-urban first nation community in coastal British Columbia, Canada: Toward a risk-benefit assessment. *Journal of Toxicology and Environmenal Health* A67(8–10):791–808.

Muckle G, Ayotte P, Dewailly E, Jacobson SW, Jacobson JL. 2001. Determinants of polychlorinated biphenyls and methylmercury exposure in Inuit women of childbearing age. *Environmental Health Perspectives* 109(9):957–963.

Naylor RL, Goldburg RJ, Primavera JH. Kautsky N, Beveridge MC, Clay J, Folke C, Lubchenco J, Mooney H, Troell M. 2000. Effect of aquaculture on world fish supplies. *Nature* 405(6790):1017–1024.

NFI (National Fisheries Institute). 2005. *Top 10 U.S. Consumption by Species Chart*. [Online]. Available: http://www.aboutseafood.com/media/top_10.cfm [accessed November 29, 2005].

NMFS (National Marine Fisheries Service). 2002. *Fisheries of the United States 2001*. Silver Spring, MD: National Oceanic and Atmospheric Administration (NOAA). [Online]. Available: http://www.st.nmfs.gov/st1/fus/fus01/2001-fus.pdf [accessed December 7, 2006].

NMFS. 2005a. *Fisheries of the United States 2004*. Silver Spring, MD: National Oceanic and Atmospheric Administration (NOAA). [Online]. Available: http://www.st.nmfs.gov/st1/fus/fus04/fus_2004.pdf [accessed December 22, 2005].

NMFS. 2005b. *A Message from the NOAA Assistant Administrator for Fisheries*. [Online]. Available: http://www.mafmc.org/mid-atlantic/StatusReport2004.pdf [accessed May 9, 2006].

NRC (National Research Council). 2000. *Toxicological Effects of Methylmercury*. Washington, DC: National Academy Press.

Nutrition Business International. 1998. $23 billion and counting: Nutrition industry braces for a competitive future. *Nutrition Business Journal* 3(9):1–5, 13, 18.

Pawlosky RJ, Hibbeln JR, Novotny JA, Salem N Jr. 2001. Physiological compartmental analysis of alpha-linolenic acid metabolism in adult humans. *Journal of Lipid Research* 42(8):1257–1265.

Ratnayake WMN, Ackman RG. 1989. Effect of redfish meal enriched diets on the taste and n-3 PUFA of 42-day-old broiler chickens. *Journal of Science and Food Agriculture* 49:59–74.

Receveur O, Boulay M, Kuhnlein HV. 1997. Decreasing traditional food use affects diet quality for adult Dene/Metis in 16 communities of the Canadian Northwest Territories. *Journal of Nutrition* 127(11):2179–2186.

Reis GJ, Silverman DI, Boucher TM, Sipperly ME, Horowitz GL, Sacks FM, Pasternak RC. 1990. Effects of two types of fish oil supplements on serum lipids and plasma phospholipid fatty acids in coronary artery disease. *American Journal of Cardiology* 66(17):1171–1175.

Rupp EM, Miller FI, Baes CF III. 1980. Some results of recent surveys of fish and shellfish consumption by age and region of U.S. residents. *Health Physics* 39(2):165–175.

SAFMC (South Atlantic Fishery Management Council). 2005. Council scheduled to approve amendment 13C for snapper grouper fishery during December Meeting. *South Atlantic Update, Fall edition*. P. 1.

Sapozhnikova Y, Bawardi O, Schlenk D. 2004. Pesticides and PCBs in sediments and fish from the Salton Sea, California, USA. *Chemosphere* 55(6):797–809.

Satoh H. 2003. Behavioral teratology of mercury and its compounds. *Tohoku Journal of Experimental Medicine* 201(1):1–9.

Scheideler SE, Froning GW. 1996. The combined influence of dietary flaxseed variety, level, form, and storage conditions on egg production and composition among vitamin E–supplemented hens. *Poultry Science* 75(10):1221–1226.

Schmitt CJ, Zajicek JL, May TW, Cowman DF. 1999. Organochlorine residues and elemental contaminants in US freshwater fish, 1976–1986: National Contaminant Biomonitoring Program. *Reviews of Environmental Contamination and Toxicology* 162.43–104.

Sechena R, Liao S, Lorenzana R, Nakano C, Polissar N, Fenske R. 2003. Asian American and Pacific Islander seafood consumption—a community-based study in King County, Washington. *Journal of Exposure Analysis and Environmental Epidemiology* 13(4):256–266.

Sharma S, Murphy SP, Wilkens LR, Shen L, Hankin JH, Henderson B, Kolonel LN. 2003. Adherence to the Food Guide Pyramid recommendations among Japanese Americans, Native Hawaiians, and whites: Results from the Multiethnic Cohort Study. *Journal of the American Dietetic Association* 103(9):1195–1198.

Sharma S, Murphy SP, Wilkens LR, Shen L, Hankin JH, Monroe KR, Henderson B, Kolonel LN. 2004. Adherence to the food guide pyramid recommendations among African Americans and Latinos: Results from the Multiethnic Cohort. *Journal of the American Dietetic Association* 104(12):1873–1877.

Sijtsma L, de Swaaf ME. 2004. Biotechnological production and applications of the omega-3 polyunsaturated fatty acid docosahexaenoic acid. *Applied Microbiology and Biotechnology* 64(2):146–153.

Sindelar CA, Scheerger SB, Plugge SL, Eskridge KM, Wander RC, Lewis NM. 2004. Serum lipids of physically active adults consuming omega-3 fatty acid-enriched eggs or conventional eggs. *Nutrition Research* 24(9):731–739.

Tocher DR, Fonseca-Madrigal J, Bell JG, Dick JR, Henderson RJ, Sargent JR. 2003. Effects of diets containing linseed oil on fatty acid desaturation and oxidation in hepatocytes and intestinal enterocytes in Atlantic salmon (*Salmo salar*). *Fish Physiology and Biochemistry* 26:157–170.

US EPA (US Environmental Protection Agency). 1997. *Mercury Study Report to Congress: Volume 1: Executive Summary.* EPA-452-R-97-003. Washington, DC: EPA. [Online]. Available: http://www.epa.gov/ttn/oarpg/t3/reports/volume1.pdf [accessed August 24, 2006].

US EPA/FDA (Food and Drug Administration). 2004. *What You Need to Know About Mercury in Fish and Shellfish.* EPA-823-R-04-005. [Online]. Available: http://www.epa.gov/waterscience/fishadvice/advice.html or http://www.cfsan.fda.gov/~dms/admehg3.html [accessed September 8, 2005].

US Tuna Foundation. 2005. *About Tuna.* [Online]. Available: http://www.tunafacts.org/abouttuna/index.html [accessed October 02, 2006].

USDA (US Department of Agriculture). 2005. *USDA National Nutrient Database for Standard Reference Release 18.* [Online]. Available: http://www.nal.usda.gov/fnic/foodcomp/Data/SR18/sr18.html [accessed October 10, 2005].

Van Elswyk ME. 1997. Comparison of n-3 fatty acid sources in laying hen rations for improvement of whole egg nutritional quality: A review. *British Journal of Nutrition* 78(Suppl 1): S61–S69.

van Leeuwen S, de Boer J. 2004. Detecting organic contaminants in food: The case of fish and shellfish. In: Watson DH, ed. *Pesticide, Veterinary and Other Residues in Foods.* Cambridge, UK: Woodhead Publishing. Pp. 536–576.

Vanschoonbeek K, de Maat MPM, Heemskerk JWM. 2003. Fish oil consumption and reduction of arterial disease. *Journal of Nutrition* 133(3):657–660.

Watson R, Pauly D. 2001. Systematic distortions in world fisheries catch trends. *Nature* 414(6863):534–536.

Wu G, Truksa M, Datla N, Vrinten P, Bauer J, Zank T, Cirpus P, Heinz E, Qiu X. 2005. Stepwise engineering to produce high yields of very long-chain polyunsaturated fatty acids in plants. *Nature Biotechnology* 23(8):1013–1017.

3

Health Benefits Associated with
Nutrients in Seafood

This chapter reviews the evidence for benefits derived from nutrients in seafood or from dietary supplementation with nutrients derived from seafood. The review of evidence related specifically to the omega-3 fatty acids eicosapentaenoic acid (EPA) and docosahexaenoic acid (DHA) from seafood is presented in two parts: Part I addresses the impact of EPA/DHA on maternal, infant, and child health outcomes and Part II addresses the impact on chronic disease, particularly coronary heart disease, in adults. The discussions that follow include a review of the literature and evaluation of the quality of the evidence for benefits.

The committee considered a broad range of evidence on potential benefits associated with nutrients from seafood and reviewed evidence from other systematic reviews, i.e., the Agency for Health Research and Quality (AHRQ) reviews (Balk et al., 2004; Schachter et al., 2004, 2005; Wang et al., 2004) and other published reports of evidence associating nutrients from seafood with specific health outcomes. In cases where benefits were not supported or were poorly supported by the literature, a statement is made to that effect.

Scientific evidence to support benefits associated with seafood intake on cardiovascular risk reduction through prevention of disease development consists mainly of observational studies of seafood consumption among the general population. Recommendations to the general population are inferred from these findings despite the fact that they have not been tested by trials in this population. Fish-oil supplementation, on the other hand, has been used in secondary prevention trials in high cardiovascular-risk populations or populations with established disease to examine its role in preventing recurrence of cardiovascular events.

Given the potential for different outcomes in general compared to high-risk populations, the committee also considered best practice guidelines for both, which take into account currently available evidence. The conclusions drawn from the evidence reviewed were the basis for decision-making about seafood selections discussed in later chapters. The literature reviewed in the chapter is summarized in tables included in Appendix B.

INTRODUCTION

Seafood is a food source comparable to other animal protein foods in nutrient composition (see Chapter 2). In addition, seafood is an important contributor of selenium to the American diet and is unique among animal protein foods as a rich source for the omega-3 fatty acids EPA and DHA, although the roles of these fatty acids in maintaining health and preventing certain chronic diseases have not been completely elucidated (IOM, 2002/2005).

Benefits to the General Population Associated with Nutrients in Seafood

As noted in Chapter 1, the US *Dietary Guidelines for Americans* (DGA) provides science-based advice to promote health and reduce risk for chronic diseases through diet and physical activity. The guidelines are targeted to the general public over 2 years of age living in the United States. But as noted in Chapter 2, general adherence to the DGA is low among the US population.

Seafood provides an array of nutrients that may have beneficial effects on health (see Chapter 2). While protein is an important macronutrient in the diet, most Americans already consume enough protein and do not need to increase their intake. Fats and oils are also part of a healthful diet, but the type of fat can be important, for example, with regard to heart disease. Many Americans consume greater than recommended amounts of saturated fat from high-fat animal protein foods such as beef and pork as well as trans fat from processed foods (Capps et al., 2002). A diet high in fat (greater than 35 percent of calories), particularly animal fat, may increase saturated fat intake, add excess calories, and increase risk for coronary heart disease. Many seafood selections, depending upon preparation method, are lower in total and saturated fat and cholesterol than some more frequently selected animal protein foods, including both lean and fatty cuts of beef, pork, and poultry (Table 3-1). By substituting seafood more often for other animal foods, consumers can decrease their overall intake of total and saturated fats while retaining the nutritional quality of other protein food choices.

TABLE 3-1 Differences in Saturated Fat Content Between Commonly Consumed Animal Food Products

Food Category	Portion Size (ounces)	Saturated Fat (grams)	Calories (kcal)
Cheese			
Regular cheddar cheese	1	6.0	114
Low-fat cheddar cheese	1	1.2	49
Ground beef			
Regular ground beef (25% fat)	3 (cooked)	6.1	236
Extra lean ground beef (5% fat)	3 (cooked)	2.5	145
Chicken			
Fried chicken (with skin)	3	3.4	229
Roasted chicken (no skin)	3	0.9	130
Fish			
Fried fish (catfish)	3	2.8	195
Baked fish (catfish)	3	1.5	129

SOURCE: USDA, Release 18.

The 1994–1996 Continuing Survey of Food Intake by Individuals (CSFII) identified several micronutrients that were consumed at levels below the Recommended Dietary Allowance (RDA), including vitamins E and B-6, calcium, iron, magnesium, and zinc. Seafood is a good source of zinc and some calcium, e.g., from canned salmon or other fish with bones, which may contribute to the total intake of these nutrients when substituted for other animal food products. For example, a 3-ounce cooked serving of beef, lamb, chicken, or pork contains approximately 10–20 mg of calcium, whereas a 3-ounce serving of canned salmon with bones contains approximately 240 mg. (Source: http://www.nal.usda.gov/fnic/foodcomp/Data/SR18/sr18.html.)

Nutritional Benefits Associated with Omega-3 Fatty Acids

Optimal Intake Levels for EPA and DHA

There are insufficient data on the distribution of requirements to set an Estimated Average Requirement (EAR) for alpha-linolenic acid (ALA), so an Adequate Intake (AI) was set instead, at approximately the level of current intakes (IOM, 2002/2005). Given that ALA conversion to EPA and DHA is low and variable (Burdge, 2004), intakes of the preformed omega-3 fatty acids may be less than desired under certain physiologic circumstances (see Chapter 2). Despite the number of studies conducted over the past two decades to assess the impact of omega-3 fatty acids in general on health outcomes, optimal intake levels for EPA and DHA are still not defined. The Dietary Reference Intakes (IOM, 2002/2005) did not establish a requirement for any omega-3 fatty acids; rather, an estimate of adequacy, the AI, was derived from the highest median intake of ALA in the United States.

Target intake goals for seafood consumption for the general population and recommended EPA/DHA intake levels for specific population subgroups have been put forward by both public agencies and private organizations (reviewed in Chapter 1). Whether there are benefits to the general population that are related specifically to EPA/DHA obtained from consuming seafood is not clear from the available evidence. A low-saturated-fat, nutrient-dense protein food such as seafood does represent a good food choice for the general population and this is reflected in the recommendations of the *Dietary Guidelines for Americans* to choose low-fat foods from among protein sources that include fish (see Chapter 1). The evidence in support of recommendations to increase EPA/DHA intake, whether from seafood or fish-oil supplements, among the population groups that would most benefit is presented in the following discussions.

It should, however, be kept in mind that the benefits of seafood consumption for health may not be limited to intake of EPA/DHA. Other nutrients present in seafood may provide specific health benefits or even facilitate the action of EPA/DHA. Additionally, substitution of seafood for other food sources may decrease exposure to nutrients that are shown to increase health risks, such as saturated fats. On the other hand, some contaminants or toxins present in seafood may decrease or negate the benefit of EPA/DHA, as illustrated by the dilemma in making recommendations for seafood consumption in pregnant women, considering the potential benefits of EPA/DHA compared to potential risks of methylmercury exposure to the fetus. Therefore, when assessing the question of benefits of seafood consumption, seafood should not be considered as equivalent to EPA/DHA. This differentiation may explain some of the inconsistencies in the findings described below. In other words, demonstrated benefits of EPA/DHA do not necessarily mean benefits of seafood, and lack of benefit from EPA/DHA does not necessarily mean lack of benefit from seafood.

Part I: Benefits to Women, Infants, and Young Children Associated with Omega-3 Fatty Acids

BENEFITS TO WOMEN DURING AND AFTER PREGNANCY

Preeclampsia

An array of studies based on supplemental intake of EPA/DHA or biochemical indicators of EPA/DHA levels has been carried out to determine whether there is an association between increased intake or blood levels of EPA/DHA and decreased incidence of or risk for preeclampsia (Olsen and Secher, 1990; Schiff et al., 1993; Williams et al., 1995; Velzing-Aarts et al., 1999; Clausen et al., 2001). Because these and other studies, including randomized clinical trials (Bultra-Ramakers et al., 1995; Onwude et al., 1995; Salvig et al., 1996) or reviews of trials (Sibai, 1998) did not show clear evidence of a beneficial effect of a broad range of intake (or biochemical indicators) of EPA/DHA levels, it does not appear likely that increased seafood intake or fish-oil supplementation will reduce the incidence of preeclampsia among US women (see Appendix Table B 1a).

Postpartum Depression

During pregnancy and lactation there is a correspondent transfer of DHA from the mother to the fetus or infant (Holman et al., 1991; Al et al., 1995). Following pregnancy and lactation, maternal DHA blood levels may require many months for recovery to pre-pregnancy levels (Otto et al., 2001). Although prior depressive illness is the best predictor of higher risk for postpartum depression, it has been proposed that low DHA levels in the brain in late pregnancy and early postpartum period may contribute to the emergence of postpartum depression (Hibbeln and Salem, 1995). Further, it has been hypothesized that increased EPA/DHA intake during pregnancy could reduce the risk for postpartum depression. To date, however, there have been no randomized controlled trials or controlled clinical studies testing whether increased omega-3 fatty acid intake by pregnant women could reduce the risk for postpartum depression.

Hibbeln (2002) conducted a cross-cultural review of 41 studies and concluded that there is an association between increased seafood consumption and higher maternal milk DHA levels (p<0.006) and that this was associated with a lower prevalence of postpartum depression (p<0.0001). Timonen et al. (2004) followed up the Northern Finland 1966 Birth Cohort prospectively from pregnancy to 31 years of age. Members of the cohort were sent questionnaires, invited to undergo a clinical examination to assess indices of depression, and asked to estimate seafood consumption in the previous six months (presumably related to the lifetime pattern of seafood consumption). The study found that females who rarely consumed fish showed greater incidences of life-time depression than regular consumers of fish, based on the Hopkins Symptom Check List (HSCL-25) depression subscale alone (cutoff-point 2.01) (OR=1.4; 95% confidence interval [CI] 1.1-1.9) and the HSCL-25 depression subscale (cutoff-point 2.01) with a doctor diagnosis (OR=2.6; 95% CI 1.4-5.1), but not based on doctor diagnosis alone (OR=1.3; 95% CI 0.9-1.9) or suicidal ideation. This study, however, did not show causation and did not address postpartum depression specifically.

Otto et al. (2003) investigated the relationship between postpartum depression and changes in maternal plasma phospholipid-associated fatty acid (DHA and docosapentaenoic acid [DPA]) status by measurement at 36 weeks of pregnancy, at delivery, and 32 weeks postpartum in women in the Netherlands. Postpartum depression was assessed using the Edinburgh Postnatal Depression Scale (EPDS), developed as a screening and monitoring tool for postpartum depression (Cox et al., 1987). Only relative plasma fatty acid levels (percent of total fatty acids, wt/wt) were reported because total absolute amounts of plasma phospholipid-associated fatty acids at delivery and changes that occurred postpartum were not significantly different between the "possibly depressed" and "non-depressed" groups. The conclusion from this study was that the ratio of 22:6 n-3 (DHA) to 22:5 n-6 (DPA) becomes reduced during pregnancy and the difference is significant ($p<0.04$) compared to increased EPDS scores, while DHA status at delivery did not correlate with depressive symptoms ($p=0.563$) (Otto et al., 2003).

In contrast to the above-mentioned studies, Llorente et al. (2003) examined a cohort of 44 women who consumed 200 mg of DHA per day during the first 4 months of lactation compared to a placebo control group (n=45) for indices of postpartum depression and information processing (cognition). Both groups were analyzed for symptoms of depression using a self-rating questionnaire, the Beck Depression Inventory (BDI). Additionally, a subgroup of the population was administered the EPDS and the Structured Clinical Interview for Diagnostic and Statistical Manual of Mental Disorders, Fourth Edition, Axis I Disorders—Clinical Version. A positive and statistically significant correlation was found between the BDI questionnaire at 4 months and the EPDS scores at 18 months ($p<0.0001$), which validated use of the BDI for assessment of symptoms. However, no difference was found between the supplemented and control groups for diagnostic measures of postpartum depression or information processing (see Appendix Table B-1b).

Summary of Evidence

Based solely on these studies, the committee cannot draw a conclusion about the effect of increased EPA/DHA on postpartum depression. Thus, there is not sufficient evidence to conclude that the health of pregnant or lactating women will benefit directly from an increase in seafood intake.

BENEFITS TO INFANTS AND CHILDREN ASSOCIATED WITH PRENATAL OMEGA-3 FATTY ACID INTAKE

Transfer of Maternal DHA to the Fetus or Breastfeeding Infant

The level of maternal DHA intake influences DHA levels in both maternal blood and milk. Blood DHA levels increase by about 50 percent in pregnancy (Al et al., 1995) and decline dramatically by 6 weeks after parturition, especially with lactation (Makrides and Gibson, 2000; Otto et al., 2001). DHA transport across the placenta is increased with higher compared to lower maternal blood DHA concentration and, compared with other fatty acids in maternal blood, DHA is selectively transferred across the placenta (Haggerty et al., 1997, 1999, 2002). Thus, increased maternal blood DHA levels in pregnancy may enhance DHA availability for placental transfer to the fetus.

Maternal DHA status could influence the DHA supply available to the fetal brain as well as other organs and tissues (Clandinin et al., 1980a). Brain DHA accumulates rapidly from approximately 22 weeks gestation until at least 2 years after birth (Clandinin et al., 1980b; Martinez, 1992). Studies that examined autopsy tissue from a limited number (n = 5) of both preterm and term infants reported that tissue from infants who consumed breast milk after birth showed greater cortical accumulation of DHA than those fed formulas that did not contain DHA, and the differences increased with duration of feeding (Farquharson et al., 1992; Makrides et al., 1994).

Duration of Gestation and Birth Weight

Infant birth weight is the result of a complex interaction involving many factors, including both biological and social mechanisms. Biological mechanisms are also variable and complex but appear to be linked to duration of gestation and fetal growth, conditional on duration of gestation (Ghosh and Daga, 1967; Villar and Belizan, 1982; Alberman et al., 1992). Higher birth weight is positively associated with cognitive ability among full-term infants in the normal birth weight range (Matte et al., 2001; Richards et al., 2001) as well as some preterm infants (Hediger et al., 2002). Low infant birth weight (less than 2500 grams or 5.2 pounds) (Juneja and Ramji, 2005), fetal growth retardation (van Wassenaer, 2005), and preterm delivery (Hediger et al., 2002) are associated with poor developmental outcomes.

Fish-Oil Supplementation

Observational and experimental studies have been carried out to determine if there is a relationship between DHA intake and increased gestation duration or birth weight. Both observational and experimental studies suggest that increased seafood consumption or DHA intake from supplements can increase gestation duration or birth weight. Any outcome correlated with a variable in an observational study can only suggest an association. In the case of the observational studies cited here showing relationships between EPA/DHA or seafood intake, the effect may be explained by these variables or by other variables that accompany diets higher in EPA/DHA or seafood intake. The People's League of Health trial (reviewed in Olsen, 2006) showed that deliveries before 40 weeks were reduced by 20.4 percent in the group that received a fish-oil/vitamin supplement compared to the group that was not supplemented ($p<0.0008$) (Olsen and Secher, 1990).

Several randomized controlled trials (RCT) have tested for an association between dietary supplementation with fish oil or the omega-3 fatty acids from fish oil (i.e., either DHA alone or EPA and DHA) and longer duration gestation. Olsen et al. (1992) conducted an RCT that administered 2.7 g/day of a fish-oil supplement beginning in the 30th week of pregnancy in a Danish cohort. The study found an average increase in gestation of 2.8 days in subjects from the fish-oil treatment group compared with control groups receiving an olive oil supplement or no supplement ($p<0.01$). In a similar study, Olsen et al. (2000) found among women who had a previous preterm delivery (delivery at <37 weeks) a significantly decreased risk for recurrent preterm delivery, a mean increase in gestation of 8.5 days ($p=0.01$), and an increase in birth weight of 209 g ($p=0.02$) in the fish oil compared to the olive-oil treatment group. In this study, however, prophylactic trials using fish-oil supplementation did not increase gestation duration and birth weight in pregnancies with intrauterine growth retardation, twins, or pregnancy-induced hypertension.

In contrast to these studies, a randomized trial conducted in Norwegian women (Helland et al., 2001) found no increase in either gestation duration or birth weight with a supplement of 2 g/day of EPA and DHA from cod-liver oil during the last two trimesters of pregnancy. However, a post hoc analysis found an increase in length of gestation of 7 days in infants in the highest quartile for plasma phospholipid DHA compared to those in the lowest quartile (Helland et al., 2001). Similarly, a post hoc analysis of results from the previously mentioned Danish trial (Olsen et al., 1992) found an increase in gestation duration of 5.7 days associated with fish-oil supplementation in a group of women who had the lowest 20 percent of seafood consumption at study entry ($p<0.05$), compared to a 2.8-day increase in gestation associated with fish-oil supplementation in all women.

The committee found that compared to women in Denmark and Norway, US women have been shown to consume less omega-3 long-chain polyunsaturated fatty acids and have lower levels of DHA in breast milk (Jensen et al., 1995). They also have, on average, shorter gestation durations and smaller infants (Smuts et al., 2003 a,b; Olsen et al., 1992; Helland et al., 2001). Birth weight depends on both length of gestation and intrauterine growth. Problematically high birth weight is not due to excessive gestation but rather to excessive intrauterine growth. No experimental trials have been conducted in the United States in which fish-oil supplements were evaluated for increasing gestation duration.

EPA/DHA Intake from Seafood and Other Food Sources

In a randomized controlled trial, Smuts et al. (2003b) evaluated the effect of feeding DHA-fortified eggs (mean 133 mg DHA/egg) to pregnant women in the United States, beginning at 24–28 weeks gestation. They reported a significant increase in gestation of 6 days among women consuming the high-DHA eggs compared to women receiving unfortified eggs (mean 33 mg DHA/egg). There was no significant increase in birth weight ($p=0.184$), birth length ($p=0.061$), or head circumference ($p=0.081$) among infants of mothers consuming high-DHA eggs. Although birth weight is frequently used as a marker for infant growth, head circumference and birth length are likely better indicators of positive pregnancy outcome.

An observational study examining an association between seafood consumption and gestational duration was conducted in a cohort of women in the Orkney Islands and Aberdeen, Scotland. This study identified a significant association between the 30 percent greater amount of seafood consumed by Orkney Island women over that consumed by women in Aberdeen, Scotland, and an increase in gestational duration of 2.5 days ($p=0.01$) (Harper et al., 1991).

Olsen et al. (1991) examined whether there was a difference in the ratio of the long-chain polyunsaturated fatty acids (LCPUFA) EPA, DPA, and DHA to arachidonic acid (AA) measured in erythrocytes obtained within 2 days of delivery between Faroese and mainland Danish women and whether there was a correlation between the LCPUFA levels and gestational duration in these populations. Among the Faroese subjects, significantly higher percentages of blood EPA and DHA were detected compared to Danish subjects, whereas DPA and AA values in both groups were similar. The Faroese subjects were found to have a gestational duration an average of 2 days longer ($p=0.3$) and a corresponding higher birth weight of 140 g (p=0.1) compared to the Danish subjects, but these differences were not significant. After making allowance for seven potential confounders, an increase in duration of gestation of 5.7 days was found for each 20 percent increase in the ratio of erythrocyte EPA and DHA to AA in the Danish women (95% CI 1.4-10.1 days; p=0.02), but not in Faroese women (95% CI −2.0 to 3.3; p=0.6).

Increased gestational duration has also been investigated using observational studies of women who consumed seafood in geographical locations where there was higher exposure to environmental contaminants. Grandjean et al. (2001) examined a birth cohort from the Faroe Islands whose mothers consumed the meat and blubber from pilot whales in addition to regional fish. In a questionnaire, the women reported that they consumed, on average, 72 g of fish, 12 g of whale meat, and 7 g of whale blubber per day (Grandjean et al., 2001). The estimated intake of polychlorinated biphenyls (PCBs) for these women was 30 μg/g of blubber, and of mercury was 2 μg/g of whale meat (Grandjean et al., 2001). In addition to the increase in contaminant concentrations, there was an approximate 10-fold molar excess of selenium over mercury in serum samples from the subjects. The concentration of EPA in the cord[1] serum from the infants of Faroese subjects was strongly associated with a maternal diet rich in marine fats. Gestational length showed a strong positive association with cord serum DHA concentration. Each 1 percent increase in the relative DHA concentration in cord serum phospholipids was associated with an increased duration of 1.5 days (95% CI 0.70-2.22), supporting the hypothesis that increased seafood intake may prolong gestation.

Lucas et al. (2004) concluded from an observational study that infants of the Inuit in Nunavik, Canada, had 2.2-fold higher omega-3 fatty acid (p<0.0001), 18.6-fold higher mercury (p<0.0001), 2.4-fold higher lead (presumably related to maternal smoking as ~85 percent of pregnant Inuit women studied smoked) (p<0.0001), and 3.6-fold higher PCB congener 153 cord blood levels (p<0.0001) compared to levels from infants in southern Québec. Despite the association of seafood intake with environmental contaminants, however, the Nunavik women whose infants were in the third compared to the first tertile of percentage of omega-3 fatty acid out of total highly unsaturated fatty acid (HUFA) cord blood values still had a mean 5.4-day longer gestation duration (95% CI 0.7-10.1; p<0.05). This study also showed a nonsignificant increase in mean adjusted birth weight in the third, compared to the first, tertile among Inuit (difference = 77 g, 95% CI −64 to 217).

---

[1]Examining the blood remaining in the umbilical cord after birth, though it is not precisely identical to that in the infant bloodstream, provides a noninvasive way to approximate the infant's blood profile.

Infants born preterm are at higher risk for neonatal complications and developmental delay. A reduction in the incidence of preterm birth (birth at <37 weeks) is desirable and could be associated with an increase in gestation duration among this at-risk population. Olsen and Secher (2002) evaluated the risk of preterm birth in relation to seafood intake in a prospective cohort study in Denmark. A questionnaire was used to evaluate intake of seafood, including roe, prawn, crab, and mussels, as well as fish-oil supplements, among participants. Quantification of fish consumption and EPA/DHA intakes was based on assumptions about the type and amount of fish reported in the questionnaire. Results of the analysis were based on seafood consumption only, since very few of the subjects took fish-oil supplements. Among the respondents, there was a trend of decreasing incidence of low birth weight, preterm birth, and intrauterine growth retardation with increasing fish consumption and increasing mean birth weight and duration of gestation among subjects. Women who were not smokers, primiparous women, teenagers, and women who had low weight, short stature, and without a high school education and cohabitant tended to fall into the low exposure group. This group had 3.57 (95% CI 1.14-11.14) times the risk of preterm birth and 3.60 (95% CI 1.15-11.20) times the risk of low birth weight (< 2500 g) delivery compared to women who consumed the highest amount of seafood. This study could be interpreted to suggest that a relatively low threshold intake of seafood EPA and DHA may increase gestation duration. However, Olsen et al. (2004) found no relationship between seafood EPA and DHA intake and duration of gestation or risk of preterm birth in US women from Massachusetts.

Summary of Evidence

In summary, observational studies suggest and several experimental studies support that EPA/DHA supplementation or higher seafood intake is associated with an increased duration of gestation. In trials that show longer gestation duration, the populations studied varied markedly in both baseline EPA and DHA blood levels and in estimated amounts of EPA and DHA provided from supplements (see Appendix Table B-1c). The clinical significance of increased duration of gestation is not clear. In general, health professionals consider that the fetus benefits from a longer time in utero up to the point that the fetus is >4500 g, although the advantage remains theoretical.

Development in Infants and Children

During pregnancy, AA and DHA are delivered to the fetus via the placenta (Crawford et al., 1997). Hornstra et al. (1995) found that maternal essential fatty acid status progressively declines during pregnancy. There appears to be a greater transplacental gradient in proportions of AA and DHA at term than midterm. Such a difference is consistent with the decline in plasma concentration of DHA between the beginning and end of pregnancy and suggests that the placenta is progressively depleting maternal DHA as the fetus grows (Crawford, 2000). Although the mechanism of transport for AA and DHA has not been elucidated, Campbell et al. (1998) proposed and Larque et al. (2003) identified a fatty acid binding protein, p-FABPpm, in placental tissue that showed a higher binding capacity for DHA and AA than linoleic acid (LA) and oleic acid (OA).

Visual Acuity and Sensory-Motor Development

Because lower visual acuity was observed in rhesus monkeys with lower brain DHA ($p < 0.001$) (Neuringer et al., 1984), this outcome has been the most studied in human infants relative to DHA intake. The first experimental studies that provided DHA, AA, and EPA to preterm infants demonstrated an increase in blood lipid content of these fatty acids as well as increases in visual acuity (Uauy et al., 1990; Carlson et al., 1993). Subsequently, DHA in cord blood and infant blood lipids has been used as an indicator of DHA exposure of the fetus or infant.

DHA status in infants is determined using blood as a biomarker because levels of DHA in the brain correlate with those in erythrocytes (Makrides et al., 1994). Previous studies have identified a correlation between dietary intake of AA, DHA, and other LCPUFAs; their respective levels in blood and erythrocyte phospholipids; and performance on tests of visual acuity and sensory-motor development in preterm infants (Uauy et al., 1990; Bjerve et al., 1993; Carlson et al., 1993). Observational studies that associate higher maternal EPA or DHA intake with higher stereoacuity or visual acuity in their infants are discussed below. Subsequently, maternal EPA/DHA supplementation or biochemical markers for their intake have been assessed as indicators of an association between increased intake levels of EPA/DHA and improved sensory-motor development in infants and young children.

Williams et al. (2001) observed that stereoacuity at 3.5 years of age in a subset of 435 healthy full-term children from the Avon Longitudinal Study of Parents and Children (ALSPAC) cohort was associated with breastfeeding, greater maternal age, and maternal antenatal consumption of fatty fish. After multiple logistic regression, only breastfeeding and maternal consumption of fatty fish at least once every 2 weeks remained significant predictors of higher stereoacuity (foveal acuity) in the children. Among 4733 women in the main ALSPAC cohort for whom both dietary intake and red blood cell DHA percentage were available, only intake of fatty fish was associated with higher red blood cell DHA levels, an indicator of higher maternal DHA status. Higher maternal DHA intake is also known to increase human milk DHA (Jensen et al., 2005). Therefore, both variables associated with significantly higher stereoacuity are themselves influenced by maternal DHA intake, and both could be expected to result in increased DHA exposure of the fetus or infant.

Innis et al. (2001) conducted a prospective observational study of 83 infants who were breastfed at least 3 months. Blood and plasma fatty acid status were determined at 2 months; visual acuity at 2, 4, 6, and 12 months; and speech perception and object search at 9 months. Maternal milk DHA content was measured as an indicator of maternal DHA status, and this was linked with higher visual acuity (p<0.01) and higher ability to discriminate nonnative retroflex and phonetic contrasts (p<0.02) in infants at 2 months of age (see Appendix Table B-1d). Both of these tasks suggest more mature sensory development; however, additional measures would be required to make a definitive determination. Placement in front of the Teller Acuity Cards (the technique employed to measure visual acuity) does not require motor development such as head turning, but it is required on the infants' performance on head-turning in response to sound. Thus, associations of DHA with motor function cannot be ruled out, particularly for the task related to hearing. Differences in cognitive development (discussed in the next section) also cannot be ruled out as a possible explanation for the association. However, factors that have been associated with cognitive development in infancy include speed, attention, and memory (Jacobson et al., 1992; Rose et al., 2004).

Cognitive Development

Cognitive developmental outcome has been assessed in a single random-ized controlled trial in children born to women supplemented with EPA and DHA during pregnancy (see Appendix Table B-1d). Helland et al. (2001, 2003) evaluated children whose mothers consumed 2 g/day of DHA and EPA from cod liver oil for the last two trimesters of pregnancy compared with children of those receiving a corn oil supplement as control and found significantly higher Mental Processing Composite scores at 4 years of age in the children of supplemented mothers (p=0.049). Women continued to consume the cod-liver oil supplements or the control oil during lactation, most of the infants were breastfed, and infants from both groups began to receive a fish-oil supplement at ~1 month of age. The analysis of results suggested that all of the increase in IQ at 4 years of age was attributed to prenatal rather than postnatal exposure to EPA and DHA. The trial was conducted in Norwegian woman, whose seafood consumption considerably exceeds that of US women.

Auestad et al. (2001) found that breast milk DHA levels between Nor-wegian women in the control group was 0.51 percent compared to DHA levels of 0.12 percent reported in breast milk of US women. Although the results of this study suggest that provision of EPA and DHA to neonates through supplemented formula might be greater than can be easily achieved through the diet, other investigators have reported higher levels of DHA in human milk than those reported by Auestad et al. (2001). Birch et al. (1998) compared visual acuity among infants who were fed DHA- and/or AA-supplemented formula with infants fed unsupplemented formula and breastfed infants. In comparing the red blood cell content of DHA among the infant groups, there was no significant difference in DHA level between the DHA-supplemented group and the breastfed group at week 0 and at week 52. However, there was a significant difference at week 17. In addition, a significant difference in the red blood cell AA concentration was found between the DHA-supplemented and breastfed groups only at week 17. As with the findings of Auestad et al. (2001), Birch et al. found that dietary supply of DHA is associated with optimal visual acuity.

Jensen and co-workers (2005) hypothesized that DHA supplementation of breastfeeding women would increase the DHA content of plasma lipids and improve visual and neuropsychological development in their infants. Women who planned to breastfeed were randomly assigned in a double-blinded manner to receive either a 200-mg algal DHA supplement or a control mixture of 50:50 soy and corn oil for the first 4 postnatal months. The results showed an increase in milk lipid and plasma phospholipid DHA levels of 75 and 35 percent, respectively, in the DHA-supplemented compared to control groups at 4 months. No differences were seen between supplemented and unsupplemented groups in either developmental indexes at 12 months or in visual acuity at 4 or 8 months. DHA-supplemented children subsequently showed higher Bayley Psychomotor Development scores at 30 months of age (p=0.005); and, in an earlier report, longer sustained attention at 5 years of age (Jensen et al., 2005). These outcomes suggest that 4 months of postnatal DHA supplementation via mother's milk is associated with long-term motor and cognitive development as defined by the Bayley Psychomotor Development score in US children. Because neither the experimental trial by Helland et al. (2003) nor that by Jensen et al. (2005) found benefits in infancy from maternal DHA supplementation, but both found benefits in early childhood, these trials suggest that studies that stopped developmental follow-up in infancy may have missed benefits to children of improving maternal omega-3 fatty acid intake. These findings also suggest that the benefit of perinatal DHA intake may only be manifested after a latency period.

Oken et al. (2005) in a prospective observational cohort study of pregnant women from Massachusetts, Project VIVA (see Box 3-1), examined associations of maternal fish intake during pregnancy and maternal hair mercury at delivery with infant cognition in a subset for which these data

BOX 3-1
Longitudinal Studies of Beneficial Outcomes to Women and Children from Seafood Consumption

Project Viva

Project Viva is a longitudinal study of women and their children, investigating the "effects of mother's diet and other factors during pregnancy on her health and the health of her child."

From 1999 to 2002, more than 2600 pregnant women were enrolled from eight different Harvard Vanguard Medical Associate sites in the greater Boston area. Participating expectant mothers completed standardized interviews (on diet, exercise, medical history, stress, societal factors, and financial support) and provided blood samples several times during and after their pregnancies.

Participating mothers were also asked to enroll their babies in the study. Research assistants interviewed the mothers and measured the newborns' body size and blood pressure in the first few days after birth (1703 women and 1203 newborns) and 6 months later (1266 mothers and 1210 babies). Hair samples from 210 women and umbilical cord blood from 1022 participants were also collected at delivery, and developmental tests were performed on the infants at 6 months of age.

At the child's first, second, and fourth birthdays, the mothers were sent a questionnaire asking about their child's health, diet, and environment, and at their third birthday, research assistants measured body size and blood pressure and performed additional developmental tests. The mother and child were also asked for another blood sample.

The Project Viva investigators hope to follow the Viva children throughout their lives, and are currently pursuing additional funding opportunities. The information provided here, along with updates, articles, facts, etc., can be accessed at http://www.dacp.org/viva/index.html [accessed November 2, 2005].

Avon Longitudinal Study of Parents and Children (ALSPAC)

"The Avon Longitudinal Study of Parents and Children (ALSPAC) also known as 'Children of the 90s' Is aimed at identifying ways in which to optimize the health and development of children. The main goal is to understand the ways in which the physical and social environments interact, over time, with the genetic inheritance to affect the child's health, behavior and development."

Over 14,500 pregnant women, resident in Avon, UK, were enrolled in this study, along with almost 14,000 of their children. Throughout their pregnancies, expectant mothers (and sometimes their partners) received various questionnaires to identify features of the early environment that might affect the fetus and to acquire information on the mother's

continued

BOX 3-1
Continued

demographic characteristics; past medical, social, and environmental history; and attitudes, activities, and emotional well-being. Maternal blood and urine samples were also obtained when the mothers gave routine samples at their respective clinics.

During delivery, cord blood and umbilical cord samples were collected, along with the placentas from births at two major hospitals. After delivery, further questionnaires were distributed to both the mothers from 4 weeks and throughout the next 9.5 years and to the children from 65 months until 9.5 years of age. During these years, samples of the child's hair and nail clippings, primary teeth, blood, and urine were also collected. For a complete list of topics covered on all questionnaires, see the ALSPAC website (http://www.ich.bristol.ac.uk/protocol/section3.htm).

"ALSPAC has the long-term aim of following the children into adulthood and thus will be set to answer questions related to prenatal and postnatal factors associated, for example, with schizophrenia, delinquency, and reproductive failure on the one hand, and realisation of full educational potential, health and happiness on the other." The information provided here, along with updates, articles, facts, etc., can be accessed at http://www.ich.bristol.ac.uk/welcome/index.shtml [accessed May 30, 2006].

---

were available. After adjusting for participant characteristics with linear regression, higher cognitive performance was associated with higher seafood intake. Each additional serving of fish per week was associated with a 4-point higher visual recognition memory (VRM) score at 6 months of age (95% CI 1.3-6.7), although an increase of 1 ppm in mercury was associated with a decrement in the VRM score of 7.5 (95% CI −13.7 to −1.2). VRM scores were highest among infants of women who consumed more than 2 servings of fish per week and had hair mercury levels less than or equal to 1.2 ppm. The study concluded that higher fish consumption was associated with better infant cognition but higher mercury levels were associated with lower cognition.

Daniels et al. (2004) studied a subset of 1054 children from the British ALSPAC cohort (see Box 3-1) for associations between maternal fish intake during pregnancy and infant development of language and communication skills in relation to mercury exposure. This study found an association between maternal fish intake during pregnancy and comprehension on the MacArthur Communicative Development Inventory (MCDI) (consumption of 1–3 or 4+ fish meals/week decreased odds of a low MCDI score, p<0.05) and the Denver Developmental Screening Test (DDST) (consumption of 1–3 or 4+ fish meals/week decreased odds of a low DDST score, p<0.05) at 15 and 18 months, respectively. In this cohort, mercury levels were low and not associated with measures of neurodevelopment. Similar findings of association between maternal DHA status and more mature attentional development in infancy (Willatts et al., 2003b; Colombo et al., 2004) and lower distractibility among toddlers (Colombo et al., 2004) were reported.

Some animal studies suggest that low brain DHA early in development produces adverse effects on behavior that are not reversible even when brain DHA content is returned to normal (Kodas et al., 2004; Levant et al., 2004). No studies have been designed to address possible programming of development in human infants, but the animal work suggests that timing of brain DHA accumulation should be considered as a variable in human studies.

Sleep Patterns

Cheruku et al. (2002) investigated whether central nervous system integrity in newborns, measured with sleep recordings, was associated with maternal DHA status. Plasma phospholipid fatty acids, including DHA, were measured in 17 women at parturition, and infant body movement and respiratory patterns were measured on postpartum days 1 and 2. Infants born to mothers in the high-DHA group had significantly lower ratios of active compared to quiet sleep patterns and less total active sleep compared to infants of low-DHA mothers. The conclusion from this study is that infants born to mothers with higher plasma DHA had more mature sleep patterns (p<0.05) compared to infants of mothers with lower plasma DHA levels (see Appendix Table B-1d).

Infant and Child Allergy

Few studies have been carried out to examine whether supplementation with fish oil is associated with reducing the inflammatory responses to allergens. Hodge et al. (1998) assessed the clinical and biochemical effects in asthmatic children of fish-oil supplementation and a diet that increases omega-3 and reduces omega-6 fatty acids. Although the supplemented group had higher plasma levels of omega-3 fatty acids and lower stimulated tumor necrosis factor-α production, there was no effect of the intervention on the clinical severity of asthma in the children. Dunstan et al. (2003) examined associations between fish-oil supplementation and levels of immune factors (cytokines and IgE) in a randomized, double-blind, placebo-controlled trial. No significant differences were found in interleukin (IL-13) (p=0.025) and cytokine levels within the treatment group, except that neonates of supplemented mothers had significantly lower levels of IL-13. In a subset of children from the ALSPAC cohort, Newson et al. (2004) found no relationship between cord and maternal red blood cell EPA/DHA and either eczema at 18 to 30 months (p>0.05) or wheezing at 30 to 42 months (p>0.05). These findings do not provide strong support for the hypothesis that exposure to omega-3 fatty acids from fish oil in utero or through breast milk could decrease the incidence of wheezing and atopic disease in early childhood (see Appendix Table B-1e).

Summary of Evidence

The strongest evidence of benefit for higher maternal seafood or EPA/ DHA intake is an increase in gestation duration, with anticipated benefits to the newborn. Populations or subgroups within populations who have the lowest baseline consumption of seafood may show the greatest benefit in duration of gestation with higher EPA/DHA intake. Observational and experimental studies offer evidence that maternal DHA intake can benefit development of the offspring; however, there are large gaps in knowledge that need to be filled by experimental studies.

The average EPA/DHA intake among US women is considerably below that of most other populations in the world and the majority of the data on benefits to infants and children from increased DHA levels comes from populations outside the United States and/or from studies using supplementation rather than seafood consumption.

BENEFITS TO INFANTS FROM POSTNATAL SUPPLEMENTATION THROUGH FORMULA

Although the focus of this report is seafood intake, the committee reviewed evidence for benefits associated with DHA-supplemented infant formulas to consider whether this data supports the previously discussed findings on benefits associated with seafood consumption or fish-oil supplementation in pregnant and lactating women. Formula-fed infants have much lower red blood cell phospholipid DHA levels than breastfed infants (Putnam et al., 1982; Carlson et al., 1986; Sanders and Naismith, 1979). DHA supplementation may increase brain DHA levels and improve visual acuity and various behavioral domains that are dependent upon brain function. Since 2002, infant formulas supplemented with DHA from algal oil in combination with a fungal source of AA have been commercially available in the United States. Randomized clinical trials have been conducted using a variety of sources of EPA/DHA including fish oil, tuna eye socket oil, egg phospholipid, total egg lipids, and algal oils to test for associations between DHA supplementation and improved developmental outcomes in formula-fed infants.

Visual Acuity

Studies by Carlson et al. (1993; 1996a,b; 1999) have tested the effect of DHA-supplemented formula on infant visual acuity using the Teller Acuity Card (TAC) procedure. The TAC procedure is subjective because it assesses an integrated behavioral response and may be influenced by nonvisual factors such as alertness, attention, and motor control (Lauritzen et al., 2001). Studies using the TAC procedure found significantly higher visual acuity in the groups receiving supplemented formula; higher visual acuity was found throughout infancy in trials that employed the sweep visual evoked potential (VEP) acuity procedure (Birch et al., 1992, p<0.025; 1998, p<0.05). VEP measures involve placing electrodes over the visual cortex to measure responses to different grating stimuli. This is not a subjective measure of visual acuity and also is more sensitive at detecting the threshold of visual acuity.

Higher VEP acuity was also found in studies on term infants that used formulas supplemented with both DHA and AA after weaning from breast milk (Hoffman et al., 2003, p<0.0005; Birch et al., 2002, p<0.003). Two trials that measured VEP acuity in preterm (Bougle et al., 1999) and term infants (Makrides et al., 2000) did not find any association between infant visual acuity and DHA-supplemented formula. However, these studies measured acuity using a flash of light rather than a sweep of high-contrast bands of graded spatial frequencies.

With the exception of Bougle et al. (1999), all of the previously discussed preterm infant trials and about half of the term infant trials that measured visual acuity have found higher visual acuity at some age. Uauy et al. (2001) in a review and San Giovanni et al. (2000a,b) in meta-analyses of previous studies concluded that DHA supplementation of infant formula was beneficial to visual acuity development in both preterm and term infants. A Cochrane systematic review of nine randomized controlled trials, however, concluded that there was no association between DHA supplementation and increased visual acuity or general development in term infants (Simmer, 2005) (see Appendix B-1f).

Cognitive and Motor Development

Many of the experimental trials that have studied postnatal DHA supplementation have also measured nonvisual developmental outcomes, most commonly global scales of development such as the Bayley Scales of Infant Mental Development Index (MDI) and Psychomotor Developmental Index (PDI) or a related test, Brunet-Lezine's developmental quotient (see Appendix Table B-1g). The majority of the extant published trials were reviewed by Gibson et al. (2001) and Uauy et al. (2001). Two trials in term infants found higher apparent motor development in infancy with DHA supplementation, as tested by the motor aspect of the Brunet-Lezine (p<0.05) (Agostoni et al., 1995) or general movement assessment (p=0.032) (Bouwstra et al., 2003). However, neither study found any benefit for movement or psychomotor development when the infants were tested again at 18 months of age. Birch et al. (2000) found higher (by 7 points) Bayley MDI scores at 18 months of age in term infants who consumed a formula supplemented with DHA and AA, compared to those who consumed the control formula (p<0.05), whereas Lucas et al. (1999) found no benefit of DHA and AA on either the Bayley MDI or PDI of term infants at 18 months of age.

It has been hypothesized that preterm infants may benefit more than term infants from DHA supplementation. Fewtrell et al. (2002, 2004) found no effect of supplementation on Bayley MDI of preterm infants in two other larger longitudinal studies.

Among smaller studies in preterm infants, however, Clandinin et al. (2005) in a randomized controlled trial found significant increases in both the Bayley MDI and PDI in preterm infants given DHA- and AA-supplemented formula (p<0.05) whereas van Wezel-Meijler et al. (2002) did not; Carlson et al. found higher Bayley MDI but not PDI at 12 months in only one of two preterm trial (Carlson et al., 1994, 1997).

Global tests such as the Bayley Scales of Infant Development and the Brunet-Lezine administered in infancy may be less related to performance on cognitive tests in childhood than more specific tests of attention and problem-solving (Carlson and Neuringer, 1999; Jacobson, 1999). While there is limited evidence from global tests of infant development (e.g., higher Bayley MDI scores in properly powered trials) to conclude there may be cognitive benefits of DHA supplementation for either preterm or term infants, evidence in support of benefits associated with DHA supplementation from specific tests in infancy that are more strongly related to several developmental parameters is mixed. O'Connor et al. (2001) assessed, among other measures, developmental outcomes in infants who received DHA- and AA-supplemented formula compared to controls. No differences were found in the Bayley MDI at 12 months, although the motor development index scores were higher among the supplemented infants who weighed less than 1250 g at birth compared to the nonsupplemented controls (p=0.007). When Spanish-speaking and twin infants were excluded from the analyses scores for the MacArthur Communicative Development Inventories, the supplemented infants had higher vocabulary comprehension at 14 months (p=0.01 for the egg triglyceride/fish group; p=0.04 for the fish/fungal group).

While there is limited evidence from global tests of infant development (e.g., higher Bayley MDI scores in properly powered trials) to conclude there may be cognitive benefits of DHA supplementation for either preterm or term infants, there is collective evidence of benefits associated with supplementation from specific tests in infancy that are better related to later cognitive function, e.g., higher novelty preference (O'Connor et al., 2001, p=0.02); duration of looking (Carlson and Werkman, 1996, p<0.05; Werkman and Carlson, 1996, p<0.05); and problem-solving (Willatts et al., 1998a, p=0.021; 1998b, p<0.02); although, excepting Willatts et al., these benefits have been found in preterm infants. Infants who received the supplemented formula had significantly more intentional solutions than infants who received the control formula (median 2 vs. 0; p=0.021). Intention scores (median 14.0 vs. 11.5; p=0.035) were also increased in this group (Willatts et al., 1998a).

Among studies assessing postnatal DHA supplementation, Willatts et al. (2003a) identified a long-term cognitive benefit, specifically, higher scores and speed on the matching familiar figures test (MFFT) at school age, in children provided DHA formula supplementation compared to unsupplemented formula as infants. Cognitive benefits reported at school age after postnatal supplementation are longer sustained attention at 5 years (Jensen et al., 2004) and higher IQ at 4 years of age noted in children exposed to higher DHA through maternal supplementation (Helland et al., 2003).

Language is highly associated with IQ, and studies that have assessed some aspect of early language are included here under the general topic of cognitive function. Scott et al. (1998) reported lower vocabulary comprehension (p=0.17) and production scores (p=0.027) with the MacArthur Communicative Development Inventories in term infants supplemented with formula containing DHA compared to control and DHA+AA formula groups, but not the human milk group. No effects of early DHA feeding on language were apparent at three years of age when children were tested again (Auestad et al., 2003). In a term study supported by Ross Laboratories, Auestad et al. (2001) found, in a randomized controlled trial among term infants, significantly higher vocabulary production in those fed DHA and AA from fish and fungal sources compared to DHA and AA from egg triglyceride (p<0.05). Neither group differed, however, from controls on this or any other MacArthur subscore.

At most, specific outcomes have been measured in only one or two individual trials and these have been measured at different ages. Even though numerous developmental outcomes have been identified that collectively suggest there are benefits associated with EPA/DHA supplementation, it is difficult to subject the studies in total to a systematic review, because of the differences in experimental design among the studies. The benefits of postnatal DHA supplementation for cognitive development need further study because of the heavy reliance on global assessments as outcomes and the limited employment of more specific developmental outcomes. Furthermore, the majority of trials stopped looking at development well before children reached school age, when more sophisticated measures of cognitive function may be employed.

Allergy and Immunity

Reviews of the effects of fatty acid supplementation on immune function in the neonate have not provided strong support for beneficial effects (Calder et al., 2001; Field et al., 2001) (see Appendix Table B-1h). One human study showed positive effects of human milk and formulas containing DHA and AA compared to formulas without DHA and AA in the form of lower CD4RO+ immune cells and IL-10 cytokine production (Field et al., 2000). However, experimental studies of DHA-supplemented lactating women have not found any effect of supplementation on milk cytokines at intakes as high as 140 mg/day EPA and 600 mg/day DHA (Hawkes et al., 2002) or 3.7 g EPA/DHA from fish oil (28 percent EPA and 56 percent DHA) in a group selected to be at high risk for allergic disease (Denburg et al., 2005).

Summary of Evidence

The strongest evidence of benefit for postnatal DHA supplementation in formula-fed preterm and term infants is higher visual acuity, an outcome that has been measured repeatedly in clinical trials. In addition, some positive effects have been found on cognitive function in infancy and childhood in both experimental and observational studies and in relation to both pre- and postnatal DHA intake. Reviews that take into account all lines of evidence have concluded that omega-3 fatty acids can be beneficial to cognitive development (Cohen et al., 2005; McCann and Ames, 2005), whereas reviews that rely strictly on published results from experimental trials limited to global assessments of cognitive development, e.g., the MDI, do not offer strong support (Simmer, 2005; Simmer and Patole, 2005).

Results of some experimental trials suggest that postnatal DHA infant formula supplementation benefits cognitive function as well. Specific behavioral domains such as novelty preference and duration of looking are more related to later function than global tests of development (Carlson and Neuringer, 1999; Jacobson, 1999). Bryan et al. (2004) and Cheatham et al. (2006) postulate that benefits associated with postnatal infant formula supplementation may have been underestimated as a result of the emphasis on global tests of infant development as well as the paucity of outcomes measured in childhood.

Animal Studies

Results from animal studies indicate a possible role for the timing of exposure to DHA in development. These studies testing variable levels of brain DHA on neurotransmitters such as dopamine and serotonin (Delion et al., 1996; de la Presa Owens and Innis, 1999; Chalon et al., 2001; Kodas et al., 2004) and responses of these neurotransmitter systems in rodent and pig models suggest there is a critical window for brain DHA accumulation for some aspects of development and that behavior remains abnormal even when brain DHA is remediated well before testing (Kodas et al., 2004; Levant et al., 2004). These animal studies, although not the subject of this review, provide suggestive evidence that the presence of DHA could be critical during early periods of human brain development.

BENEFITS TO CHILDREN

The few studies that exist of EPA/DHA supplementation in children have focused on the potential for EPA/DHA to modify diseases, i.e., they have not been designed to evaluate if DHA is needed in healthy children after infancy for optimal neurological development or physiological function. The majority of studies in children relate to diseases and disorders that involve brain and behavior, especially attention deficit hyperactivity disorder (ADHD) or dyslexia, though one experimental study evaluated possible effects of supplementation on symptoms of allergy. Few randomized trials have been carried out to test whether EPA/DHA supplementation in children reduced symptoms of ADHD, and there is little evidence for benefits. Neither can any conclusions yet be drawn about the possible role of seafood or EPA/DHA supplementation in the prevention of asthma. There is interest in the clinical benefits of EPA/DHA in certain childhood diseases and it is being actively studied, but such therapeutic interventions are beyond the scope of this report (see Appendix Table B-1i and B-1j).

FINDINGS

1. Seafood is a nutrient-rich food that makes a positive contribution to a healthful diet. It is a good source of protein, and relative to other protein foods, e.g., meat, poultry, and eggs, is generally lower in saturated fatty acids and higher in the omega-3 fatty acids EPA and DHA as well as selenium;

2. The evidence to support benefits to pregnancy outcome in females who consume seafood or fish-oil supplements as part of their diet during pregnancy is derived largely from observational studies. Clinical trials and epidemiological studies have also shown an association between increased duration of gestation and intake of seafood or fish-oil supplements. Evidence

that the infants and children of mothers who consume seafood or EPA/DHA supplements during pregnancy and/or lactation may have improved developmental outcomes is also supported largely by observational studies;

3. Increased EPA/DHA intake by pregnant and lactating women is associated with increased transfer to the fetus and breastfed infant.

a. A number of observational studies show a positive association between maternal blood or breast milk DHA levels and a range of developmental outcomes in infants and children.

b. Two experimental studies of maternal EPA/DHA supplementation found cognitive benefits for the children when they were 4 or 5 years of age.

c. Because these two studies differed dramatically in timing of EPA/DHA supplementation (pre- and postnatally or postnatally), source (cod-liver oil or algal DHA), and amount (2 g or 200 mg EPA/DHA) and, likely, in usual seafood intake (Norway or US residents), insufficient data are available to define an ideal level of EPA/DHA intake from seafood in pregnant and lactating women;

4. A large number of experimental trials have provided DHA directly to human infants through infant formula and have found benefits for infant and child neurological development. These trials offer the best evidence that infants/children would benefit from increased DHA in breast milk and increased maternal seafood intake.

a. Visual acuity has been measured in the most trials and is increased by DHA supplementation, with preterm infants more likely to benefit than term infants.

b. Cognitive benefits of postnatal DHA supplementation with formula have also been found in infancy and early childhood. However, the number of trials has been limited and the specific outcomes varied, precluding a systematic review;

5. At present there is no convincing evidence that ADHD, other behavioral disorders, and asthma in children can be prevented or treated with seafood or EPA/DHA consumption.

Part II: Benefits for Prevention of Adult Chronic Disease

CARDIOVASCULAR DISEASE, CARDIOVASCULAR MORTALITY, AND ALL-CAUSE MORBIDITY AND MORTALITY

Most evidence for benefits of seafood consumption and EPA/DHA supplementation associated with coronary heart disease (CHD) mortality is inferred from interventional studies of populations at risk, observational studies in the general population, and mechanistic studies. Early investigations of the association between diet and cardiovascular disease led to the recommendations to restrict dietary fat and cholesterol as a public health intervention to prevent CHD. However, subsequent observations suggest a more complex association between dietary fat intake and cardiovascular pathophysiology (Howard et al., 2006).

Cardiovascular Benefits to Specific Population Groups

Certain populations in the Mediterranean region consuming a diet relatively high in monounsaturated fat from olive oil enjoyed some of the lowest cardiovascular disease rates in the world. Another intriguing observation came from the comparison of Greenland Eskimo populations that had low mortality rates from CHD compared to the mainland Danish population, despite having a diet rich in fat (Bang et al., 1971). Bang et al. (1971) hypothesized that genetics, lifestyle, and the high content of EPA/DHA in the diet (which consisted primarily of fish, sea birds, seal, and whale) may account for the low cardiovascular mortality rate observed in this population. Plasma lipid patterns examined in this study showed that most types of lipids were decreased compared to a Danish cohort control and Eskimos living in Denmark (p<0.001). Remarkably, the levels of pre-β lipoprotein (p<0.001) and, consequently, plasma triglycerides (p<0.001) were much lower among the Greenland Eskimos than the Danish controls. As a result of this and related studies, seafood consumption, including or even especially of seafood rich in fat, has received increased attention as a public health means to decrease the burden of cardiovascular disease.

Several observational studies have shown an inverse association between seafood consumption and the risk of cardiovascular disease, most probably due to reductions of sudden death (reviewed in Wang et al., 2006). Some studies, however, have not found a significant association between seafood consumption and cardiovascular disease. These discrepancies may be due to differences among study populations and the type, amount, or preparation method of seafood consumed. For example, among studies reviewed, it has been hypothesized that the benefit of greater amounts of seafood may be more apparent in populations that have low seafood intakes and are at higher risk for cardiovascular disease (Marckmann and Gronbaek, 1999). Although initial studies suggested an optimal level of seafood consumption, more recent analyses have brought this observation into question and have suggested a more continuous association between seafood consumption and prevention of cardiovascular disease (p for trend = 0.03) (He et al., 2004b).

The possible mechanisms by which seafood or EPA/DHA supplements are cardioprotective include demonstrated antiarrhythmic, antithrombotic, antiatherosclerotic, and anti-inflammatory effects. Ismail (2005) and Calder (2004) linked the consumption of EPA/DHA to improved endothelial function, lower blood pressure, and lower fasting and postprandial triglyceride concentrations. Furthermore, populations and individuals who consume large amounts of seafood also tend to consume smaller amounts of alternative protein sources, such as beef, that are rich in saturated fats that are known to increase blood cholesterol levels and to elicit a proinflammatory state (Weisberger, 1997; Baer et al., 2004; Miller, 2005). Any one or a combination of these effects may explain the association between seafood intake and cardiovascular protection observed in some studies.

It is important to note that supplementation trials have been mostly conducted in individuals with existing cardiovascular disease for secondary prevention. Therefore, these findings are relevant to the progression of existing cardiovascular disease, but may not be relevant to the development of new cardiovascular disease in the general population, as these two processes may have different biological determinants. On the other hand, many observational studies of seafood consumption have been conducted in the general population and are relevant to primary prevention and the development of cardiovascular disease in the first place. Again, as determinants of cardiovascular disease development may be different from those of disease progression, the pertinence of these observational studies to secondary prevention is limited. These studies are, however, more informative than supplementation studies to assess the role of seafood in a healthy diet. The committee has tried to clearly differentiate these two types of studies and the conclusions that can be derived from them in the discussions that follow.

Seafood or Omega-3 Fatty Acid Consumption and Coronary Heart Disease

Randomized Controlled Trials in High Risk Populations

No randomized controlled trials have been carried out on subjects representative of the general population, as the small expected number of cardiovascular events would require large and perhaps impractical sample sizes and/or follow-up periods. In an early randomized trial of men who had already experienced a myocardial infarction (MI), Burr et al. (1989) reported that dietary advice, including advice to increase consumption of seafood, was associated with a significant reduction (29 percent) in 2-year all-cause mortality (p<0.05). An extended follow-up of these subjects, however, did not suggest any substantial long-term survival benefit (Ness et al., 2002). In contrast, in a separate study of male subjects over age 70 with stable angina, Burr et al. (2003) reported higher, and not lower, cardiovascular mortality in the group assigned to receive advice to consume seafood or n-3 fatty acid supplements (p=0.02). The reports by Burr et al. (2003) and Ness et al. (2002) seemed to some researchers a serious challenge to the idea that patients with coronary artery disease (CAD) and those at increased risk for heart disease should be advised to increase consumption of seafood rich in EPA/DHA or to take fish-oil supplements (Marckmann, 2003). A more detailed review of the literature considered by the committee is provided in Appendix B-2.

The Gruppo Italiano per lo Studio della Sopravvivenza nell'Infarto Miocardico (GISSI-Prevenzione) trial (GISSI Prevenzione Investigators, 1999) examined associations between dietary supplementation with EPA/DHA from fish oil, vitamin E, or combined treatment, and incidence of a second MI. From October 1993 to September 1995, 11,324 Italian patients surviving recent ($\leq$ 3 months) MI were randomly assigned supplements of EPA/DHA (1 g daily, n=2836), vitamin E (300 mg daily, n=2830), both (n=2830), or none (control, n=2828) for 3.5 years. The primary combined efficacy measurement endpoints of death, nonfatal MI, and nonfatal stroke were significantly reduced by EPA/DHA treatment; the relative risk reduction (RRR) was 15 percent for death, nonfatal MI, or nonfatal stroke (RR=0.85; 95% CI 0.74-0.98). Intention-to-treat analyses were done according to a (two-way) factorial design and by a (four-way) treatment group.

Results showed that EPA/DHA, but not vitamin E supplementation, significantly reduced risk of death, nonfatal MI, and nonfatal stroke (RR=0.90, 95% CI 0.82-0.99, two-way analysis; RR=0.85, 95% CI 0.74-0.98, four-way analysis). A decrease was found in the risk of all-cause mortality (14 percent [95% CI 3-24] two-way, 20 percent [95% CI 6-33] four-way) and cardiovascular death (17 percent [95% CI 3-29] two-way, 30 percent [95% CI 13-44] four-way). There was no significant effect between the combined treatment and EPA/DHA for the primary endpoints listed above. This study showed that dietary supplementation with fish oil as a source of EPA/DHA led to a statistically significant benefit in people with a history of MI; however, effects on fatal cardiovascular events require further exploration.

The percentage of patients who experienced at least one cardiac event (cardiac death, resuscitation, recurrent MI, or unstable angina) was 28 in the EPA/DHA group and 24 in the corn oil (control) group. There was no significant difference in prognosis between the groups for either single or combined cardiac events. Total cholesterol concentrations decreased in both groups, although intergroup differences were not significant. On average, high density lipoprotein (HDL) cholesterol increased by 1.1 percent in the EPA/DHA group and by 0.55 percent in the corn oil group (p=0.0016) per month. In the same time period, triacylglycerol concentrations decreased by 1.3 percent in the EPA/DHA group, whereas they increased by 0.35 percent in the corn oil group per month (p<0.0001). Thus, no clear clinical benefit of a high-dose concentrate of EPA/DHA acids compared with corn oil was shown, despite a favorable effect on serum lipids.

In addition to the randomized clinical trials described above, another commonly cited study in support of the benefits of fish oil consumption comes from the Indian Study on Infarct Survival. This was reported by Singh et al. (1997) as a randomized, placebo-controlled study of 360 Indian patients enrolled within 1 day after MI into one of three groups: a group receiving fish oil (1.08 g/day EPA and 0.72 g/day DHA), a group receiving mustard seed oil (20.0 g/day, ALA content 2.9 g/day), and a placebo (control) group receiving aluminum hydroxide (100 mg/day). The combined primary end point was total cardiac events (sudden cardiac death plus total cardiac deaths plus nonfatal reinfarction). According to the authors, the fish oil group had a 30 percent lower risk in total cardiac events after 1 year, compared to the placebo group (RR=0.70; 95% CI 0.29-0.90). However, serious concerns have been raised about the performance and conclusions of this trial and other related publications from this investigator (White, 2005; Al-Marzouki et al., 2005) and therefore, based on these caveats, the evidence in support of EPA/DHA consumption should be considered after exclusion of this widely used report.

Taken together, these randomized trials showed conflicting results for an effect of EPA/DHA on cardiovascular events and no long-term protective effect of seafood intake in subjects with a previous history of CHD. These findings are consistent with a systematic Cochrane review that concluded that "It is not clear that dietary or supplemental omega-3 fats alter total mortality, combined cardiovascular events, or cancers in people with, or at high risk of, cardiovascular disease or in the general population" (Hooper et al., 2005) and with the more recent work of Hooper et al. (2006).

Observational Studies of Seafood or EPA/DHA Intake in the General Population

Several studies have addressed a possible association of seafood or EPA/DHA intake with cardiovascular deaths or events in the general population, including individuals with a previous history of CHD. Whelton et al. (2004)

conducted a meta-analysis of observational studies to determine if seafood consumption was associated with lower fatal and total CHD in people with and without a history of heart disease. The analysis included English-language articles published before May 2003. A total of 19 observational studies (14 cohort and 5 case-control) met the prestated inclusion criteria that the studies were conducted in adult humans, used an observational case-control or cohort design, compared a group that consumed seafood regularly with one that did not, used CHD as an outcome, and reported an association as a relative risk (RR), hazard ratio (HR), or odds ratio (OR) of CHD by category of seafood consumption. A random effects model was used to pool data from each study. The analysis found that regular fish consumption compared to little to no fish consumption was associated with a relative risk of 0.83 (95% CI 0.76-0.90; p<0.005) for fatal CHD and 0.86 (95% CI 0.81-0.92; p<0.005) for total CHD.

He et al. (2004b) also examined associations between seafood consumption and CHD mortality in people with or without a history of heart disease using a meta-analysis design. A database was developed based on 11 eligible studies that included 13 cohorts consisting of a total of 222,364 individuals and an average follow-up of 11.8 years. Pooled RR and 95 percent CI for CHD mortality were calculated by using both fixed-effect and random-effect models. Possible dose-response relationships were assessed using a linear regression analysis of the log RR weighted by the inverse of variance. The results of the analysis found a consistent inverse association between sea food consumption and CHD mortality rates and suggested a dose-response association. The pooled multivariate RRs for CHD mortality, compared to seafood intake less than once per month, were 0.89 (95% CI 0.79-1.01) for seafood intake one to three times per month, 0.85 (95% CI 0.76-0.96) for once per week, 0.77 (95% CI 0.66-0.89) for two to four times per week, and 0.62 (95% CI 0.46-0.82) for five or more times per week.

Each 20 g/day increase in seafood intake lowered the risk of CHD mortality by 7 percent (p for trend = 0.03). These results indicate that mortality from CHD may be significantly reduced by eating seafood as infrequently as once per week, with increasing benefit with increasing intake. This meta-analysis does not provide subgroup analyses and does not include case-control studies.

The most recent meta-analysis by König et al. (2005) provides another quantitative assessment of the association between seafood consumption and CHD. In this meta-analysis, all studies identified of primary prevention, i.e., incidence of CHD in people without a history of CHD, were observational studies that assessed seafood intake, while all studies of secondary prevention, i.e., in people with a history of CHD, were randomized trials using EPA/DHA supplements at doses difficult to achieve with seafood consumption. The authors of this meta-analysis were able to provide a quantitative assessment of the association of seafood consumption with CHD mortality and nonfatal MI in people without a history of CHD, but concluded that insufficient evidence supported a quantitative assessment of seafood consumption for secondary prevention. From this study, it was estimated that, compared to not eating seafood, eating a small amount of seafood—as little as half a serving per week—was associated with a reduction in risk of cardiovascular death of 17 percent (95% CI 8.8-25.0) and a reduction in risk of nonfatal MI of 27 percent (95% CI 21-34). Each additional weekly serving of seafood was associated with a further decrease in the risk of cardiovascular death of 3.9 percent (95% CI 1.1-6.6), but no additional benefit was statistically significant for the risk of nonfatal MI. The Agency for Healthcare Research and Quality (AHRQ) reviews are systematic reviews that synthesize observational and experimental studies in a qualitative way (see Appendix B). The conclusions of the AHRQ reviews are also based on intervention studies in groups at risk. In contrast, the studies by Whelton et al., He et al., and Konig et al. are meta-analyses that quantitatively combined observational studies. Meta-analyses are usually considered stronger evidence than systematic reviews.

Taken together, these meta-analyses of observational studies suggest a negative association between seafood consumption and CHD or death, particularly in individuals without a prior history of CHD. Recent data suggest that even small amounts of seafood consumption may be associated with a decreased risk for CHD or death (Schmidt et al., 2005a,b). These results should, however, be interpreted with caution, as they are based on observational studies and are thus subject to residual confounding. In other words, based on observational studies only, it is difficult to exclude the possibility that seafood intake may just be a marker for healthier lifestyle, and that no causal association exists between seafood consumption and cardiovascular protection (see Appendix Tables B-2a and B-2b).

Stroke

The only reported studies of the association between seafood consumption and stroke have been observational (see Appendix Table B-2b). He et al. (2004a) quantitatively assessed the relationship between seafood consumption and risk of stroke using a meta-analysis of nine cohorts from eight studies. Pooled RR and 95 percent CI of risk for stroke were estimated by variance-based meta-analysis. These results demonstrated that consumption of seafood was inversely related to stroke risk, particularly ischemic stroke. Even infrequent seafood consumption (as seldom as 1 to 3 times per month) may be protective against the incidence of ischemic stroke compared to seafood consumption less than once per month. The pooled RRs for *all* stroke, compared to individuals who consumed seafood less than once a month, were 0.91 (95% CI 0.79-1.06) for individuals with seafood intake one to three times/month, 0.87 (95% CI 0.77-0.98) for once/week, 0.82 (95% CI 0.72-0.94) for two to four times/week; and 0.69 (95% CI 0.54-0.88) for five or more times/week (p for trend = 0.06).

Three large cohort studies with data on stroke subtypes were used in a stratified meta-analysis to determine pooled RRs across five categories of seafood intake for ischemic stroke. Compared to individuals who consumed seafood less than once a month, the RRs were 0.69 (95% CI 0.48-0.99) for individuals with seafood intake one to three times/month, 0.68 (95% CI 0.52-0.88) for once/week, 0.66 (95% CI 0.51-0.87) for two to four times/week; and 0.65 (95% CI 0.46-0.93) for five or more times/week (p for trend = 0.24) (He et al., 2004a).

For hemorrhagic stroke, compared to individuals who consumed seafood less than once a month, the RRs were 1.47 (95% CI 0.81-2.69) for individuals with seafood intake one to three times/month, 1.21 (95% CI 0.78-1.85) for once/week, 0.89 (95% CI 0.56-1.40) for two to four times/week, and 0.80 (95% CI 0.44-1.47) for five or more times/week (p for trend = 0.31) (He et al., 2004a). In a separate recent meta-analysis, Bouzan et al. (2005) quantified the association of seafood consumption with stroke risk, based on five cohort studies and one case-control study. Although a decrease of 12 percent in the risk of both ischemic and hemorrhagic strokes was observed with a small amount of seafood consumption compared to no seafood consumption, this result was not statistically significant (95%CI: increased risk of 1 percent to decreased risk of 25 percent). Furthermore, there was no evidence for further decrease in the risk of strokes with increasing seafood intake above a small amount: 2 percent decrease in risk per serving per week (95%CI: increased risk of 2.7 percent to decreased risk of 6.6 percent).

Skerrett and Hannekens (2003) reviewed ecologic/cross-sectional and case-control studies of associations between consumption of seafood or EPA/DHA and stroke risk. Five prospective studies showed inconsistent results: no association, a possible inverse association, and three significant inverse associations. In the most recent Nurses' Health Study, the relative risk for total stroke was somewhat lower among women who regularly ate seafood compared to those who did not, although there was no significant difference. After adjusting for age, smoking, and other cardiovascular risk factors, a significant decrease in the risk for thrombotic stroke was observed among women who ate seafood at least two times per week compared with those who ate seafood less than once per month (RR=0.49; 95% CI 0.26-0.93). The decrease observed among women in the highest quintile of EPA/DHA intake was not significant nor was an association observed between consumption of seafood or fish oil and hemorrhagic stroke.

Data from Mozaffarian et al. (2005) suggest that the type of seafood meal may be an influential variable. Mozaffarian and collaborators investigated the association between seafood consumption and stroke risk in the Cardiovascular Health Study, an older population in whom the disease burden is high. Dietary intakes were assessed in 4775 adults aged ≥65 years (range, 65–98 years) and free of known cerebrovascular disease at baseline in 1989–1990 using a food frequency questionnaire. In a subset of this population, consumption of tuna or other broiled or baked seafood, but not fried seafood or fish sandwiches (fish burgers), correlated with plasma phospholipid long-chain omega-3 fatty acid levels. During 12 years of follow-up, participants experienced 626 incident strokes, of which 529 were ischemic strokes. Tuna/other seafood consumption was associated with a 27 percent lower risk of ischemic stroke when consumed one to four times per week (HR=0.73; 95% CI 0.55-0.98), and with a 30 percent lower risk when consumed five or more times per week (HR=0.70, 95% CI 0.50-0.99) compared with consumption of less than once per month.

Conversely, consumption of fried fish/fish sandwiches was associated with a 44 percent higher risk of ischemic stroke when consumed once per week compared with less than once per month (HR=1.44; 95% CI 1.12-1.85). Seafood consumption was not associated with hemorrhagic stroke. Consumption of tuna or other broiled or baked seafood was associated with lower risk of ischemic stroke while intake of fried seafood/fish sandwiches was associated with higher risk among elderly individuals.

Taken together, these observational studies provided inconclusive results for an association between seafood intake and stroke. These results suggest that seafood consumption may influence stroke risk; however, identification of mechanisms or alternate explanations for the results requires further study. The type of seafood meal, particularly the method of preparation, is not recorded in most observational studies but may be a major effect modifier.

Lipid Profiles

The effects of seafood or EPA/DHA on serum lipid profiles have been extensively studied to determine if intake influences indicators of cardiovascular disease risk (see Appendix Table B-2c). In AHRQ Evidence Report/Technology Assessment No. 93 (2004), Balk et al. showed that with few exceptions, serum triglyceride levels were found to decrease with increasing intake of EPA/DHA, and this change was statistically and biologically significant. Moreover, the effect appears to be dose-dependent regardless of the EPA/DHA source. Most of the studies reviewed reported net decreases of approximately 10–33 percent in triglyceride levels. Effects were dose-dependent among subjects that were healthy, had cardiovascular disease, or were at increased risk for cardiovascular disease or dyslipidemia, and were greatest among subjects who had higher mean baseline triglyceride levels.

EPA/DHA intake was only weakly associated with levels of other serum lipids, including total, high-density lipoprotein (HDL), and low-density lipoprotein (LDL) cholesterol and lipoprotein (a) (Lp(a)). Balk et al. (2004) reviewed 65 randomized controlled trials and found a wide range of effects of EPA/DHA on total cholesterol. Most studies achieved a small net effect and the trend was towards increased total cholesterol; however, the direction of the effect was not consistent across studies. For example, two studies (Hanninen et al., 1989; Mori et al., 1994) used seafood-based diets as part of the intervention protocol, and neither of them reported significant effects of seafood consumption on total cholesterol levels. Further, Mori et al. (1994) found that LDL cholesterol levels were not changed in subjects consuming EPA/DHA-enriched diets. No significant differences were found in men who consumed various doses of EPA and DHA either from seafood or fish oil.

Balk et al. (2004) reviewed 19 reports of effects of EPA/DHA on HDL cholesterol. Most studies reported small increases in HDL cholesterol, and in about one-third of the studies, the effects were statistically significant. One study conducted in men using intervention with a seafood-enriched diet (Mori et al., 1994) found no difference among those consuming various doses of EPA and DHA either as supplements or from seafood in a diet regimen. In a randomized controlled trial, Vandongen et al. (1993) found that the effect of EPA/DHA on HDL cholesterol was independent of the source of the EPA/DHA.

Consistent effects of EPA/DHA on Lp(a) levels have not been found (Balk et al., 2004). In approximately one-third of the 14 studies reviewed, EPA/DHA intakes were associated with a net increase in Lp(a) compared to controls. In the remaining studies reviewed, the net decrease in Lp(a) level was generally small and nonsignificant. Only two studies (Eritsland et al., 1995; Luo et al., 1998) reported a statistically significant difference between the effect of EPA/DHA intake and control. Both found a net decrease in Lp(a) (p=0.023; only for those with a baseline Lp(a) of ≥ 20 mg d/l). However, the large interindividual variability in Lp(a) levels resulted in wide confidence intervals in all studies reviewed by Balk et al. (2004). One study examined a diet enriched with seafood, but found no significant effect on Lp(a) levels (Schaefer et al., 1996).

Blood Pressure

Increased consumption of seafood is one of several dietary recommendations in studies examining dietary effects on blood pressure. Thus, the effect of EPA/DHA from seafood is difficult to isolate from benefits provided by other dietary changes.

Randomized Controlled Trials

The effect of fish-oil supplementation has been studied in a meta-analysis of experimental studies (Geleijnse et al., 2002). The overall results of 36 trials examined indicate that the mean adjusted net reduction in systolic and diastolic blood pressure was –2.1 mmHg (95% CI –3.2 to –1.0), and –1.6 mmHg (95% CI –2.2 to –1.0), respectively. Moreover, systolic and diastolic blood pressure reductions were significantly greater in older (mean age ≥45 years) than younger populations, and in hypertensive (blood pressure ≥140/90 mmHg) compared to normotensive populations. Inconsistent results among studies in women precluded adequate analysis based on sex. Body mass index, trial duration, and seafood dose did not affect the blood pressure response noted with fish-oil supplementation. Studies conducted in diabetic patients were not included in the meta-analysis. The review by Balk et al. (2004) found only small and inconsistent net effects of EPA/DHA on blood pressure levels of diabetic patients.

A single RCT with advice to increase seafood intake has been reported. The Diet and Reinfarction Trial (DART) examined the effect of advice to consume seafood on blood pressure outcomes at 6 and 24 months in over 2000 men with a history of MI (Ness et al., 1999). The average intake of the group advised to consume fish was 330 mg of EPA compared to 100 mg in the control group. There were no significant differences in blood pressure detected between the groups at either 6 or 24 months.

Observational Studies

Appleby et al. (2002) examined the effect of diet and lifestyle factors on differences between meat eaters, seafood eaters, vegetarians, and vegans on the prevalence of self-reported hypertension, and mean systolic and diastolic blood pressure. Data for the analysis was obtained from the Oxford cohort of the European Prospective Investigation into Cancer and Nutrition (EPIC-Oxford). More than 11,000 adult men and women were classified into the four diet groups for analysis. Results showed that age-adjusted prevalence of self-reported hypertension in men was 15 percent in meat eaters, 9.8 percent in both seafood eaters and vegetarians, and 5.8 percent in vegans. In women, the prevalence was 12.1, 9.6, 8.9, and 7.7 percent in the respective diet groups. After adjustment for body mass index (BMI), the group differences decreased in both men and women. When seafood eaters were compared to vegetarians, no benefit was seen that could be attributed to seafood consumption per se.

Dewailly et al. (2001) examined the relationship between plasma phospholipid concentrations of EPA/DHA and various cardiovascular disease risk factors among the Inuit of Nunavik, Canada, whose traditional high-seafood diet contains very large amounts of EPA/DHA. Over 400 Inuit adults participated in a health survey that included home interviews and clinical visits. Plasma samples were obtained from participants and analyzed for phospholipid fatty acid composition. No association was found between phospholipid content of EPA/DHA and blood pressure in this population of high seafood consumers.

It is unclear from these studies whether seafood consumption, in the range consumed by most Americans, is an effective means to reduce blood pressure (see Appendix Table B-2d). Further, it is not known if the association between EPA/DHA consumption and blood pressure is linear or if there is a threshold below which no benefit is detectable.

Arrhythmia

Leaf et al. (2003) reviewed studies of prevention of arrhythmic deaths correlated with EPA/DHA intake, summarizing clinical evidence for the antiarrhythmic effect of EPA/DHA and reviewing possible mechanisms of action through modulation of ion channels in cardiomyocytes. Based on the evidence from human and experimental data (see Appendix B-2e) the authors suggest that in the presence of family history of sudden cardiac death, supplementation with EPA and DHA should be of 1 to 2 grams/day.

Christensen et al. (1999) examined the effect of EPA/DHA on heart rate variability in healthy subjects by randomized controlled trial. Treatment groups received either low- or high-dose EPA/DHA from fish-oil supplements and control groups received olive oil for 12 weeks. No significant effect of the fish-oil supplements was found on heart rate variability. In an earlier study, Christensen et al. (1996) examined the effect of EPA/DHA supplementation on subjects who had a recent MI and found significant improvement in heart rate variability among the fish-oil supplemented group (p=0.04); however, when those subjects were segregated by level of seafood consumption (Christensen, 1997), the groups who consumed one or more seafood meals per week had somewhat higher heart rate variability that was not statistically significant.

More recently, Frost and Vestergaard (2005) examined the association between consumption of EPA/DHA from fish and risk of atrial fibrillation or flutter on the prospective cohort study of 47,949 participants (mean age: 56 years) in the Danish Diet, Cancer, and Health Study. During a follow-up of 5.7 years, atrial fibrillation or flutter had developed in 556 subjects (374 men and 182 women). Using the lowest quintile of omega-3 fatty acid intake from fish as a reference, the unadjusted hazard rate ratios in quintiles 2–5 were 0.93 (95% CI 0.70-1.23), 1.11 (95% CI 0.85-1.46), 1.10 (95% CI 0.84-1.45), and 1.44 (95% CI 1.12-1.86), respectively (p for trend=0.001). The corresponding adjusted hazard rate ratios were 0.86 (95% CI 0.65-1.15), 1.08 (95% CI 0.82-1.42), 1.01 (95% CI 0.77-1.34), and 1.34 (95% CI 1.02-1.76) (p for trend = 0.006). In conclusion, there was no association between n-3 fatty acid intake from fish and a reduction in risk of atrial fibrillation or flutter. Surprisingly, the risk was significantly higher at increased EPA/DHA intake. The authors, however, were unable to exclude the possibility of residual confounding caused by a lack of information on intake of fish-oil supplements.

Other Cardiovascular Indicators

Fibrinogen

Balk et al. (2004) found no consistent effect of EPA/DHA on fibrinogen levels, and the studies reviewed were equally divided among those showing increases, no change, or decreases in fibrinogen levels compared to controls. Most of the study results were not significant. However, for those that did show statistically significant differences between omega-3 treatment and controls, three showed decreases ranging from 5–20 percent, and one showed an increase of 11 percent in fibrinogen levels. Cobiac et al. (1991) reported that seafood consumption may be associated with a small decrease in fibrinogen level (change = 0.15±0.12), which was significantly different than the change in the controls (p<0.05). Overall, however, no significant differences in effect of EPA/DHA on fibrinogen level have been shown (see Appendix Table B-2f).

Clotting Factors

Most studies reviewed by Balk et al. (2004) found a net decrease in von Willebrand factor with increased EPA/DHA intake. However, only one study reported statistical significance in the association. None of the studies reviewed examined the effects of regular consumption of seafood meals on von Willebrand factor levels.

Other clotting factors were also reviewed by Balk et al. (2004). Factor VII showed no consistency in effects across studies, with equal numbers of subjects reporting increases and decreases of factor VII activity in relation to EPA/DHA intake. Agren et al. (1997) reported that the effects of EPA/DHA levels from seafood consumption were not significant and were similar to those observed for fish-oil supplementation and an algal source of DHA oil supplementation in the same study. Findings from studies on EPA/DHA on factor VIII are similar to those for factor VII with some studies showing a net increase and others a net decrease. None of the studies investigated specify the effect of increased seafood consumption on factor VIII levels (Balk et al., 2004) (see Appendix Table B-2f).

Platelet Aggregation

Platelet aggregation is a very complex measurement, depending on the aggregating agent, the dose of the agent, and the measurement metric used. As a result, findings of studies on the effects of EPA/DHA on platelet aggregation are inconsistent and difficult to interpret (Balk et al., 2004). Agren et al. (1997) examined the effects of a seafood-based diet, fish-oil supplementation, and algal DHA oil on platelet aggregation and showed that collagen aggregation was reduced more in subjects on both the seafood diet and fish-oil supplementation regimens, but not the algal DHA oil treatment, compared to the controls ($p<0.05$). No significant association was found for EPA/DHA impairment of platelet aggregation, although algal DHA oil is less potent than either fish oil or seafood (which are sources of both EPA and DHA) (see Appendix Table B-2f).

Indicators of Glucose Tolerance in Diabetes

Although EPA/DHA consumption has been shown to improve lipid profiles and other indicators of cardiovascular risk in those with type II diabetes, there is currently no evidence that intakes of 2–4 g/day of EPA/DHA can improve glycemic control (Grundt et al., 1995; Sirtori et al., 1998; Kesavulu et al., 2002). Consistent with this finding, a review (Balk et al., 2004) concluded that there was no clear evidence that EPA/DHA had an effect on moderating glucose tolerance or hemoglobin A_{1c} levels, fasting blood sugar, and fasting insulin levels (see Appendix Table B-2g).

Allergy and Asthma

The Nurses' Health Study's prospective cohort was evaluated by Troisi et al. (1995) for a possible association of risk for adult-onset asthma and frequency of intake of various types of food. A semi-quantitative food frequency questionnaire was employed to index food intake over the previous year (e.g., "dark meat" seafood vs. other seafood). Over 1200 cases of adult-onset asthma were identified. Data from this study showed that the 6-year risk of adult-onset asthma was unrelated to the frequency of intake of dark meat seafood, tuna, or shrimp. This nonsignificant association was maintained when results were adjusted for age and smoking status, and also when other factors (body mass index, residential area, number of physician visits, and energy intake) were adjusted for (see Appendix Table B-2h; see also Schachter et al., 2004, AHRQ Report No. 91).

Cancer

The biological functions associated with consumption of omega-3 fatty acids suggest that it may have some impact on cancer risk (Larsson, 2004). Available evidence comes primarily from observational studies rather than randomized controlled trials (Terry, 2003; MacLean, 2006) (see Appendix Table B-2i; see also MacLean et al., 2005b, AHRQ Report No. 113). A small number of these studies show some protection for certain types of cancer (i.e., breast, colorectal, and lung), whereas others support an increase in risk (e.g., breast). The majority of the studies, however, conclude there is no significant effect on risk for cancer associated with seafood consumption or intake of other sources of EPA/DHA. Overall, the consumption of seafood, ALA, or EPA/DHA from all sources does not appear to decrease cancer risk (MacLean, 2006).

Aging and Other Neurological Outcomes

Consumption of EPA/DHA, specifically from seafood consumption, may provide some protection in terms of age-related cognitive decline as well as risk for Alzheimer's and other neurological diseases (Kalmijn et al., 1997; Gharirian et al., 1998; Barberger-Gateau et al., 2002; Morris et al., 2003). It should be noted that, as discussed above for cancer, evidence for reduced risk for these diseases comes primarily from observational studies. The beneficial effects appear to be more closely related to the consumption of seafood and/or global intake of DHA rather than EPA or ALA. Overall, the evidence is tenuous and counterbalanced by a number of studies that did not find significant benefits (see Appendix Table B-2j; see also MacLean et al., 2005a, AHRQ Report No. 114).

Summary of Evidence

Results from individual studies are not consistent and results from critical reviews are not clearly supportive of a cardioprotective effect of EPA/DHA. Furthermore, evidence for an effect on other adult chronic disease is controversial. Tables that summarize the committee's assessment of levels of evidence and reports from individual studies are shown in Table 3-2 and Appendix Tables B-1 through B-2. The level of evidence identified as "Contradictory or insufficient evidence to base recommendations" includes outcomes where a large body of literature exist, but leads to contradictory conclusions, as well as outcomes where the body of literature is too small to lead to recommendations. The committee's assessment of level of evidence summarized in Table 3-2 has its limitations. The Oxford Centre for Evidence-based Medicine's levels of evidence may not be ideal to assess nutrition studies. The quality of the various studies cannot be summarized

TABLE 3-2 Level of Evidence for Benefits of Increasing Seafood or EPA/ DHA Intake in the General Population[a] and Specific Subgroups Reviewed

Level of Evidence[b]		Higher Seafood Intake	Increase in EPA/DHA Intake
1a	Meta-analyses of randomized controlled trials		• Blood pressure • Triglyceride levels • Infant neurological development
1b	Randomized controlled trial(s)		• Gestational duration • Mortality and cardiovascular events in people with a history of MI • Infant neurological development
2a/3a	Meta-analyses of observational studies	• Cardiovascular mortality and events	
2b	Cohort study(ies)	• Fetal neurological development • Gestational duration • Postpartum depression in women	
3b	Case-control study(ies) Cross-sectional study(ies)		
	Contradictory evidence or insufficient evidence on which to base recommendations	• Blood pressure • Stroke • Allergy and asthma • Cancer • Alzheimer's disease • Glycemic control in type II diabetes	• Cardiovascular mortality and events • Arrhythmia • Cancer • Alzheimer's disease • Glycemic control in type II diabetes • Allergy and asthma • Preeclampsia • Postpartum depression • HDL, LDL, Lp(a) levels

[a]Unless otherwise noted.
[b]The level of evidence is based on the Oxford Centre for Evidence based Medicine's Levels of Evidence (http://www.cebm.net/levels_of_evidence.asp#top). When several levels of evidence existed, only the highest level of evidence was reported.

using this approach, but is described in more detail in the preceding discussions. Furthermore, the committee's selection of studies reflects its subjective assessment of quality and importance, and is therefore subject to limitations. Only the highest level of evidence is provided in the table, and studies with a lower level of evidence are omitted. For an alternative approach to the assessment and synthesis of evidence, refer to the recent and comprehensive

AHRQ systematic reviews addressing these questions (Balk et al., 2004, AHRQ Report No. 93; Jordan et al., 2004, AHRQ Report No. 92; MacLean et al., 2004, AHRQ Report No. 89; Schachter et al., 2004, AHRQ Report No. 91; Wang et al., 2004, AHRQ Report No. 94; MacLean et al., 2005b, AHRQ Report No. 113; MacLean et al., 2005a, AHRQ Report No. 114.)

FINDINGS

1. Observational evidence suggests that increased seafood consumption is associated with a decreased risk of cardiovascular deaths and cardiovascular events in the general population. Evidence is insufficient to assess if this association is mediated through an increase in EPA and DHA consumption and/or a decrease in saturated fat consumption and/or other correlates of seafood consumption.

2. Experimental studies of the effect of EPA/DHA supplements on cardiovascular mortality or cardiovascular disease have not been conducted in the general population.

3. There is mixed evidence suggesting that consumption of fish-oil supplements for individuals with a history of MI will protect them from further coronary events. Meta-analyses have also led to mixed conclusions, with most recent analyses suggesting no benefits. Experimental evidence from in vitro and other types of mechanistic studies suggests that EPA/DHA intake should be associated with positive cardiovascular outcomes. However, this prediction has not been borne out in results of human studies.

4. In the general population, the effect from increased seafood consumption on the lipid profile is unclear. However, experimental studies of EPA/DHA supplementation at levels >1 g per day showed decreased triglyceride levels; the effect on other components of the lipid profile is less clear.

5. Evidence is inconsistent for protection against further cardiovascular events in individuals with a history of myocardial infarction from consumption of EPA/DHA-containing seafood or fish-oil supplements. The protection evidenced by population (observational) studies has not been consistently observed in randomized clinical trials.

6. Evidence for a benefit associated with seafood consumption or fish-oil supplements on blood pressure, stroke, cancer, asthma, type II diabetes, or Alzheimer's disease is inconclusive. Whereas observational studies have suggested a protective role of EPA/DHA for each of these diseases, supportive evidence from randomized clinical trials is either nonexistent or inconclusive.

7. Based on the three recent meta-analyses of observational studies (Table 3-2), there appears to be a linear association between seafood consumption and primary prevention of cardiovascular disease; the committee did not find strong scientific evidence to suggest a threshold of consumption,

such as two servings per week, below which seafood consumption provides no benefit and above which increasing consumption provides no additional benefits.

RECOMMENDATIONS

Recommendation 1: Dietary advice to the general population from federal agencies should emphasize that seafood is a component of a healthy diet, particularly as it can displace other protein sources higher in saturated fat. Seafood can favorably substitute for other high biologic value protein sources while often improving the overall nutrient profile of the diet.

Recommendation 2: Although advice from federal agencies should also support inclusion of seafood in the diets of pregnant females or those who may become pregnant, any consumption advice should stay within federal advisories for specific seafood types and state advisories for locally caught fish.

RESEARCH RECOMMENDATIONS

Pregnant and Lactating Women

Recommendation 1: Better data are needed to determine if outcomes of increasing consumption of seafood or increasing EPA/DHA intake levels in US women would be comparable to outcomes of populations in other countries. Such studies should be encouraged to include populations of high fish-consumers outside the United States to determine if there are differences in risks for these populations compared to US populations.

Recommendation 2: Dose-response studies of EPA/DHA in pregnant and lactating women are needed. This information will help determine if higher intakes can further increase gestation duration, reduce premature births, and benefit infant development. Other studies should include assessing whether DHA alone can act independently of EPA to increase duration of gestation.

Infants and Toddlers

Recommendation 3: Research is needed to determine if cognitive and developmental outcomes in infants are correlated with performance later in childhood. This should include:

- Evaluating preschool and school-age children exposed to EPA/DHA in utero and postnatally, at ages beginning around 4 years when executive function is more developed, and;

- Evaluating development of school-age children exposed to variable EPA/DHA levels in utero and postnatally with measures of distractibility, disruptive behavior, and oppositional defiant behavior, as well as more commonly assessed cognitive outcomes and more sophisticated tests of visual function.

Recommendation 4: Additional data is needed to better define optimum intake levels of EPA/DHA for infants and toddlers.

Children

Recommendation 5: Better-designed studies about EPA/DHA supplementation in children with behavioral disorders are needed.

Adults at Risk for Chronic Disease

Recommendation 6: In the absence of meta-analyses that systematically combine quantitative data from multiple studies, further meta-analyses and larger randomized trials are needed to assess outcomes other than cardiovascular, in particular total mortality, in order to explore possible adverse health effects of EPA/DHA supplementation.

Recommendation 7: Additional clinical research is needed to assess a potential effect of seafood consumption and/or EPA/DHA supplementation on stroke, cancer, Alzheimer's disease, and depression.

Recommendation 8: Future epidemiological studies should assess intake of specific species of seafood and/or biomarkers, in order to differentiate the health effects of EPA/DHA from those of contaminants, such as methylmercury.

REFERENCES

Agostoni C, Trojan S, Bellu R, Riva E, Giovannini M. 1995. Neurodevelopmental quotient of healthy term infants at 4 months and feeding practice: The role of long-chain polyunsaturated fatty acids. *Pediatric Research* 38(2):262–266.

Agren JJ, Vaisanen S, Hanninen O. 1997. Hemostatic factors and platelet aggregation after a fish-enriched diet or fish oil or docosahexaenoic acid supplementation. *Prostaglandins Leukotrienes & Essential Fatty Acids* 57(4–5):419–421.

Al MDM, van Houwelingen AC, Kester ADM, Hasaart THM, de Jong AEP, Hornstra G. 1995. Maternal essential fatty acid patterns during normal pregnancy and their relationship to the neonatal essential fatty acid status. *British Journal of Nutrition* 74(1):55–68.

Alberman E, Emanuel I, Filakti H, Evans SJ. 1992. The contrasting effects of parental birthweight and gestational age on the birthweight of offspring. *Paediatric and Perinatal Epidemiology* 6(2):134–144.

Al-Marzouki S, Evans S, Marshall T, Roberts I. 2005. Are these data real? Statistical methods for the detection of data fabrication in clinical trials. *British Medical Journal* 331(7511):267–270.

Appleby PN, Davey GK, Key TJ. 2002. Hypertension and blood pressure among meat eaters, fish eaters, vegetarians and vegans in EPIC-Oxford. *Public Health Nutrition* 5(5):645–654.

Auestad N, Halter R, Hall RT, Blatter M, Bogle ML, Burks W, Erickson JR, Fitzgerald KM, Dobson V, Innis SM, Singer LT, Montalto MB, Jacobs JR, Qiu W, Bornstein MH. 2001. Growth and development in term infants fed long-chain polyunsaturated fatty acids: A double-masked, randomized, parallel, prospective, multivariate study. *Pediatrics* 108(2):372–381.

Auestad N, Scott DT, Janowsky JS, Jacobsen C, Carroll RE, Montalto MB, Halter R, Qiu W, Jacobs JR, Connor WE, Connor SL, Taylor JA, Neuringer M, Fitzgerald KM, Hall RT. 2003. Visual, cognitive, and language assessments at 39 months: A follow-up study of children fed formulas containing long-chain polyunsaturated fatty acids to 1 year of age. *Pediatrics* 112(3 Part 1):e177–e183.

Baer DJ, Judd JT, Clevidence BA, Tracy RP. 2004. Dietary fatty acids affect plasma markers of inflammation in healthy men fed controlled diets: A randomized crossover study. *American Journal of Clinical Nutrition* 79(6):969–973.

Balk E, Chung M, Lichtenstein A, Chew P, Kupelnick B, Lawrence A, DeVine D, Lau J. 2004. *Effects of Omega-3 Fatty Acids on Cardiovascular Risk Factors and Intermediate Markers of Cardiovascular Disease.* Summary, Evidence Report/Technology Assessment No. 93 (Prepared by the Tufts-New England Medical Center Evidence-based Practice Center, Boston, MA). AHRQ Publication No. 04-E010-1. Rockville, MD: Agency for Healthcare Research and Quality.

Bang HO, Dyerberg J, Nielsen AB. 1971. Plasma lipid and lipoprotein pattern in Greenlandic West-coast Eskimos. *Lancet* 1(7710):1143–1145.

Barberger-Gateau P, Letenneur L, Deschamps V, Peres K, Dartigues J-F, Renaud S. 2002. Fish, meat, and risk of dementia: A cohort study. *British Medical Journal* 325(7370): 932–933.

Birch EE, Birch DG, Hoffman DR, Uauy R. 1992. Dietary essential fatty acid supply and visual acuity development. *Investigations in Ophthalmology and Visual Science* 33(11): 3242–3253.

Birch EE, Hoffman DR, Uauy R, Birch DG, Prestidge C. 1998. Visual acuity and the essentiality of docosahexaenoic acid and arachidonic acid in the diet of term infants. *Pediatric Research* 44(2):201–209.

Birch EE, Garfield S, Hoffman DR, Uauy R, Birch DG. 2000. A randomized controlled trial of early dietary supply of long-chain polyunsaturated fatty acids and mental development in term infants. *Developmental Medicine and Child Neurology* 42(3):174–181.

Birch EE, Hoffman DR, Castaneda YS, Fawcett SL, Birch DG, Uauy RD. 2002. A randomized controlled trial of long-chain polyunsaturated fatty acid supplementation of formula in term infants after weaning at 6 wk of age. *American Journal of Clinical Nutrition* 75(3):570–580.

Bjerve KS, Brubakk AM, Fougner KJ, Johnsen H, Midthjell K, Vik T. 1993. Omega-3 fatty acids: Essential fatty acids with important biological effects, and serum phospholipid fatty acids as markers of dietary omega 3-fatty acid intake. *American Journal of Clinical Nutrition* 57(Suppl 5):801S–805S.

Bougle D, Denise P, Vimard F, Nouvelot A, Penneillo MJ, Guillois B. 1999. Early neurological and neuropsychological development of the preterm infant and polyunsaturated fatty acids supply. *Clinical Neurophysiology* 110(8):1363–1370.

Bouwstra H, Dijck-Brouwer DA, Wildeman JA, Tjoonk HM, van der Heide JC, Boersma ER, Muskiet FA, Hadders-Algra M. 2003. Long-chain polyunsaturated fatty acids have a positive effect on the quality of general movements of healthy term infants. *American Journal of Clinical Nutrition* 78(2):313–318.

Bouzan C, Cohen JT, Connor WE, Kris-Etherton PM, Gray GM, Konig A, Lawrence RS, Savitz DA, Teutsch SM. 2005. A quantitative analysis of fish consumption and stroke risk. *American Journal of Preventive Medicine* 29(4):347–352.

Bryan J, Osendarp S, Hughes D, Calvaresi E, Baghurst K, van Klinken J-W. 2004. Nutrients for cognitive development in school-aged children. *Nutrition Reviews* 62(8):295–306.

Bulstra-Ramakers MT, Huisjes HJ, Visser GH. 1995. The effects of 3g eicosapentaenoic acid daily on recurrence of intrauterine growth retardation and pregnancy induced hypertension. *British Journal of Obstetrics and Gynaecology* 102(2):123–126.

Burdge G. 2004. Alpha-linolenic acid metabolism in men and women: Nutritional and biological implications. *Current Opinion in Clinical Nutrition and Metabolic Care* 7(2):137–144.

Burr ML, Fehily AM, Gilbert JF, Rogers S, Holliday RM, Sweetnam PM, Elwood PC, Deadman NM. 1989. Effects of changes in fat, fish, and fibre intakes on death and myocardial reinfarction: Diet and reinfarction trial (DART). *Lancet* 2(8666):757–761.

Burr ML, Ashfield-Watt PAL, Dunstan FDJ, Fehily AM, Breay P, Ashton T, Zotos PC, Haboubi NAA, Elwood PC. 2003. Lack of benefit of dietary advice to men with angina: Results of a controlled trial. *European Journal of Clinical Nutrition* 57(2):193–200.

Calder PC. 2001. Polyunsaturated fatty acids, inflammation, and immunity. *Lipids* 36(9): 1007–1024.

Calder PC. 2004. n-3 fatty acids and cardiovascular disease: Evidence explained and mechanisms explored. *Clinical Science* (London, England) 107(1):1–11.

Campbell FM, Gordon MJ, Dutta-Row AK. 1998. Placental membrane fatty acid-binding protein preferentially binds arachidonic and docosahexaenoic acids. *Life Sciences* 63:235–240.

Capps O Jr, Cleveland L, Park J. 2002. Dietary behaviors associated with total fat and saturated fat intake. *Journal of the American Dietetic Association* 102(4):490–502, 612.

Carlson SE. 1997. Long chain polyunsaturated fatty acid supplementation of preterm infants. In: Dobbing J, ed. *Developing Brain Behavior: The Role of Lipids in Infant Formula.* London, England: Academic Press Limited. Pp. 41–102.

Carlson SE, Neuringer M. 1999. Polyunsaturated fatty acid status and neurodevelopment: A summary and critical analysis of the literature. *Lipids* 34(2):171–178.

Carlson SE, Werkman SH. 1996. A randomized trial of visual attention of preterm infants fed docosahexaenoic acid until two months. *Lipids* 31(1):85–90.

Carlson SE, Rhodes PG, Ferguson MG. 1986. Docosahexaenoic acid status of preterm infants at birth and following feeding with human milk or formula. *American Journal of Clinical Nutrition* 44(6):798–804.

Carlson SE, Werkman SH, Rhodes PG, Tolley EA. 1993. Visual-acuity development in healthy preterm infants: Effect of marine-oil supplementation. *American Journal of Clinical Nutrition* 58(1):35–42.

Carlson SE, Werkman SH, Peeples JM, Wilson WM. 1994. Long-chain fatty acids and early visual and cognitive development of preterm infants. *European Journal of Clinical Nutrition* 48(Suppl 2):S27–S30.

Carlson SE, Ford AJ, Werkman SH, Peeples JM, Koo WW. 1996a. Visual acuity and fatty acid status of term infants fed human milk and formulas with and without docosahexaenoate and arachidonate from egg yolk lecithin. *Pediatric Research* 39(5):882–888.

Carlson SE, Werkman SH, Tolley EA. 1996b. Effect of long-chain n-3 fatty acid supplementation on visual acuity and growth of preterm infants with and without bronchopulmonary dysplasia. *American Journal of Clinical Nutrition* 63(5):687–697.

Carlson SE, Werkman SH, Montalto MB, Tolley EA. 1999. Visual acuity development of preterm (PT) infants fed docosahexaenoic acid (DHA) and arachidonic acid (ARA): Effect of age at supplementation. *Pediatric Research* 45:279A.

Chalon S, Vancassel S, Zimmer L, Guilloteau D, Durand G. 2001. Polyunsaturated fatty acids and cerebral function: Focus on monoaminergic neurotransmission. *Lipids* 36(9): 937–944.

Cheatham C, Colombo J, Carlson SE. 2006. N-3 fatty acids and cognitive and visual acuity development: Methodologic and conceptual considerations. *American Journal of Clinical Nutrition* 83(Suppl 6):1458S–1466S.

Cheruku SR, Montgomery-Downs HE, Farkas SL, Thoman EB, Lammi-Keefe CJ. 2002. Higher maternal plasma docosahexaenoic acid during pregnancy is associated with more mature neonatal sleep-state patterning. *American Journal of Clinical Nutrition* 76(3):608–613.

Christensen JH, Gustenhoff P, Korup E, Aaroe, J, Toft E, Moller J, Rasmussen K, Dyerberg J, Schmidt EB. 1996. Effect of fish oil on heart rate variability in survivors of myocardial infarction: A double blind randomised controlled trial. *British Medical Journal* 312(7032):677–678.

Christensen JH, Korup E, Aaroe J, Toft E, Moller J, Rasmussen K, Dyerberg J, Schmidt EB. 1997. Fish consumption, n-3 fatty acids in cell membranes, and heart rate variability in survivors of myocardial infarction with left ventricular dysfunction. *American Journal of Cardiology* 79(12):1670–1673.

Christensen JH, Christensen MS, Dyerberg J, Schmidt EB. 1999. Heart rate variability and fatty acid content of blood cell membranes: A dose-response study with n-3 fatty acids. *American Journal of Clinical Nutrition* 70(3):331–337.

Clandinin MT, Chappell JE, Leong S, Heim T, Swyer PR, Chance GW. 1980a. Intrauterine fatty acid accretion rates in human brain: Implications for fatty acid requirements. *Early Human Development* 4(2):121–129.

Clandinin MT, Chappell JE, Leong S, Heim T, Swyer PR, Change GW. 1980b. Extrauterine fatty acid accretion in infant brain: Implications for fatty acid requirements. *Early Human Development* 4(2):131–138.

Clandinin MT, Van Aerde JE, Merkel KL, Harris CL, Springer MA, Hansen JW, Diersen-Schade DA. 2005. Growth and development of preterm infants fed infant formulas containing docosahexaenoic acid and arachidonic acid. *Journal of Pediatrics* 146(4):461–468.

Clausen T, Slott M, Solvoll K, Drevon CA, Vollset SE, Henriksen T. 2001. High intake of energy, sucrose, and polyunsaturated fatty acids is associated with increased risk of preeclampsia. *American Journal of Obstetrics and Gynecology* 185(2):451–458.

Cobiac L, Clifton PM, Abbey M, Belling GB, Nestel PJ. 1991. Lipid, lipoprotein, and hemostatic effects of fish vs. fish-oil n-3 fatty acids in mildly hyperlipidemic males. *American Journal of Clinical Nutrition* 53(5):1210–1216.

Cohen JT, Bellinger DC, Connor WE, Shaywitz BA. 2005. A quantitative analysis of prenatal intake of n-3 polyunsaturated fatty acids and cognitive development. *American Journal of Preventive Medicine* 29(4):366–374.

Colombo J, Kannass KN, Shaddy DJ, Kundurthi S, Maikranz JM, Anderson CJ, Blaga OM, Carlson SE. 2004. Maternal DHA and the development of attention in infancy and toddlerhood. *Child Development* 75(4):1254–1267.

Cox JL, Holden JM, Sagovsky R. 1987. Detection of postnatal depression. Development of the 10-item Edinburgh Postnatal Depression Scale. *British Journal of Psychiatry* 150:782–786.

Crawford MA. 2000. Placental delivery of arachidonic and docosahexaenoic acids: Implications for the lipid nutrition of preterm infants. *American Journal of Clinical Nutrition* 71(Suppl 1):275S–284S.

Crawford MA, Costeloe K, Ghebremeskel K, Phylactos A, Skirvin L, Stacey F. 1997. Are deficits of arachidonic and docosahexaenoic acids responsible for the neural and vascular complications of preterm babies? *American Journal of Clinical Nutrition* 66(Suppl): 1032S–1041S.

DACP (Department of Ambulatory Care and Prevention). 2005. *Project Viva.* [Online]. Available: http://www.dacp.org/viva/index.html [accessed February 23, 2006].

Daniels JL, Longnecker MP, Rowland AS, Golding J, the ALSPAC Study Team. 2004. Fish intake during pregnancy and early cognitive development of offspring. *Epidemiology* 15(4):394–402.

de la Presa Owens S, Innis SM. 1999. Docosahexaenoic and arachidonic acid prevent a decrease in dopaminergic and serotoninergic neurotransmitters in frontal cortex caused by a linoleic and α-linolenic acid deficient diet in formula-fed piglets. *Journal of Nutrition* 129(11):2088–2093.

Delion S, Chalon S, Guilloteau D, Besnard J-C, Durand G. 1996. α-linolenic acid dietary deficiency alters age-related changes of dopaminergic and serotoninergic neurotransmission in the rat frontal cortex. *Journal of Neurochemistry* 66(4):1582–1591.

Denburg JA, Hatfield HM, Cyr MM, Hayes L, Holt PG, Sehmi R, Dunstan JA, Prescott SL. 2005. Fish oil supplementation in pregnancy modifies neonatal progenitors at birth in infants at risk of atopy. *Pediatric Research* 57(2):276–281.

Denny SI, Thompson RL, Margetts BM. 2003. Dietary factors in the pathogenesis of asthma and chronic obstructive pulmonary disease. *Current Allergy and Asthma Reports* 3(2): 130–136.

Dewailley E, Blanchet C, Lemieux S, Sauve L, Gingras S, Ayotte P, Holub BJ. 2001. N-3 fatty acids and cardiovascular disease risk factors among the Inuit of Nunavik. *American Journal of Clinical Nutrition* 74(4):464–473.

Dunstan JA, Mori TA, Barden A. 2003. Maternal fish oil supplementation in pregnancy reduces interleukin-13 levels in cord blood of infants at high risk of atopy. *Clinical and Experimental Allergy* 33(4):442–448.

Eritsland J, Arnesen H, Berg K. 1995. Serum Lp(a) lipoprotein levels in patients with coronary artery disease and the influence of long-term n-3 fatty acid supplementation. *Scandinavian Journal of Clinical & Laboratory Investigation* 55(4):295–300.

Farquharson J, Jamieson EC, Logan RW, Cockburn MD, Patrick WA. 1992. Infant cerebral cortex phospholipid fatty-acid composition and diet. *Lancet* 340(8823):810–813.

Fewtrell MS, Morley R, Abbott A, Singhal A, Isaacs EB, Stephenson T, MacFadyen U, Lucas A. 2002. Double-blind, randomized trial of long-chain polyunsaturated fatty acid supplementation in formula fed to preterm infants. *Pediatrics* 110(1):73–82.

Fewtrell MS, Abbott RA, Kennedy K, Singhal A, Morley R, Caine E, Jamieson C, Cockburn F, Lucas A. 2004. Randomized, double-blind trial of long-chain polyunsaturated fatty acid supplementation with fish oil and borage oil in preterm infants. *Journal of Pediatrics* 144(4):471–479.

Field CJ, Thomson CA, Van Aerde JE, Parrott A, Euler A, Lien E, Clandinin MT. 2000. Lower proportion of CD45R0+ cells and deficient interleukin-10 production by formula-fed infants, compared with human-fed, is corrected with supplementation of long-chain polyunsaturated fatty acids. *Journal of Pediatric Gastroenterology and Nutrition* 31(3):291–299.

Field CJ, Clandinin MT, Van Aerde JE. 2001. Polyunsaturated fatty acids and T-cell function: Implications for the neonate. *Lipids* 36(9):1025–1032.

Frost L, Vestergaard P. 2005. n-3 fatty acids consumed from fish and risk of atrial fibrillation or flutter: The Danish Diet, Cancer, and Health Study. *American Journal of Clinical Nutrition* 81(1):50–54.

Geleijnse JM, Giltay EJ, Grobbe DE, Donders AR, Kok FJ. 2002. Blood pressure response to fish oil supplementation: Metaregression analysis of randomized trials. *Journal of Hypertension* 20(8):1493–1499.

Ghadirian P, Jain M, Ducic S, Shatenstein B, Morisset R. 1998. Nutritional factors in the aetiology of multiple sclerosis: A case-control study in Montreal, Canada. *International Journal of Epidemiology* 27(5):845–852.

Ghosh S, Daga S. 1967. Comparison of gestational age and weight as standards of prematurity. *Journal of Pediatrics* 71(2):173–175.

Gibson RA, Chen W, Makrides M. 2001. Randomized trials with polyunsaturated fatty acid interventions in preterm and term infants: Functional and clinical outcomes. *Lipids* 36(9):873–883.

GISSI Study Investigators. 1999. Dietary supplementation with n-3 polyunsaturated fatty acids and vitamin E after myocardial infarction: Results of the GISSI-Prevenzione trial. Gruppo Italiano per lo Studio della Sopravvivenza nell'Infarto miocardico. *Lancet* 354(9177):447–455.

Grandjean P, Bjerve KS, Weihe P, Steuerwald U. 2001. Birthweight in a fishing community: Significance of essential fatty acids and marine food contaminants. *International Journal of Epidemiology* 30(6):1272–1278.

Grundt H, Nilsen DW, Hetland O, Aarsland T, Baksaas I, Grande T, Woie L. 1995. Improvement of serum lipids and blood pressure during intervention with n-3 fatty acids was not associated with changes in insulin levels in subjects with combined hyperlipidaemia. *Journal of Internal Medicine* 237(3):249–259.

Haggarty P, Page K, Abramovich DR, Ashton J, Brown D. 1997. Long-chain polyunsaturated fatty acid transport across the perfused human placenta. *Placenta* 18(8):635–642.

Haggarty P, Ashton J, Joynson M, Abramovich DR, Page K. 1999. Effect of maternal polyunsaturated fatty acid concentration on transport by the human placenta. *Biology of the Neonate* 75(6):350–359.

Haggarty P, Abramovich DR, Page K. 2002. The effect of maternal smoking and ethanol on fatty acid transport by the human placenta. *British Journal of Nutrition* 87(3):247–252.

Hanninen OO, Agren JJ, Laitinen MV, Jaaskelainen IO, Penttila IM. 1989. Dose response relationships in blood lipids during moderate freshwater fish diet. *Annals of Medicine* 21(3):203–207.

Harper V, MacInnes R, Campbell D, Hall M. 1991. Increased birth weight in northerly islands: Is fish consumption a red herring? *British Medical Journal* 303(6795):166.

Hawkes JS, Bryan D-L, Makrides M, Neumann MA, Gibson RA. 2002. A randomized trial of supplementation with docosahexaenoic acid–rich tuna oil and its effects on the human milk cytokines interleukin 1ß, interleukin 6, and tumor necrosis factor. *American Journal of Clinical Nutrition* 75(4):754–760.

He K, Song Y, Daviglus ML, Liu K, Van Horn L, Dyer AR, Goldbourt U, Greenland P. 2004a. Fish consumption and incidence of stroke: A meta-analysis of cohort studies. *Stroke* 35(7):1538–1542.

He K, Song Y, Daviglus ML, Liu K, Van Horn L, Dyer AR, Greenland P. 2004b. Accumulated evidence on fish consumption and coronary heart disease mortality: A meta-analysis of cohort studies. *Circulation* 109(22):2705–2711.

Hediger ML, Overpeck MD, Ruan WJ, Troendle JF. 2002. Birthweight and gestational age effects on motor and social development. *Paediatric Perinatal Epidemiology* 16(1):33–46.

Helland IB, Saugstad OD, Smith L, Saarem K, Solvoll K, Ganes T, Drevon CA. 2001. Similar effects on infants of n-3 and n-6 fatty acids supplementation to pregnant and lactating women. *Pediatrics* 108(5):e82. [Online]. Available: http://www.pediatrics.org/cgi/content/full/108/5/e82/ [accessed August 22, 2005].

Helland IB, Smith L, Saarem K, Saugstad OD, Drevon CA. 2003. Maternal supplementation with very-long-chain n-3 fatty acids during pregnancy and lactation augments children's IQ at 4 years of age. *Pediatrics* 111(1):39–44.

Hibbeln JR. 2002. Seafood consumption, the DHA content of mothers' milk and prevalence rates of postpartum depression: A cross-national, ecological analysis. *Journal of Affective Disorders* 69(1–3):15–29.

Hibbeln JR, Salem N Jr. 1995. Dietary polyunsaturated fatty acids and depression: When cholesterol does not satisfy. *American Journal of Clinical Nutrition* 62(1):1–9.

Hodge L, Salome CM, Hughes JM, Liu-Brennan D, Rimmer J, Allman M, Pang D, Armour C, Woolcock AJ. 1998. Effect of dietary intake of omega-3 and omega-6 fatty acids on severity of asthma in children. *European Respiratory Journal* 11(2):361–365.

Hoffman DR, Birch EE, Castaneda YS, Fawcett SL, Wheaton DH, Birch DG, Uauy R. 2003. Visual function in breast-fed term infants weaned to formula with or without long-chain polyunsaturated at 4 to 6 months: A randomized clinical trial. *Journal of Pediatrics* 142(6):669–677.

Holman RT, Johnson SB, Ogburn PL. 1991. Deficiency of essential fatty acids and membrane fluidity during pregnancy and lactation. *Proceedings of the National Academy of Sciences of the United States of America* 88(11):4835–4839.

Hooper L, Thompson RL, Harrison RA, Summerbell CD, Moore H, Worthington HV, Durrington PN, Ness AR, Capps NE, Davey Smith G, Riemersma RA, Ebrahim SB. 2005. Omega 3 fatty acids for prevention and treatment of cardiovascular disease. *Cochrane Database of Systematic Reviews* (4):CD003177.

Hooper L, Thompson RL, Harrison RA, Summerbell CD, Ness AR, Moore HJ, Worthington HV, Durrington PN, Higgins JPT, Capps NE, Riemersma RA, Ebrahim SBJ, Davey-Smith G. 2006. Risks and benefits of omega 3 fats for mortality, cardiovascular disease, and cancer: Systematic review. *British Medical Journal* 332(7544):752–760.

Hornstra G, Al MD, van Houwelingen AC, Foreman-van Drongelen MM. 1995. Essential fatty acids in pregnancy and early human development. *European Journal of Obstetrics, Gynecology and Reproductive Biology* 61(1):57–62.

Howard BV, Van Horn L, Hsia J, Manson JE, Stefanick ML, Wassertheil-Smoller S, Kuller LH, LaCroix AZ, Langer RD, Lasser NL, Lewis CE, Limacher MC, Margolis KL, Mysiw WJ, Ockene JK, Parker LM, Perri MG, Phillips L, Prentice RL, Robbins J, Rossouw JE, Sarto GE, Schatz IJ, Snetselaar LG, Stevens VJ, Tinker LF, Trevisan M, Vitolins MZ, Anderson GL, Assaf AR, Bassford T, Beresford SA, Black HR, Brunner RL, Brzyski RG, Caan B, Chlebowski RT, Gass M, Granek I, Greenland P, Hays J, Heber D, Heiss G, Hendrix SL, Hubbell FA, Johnson KC, Kotchen JM. 2006. Low-fat dietary pattern and risk of cardiovascular disease: The Women's Health Initiative Randomized Controlled Dietary Modification Trial. *Journal of the American Medical Association* 295(6):655–666.

Innis SM, Gilley J, Werker J. 2001. Are human milk long-chain polyunsaturated fatty acids related to visual and neural development in breast-fed term infants? *Journal of Pediatrics* 139(4):532–538.

IOM (Institute of Medicine). 2002/2005. *Dietary Reference Intakes for Energy, Carbohydrate, Fiber, Fat, Fatty Acids, Cholesterol, Protein, and Amino Acids.* Washington, DC: The National Academies Press.

Ismail HM. 2005. The role of omega-3 fatty acids in cardiac protection: An overview. *Frontiers in Bioscience: A Journal and Virtual Library* 10:1079–1788.

Jacobson SW. 1999. Assessment of long-chain polyunsaturated fatty acid nutritional supplementation on infant neurobehavioral development and visual acuity. *Lipids* 34(2):151–160.

Jacobson SW, Jacobson JL, O'Neill JM, Padgett RJ, Frankowski JJ, Bihun JT. 1992. Visual expectation and dimensions of infant information processing. *Child Development* 63(3):711–724.

Jensen RG, Bitman J, Carlson SE, Couch SC, Hamosh M, Newburg DS. 1995. Milk lipids; A. Human milk lipids. In: Jensen RG, ed. *Handbook of Milk Composition.* San Diego, CA: Academic Press. Pp. 495–542.

Jensen CL, Voigt RG, Llorente AM, Peters SU, Prager TC, Zou Y, Fraley JK, Heird WC. 2004. Effect of maternal docosahexaenoic acid (DHA) supplementation on neuropsychological and visual status of former breast-fed infants at five years of age. *Pediatric Research* (abstract) 55:181A.

Jensen CL, Voigt RG, Prager TC, Zou YL, Fraley JK, Rozelle JC, Turcich MR, Llorente AM, Anderson RE, Heird WC. 2005. Effects of maternal docosahexaenoic acid intake on visual function and neurodevelopment in breastfed term infants. *American Journal of Clinical Nutrition* 82(1):125–132.

Jordan H, Matthan N, Chung M, Balk E, Chew P, Kupelnick B, DeVine D, Lawrence A, Lichtenstein A, Lau J. 2004. *Effects of Omega-3 Fatty Acids on Arrhythmogenic Mechanisms in Animal and Isolated Organ/Cell Culture Studies.* Evidence Report/Technology Assessment No. 92 (Prepared by the Tufts-New England Medical Center Evidence-based Practice Center, under Contract No. 290-02-0022). AHRQ Publication No 04-E011-2. Rockville, MD: Agency for Healthcare Research and Quality.

Juneja M, Shankar A, Ramji. 2005. Neurodevelopmental, functional and growth status of term low birthweight infants at eighteen months. *Indian Pediatrics* 42(11):1134–1140.

Kalmijn S, Feskens EJ, Launer LJ, Kromhout D. 1997. Polyunsaturated fatty acids, antioxidants, and cognitive function in very old men. *American Journal of Epidemiology* 154(1):33–41.

Kesavulu MM, Kameswararao B, Apparao CH, Kumar EG, Harinarayan CV. 2002. Effect of omega-3 fatty acids on lipid peroxidation and antioxidant enzyme status in type 2 diabetic patients. *Diabetes and Metabolism* 28(1):20–26.

Kodas E, Galineau L, Bodard S, Vancassel S, Guilloteau D, Besnard J-C, Chalon S. 2004. Serotoninergic neurotransmission is affected by n-3 polyunsaturated fatty acids in the rat. *Journal of Neurochemistry* 89(3):695–702.

Konig A, Bouzan C, Cohen JT, Connor WE, Kris-Etherton PM, Gray GM, Lawrence RS, Savitz DA, Teutsch SM. 2005. A quantitative analysis of fish consumption and coronary heart disease mortality. *American Journal of Preventive Medicine* 29(4):335–346.

Larque E, Demmelmair H, Berger B, Hasbargen U, Koletzko B. 2003. In vivo investigation of the placental transfer of 13C-labeled fatty acids in humans. *Journal of Lipid Research* 44:49–55.

Larsson SC, Kumlin M, Ingelman-Sundberg M, Wolk A. 2004. Dietary long-chain n-3 fatty acids for the prevention of cancer: A review of potential mechanisms. *American Journal of Clinical Nutrition* 79(6):935–945.

Lauritzen L, Hansen HS, Jorgensen MH, Michaelsen KF. 2001. The essentiality of long chain n-3 fatty acids in relation to development and function of the brain and retina. *Progress in Lipid Research* 40(1–2):1–94.

Leaf A, Kang JX, Xiao Y-F, Billman GE. 2003. Clinical prevention of sudden cardiac death by n-3 polyunsaturated fatty acids and mechanism of prevention of arrhythmias by n-3 fish oils. *Circulation* 107(21):2646–2652.

Levant B, Radel JD, Carlson SE. 2004. Decreased brain docosahexaenoic acid during development alters dopamine-related behaviors in adult rats that are differentially affected by dietary remediation. *Behavioural Brain Research* 152(1):49–57.

Llorente AM, Jensen CL, Voigt RG, Fraley JK, Berretta MC, Heird WC. 2003. Effect of maternal docosahexaenoic acid supplementation on postpartum depression and information processing. *American Journal of Obstetrics and Gynecology* 188(5):1348–1353.

Lucas A, Stafford M, Morley R, Abbott R, Stephenson T, MacFadyen U, Elias A, Clements H. 1999. Efficacy and safety of long-chain polyunsaturated fatty acid supplementation of infant-formula milk: A randomised trial. *Lancet* 354(9194):1948–1954.

Lucas M, Dewailly E, Muckle G, Ayotte P, Bruneau S, Gingras S, Rhainds M, Holub BJ. 2004. Gestational age and birth weight in relation to n-3 fatty acids among Inuit (Canada). *Lipids* 39(7):617–626.

MacLean CH, Mojica, WA, Morton SC, Pencharz J, Hasenfeld Garland R, Tu W, Newberry SJ, Jungvig LK, Grossman J, Khanna P, Rhodes S, Shekelle P. 2004. *Effects of Omega-3 Fatty Acids on Lipids and Glycemic Control in Type II Diabetes and the Metabolic Syndrome and on Inflammatory Bowel Disease, Rheumatoid Arthritis, Renal Disease, Systemic Lupus Erythematosus, and Osteoporosis.* Evidence Report/Technology Assessment. No. 89 (Prepared by the Southern California/RAND Evidence-based Practice Center, under Contract No. 290-02-0003). AHRQ Publication No. 04-E012-2. Rockville, MD: Agency for Healthcare Research and Quality.

MacLean CH, Issa AM, Newberry SJ, Mojica WA, Morton SC, Garland RH, Hilton LG, Traina SB, Shekelle PG. 2005a. *Effects of Omega-3 Fatty Acids on Cognitive Function with Aging, Dementia, and Neurological Diseases.* Evidence Report/Technology Assessment No. 114 (Prepared by the Southern California/RAND Evidence-based Practice Center, under Contract No. 290-02-0003.) AHRQ Publication No. 05-E011-2. Rockville, MD: Agency for Healthcare Research and Quality.

MacLean CH, Newberry SJ, Mojica, WA, Issa A, Khanna P, Lim YW, Morton SC, Suttorp M, Tu W, Hilton LG, Garland RH, Traina SB, Shekelle PG. 2005b. *Effects of Omega-3 Fatty Acids on Cancer.* Evidence Report/Technology Assessment No. 113 (Prepared by the Southern California/RAND Evidence-based Practice Center, under Contract No. 290-02-0003). AHRQ Publication No. 05-E010-2. Rockville, MD: Agency for Healthcare Research and Quality.

MacLean CH, Newberry SJ, Mojica WA, Khanna P, Issa AM, Suttorp MJ, Lim YW, Traina SB, Hilton L, Garland R, Morton SC. 2006. Effects of omega-3 fatty acids on cancer risk: A systematic review. *Journal of the American Medical Association* 295(4):403–415.

Makrides M, Gibson RA. 2000. Long-chain polyunsaturated fatty acid requirements during pregnancy and lactation. *American Journal of Clinical Nutrition* 71(1 Suppl): 307S–311S.

Makrides M, Neumann MA, Byard RW, Simmer K, Gibson RA. 1994. Fatty acid composition of brain, retina, and erythrocytes in breast- and formula-fed infants. *American Journal of Clinical Nutrition* 60(2):189–194.

Makrides M, Neumann MA, Simmer K, Gibson RA. 2000. A critical appraisal of the role of dietary long-chain polyunsaturated fatty acids on neural indices of term infants: A randomized, controlled trial. *Pediatrics* 105(1 Part 1):32–38.

Marckmann P. 2003. Fishing for heart protection. *American Journal of Clinical Nutrition* 78(1):1–2.

Marckmann P, Gronbaek M. 1999. Fish consumption and coronary heart disease mortality. A systematic review of prospective cohort studies. *European Journal of Clinical Nutrition* 53(8):585–590.

Martinez M. 1992. Tissue levels of polyunsaturated fatty acids during early human development. *Journal of Pediatrics* 120(3 Part 2):S129–S138.

McCann JC, Ames BN. 2005. Is docosahexaenoic acid, an n-3 long-chain polyunsaturated fatty acid, required for development of normal brain function? An overview of evidence from cognitive and behavioral tests in humans and animals. *American Journal of Clinical Nutrition* 82(2):281–295.

Miller GJ. 2005. Dietary fatty acids and the haemostatic system. *Atherosclerosis* 179(2): 213–227.

Mori TA,Vandongen R, Beilin LJ, Burke V, Morris J, Ritchie J.1994. Effects of varying dietary fat, fish and fish oils on blood lipids in a randomized controlled trial in men at risk of heart disease. *American Journal of Clinical Nutrition* 59(5):1060–1068.

Morris MC, Evans DA, Bienias JL, Tangney CC, Bennett DA, Wilson RS, Aggarwal N, Schneider J. 2003. Consumption of fish and n-3 fatty acids and risk of incident Alzheimer disease. *Archives of Neurology* 60(7):940–946.

Mozaffarian D, Longstreth WT Jr, Lemaitre RN, Manolio TA, Kuller LH, Burke GL, Siscovick DS. 2005. Fish consumption and stroke risk in elderly individuals: The cardiovascular health study. *Archives of Internal Medicine* 165(2):200–206. Erratum in: *Archives of Internal Medicine* 165(6):683.

Ness AR, Whitley E, Burr ML, Elwood PC, Smith GD, Ebrahim S. 1999. The long-term effect of advice to eat more fish on blood pressure in men with coronary disease: Results from the Diet and Reinfarction Trial. *Journal of Human Hypertension* 13(11):729–733.

Ness AR, Hughes J, Elwood PC, Whitley E, Smith GD, Burr ML. 2002. The long-term effect of dietary advice in men with coronary disease: Follow-up of the Diet and Reinfarction trial (DART). *European Journal of Clinical Nutrition* 56(6):512–518.

Neuringer M, Connor WE, Van Petten C, Barstad L. 1984. Dietary omega-3 fatty acid deficiency and visual loss in infant rhesus monkeys. *Journal of Clinical Investigations* 73(1):272–276.

Newson RB, Shaheen SO, Henderson AJ, Emmett PM, Sherriff A, Calder PC. 2004. Umbilical cord and maternal blood red cell fatty acids and early childhood wheezing and eczema. *Journal of Allergy and Clinical Immunology* 114(3):531–537.

O'Connor DL, Hall R, Adamkin D, Auestad N, Castillo M, Connor WE, Connor SL, Fitzgerald K, Groh-Wargo S, Hartman EE, Jacobs J, Janowsky J, Lucas A, Margeson D, Mena P, Neuringer M, Nesin M, Singer L, Stephenson T, Szabo J, Zemon V. 2001. Growth and development in preterm infants fed long-chain polyunsaturated fatty acids: A prospective, randomized controlled trial. *Pediatrics* 108(2):259–371.

Oken E, Kleinman KP, Olsen SF, Rich-Edwards JW, Gillman MW. 2004. Associations of seafood and elongated n-3 fatty acid intake with fetal growth and length of gestation: Results from a US pregnancy cohort. *American Journal of Epidemiology* 160(8):774–783.

Oken E, Wright RO, Kleinman KP, Bellinger D, Hu H, Rich-Edwards JW, Gillman MW. 2005. Maternal fish consumption, hair mercury, and infant cognition in a US cohort. *Environmental Health Perspectives* 113(10):1376–1380.

Olsen SF. 2006. The People's League of Health trial. *Journal of the Royal Society of Medicine* 99(1):44–45.

Olsen SF, Secher NJ. 1990. A possible preventive effect of low-dose fish oil on early delivery and pre-eclampsia: Indications from a 50-year-old controlled trial. *British Journal of Nutrition* 64(3):599–609.

Olsen SF, Secher NJ. 2002. Low consumption of seafood in early pregnancy as a risk factor for preterm delivery: Prospective cohort study. *British Medical Journal* 324(7335): 447–450.

Olsen SF, Hansen HS, Sommer S, Jensen B, Sorensen TI, Secher NJ, Zachariassen P. 1991. Gestational age in relation to marine n-3 fatty acids in maternal erythrocytes: A study of women in the Faroe Islands and Denmark. *American Journal of Obstetrics and Gynecology* 164(5 Part 1):1203–1209.

Olsen SF, Sorensen JD, Secher NJ, Hedegaard M, Henriksen TB, Hansen HS, Grant A. 1992. Randomised controlled trial of effect of fish-oil supplementation on pregnancy duration. *Lancet* 339(8800):1003–1007.

Olsen SF, Secher NJ, Tabor A, Weber T, Walker JJ, Gluud C, Fish Oil Trials In Pregnancy (FOTIP) Team. 2000. Randomised clinical trials of fish oil supplementation in high risk pregnancies. *British Journal of Obstetrics and Gynecology* 107(3):382–395.

Onwude JL, Lilford RJ, Hjartardottir H, Staines A, Tuffnell D. 1995. A randomized double blinded placebo controlled trial of fish oil in high risk pregnancy. *British Journal of Obstetrics and Gynaecology* 102(2):95–100.

Otto SJ, van Houwelingen AC, Badart-Smook A, and Hornstra G. 2001. Comparison of the peripartum and postpartum phospholipid polyunsaturated fatty acid profiles of lactating and nonlactating women. *American Journal of Clinical Nutrition* 73(6):1074–1079.

Otto SJ, de Groot RH, Hornstra G. 2003. Increased risk of postpartum depressive symptoms is associated with slower normalization after pregnancy of the functional docosahexaenoic acid status. *Prostaglandins, Leukotrienes and Essential Fatty Acids* 69(4):237–243.

Putnam JC, Carlson SE, DeVoe PW, Barness LA. 1982. The effect of variations in dietary fatty acids on the fatty acid composition of erythrocyte phosphatidylcholine and phosphatidyl-ethanolamine in human infants. *American Journal of Clinical Nutrition* 36(1):106–114.

Rose SA, Feldman JF, Jankowski JJ. 2004. Dimensions of cognition in infancy. *Intelligence* 32(3):245–262.

Salvig JD, Olsen SF, Secher NJ. 1996. Effects of fish oil supplementation in late pregnancy on blood pressure: A randomised controlled trial. *British Journal of Obstetrics and Gynae-cology* 103(6):529–533.

Sanders TA, Naismith DJ. 1979. A comparison of the influence of breast-feeding and bottle-feeding on the fatty acid composition of the erythrocytes. *British Journal of Nutrition* 41(3):619–623.

SanGiovanni JP, Berkey CS, Dwyer JT, Colditz GA. 2000a. Dietary essential fatty acids, long-chain polyunsaturated fatty acids, and visual resolution acuity in healthy fullterm infants: A systematic review. *Early Human Development* 57(3):165–188.

SanGiovanni JP, Parra-Cabrera S, Colditz GA, Berkey CS, Dwyer JT. 2000b. Meta-analysis of dietary essential fatty acids and long-chain polyunsaturated fatty acids as they relate to visual resolution acuity in healthy preterm infants. *Pediatrics* 105(6):1292–1298.

Schachter HM, Reisman J, Tran K, Dales B, Kourad K, Barnes D, Sampson M, Morrison A, Gaboury I, Blackman J. 2004. *Health Effects of Omega-3 Fatty Acids on Asthma*. Summary, Evidence Report/Technology Assessment No. 91. (Prepared by the University of Ottawa Evidence-based Practice Center, Ottawa, Canada). AHRQ Publication No. 04-E013-1. Rockville, MD: Agency for Healthcare Research and Quality.

Schachter HM, Kourad K, Merali Z, Lumb A, Tran K, Miguelez M, et al. 2005. *Effects of Omega-3 Fatty Acids on Mental Health*. Summary, Evidence Report/Technology Assessment #116 (Prepared by the University of Ottawa Evidence-based Practice Center, under Contract No. 290-02-0021). AHRQ Publication No. 05-E022-1. Rockville, MD: Agency for Healthcare Research and Quality.

Schaefer EJ, Lichtenstein AH, Lamon-Fava S. 1996. Effects of National Cholesterol Education Program Step 2 diets relatively high or relatively low in fish derived fatty acids on plasma lipoproteins in middle aged and elderly subjects. *American Journal of Clinical Nutrition* 63(2):234–241.

Schiff E, Ben-Baruch G, Barkai G, Peleg E, Rosenthal T, Mashiach S. 1993. Reduction of throm-boxane A2 synthesis in pregnancy by polyunsaturated fatty acid supplements. *American Journal of Obstetrics and Gynecology* 168(1 Part 1):122–124.

Schmidt EB, Arnesen H, Christensen JH, Rasmussen LH, Kristensen SD, De Caterina R. 2005a. Marine n-3 polyunsaturated fatty acids and coronary heart disease. Part II: clinical trials and recommendations. *Thrombosis Research* 115(4):257–262.

Schmidt EB, Arnesen H, de Caterina R, Rasmussen LH, Kristensen SD. 2005b. Marine n-3 polyunsaturated fatty acids and coronary heart disease. Part I: background, epidemiology, animal data, effects on risk factors and safety. *Thrombosis Research* 115(3):163–170.

Scott DT, Janowsky JS, Carroll RE, Taylor JA, Auestad N, Montalto MB. 1998. Formula supplementation with long-chain polyunsaturated fatty acids: Are there developmental benefits? *Pediatrics* 102(5):E59.

Sibai BM. 1998. Prevention of preeclampsia: A big disappointment. *American Journal of Obstetrics and Gynecology* 179(5):1275–1278.

Simmer K. 2005. Longchain polyunsaturated fatty acid supplementation in infants born at term. *Cochrane Library* Issue 2. [Online]. Available: http://www.cochrane.org/cochrane/revabstr/AB000376.htm [accessed October 18, 2005].

Simmer K, Patole S. 2005. Longchain polyunsaturated fatty acid supplementation in pre-term infants. *Cochrane Library* Issue 2. [Online]. Available: http://www.cochrane.org/cochrane/revabstr/AB000375.htm [accessed October 18, 2005].

Singh RB, Niaz MA, Sharma JP, Kumar R, Rastogi V, Moshiri M. 1997. Randomized, double-blind, placebo-controlled trial of fish oil and mustard oil in patients with suspected acute myocardial infarction: The Indian experiment of infarct survival—4. *Cardiovascular Drugs Therapy* 11(3):485–491.

Sirtori CR, Crepaldi G, Manzato E, Mancini M, Rivellese A, Paoletti R, Pazzucconi F, Pamparana F, Stragliotto E. 1998. One-year treatment with ethyl esters of n-3 fatty acids in patients with hypertriglyceridemia and glucose tolerance: Reduced triglyceride, total cholesterol and increased HDL-C without glycemic alterations. *Atherosclerosis* 137(2):419–427.

Skerrett PJ, Hennekens CH. 2003. Consumption of fish and fish oils and decreased risk of stroke. *Preventive Cardiology* 6(1):38–41.

Smuts CM, Borod E, Peeples JM, Carlson SE. 2003a. High-DHA eggs: Feasibility as a means to enhance circulating DHA in mother and infant. *Lipids* 38(4):407–414.

Smuts CM, Huang M, Mundy D, Plasse T, Major S, Carlson SE. 2003b. A randomized trial of docosahexaenoic acid supplementation during the third trimester of pregnancy. *Obstetrics and Gynecology* 101(3):469–479.

Terry PD, Rohan TE, Wolk A. 2003. Intakes of fish and marine fatty acids and the risks of cancers of the breast and prostate and of other hormone-related cancers: A review of the epidemiologic evidence. *American Journal of Clinical Nutrition* 77(3):532–543.

Timonen M, Horrobin D, Jokelainen J, Laitinen J, Herva A, Rasanen P. 2004. Fish consumption and depression: The Northern Finland 1966 birth cohort study. *Journal of Affective Disorders* 82(3):447–452.

Troisi RJ, Willett WC, Weiss ST. 1995. A prospective study of diet and adult-onset asthma. *American Journal of Respiratory Critical Care* 151(5):1401–1408.

Uauy Rm Birch DG, Birch EE, Tyson JE, Hoffman. 1990. Effect of dietary omega-3 fatty acids on retinal function of very-low-birth-weight neonates. *Pediatric Research* 28(5):485–492.

Uauy R, Hoffman DR, Peirano P, Birch DG, Birch EE. 2001. Essential fatty acids in visual and brain development. *Lipids* 36(9):885–895.

University of Bristol. 2001. *ALSPAC: Parental Involvement and Questionnaire Administration.* [Online]. Available: http://www.ich.bristol.ac.uk/protocol/section3.htm [accessed February 23, 2006].

University of Bristol. 2006. *Avon Longitudinal Student of Parents and Children (ALSPAC).* [Online]. Available: http://www.ich.bristol.ac.uk/welcome/index.shtml [accessed February 23, 2006].

USDA. 2005. *USDA National Nutrient Database for Standard Reference Release 18.* [Online]. Available: http://www.nal.usda.gov/fnic/foodcomp/Data/SR18/sr18.html [accessed March 1, 2006].

Van Wassenaer A. 2005. Neurodevelopmental consequences of being born SGA. *Pediatric Endocrinology Reviews* 2(3):372–377.

van Wezel-Meijler G, Van Der Knaap MS, Huisman J, Jonkman EJ, Valk J, Lafeber HN. 2002. Dietary supplementation of long-chain polyunsaturated fatty acids in preterm infants: Effects on cerebral maturation. *Acta Paediatrica* 91(9):942–950.

Vandongen R, Mori TA, Burke V, Beilin LJ, Morris J, Ritchie J. 1993. Effects on blood pressure of omega 3 fats in subjects at increased risk of cardiovascular disease. *Hypertension* 22(3):371–379.

Velzing-Aarts FV, van der Klis FRM, Muskiet FAJ. 1999. Umbilical vessels of preeclamptic women have low contents of both n-3 and n-6 long-chain polyunsaturated fatty acids. *American Journal of Clinical Nutrition* 69(2):293–298.

Villar J, Belizan JM. 1982. The relative contribution of prematurity and fetal growth retardation to low birth weight in developing and developed societies. *American Journal of Obstetrics and Gynecology* 143(7):793–798.

Wang C, Chung M, Balk E, Kupelnick B, DeVine D, et al. 2004. *Effects of Omega-3 Fatty Acids on Cardiovascular Disease.* Evidence Report/Technology Assessment No. 94 (Prepared by the Tufts-New England Medical Center Evidence-based Practice Center, Boston, MA, under Contract No. 290-02-0022). AHRQ Publication No. 04-E009-2. Rockville, MD: Agency for Healthcare Research and Quality.

Wang C, Harris WS, Chung M, Lichtenstein AH, Balk EM, Kupelnick B, Jordan HS, Lau J. 2006. n-3 fatty acids from fish or fish-oil supplements, but not α-linolenic acid, benefit cardiovascular disease outcomes in primary- and secondary-prevention studies: A systematic review. *American Journal of Clinical Nutrition* 84(1):5–17.

Weisburger JH. 1997. Dietary fat and risk of chronic disease: Mechanistic insights from experimental studies. *Journal of the American Dietetic Association* 97(Suppl 7):S16–S23.

Werkman SH, Carlson SE. 1996. A randomized trial of visual attention of preterm infants fed docosahexaenoic acid until nine months. *Lipids* 31(1):91–97.

Whelton SP, He J, Whelton PK, Muntner P. 2004. Meta-analysis of observational studies on fish intake and coronary heart disease. *American Journal of Cardiology* 93(9):1119–1123.

White. 2005. Suspected research fraud: Difficulties of getting at the truth. *British Medical Journal* 331(7511):281–288.

Willatts P, Forsyth JS, DiModugno MK, Varma S, Colvin M. 1998a. Effect of long-chain polyunsaturated fatty acids in infant formula on problem solving at 10 months of age. *Lancet* 352(9129):688–691.

Willatts P, Forsyth JS, DiModugno MK, Varma S, Colvin M. 1998b. Influence of long-chain polyunsaturated fatty acids on infant cognitive function. *Lipids* 33(10):973–980.

Willatts P, Forsyth J, Agostoni C, Bissenden J, Casaear P, and Behm G. 2003a. *Effects of Long-Chain Polyunsaturated Fatty Aid Supplementation in Infancy on Cognitive Function in Later Childhood.* Maternal and Infant LCPUFA Workshop. Kansas City, MO: AOCS.

Willatts P, Forsyth S, Mires G, Ross P. 2003b. *Maternal DHA Status in Late Pregnancy Is Related to Infant Look Duration and Acuity at Age 4 Months.* Poster presented at the meeting of the Society for Research in Child Development, Tampa, FL.

Williams MA, Zingheim RW, King IB, Zebelman AM. 1995. Omega-3 fatty acids in maternal erythrocytes and risk of preeclampsia. *Epidemiology* 6(3):232–237.

Williams C, Birch EE, Emmett PM, Northstone K. 2001. Stereoacuity at age 3.5 y in children born full-term is associated with prenatal and postnatal dietary factors: A report from a population-based cohort study. *American Journal of Clinical Nutrition* 73(2):316–322.

4

Health Risks Associated
with Seafood Consumption

This chapter reviews the potential risks associated with chronic exposure to particular seafoodborne contaminants and risks associated with certain more acute seafoodborne hazards. The discussion includes consideration of the extent to which seafood consumption might increase consumers' risk of adverse health impacts due to exposure to toxicants, depending upon the critical dose-response relationships for the contaminant, the distribution of contaminant body burden in the population, and the extent to which the body burden is due to seafood consumption rather than to other sources and pathways of exposure. The chapter concludes with a discussion of the interaction between nutrients and contaminants—in particular, selenium and methylmercury—in seafood, and measures that consumers can take to reduce exposure to contaminants that may be present in seafood.

ENVIRONMENTAL CHEMICALS

Consumers seeking the health benefits associated with the consumption of seafood are concerned about potential health risks associated with the presence of chemical contaminants, both those occurring naturally and those resulting from human activities, in seafood. These contaminants include inorganic compounds such as methylmercury and other metals, as well as persistent organic pollutants (POPs) such as dioxins and polychlorinated biphenyls (PCBs). Of these, methylmercury is the contaminant that has elicited the most concern among consumers.

Methylmercury

Mercury is a heavy metal that is present in the environment as a result of both human activities (referred to as anthropogenic sources) and natural processes. The primary anthropogenic source is the combustion of fossil carbon fuels, particulary from coal-fired utility boilers; other sources include municipal, medical, and hazardous waste incineration (NRC, 2000). The natural sources include volcanic emissions and the weathering of rock containing mercury ore. Mercury can be deposited locally or travel long distances in the atmosphere and contaminate sites far from its point of release. Further, the complex biogeochemistry of mercury fate and transport creates uncertainty in efforts to apportion the relative contributions of these processes to global mercury pollution. The US Environmental Protection Agency (US EPA) estimated that 50 to 75 percent of the total yearly input of mercury into the environment is anthropogenic (US EPA, 1997), while the United Nations Environment Programme (UNEP) suggests that this source accounts for more than half of the inputs (UNEP, 2002).

Mercury exists in the environment in several different forms, including metallic, inorganic, and organic, and interconversion between forms can occur. The form of mercury of greatest concern with regard to seafood consumption is methylmercury (MeHg). Methylmercury results when mercury in other forms is deposited in water bodies and biotransformed through the process of methylation by microorganisms. It bioaccumulates up the aquatic trophic food chain as smaller organisms are consumed by larger organisms. Because methylmercury is persistent, this bioaccumulation process results in large long-lived predatory species, such as certain sharks, swordfish, and tuna, or freshwater species such as bass, walleye, and pickerel having the highest concentrations (Kraepiel et al., 2003). Methylmercury levels can also be high in marine mammals such as whales, and in animals that feed on marine life, such as polar bears and sea birds. Consumption of aquatic life is the major route of human exposure to methylmercury. The seafood choices a consumer makes, and the frequency with which different species are consumed, are thus important determinants of methylmercury intake. Because of the global dispersion of methylmercury and migration of species, the extent of regional variation in body burdens among different aquatic animals is less striking than the regional variations in certain other water contaminants, such as PCBs or dioxin-like compounds (DLCs). This implies that the location in which an aquatic animal was caught might provide relatively little information about its methylmercury content.

Methylmercury is not lipophilic (lipid soluble) and is thus present in the largest concentrations in the muscle tissue of aquatic animals rather than in fat or oils. Approximately 95 percent of ingested methylmercury is absorbed across the gastrointestinal tract into the blood. The half-life of methylmercury in blood in humans is estimated to be 50 days, and the whole-body half-life to be 70–80 days, although the residence time of mercury in the brain appears to be considerably longer (NRC, 2000). Hair is frequently used as an exposure biomarker for methylmercury. Hair is a route of methylmercury excretion, and approximately 80 to 90 percent of the total mercury found in hair is in the methylated form. Hair mercury is a good biomarker in fish-consuming populations. Autopsy studies suggest that maternal hair mercury level correlates reasonably well with the level of mercury in the fetal brain (Cernichiari et al., 1995).

Mercury Burdens in the US Population

The first nationally representative estimates of blood and hair mercury levels were provided by the National Health and Nutrition Examination Survey (NHANES) of 1999–2000. Among women 16–49 years old, the geometric mean hair mercury level was 0.2 parts per million (ppm), with 75th, 90th, and 95th percentiles of 0.42, 1.11, and 1.73 ppm, respectively (McDowell et al., 2004). The geometric mean blood mercury level was 1.02, with 75th, 90th, and 95th percentiles of 2.07, 4.84, and 7.13 ppm, respectively (Mahaffey et al., 2004). The prevalence of levels in excess of 5.8 µg/L (benchmark dose lower bound [BMDL] adjusted for uncertainty and for population variability) was 5.66 percent. Levels were 50 percent higher among older women (30–49 years) compared to younger women, and levels were highest among women who self-identified as "Other" racial/ethnic category (Asians, Native Americans, Pacific Islanders). Mercury burdens were strongly associated with the amount of self-reported fish consumption (Mahaffey et al., 2004). Among women reporting eating 5–8 fish meals per month, these figures were 2.56, 4.54, 8.80, and 11.60 ppm, respectively. Levels were seven times greater among women who reported eating nine or more fish meals in the previous 30 days, compared to women who reported no consumption. Among these relatively high fish-consumers, the 50th, 75th, 90th, and 95th percentiles for blood mercury were 3.02, 6.68, 12.00, and 13.40 ppm, respectively.

Data on blood and hair mercury levels in adult men in the United States were not collected as part of NHANES until 2003, and no data for this group has been reported. Therefore, estimates must be made based on mercury biomarker data reported as part of large cohort studies. Urine and blood mercury levels of 1127 Vietnam-era pilots were measured for a study of the health effects of exposure to dental amalgam (Kingman et al., 1998). The mean blood mercury level in this group of men was 3.1 ppm, with a range up to 44 ppm, but the contribution of fish consumption to blood mercury levels is unknown because data were not collected on fish intake.

An important limitation of NHANES as a source of data on population exposures to methylmercury is that the sampling plan used to identify the 3637 women who contributed data in the 1999–2002 survey is likely to have missed subgroups of high fish-consumers, including sport fishers and subsistence fishers. Examples of such groups include individuals living in areas that provide ready access to seafood (e.g., island populations) (Ortiz-Roque and Lopez-Rivera, 2004), fishers (Burge and Evans, 1994; Bellanger et al., 2000), groups for whom fish or marine mammals are an especially important component of overall diet, and individuals who consume a high-fish diet for its cardioprotective effects. For example, one report described a case series of 116 patients who consumed large quantities of fish and had their blood tested; almost all (89 percent) had blood mercury levels greater than 5 µg/L, ranging up to 89 µg/L (Hightower and Moore, 2003). Evidence from the Third National Report on Human Exposure to Environmental Chemicals (CDC, 2005b) suggests that population exposures to mercury might have decreased between 1999–2000 and 2001–2002. Among women 16–49 years of age, the geometric mean declined from 1.02 µg/L (95% CI 0.825-1.270) to 0.833 (95% CI 0.738-0.940). An even greater decline was evident at the high end of the distribution, as the level corresponding to the 95th percentile in the earlier survey was 7.10 (95% CI 5.30-11.30) compared to 4.6 (95% CI 3.7-5.9) in the later survey. Because of the short time period covered by these data, however, the possibility that the observed time trend reflects sampling variability cannot be rejected.

Health Effects in Critical Target Organs

Organs of the central nervous and cardiovascular systems are considered to be the critical target organs with regard to methylmercury.

Neurological Toxicity The tragic epidemic of frank neurological disease that was identified in the late 1950s in Minamata, Japan, first brought to the world's attention the devastating effects of methylmercury on the developing fetal brain. Children exposed in utero to high levels of MeHg presented with cerebral palsy, mental retardation, movement and coordination disorders, dysarthria, and sensory impairments.The neuropathological lesions associated with Congenital Minamata Disease (mercury poisoning) were diffuse, occurring throughout the brain. In individuals exposed only in adulthood, the lesions were highly focal, clustering in regions that matched clinical presentation (e.g., motor disorders = precentral gyrus and cerebellum, constriction of visual fields = calcarine fissure of occipital cortex). The major molecular mechanisms of MeHg neurotoxicity include inhibition of protein and macromolecular synthesis, mitochondrial dysfunction, defective calcium and ion flux, disruption of neurotransmitter homeostasis, initiation of oxidative stress injury, microtubule disaggregation, and post-translational phosphorylation (Verity, 1997). The diffuse injury associated with prenatal exposure is attributable to the ability of MeHg to arrest mitotic cells in metaphase, disrupting the exquisitely choreographed processes of cell proliferation, differentiation, and migration. The result is a brain in which there are reduced cortical cell densities, islands of heterotopic neurons in cerebral and cerebellar white matter, anomalous cytoarchitecture, disturbance in laminar pattern of cerebral cortex, absence of granule and Purkinje cells in the cerebellum, incomplete myelination in the hypoplastic corpus callosum, glial proliferation ("bizarre astrocytes in the white matter"), and limited gyral differentiation (Choi, 1989).

No cases of Congenital Minamata Disease have been reported in the United States, where the primary concern has been whether chronic exposure to MeHg, as the result of seafood consumption among the general population, is associated with subtle adverse health outcomes. Therefore, several risk assessments have been conducted in the past decade in which the goal was to identify a fetal mercury burden that can be interpreted as being without appreciable risk. The basis for most risk assessments for MeHg exposure has been one or more of the three major epidemiologic studies available: the New Zealand study (Kjellstrom et al., 1986), the Faroe Islands study (Grandjean et al., 2001), and the Seychelles study (Myers et al., 2003) (see Box 4-1).

The New Zealand and Faroe Islands studies, but not the Seychelles study, have generally been regarded as providing evidence of harm from MeHg exposures at which clinical effects are not evident, although it should be noted that benchmark dose analyses of the data from the 9-year evaluation of children in the Seychelles study cohort produced BMDLs in the range of 17–23 ppm (Van Wijngaarden et al., 2006), only slightly higher than the BMDLs based on the New Zealand and Faroe Islands studies data. In view of the perceived discrepancies in the findings of the three studies, the choice of critical study has stimulated considerable controversy. Some risk assessors chose the Faroe Islands study (US EPA, 2001; NRC, 2000), while others chose the Seychelles study (ATSDR, 1999). In an effort to use all of the best available data, the Joint Expert Committee on Food Additives and Contaminants (JECFA), a joint committee of the World Health Organization (WHO) and the Food and Agricultural Organization of the United Nations (FAO), averaged the effect estimates reported for the Faroes and Seychelles studies; including the New Zealand study did not significantly change the results (FAO/WHO JECFA, 2003). In all these assessments, however, the final result was a single number interpreted as a reference level for intake for the most sensitive subgroup, the fetus, as shown in Table 4-1. These reference levels differ largely because of differences in the uncertainty factors applied. These levels were derived on the basis of health effects observed, rather than

BOX 4-1
Three Major Epidemiological Studies on Methylmercury

These three studies were conducted among geographically disparate island populations with a high availability of seafood (tuna is an important export product of Seychelles, approximately one-third of the Faroese workforce is employed in the fishing industry, and both aquaculture and marine fishing feature in the economy of New Zealand). Cohen (2004) summarized these three cohorts in reviews.

Seychelles Child Development Study

The Seychelles Child Development Study (SCDS) is an ongoing collaboration between the Ministry of Health of Seychelles, a small archipelago country in the Indian Ocean, and the University of Rochester, New York. "Initially the objectives focused on two primary questions. Firstly, could clinical neuro-development effects be found in children after exposure to methylmercury (MeHg) in utero from a maternal diet high in fish and, secondly, what is the lowest level of foetal [sic] exposure to cause such effects?" (Shamlaye, 2004). Seychelles was determined to be a favorable location for this study for a number of reasons: the Seychellois regularly consume fish (an average of 12 meals per week), and the number of annual births allowed for recruitment of a large cohort of mothers and children in a short period of time (Shamlaye, 2004; Myers et al., 2003). The Seychelles Child Development Study enrolled 779 mother-infant pairs between 1989 and 1990, of which 717 were eligible for analysis. Among the tests administered at 107 months were the Wechsler Intelligence Scale for Children—Third Edition, the Boston Naming Test, the California Verbal Learning Test, the Bruininks-Oseretsky Test of Motor Proficiency, a Continuous Performance Test, the Developmental Test of Visual-Motor Integration, the Grooved Pegboard, and selected subtests of the Woodcock-Johnson Tests of Achievement. The children were evaluated (i.e., cognitive, language, motor, adaptive behavior, and social-emotional development) at 6, 19, 29, 66, and 107 months. Maternal hair samples were also collected at enrollment. The information provided here, along with the results from the study, can be accessed in the Special Issue of the *Seychelles Medical and Dental Journal,* Volume 7, Issue 1, 2004. [Online]. Available: http://www.seychelles. net/smdj/ [accessed July 7, 2005]. Also, in 2000, Clarkson et al. recruited a new cohort of mother-infant pairs in Seychelles, and this project is due for completion in 2006.

Faroe Islands Study

The Faroe Islands Study, conducted in this North Atlantic Ocean archipelago located between Scotland, Norway, and Iceland, consisted of a cohort of

1022 consecutive singleton births from 1986–1987. The objective of this study was to investigate possible neurobehavioral effects of prenatal exposure to neurotoxicants, such as methylmercury. The Faroese are high consumers of seafood, including pilot whale, which exposes them to high levels of methylmercury. The study team analyzed maternal hair mercury concentrations and cord blood mercury concentrations at birth and conducted neurobehavioral examinations on 917 of the children just before school entry (about 7 years of age) and at 14 years of age. The detailed examinations, which lasted about 5 hours for each child, took place mostly in the National Hospital in Torshavn, the capital of the Faroes Island. The examination included finger tapping; hand-eye coordination; reaction time on a continuous performance test; Wechsler Intelligence Scale for Children—Revised Digit Span, Similarities, and Block Design; Bender Visual Motor Gestalt Test; Boston Naming Test; and California Verbal Learning Test. The parent accompanying the child (usually the mother) was also asked to fill out a self-administered questionnaire on the child's past medical history, current health status, and social factors (Grandjean, 1997).

New Zealand Study
The New Zealand Study involved the screening of 11,000 children born in 1978, over 900 of whose mothers consumed fish more than four times per week during pregnancy. As with the other cohorts, the objective of this study was to investigate the association between prenatal mercury exposure and subsequent development during childhood (Crump, 1998). Maternal hair samples were collected at birth to assess mercury exposure during pregnancy. At 4 years of age, the Denver Developmental Screening Test and a set of neurological screening tests were completed on 74 children, 38 with "high" maternal hair mercury levels (> 6µg/g) and 36 with "low" maternal hair mercury levels, matched on maternal demographic characteristics, age, hospital where the birth took place, and date of birth. Maternal interviews about the ages at which the child achieved developmental milestones were also conducted (Kjellstrom et al., 1986). At 6 years of age, 238 children were evaluated. A child with a high maternal hair mercury was matched with three children with low hair mercury levels, but similar in gender, maternal ethnic group, age, smoking habits, location of residence, and number of years living in New Zealand (Kjellstrom et al., 1989). The tests administered included the Test of Oral Language Development, the Weschlar Intelligence Scale for Children-Revised, and the McCarthy Scales of Children's Abilities.

TABLE 4-1 Reference Levels for Fetal Exposure to Methylmercury

Source	Reference Level
JECFA provisional tolerable weekly intake	1.6 µg/kg body weight/week
US EPA reference dose	0.1 µg/kg body weight/day
Agency for Toxic Substances and Disease Registry minimal risk level	0.3 µg/kg body weight/day

SOURCES: FAO/WHO JECFA, 2003; US EPA, 2001; ATSDR, 1999.

the general population, and are risk management guidelines rather than estimates of threshold of effect. While such numbers can be used to estimate the number of individuals at potential risk (i.e., for whom the margin of exposure is less than 10-fold), they convey nothing about the quantitative characteristics of the dose-response relationship, i.e., for the risk associated with each unit increase in mercury burden above the reference level.

A variety of hypotheses have been proposed to explain the apparent discrepancy between the results of the Seychelles and Faroe Islands studies. The National Research Council (NRC) committee did not consider that any of them is clearly supported by the evidence, however. The issues evaluated include differences between populations in the temporal characteristics of exposure (presumed to be stable among the Seychellois, but potentially episodic among the Faroese due to occasional consumption of pilot whale), reliance on different biomarkers of exposure (cord blood mercury vs. maternal hair mercury), population differences in vulnerability to methylmercury, the influence of other aspects of nutrition on methylmercury toxicity, and differences in the neuropsychological tests administered and the ages at which children were assessed. Consideration has also been given to the possibility of residual confounding in one or both studies, particularly with regard to the high exposures of the Faroese to PCBs and other POPs.

Although considerable debate has ensued seeking to identify the reasons for the apparent discrepancies among the three major studies of fetal MeHg neurotoxicity, their magnitude might be less dramatic than commonly supposed. As the analyses of the National Research Council Committee on the Toxicological Effects of Methylmercury showed, the BMDLs calculated for the three major studies vary by much less than the 10-fold (one order of magnitude) uncertainty factor applied to the BMDL to achieve the Reference Dose (RfD) (NRC, 2000). Figure 4-1 shows a qualitative effort to assess the degree of concordance among studies of the "no observed adverse effect levels" (NOAEL) estimated for each study on the basis of benchmark dose analysis. An estimate of 10 to 20 ppm appears to be reasonably accurate. Interestingly, this is the range identified by WHO (1990) based solely on the relatively poor-quality data available from a mass poisoning episode

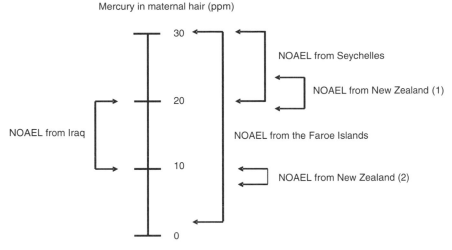

FIGURE 4-1 Integration of data from the New Zealand, Faroe Islands, and Seychelles studies of prenatal methylmercury neurotoxicity. Two ranges are provided for the NOAEL from the New Zealand study. The estimate labeled (1) was derived when the data for a child with a very high maternal hair mercury level (86 ppm) were included in the analyses. The estimate labeled 2 was derived when the data for this child were excluded. This child's mercury level was more than fourfold higher than the level for any of the 236 other children in this cohort.

NOTE: NOAEL = No observed adverse effect level.

SOURCE: Personal communication, Clarkson et al., University of Rochester, March 2005.

that occurred in Iraq in the 1970s (Personal communication, Clarkson and colleagues, University of Rochester, March 2005).

Ryan (2005) conducted an analysis of data from the three previously described studies using maximum likelihood and Bayesian hierarchical models to derive an estimate of the slope of the dose-response relationship between children's neurodevelopment and their prenatal methylmercury exposure. This analysis, presented to the Committee on Nutrient Relationships in Seafood (Ryan, 2005), suggested that children's IQ scores decline by 0.1 to 0.25 points for each ppm increase in maternal hair mercury level. The point estimates were nearly identical in the three studies (results for the New Zealand study differed considerably depending on whether one particular observation was included or excluded) (see Figure 4-2).

The point estimates of the slopes for the other neurodevelopmental endpoints measured in the three studies, some of which were common across studies, were also surprisingly similar (Figure 4-3).

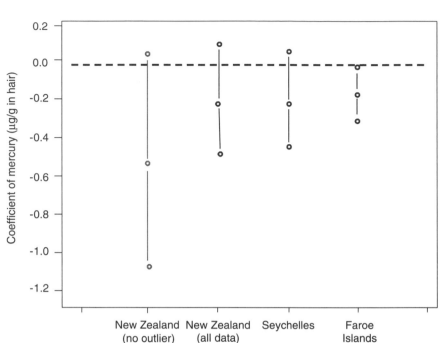

FIGURE 4-2 Point estimates and 95 percent confidence intervals, based on regression analyses, for the changes in full scale IQ ("coefficients") associated with each ppm increase in maternal hair mercury reported in the three studies. A coefficient with a negative sign indicates that the IQ scores for children within a study cohort decreased with increasing hair mercury level. Two estimates are provided for the New Zealand study, one based on the inclusion of the child with a maternal hair mercury level of 86 ppm and one based on the exclusion of this child.
SOURCE: Ryan, 2005.

These analyses, therefore, suggest that although the findings of the Seychelles study appear discrepant from those of the Faroe Islands and New Zealand studies if one focuses only on the p-values of the reported analyses, at a deeper, quantitative level that focuses on the rates of decline in scores as mercury burden increases, the findings of the three studies are remarkably concordant.

Part of the challenge in characterizing the health risks associated with increased MeHg exposure in seafood is related to the fact that this source also provides nutrients that might have health effects which mitigate those of MeHg. Thus, studies tend not to provide a "pure" estimate of MeHg toxicity but an estimate that represents the balance between the putative harm caused by the contaminant and the putative benefits provided by the

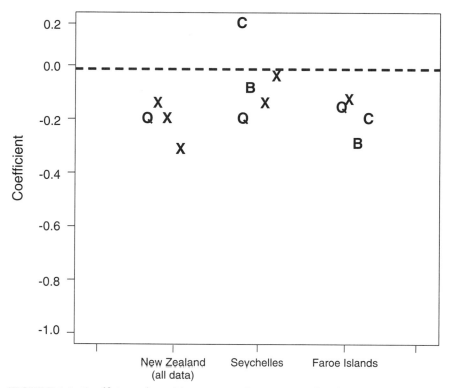

FIGURE 4-3 Coefficients for achievement and cognition-related endpoints from the three studies. The symbols Q, C, and B denote the three endpoints that are common to two or more studies, namely IQ (Q), California Verbal Learning Test (C), and Boston Naming Test (B), respectively. X's indicate endpoints that were unique to one of the studies. Coefficients reflect the change in test score for each ppm increase in maternal hair mercury. A coefficient with a negative sign indicates that a test score decreased as maternal hair mercury level increased. New Zealand estimates are based on including the child with a maternal hair mercury level of 86 ppm. The Faroe Islands median hair:cord blood ratio of 200 (Budtz-Jorgensen, 2004b) was used to convert the Faroe Islands results to units of hair mercury.
SOURCE: Ryan, 2005.

nutrients in seafood. This issue is critical, however, because the goal in giving advice regarding seafood consumption should be to enable people to obtain the greatest benefit for the least risk.

An illustration of the delicacy of this balance is provided by a study of 135 mother-infant pairs in Boston (Oken et al., 2005). Mothers reported consuming an average of 1.2 fish servings per week during the second trimester of pregnancy (range 0–5.5 servings/week), and had a mean hair mercury level at delivery of 0.55 ppm (range 0.02–2.38; 10 percent had levels >1.2 ppm). At 6 months of age, infants' scores on a visual recognition memory task were positively associated with maternal fish intake during the second trimester (4 points for each additional weekly serving), but inversely associated with maternal hair mercury level (7.5 points per ppm). Performance was best among infants whose mother consumed more than two servings of fish per week but whose hair mercury level was less than 1.2 ppm. This study was designed as a study of nutrition rather than of methylmercury intake, however, so women were asked about their fish intake using categories (canned tuna, shellfish, "dark meat" fish, other fish) that relate more directly to omega-3 fatty acid levels than to MeHg levels (see Box 3-1).

Data germane to the balance between the benefits and risks associated with consumption of fish and development in children were also reported from the Avon Longitudinal Study of Parents and Children (ALSPAC), a large ongoing birth cohort study in the UK (Daniels et al., 2004). In a subsample of 1054 of 10,092 eligible children, associations were evaluated between maternal fish consumption during week 32 of gestation, reported on a food frequency questionnaire, and maternal reports of children's language development at 15 months and general development at 18 months. The categories used in collecting data on the types of fish consumed were "white fish" (cod, haddock, plaice, fish sticks, etc.) and "oily fish" (pilchards, sardines, mackerel, tuna, herring, kippers, trout, salmon, etc.). Most women (88 percent) reported eating fish during pregnancy. Of these, 65 percent reported eating fish from both categories. Unfortunately, this way of classifying fish results in groupings that differ from those that would result if classification were based on mercury levels. Overall, children's developmental abilities, as reported by mothers, increased modestly with increased maternal fish intake during pregnancy. Most of the benefit appeared to be associated with any fish consumption, compared to none, as maternal consumption of fish more than one to three times per week did not seem to confer additional benefits, at least with regard to the child development outcomes assessed. Higher mercury concentration in umbilical tissue, for which the median was 0.01 µg/g wet weight, was not associated with adverse developmental outcomes in children, although cord tissue mercury is not a well-established biomarker of exposure. Cord mercury level did increase across strata of maternal fish intake, although the greatest increase was between the "none" and "1 per 2 weeks" strata, with little increase evident in the two strata representing greater fish intake ("1–3 per week" and "4+ per week") (see Box 3-1).

Jensen et al. (2005) reported that the usual substantial neuropsychological benefits associated with breastfeeding were not evident among the children in the Faroe Islands cohort. The authors speculated that contaminants present in the breast milk of the Faroese women mitigated the benefits to their children.

Increasing attention is being paid to the neurotoxicities observed in adults exposed to MeHg, although the findings are mixed and do not support firm conclusions about the dose-response/dose-effect relationships. In a small case series report, patients who were clinically referred for paresthesias, in 50 percent of whom mixed peripheral neuropathy with axonal loss was confirmed by electrodiagnostic studies, blood mercury levels ranged from 27 to 96 μg/L (Saint-Phard et al., 2004). Most of the patients reported consuming fish at least twice weekly. These blood mercury levels are considerably higher than those of the general US population. As noted earlier, the geometric mean among US women of child-bearing age is 0.833 μg/L (95% CI 0.738-0.94). In a study involving 129 residents of Brazilian fishing communities, in whom the mean hair mercury level was 4.2 μg/g (range 0.56–13.6), dose-dependent reductions in performance on tests of fine motor speed, dexterity, and concentration were found (Yokoo et al., 2003). In reanalyses of data from a 1977 study of 366 Québec Cree (First Nation) adults, Auger et al. (2005) reported that a 6 ppm increase in hair mercury level was associated with an odds ratio of 2.2 (95% CI 1.15-4.26) for tremor in a proportional odds ordinal regression model. Scalp hair mercury levels ranged from 0.5 to 46.1 ppm. Blood mercury level (mean 37.7 μg/L, range 1–150) was not associated with an increased risk of tremor, however. In a cross-sectional study of 106 elderly ($\geq$ 75 years) Swedes with mercury levels of 2–80 nmol/L (mean 17, standard deviation 11; values for 101 subjects were $\leq$28 nmol/L), blood mercury level was not associated with scores on the Mini-Mental Status Examination (Johansson et al., 2002). In the only large study conducted on US adults, among 474 adults aged 50 to 70 years, blood mercury level (median 2.1 μg/L; range 0–16) was not consistently associated with performance on a battery of 12 neuropsychological tests (Weil et al., 2005).

Cardiovascular Toxicity The hypothesis that elevated exposures to methylmercury might impair cardiovascular health was suggested by a series of observational studies conducted by Finnish investigators. Men with the highest level of hair mercury (>2 μg/g) had a twofold increase in risk (95% CI 1.2-3.1) (adjusted for age, examination year, ischemic exercise electrocardiogram (ECG) and maximal oxygen uptake) of an acute (fatal or nonfatal) myocardial infarction (MI) and had a 2.3-fold increased risk (95% CI 0.9-5.8) (adjusted for age, examination year, ischemic exercise ECG and maximal oxygen uptake) of death from coronary heart disease (CHD) (Salonen et al., 1995). In addition, self-reported fish consumption of 30 g per day or more was associated with a doubling of risk of an acute MI. Mercury burden was more strongly related to the amounts of nonfatty freshwater fish (turbot, vendace, northern pike, whitefish) consumed rather than fatty fish (salmon, herring, domestic rainbow trout, tuna) (Salonen et al., 1995). Follow-up examinations of this cohort conducted 4 years later indicated that high hair mercury level at baseline was a significant predictor of the increase in the common carotid intima-media thickness (IMT), suggesting accelerated carotid atherosclerosis (Salonen et al., 2000). Among men in the highest quintile of hair mercury level (>2.81 ppm), the IMT increase was 32 percent greater than among men in the rest of the cohort. The increased cardiovascular risk associated with higher fish consumption reported by Salonen et al. (1995, 2000) and Virtanen et al. (2005) might, for example, be associated with food preparation techniques (see Chapter 5) rather than methylmercury levels in the fish consumed by Finnish men, although this variable was not addressed in these reports.

In a case-control study conducted in nine countries involving 684 men less than 70 years of age with a first diagnosis of MI (Guallar et al., 2002), the adjusted (including docosahexaenoic acid [DHA]) odds ratio for men in the highest, compared to the lowest, quintile of toenail mercury level was 2.16 (95% CI 1.09-4.29). Adjusting for toenail mercury level, the risk of MI was inversely related to adipose tissue DHA level (OR=0.59, 95% CI 0.30-1.19, for highest vs. lowest quintile).

In contrast to the findings of the Finnish studies and the Guallar et al. (2002) study, essentially null findings were reported in a nested case-control study of toenail mercury levels (an alternative biomarker) and coronary heart disease (coronary artery surgery, nonfatal MI, fatal coronary heart disease) in 33,737 male health professionals (Yoshizawa et al., 2002). In the highest, compared to the lowest, quintile of mercury level, the relative risk of coronary heart disease was 0.97 (95% CI 0.63-1.50). Adjustment for omega-3 fatty acid intake did not alter this. A major uncertainty about the interpretation of these two studies is the status of toenail mercury level as a biomarker of mercury burden attributable to fish consumption. In the Yoshizawa et al. study, more than half of the study cohort consisted of dentists, and the mean toenail mercury level in dentists was more than twice the mean among the nondentist health professionals. Although toenail mercury level was modestly correlated with reported fish consumption (correlation of 0.42), toenail mercury level apparently also reflects exposures to mercury from nonfish sources, such as elemental mercury from dental amalgams and dental amalgam preparation. In this regard, it is noteworthy that when the dentists were excluded from analyses in the Yoshizawa et al. (2002) study, increased toenail mercury was associated with increased risk of coronary heart disease. The increase in risk was not statistically significant, however, at least in part because of the reduced sample size.

As noted, because the primary vehicle in which methylmercury is delivered is a food that also contains nutrients that might have health effects that are antagonistic to those of methylmercury, it is difficult to obtain "pure" estimates of methylmercury toxicities. For example, a follow-up study of the Finnish men reported on by Salonen et al. (1995) showed that men in the highest quintile of docosapentaenoic acid and docosahexaenoic acid intake, compared to men in the lowest quintile, had a 44 percent lower risk of CHD over a 4-year period (Rissanen et al., 2000). Analyses stratified by hair mercury level suggested, however, that the reduction was greater (52 percent) for men with hair mercury (Hg) levels <2 ppm than among men with hair Hg levels >2 ppm (only 24 percent). A similar shift in the balance of the risks of methylmercury and the benefits of omega-3 fatty acids was found in a study of blood mercury level and blood pressure among US women (NHANES 1999–2000; Vupputuri et al., 2005). In the entire cohort of 1240 women aged 16–49 years, blood mercury level was not significantly associated with either systolic or diastolic blood pressure. When analyses were stratified by reported fish intake (759 consumers, 481 nonconsumers), systolic blood pressure increased significantly with blood mercury level among nonconsumers, corresponding to an approximately 5 mmHg difference between the lowest quintile (0.1–0.4 µg/L) and the highest quintile (2.1–21.4). Among the fish-consumers, systolic blood pressure declined (nonsignificantly) with increasing blood mercury level. The findings were similar for changes in diastolic blood pressure with increasing blood mercury level. Overall, this pattern suggests that increased exposure to mercury, obtained from sources other than fish consumption, is associated with higher blood pressure. When mercury exposure occurs in conjunction with fish consumption, however, the effects on blood pressure are blunted and, at the levels in most US women, may be counteracted by protective factors in fish. This interpretation is consistent with the null findings of a study of hair mercury levels and blood pressure in fish-consuming Indian tribes of the Amazon rain forest (Dorea et al., 2005).

Methylmercury Reference Dose

A report from the National Research Council of the National Academies reviewed the US EPA's process in deriving the RfD (see Box 4-2). It concluded that the existing RfD of 0.1 µg/kg per day was a "scientifically justifiable level for the protection of public health," although it recommended that it be derived on the basis of the findings of the newer epidemiological studies rather than of the Iraqi study (NRC, 2000). Such a calculation is subject to numerous uncertainties, however. Among these are the choice of the functional form of the statistical model used to identify the methylmercury dose at which a doubling of the target response occurs (e.g., linear vs. supralinear vs. sublinear models), the choice of the adverse health effect, the choice of the point estimate for the excess prevalence to be prevented,

BOX 4-2
Reference Dose for Methylmercury

The US Environmental Protection Agency (US EPA, 2001) established a Reference Dose (RfD) for methylmercury (MeHg) that it defines as "...an estimate of a daily exposure to the human population (including sensitive subgroups) that is likely to be without an appreciable risk of deleterious effects during a lifetime." To derive the RfD for MeHg, the US EPA applied benchmark dose modeling. In this approach, the benchmark dose (BMD) is identified at which the prevalence of a defined health abnormality exceeds the background prevalence of the abnormality by a specified amount. The abnormality can be defined distributionally (e.g., scores more than 2 standard deviations below the mean) or clinically (e.g., the presence of a particular abnormal finding on neurologic examination). Once the critical dose is identified, the dose corresponding to the lower bound of its 95 percent confidence interval (the Benchmark Dose lower bound [BMDL]) is taken as the "point of departure" for calculating the Hg intake that would result in that dose. In other words, the BMDL is the lowest hair mercury (Hg) level that is statistically consistent with the observed increased in the prevalence of the target outcome. Although the US EPA used the Boston Naming Test results from the Faroe Islands study to illustrate the process by which it derived the RfD for Hg, it considered all of the data from the Faroe Islands and New Zealand studies and an integrative analysis that included the Seychelles study. A test score at the 5th percentile or below was selected as the critical health effect, and a doubling of the prevalence of such scores to be prevented (Rice, 2004). The US EPA selected 12 ppm in maternal hair as the critical BMDL (or 58 µg/L in cord blood). A one-compartment pharmacokinetic model, involving assumptions about factors such as the elimination constant, blood volume, MeHg absorption, fraction of absorbed dose in the blood, and the ratio of cord blood mercury to maternal blood mercury, was used to determine that an MeHg intake of 0.1 µg/kg/day over a lifetime would not result in a hair Hg level exceeding 1.2 ppm.

the choices of the point estimates for the assumptions made in fitting the one-compartment model, and the size of the aggregate uncertainty factor that should be applied to take account of all these unknowns (Rice, 2004). Reference Dose calculations are sensitive to the assumptions made about factors such as the ratio of cord blood Hg:maternal blood Hg. Although the RfD is intended to address a pregnant woman's MeHg intake, the fetal risk estimates for the Faroe Islands study, the critical study, were expressed as cord blood Hg levels. The US EPA assumed a ratio of 1:1, but recent Monte Carlo analyses suggest that the Hg level in cord blood might be as much as 70 percent higher than the Hg level in maternal blood (Stern and Smith, 2003). The results of these analyses suggest that reducing the RfD so that maternal blood Hg levels do not exceed 3.4 µg/L would prevent cord blood Hg levels from exceeding 5.8 µg/L.

The NRC (2000) study identified several other important data gaps that contribute to uncertainty, e.g., the possibility of interindividual variation in susceptibility to MeHg. Factors that might affect susceptibility include age, sex, genetics, health status, nutritional status, and toxicokinetic and toxicodynamic processes. The role of nutritional factors as potential confounders or effect modifiers of MeHg neurotoxicity is particularly important (Chapman and Chan, 2000). The many differences between the diets of the Faroese and Seychellois have been suggested as a possible explanation for apparent differences between findings. The specific dietary components suggested as possibly important are DHA, iodine, choline, and iron (Clarkson and Strain, 2003). One study found that greater consumption of tropical fruit is associated with lower hair Hg levels, although it could not be determined whether this reflected altered absorption, distribution, or excretion (Passos et al., 2003). Other data gaps pertain to the lack of information about possible late-emerging neurodevelopmental effects as children mature and the lack of dose-response analyses for other potential adverse health effects of MeHg, such as cardiovascular disease. A third class of data gaps pertains to the characterization of exposure. Factors that contribute to this are a lack of dietary intake data, the extrapolation from a biomarker such as maternal hair Hg to maternal MeHg intake, confounding by coexposures to other neurotoxic contaminants (e.g., PCBs), and the impracticality of characterizing short-term temporal variations in exposure using currently available biomarkers, particularly during potentially critical windows of brain vulnerability. Using bootstrap analyses, Budtz-Jorgensen et al. (2004b) showed that the BMDL is overestimated by 25 percent if it is not adjusted for error in measuring cord blood Hg and by 40 percent if it is not adjusted for error in measuring hair Hg. The authors argued that a failure to take these sources of error into account would result in a reference dose that is too high, and thus insufficiently protective.

Summary of Evidence

Interpretations of data from the three major epidemiologic methylmercury studies are not entirely concordant. The Faroe Islands and New Zealand studies are regarded as providing evidence that children prenatally exposed to methylmercury as the result of maternal seafood consumption during pregnancy are at increased risk of manifesting subtle neurodevelopmental deficits. The Seychelles study is regarded as not providing such evidence. A new statistical approach revealed similarities between the three studies not previously evident in published analyses. Results of this approach reduced the degree of discordance, which might have been overestimated due to a focus on p-values. This yielded greater consistency between findings of the three studies, indicating a decline of 0.1 to 0.25 points, on a scale of IQ-like measurement, for each part-per-million increase in maternal hair mercury level during pregnancy.

Observational studies in adult men from the general population have produced mixed results regarding the associations between fish consumption, mercury level, and cardiovascular health. Overall, the data considered suggests an increased risk of myocardial infarction among men with higher hair Hg levels. For both child neurodevelopment and adult cardiovascular health, emerging evidence suggests that the health benefits of seafood consumption are greater among individuals whose body burden of methylmercury is lower.

Other Metals

Metal contaminants other than mercury, including lead, manganese, chromium, cadmium, and arsenic may be present in seafood, although on a population basis, seafood consumption does not appear to be a major route of exposure to these metals. In analyses of farmed Atlantic and wild salmon, Foran et al. (2004) found that for none of nine metals measured did the levels exceed federal standards. For three of the metals measured (cobalt, copper, and cadmium), levels were significantly higher in wild than farmed salmon. Burger and Gochfeld (2005) measured the levels of seven metals (arsenic, cadmium, chromium, lead, manganese, mercury, selenium) in fish obtained from New Jersey markets. Although these levels sometimes exceeded health-based standards, the intercorrelations among the different metals were low, leading the authors to conclude that consuming a variety of fish species will reduce a consumer's risk. The source of fish is an important consideration, however. Kong et al. (2005) found levels of lead and chromium in farmed tilapia from China that exceeded local guidelines.

Persistent Organic Pollutants

Persistent organic pollutants are defined as organic chemicals that remain intact in the environment for long periods, become widely distributed geographically, bioaccumulate up the food chain by amassing in fatty tissues of animals, and are toxic to humans, wildlife, and the environment (Bidleman and Harner, 2000; IOM, 2003; UNEP Global Environmental Facility, 2003; Robson and Hamilton, 2005). Many POPs are chlorinated compounds, but brominated and fluorinated compounds also exist (e.g., brominated flame retardants and Freon) and may have a detrimental impact on the environment.

Evidence for long-range transport (to regions distant from the original source) and the threats posed to the environment (Fries, 1995a,b; UNEP Global Environmental Facility, 2003) has prompted regulatory action to reduce emissions (CFSAN, 2001; also reviewed in IOM, 2003). As a result of concerns about global circulation through the atmosphere, oceans, and other pathways, the US signed an agreement on POPs at a diplomatic conference in Stockholm, Sweden (UNEP Global Environmental Facility, 2003). Under this Convention, signatory countries were committed to reduce and/or eliminate the production, use, and/or release of the 12 POPs of greatest concern to the global community and to establish a mechanism by which additional chemicals may be added to the treaty in the future. The POPs initially targeted by the agreement, informally called the "dirty dozen" (Table 4-2), include:

- Certain insecticides, such as DDT and chlordane, once commonly used to control pests in agriculture and building materials;
- Polychlorinated biphenyls, used in electrical, heat transfer, and hydraulic equipment and as plasticizers in paints, plastics, and rubber products;
- Certain chemical byproducts, such as dioxins and furans, which are produced unintentionally from most forms of combustion, including municipal and medical waste incinerators, open barrel burning, and industrial processing.

The POPs to which seafood consumers are most likely exposed are the dioxins, dioxin-like compounds (DLCs), and PCBs.

Dioxins and Dioxin-like Compounds

Dioxins and DLCs are unintentional by products of combustion of organic material. Sources of dioxins include herbicides (2,4,5-T), wood preservatives, diesel and gasoline fuel combustion, and industrial combustion and backyard barrel burning. Currently, new dioxin releases into the environment are mostly from backyard and agricultural burning (IOM, 2003). Because of the long half-life of dioxins, they will persist in the environment. Furthermore, even if all anthropogenic sources could be eliminated, low levels of naturally occurring dioxins will continue to be produced (US EPA, 2003).

Since 1987, the US EPA has been taking action to effectively reduce environmental release of dioxins and furans to land, air, and water from

TABLE 4-2 The "Dirty Dozen" Identified
in United Nations Environment Programme

The "Dirty Dozen"
Aldrin[a]
Chlordane[a]
DDT[a]
Dieldrin[a]
Endrin[a]
Heptachlor[a]
Hexachlorobenzene[a,b,c]
Mirex[a]
Toxaphene[a]
Polychlorinated biphenyls (PCBs)[b,c]
Polychlorinated dibenzo-*p*-dioxins (Dioxins)[c]
Polychlorinated dibenzo-*p*-furans (Furans)[c]

NOTES: The United States has taken strong domestic
action to reduce emissions of POPs. Currently, none of
the pesticide POPs are registered for sale and distribution
in the United States. In 1978, the US Congress prohibited
the manufacture of any new PCBs and severely restricted
the use of remaining stocks.

[a]Pesticides.
[b]Industrial Chemical.
[c]By-products.

SOURCES: UNEP Global Environmental Facility, 2003;
IISD, 1998.

sources within the continental United States. Regulatory action has resulted
in a 77 percent decline in total dioxin and furan releases between 1987 and
1995 (US EPA, 2005) (for more information see also US EPA 1987, 1991,
1994, 1995). Overall, levels of dioxins and DLCs in the environment have
been declining for the past three decades. However, since dioxins are persistent compounds, they can be expected to remain in the environment and
the food supply for many years to come (IOM, 2003).

Toxic Equivalency Factors (TEFs) are a convenient method for assessing the toxicity of mixtures containing dioxins and DLCs but there are
uncertainties associated with calculating TEF values for individual congeners because of variability in their half-lives and differences in toxicity
to humans. The reference compound for the TEF is the dioxin compound
2,3,7,8-tetrachlorodibenzo-*p*-dioxin (TCDD). WHO recommends a tolerable daily intake of DLCs and PCBs of 1–4 pg/TEQ/kg/day (IOM, 2003).
The US EPA has estimated 0.001 pg/kg/day of TCDD as the level associated
with a 1 in 1 million excess risk for human health effects from exposure to
DLCs and PCBs (IOM, 2003). The NRC committee on EPA's Exposure and

Human Health Reassessment of TCDD and Related Compounds (NRC, 2006) noted that the classification of DLCs as "carcinogenic to humans" vs. "likely to be carcinogenic to humans" is dependent on "the definition and interpretation of the specific criteria used for classification, with the explicit recognition that the true weight of evidence lies on a continuum with no bright line that easily distinguishes between these two categories."

Bioaccumulation of Dioxins in Seafood Exposure to dioxins and DLCs occurs when fish consume aquatic invertebrates that come in direct contact with dioxin particles that settle in sediment; through direct absorption through the gills; or by eating contaminated sediment, insects, and smaller fish (Evans, 1991). Because of their lipophilic character, dioxins and DLCs are distributed to fatty tissues in fish, including the liver and gonads. Muscle tissue is less contaminated, depending on the fat content of the muscle, which is likely to be greater in the older, larger, and oily fish.

Adverse Health Effects TCDD is used as the reference congener as a measure of toxicity for all dioxin-like compounds. Adverse health effects associated with exposure to dioxins have been identified in populations exposed through unintended industrial releases. One of the largest population exposures to TCDD occurred from an unintended industrial release in Seveso, Italy. Those who were exposed to the highest doses, primarily children, exhibited chloracne (Mocarelli et al., 1999), a severe skin disease with acne-like lesions that occur mainly on the face and upper body. Other adverse health outcomes included an increased risk for cancer. When compared to the nonexposed general population, the exposed population did not show an increased overall cancer mortality, but did have a significant excess mortality risk for esophageal cancer in males and bone cancer in females among those who were exposed to the lowest doses (Bertazzi et al., 1997). The US EPA (2000a) concluded that the cancer data on the Seveso population was difficult to interpret because of the small number of cases, exposure classification problems, and limited follow-up.

In 1997, the International Agency for Research on Cancer (IARC) placed TCDD in a Group I (agents with sufficient evidence of carcinogenicity for humans) designation, but weaknesses and inconsistencies among the positive studies published have made this designation controversial (Cole et al., 2003). The US EPA (2000a) considers TCDD to be a human carcinogen and other DLCs likely carcinogens, based on epidemiological and animal studies. Although epidemiological evidence alone does not support a causal relationship between dioxin exposure and cancer, US EPA (2000a) describes TCDD as a non-genotoxic carcinogen and a potent tumor promoter.

Polychlorinated Biphenyls

Polychlorinated biphenyls are also long-lived chlorinated aromatic compounds. They include over 200 chemical compounds in the form of oily fluids to heavier grease or waxy substances. Production of PCBs began in 1929, and the compounds were used as coolants and lubricants in transformers and other electrical equipment. Because of their noncombustible insulating characteristics, PCBs were used to reduce the flammability of materials used in schools, hospitals, factories, and office buildings. A variety of commercial products, including paints, plastics, newsprint, fluorescent light ballasts, and caulking materials contained PCBs until production was banned in the 1970s.

Local sources of PCBs may be more important than local sources of dioxins and DLCs for contamination of aquatic organisms. PCBs were legally widely discharged into rivers, streams, and open landfills between 1940 and the early 1970s. In 1976, the Toxic Substance Control Act (TSCA) was passed, calling for a ban on the manufacture, processing, distribution, and use of PCBs in all products in which the PCBs were not totally enclosed. The TSCA was based on three concerns: first, PCBs persist in the environment and resist biodegradation; second, a population-wide incident of human poisoning in Japan in 1968 was attributed to introduction of PCB-contaminated oil into a community; and third, in 1975 the CDC reported that, in rat experiments, oral gavage with Aroclor 1260 (a mixture of PCBs) caused liver cancer (Kimbrough et al., 1975). As a result of the TSCA, transformers and electrical capacitors that contained PCB compartments were sealed. Such transformers remain in place unless the seals leaked or were damaged, and by 1990, any PCB transformer within 30 meters of a commercial or public access building should have been replaced, registered, or provided with protection (US EPA, 1994).

Bioaccumulation of PCBs A significant correlation has been observed between blood PCB levels and the quantity of fish consumed by humans (Fein et al., 1984; Humpfrey, 1988; Jacobson et al., 1990; Smith and Gangolli, 2002). Bioaccumulation of dioxins and PCBs in the fatty tissues of food animals contributes to human body burdens through ingestion of animal fats in foods such as meat and full-fat dairy products. These foods are the largest contributors of dioxins and DLCs from the US food supply. The levels of dioxins, DLCs, and PCBs in seafood are generally greater than those in meat; however, actual exposure levels are far lower because of the lower consumption of fish among the general population (IOM, 2003). Fish oils that are used for supplements tend to have lower levels of dioxins, DLCs, and PCBs than fatty or oily fish as a result of processing methods that remove these compounds from the final product (Source: http://www.ocean-nutrition.com/inside.asp?cmPageID=158).

Adverse Health Effects An extensive experimental literature on rodent and nonhuman primate models demonstrates that prenatal exposure to PCBs can interfere with neurodevelopment (Rice, 2000; Faroon et al., 2001; Bowers et al., 2004; Nguon et al., 2005). This literature is complemented by numerous prospective epidemiological studies of children conducted in Michigan; North Carolina; Oswego, NY; Germany; Faroe Islands; and the Netherlands (Schantz et al., 2003). The cohorts were often chosen to include children born to women who consumed fish from waters known to be contaminated with PCBs. The results of these epidemiological studies are generally congruent with those using animal models, although, as in most areas of observational research in humans, results are not always consistent across studies or consistent over time in a particular study.

Higher prenatal exposures have been associated with deficits in various functional domains including intelligence, attention, response inhibition, activity, and play behaviors (Jacobson and Jacobson, 1996; Patandin et al., 1999; Walkowiak et al., 2001; Vreugdenhil et al., 2002a,b; 2004; Jacobson and Jacobson, 2003; Stewart et al., 2003). However, there are some uncertainties about many key issues. One issue is the shape of the dose-effect relationship curve and, specifically, whether a threshold exists. A second is whether PCB exposure leading to adverse effects occurs prenatally or postnatally. Although most of the focus has been on prenatal exposures, some recent studies suggest that early postnatal exposures are also associated with neurotoxicities (Huisman et al., 1995; Walkowiak et al., 2001; Winneke et al., 2002). A third issue is the relative potency of the different congeners. For some neurodevelopmental outcomes, it is exposure to the dioxin-like congeners that is most strongly associated with deficits. A fourth issue is the impact of synergism between PCBs and other toxicants. Some studies suggest that adverse effects arise only when PCB exposure occurs in the presence of methylmercury or in environments in which individuals may be exposed to increased levels or multiple exposures (Grandjean et al., 2001; Roegge et al., 2004; Roegge and Schantz, 2006).

The PCB exposures identified in these study samples were considerably greater than those of the general US population. The median concentration of PCB 153 in the 10 studies, the only basis for direct comparison, ranged from 30 to 450 ng/g serum lipid, and the median of the 10 medians was 110 ng/g. The exposure levels in the two recent US studies were about one-third of those in the four earlier US studies or recent Dutch, German, and northern Québec studies (Longneker et al., 2003), consistent with exposure surveys indicating that PCB levels in human tissues in the United States have declined in recent decades (Sjodin et al., 2004a). In the most recent

Centers for Disease Control and Prevention (CDC) National Report of Human Exposure to Environmental Chemicals, the 95th percentile of the distribution of PCB 153 levels in the US population was 126 ng/g serum lipid (CDC, 2005d).

Animal studies carried out by CDC suggest that it is likely cancer risks were overstated and animal-specific. PCBs have been associated with health effects in laboratory animals, but typically at very high doses, possibly not relevant to noncatastrophic exposure for humans. Similar conclusions have been derived from looking at animal studies of exposure to high levels of PCBs resulting in tumor formation. Although there is evidence to substantiate PCB-associated health problems, several epidemiological studies of occupational workers exposed to PCBs found no evidence of ill health associated with their exposure. Even the PCB-chloracne association may be due to co-exposure to DLCs, and there is concern that multiple confounding factors make it difficult to interpret epidemiological studies in the workplace. Some studies of PCB workers found increases in rare liver cancers and malignant melanoma (US EPA, 2006). Thus, the US EPA found that the epidemiological studies are inconclusive; based on animal and recent human studies, PCBs are probable human carcinogens.

The earliest reported incidents of adverse effects from PCB poisoning occurred in Japan and Taiwan following widespread consumption of contaminated rice oil. The high-level exposure to PCBs resulted in skin lesions (acneform dermatitis) and peripheral nerve damage among adults, and similar effects among their offspring. Children born to exposed mothers also showed inhibition of growth and tissue maintenance (Kimbrough, 1987; Erickson, 1997). NRC (1999) also identified low birth weight and shorter gestation, and both neurological and neuromuscular deficits as adverse outcomes associated with prenatal PCB exposure.

Reports from occupational exposure to PCBs have identified several subclinical adverse health effects. The US EPA reviewed and identified many potentially serious noncancer adverse health effects associated with PCB exposure. These adverse effects included impairment of immune, reproductive, and neurological systems. The long-term impact of low-level exposure to PCBs is unclear, particularly on the endocrine system (US EPA, 2006) and will require further research to understand.

As PCB exposure levels continue to decline subsequent to federal laws banning PCB production, it may be difficult to characterize adverse health effects from low-level exposure (WHO Consultation on Risk Assessment of Non-Dioxin-Like PCBs, 2001; Ross, 2004) and to determine the significance of these exposure levels to health outcomes among the general population. Advances in analytic techniques may enhance data gathering and analysis efforts and improve our understanding of risks associated with low-level

TABLE 4-3 TEF Values from WHO (1998)

Compound	TEF value[a]
2,3,7,8-TCDD	1
Octachlorodibenzo-p-dioxins	0.0001
1,2,3,4,6,7,8,9-octachlorodibenzofuran	0.0001
3,3',4,4'-tetrachlorobiphenyl (PCB 77)	0.0001

[a]TEF = Toxicity Equivalency Factor, a numerical index that is used to compare the toxicity of different congeners and substances.

SOURCE: Van den Berg et al., 1998.

exposure as well as the role of specific PCB congeners or classes of congeners in health outcomes (Schantz et al., 2003; Ulbrick and Stahlmann, 2004).

Toxicity and Recommended Intake Limits for Dioxins, DLCs, and PCBs

Toxicity and Estimates of Risk The biological activity of dioxins, DLCs, and PCBs varies due to differences in toxicity and half-life of the various congeners. Variations in toxicity among congeners are related to a number of factors, including binding interaction at the cellular level with the arylhydrocarbon receptor (AhR) and variability in pharmacokinetics in vivo. Not all factors apply to all congeners; for example, many PCBs that do not have dioxin-like characteristics do not bind to the AhR. Van den Berg et al. (1998) describes factors used to determine the TEF values for dioxins, DLCs, and PCBs that include (but are not universal to all congeners):

- Structural relationships between congeners;
- Binding to the AhR;
- Toxic responses mediated through AhR activation; and
- Persistence and bioaccumulation.

The TEF value expresses the activity or toxicity of a specific congener relative to the toxicity of reference congeners, 2,3,7,8-TCDD; it is assigned a TEF of 1 and the toxicity of other congeners is expressed relative to TCDD (Van den Berg et al., 1998; IOM, 2003; SACN, 2004). Examples of some TEF values established by WHO are shown in Table 4-3. Toxicity can be additive in a mixture of congeners and so the Toxicity Equivalency (TEQ) of a mixture of DLCs is calculated by multiplying the concentration of each congener by its TEF, and summing across all DLCs in the mixture.

The Toxic Equivalency system is difficult to use, but it does permit extrapolation from 2,3,7,8-TCDD, a congener for which much is known.

WHO has recommended a Tolerable Daily Intake (TDI) of 1–4 pg/kg body weight per day for TCDD, and the TDI is applied to mixtures of dioxins and PCBs (IOM, 2003). Based on its estimate of cancer potency for DLCs, the US EPA concludes that intakes should not exceed 1–4 pg TEQ/kg/day in the general population (IOM, 2003).

DLC Exposure Limits in Foods With the exception of Canada and the United States, most countries utilize the TDI for assessing adverse health effects from exposure to DLCs and for setting acceptable limits in foods. The TDI represents an index for a contaminant similar to the adequate dietary intake (ADI) used for food additives. These limits are based on the assumption of an experimental threshold dose level below which no toxic effect is found in animal models, and include an additional uncertainty factor for extrapolation to humans.

The FDA and US EPA utilize probabilistic models to derive a Risk Specific Dose (RsD) for a contaminant. This model assumes the lowest dose that could result in a specific risk to humans, i.e., the dose with a lifetime cancer risk of 1 in 1 million. The use of the RfD, as previously described for methylmercury, was not applied to DLCs by the US EPA in its Draft Reassessment; the margins of exposure in the range of 100–1000 are generally considered inadequate to rule out the likelihood of significant effects occurring in humans, based on sensitive animal responses within the TEQ (US EPA, 1994; Foran et al., 2005a). Guidance on the development of risk-based meal consumption limits for 25 high-priority contaminants and analytes has been described by the US EPA (US EPA, 2000b). As described by the US EPA, a cancer slope factor (CSF) for carcinogenic risk can be calculated for DLC exposure of 1×10^{-3}/pg TEQ/kg/day (US EPA, 2000c). These risks are described later for analyzing benefits and risks associated with consuming farmed salmon (Foran et al., 2005b).

Exposure to DLCs from Seafood In 2002, the IOM Committee on the Implications of Dioxin in the Food Supply commissioned an exposure estimate for DLCs using intake estimates from the Continuing Survey of Food Intake by Individuals (CSFII) imputed to data from the FDA's Total Diet Study (Source: http://www.cfsan.fda.gov/~lrd/dioxdata.html). This analysis estimated that for all males and females in the general population, 1 year of age and older, the percentage contribution of fish and fish mixtures to the total DLC exposure from all foods was approximately 8 percent (IOM, 2003). When the data was analyzed for specific subgroups within the general population, the estimated contribution from fish and fish mixtures for pregnant and lactating women and for children (both males and females) aged 1 to 5 years was approximately 4 percent. By comparison, the estimated contribution of meat and meat mixtures to the total DLC exposure for these groups was approximately 37 and 35 percent, respectively, for pregnant and lactating women compared to children aged 1–5 years (IOM, 2003).

Polybrominated Diphenyl Ethers

Polybrominated diphenyl ethers (PBDEs) are synthetic compounds that are added to a variety of materials to increase their fire resistance. PBDEs are structurally similar to PCBs, and can exist, theoretically, as 209 distinct isomers. PBDEs are released into the environment as emissions from facilities manufacturing them and as a result of degradation, recycling, or disposal of products that contain them. The patterns of use of PBDEs are changing rapidly.

Bioaccumulation of PBDEs As with other persistent organic pollutants, PBDEs are cycled globally (de Wit et al., 2004). PBDE levels in aquatic wildlife have increased rapidly in recent decades (Ikonomou et al., 2002; Law et al., 2003), with doubling times of between 1.6 years and 6.0 years (Lunder and Sharp, 2003; Rayne et al., 2003; Hites et al., 2004a). PBDE tissue (blood, milk, and adipose) levels in humans have followed a time course similar to that in wildlife. The concentrations in human milk samples in Sweden, British Columbia, and the United States have increased manyfold over recent decades (Darnerud et al., 2001; Ryan et al., 2002; Hites, 2004; Sjodin et al., 2004a; Schecter et al., 2005), with doubling times of 10 years or less (Meironyte et al., 1999; Ryan et al., 2002). For reasons that are not known, the concentrations of PBDEs in biological tissues collected in North America are at least 10 times greater than those collected in Europe or Japan (Peele, 2004). Although ingestion is considered to be an important route of exposure to PBDEs, the importance of other routes, such as indoor air and dust, are poorly characterized and could be important in certain settings (Sjodin et al., 2004b).

Although the concentrations of PBDEs have been found to vary widely across countries, market basket surveys, total diet studies, duplicate diet studies, and commodity-specific surveys have repeatedly shown that, within a region, fish and shellfish tend to have PBDE concentrations that are greater than those found in dairy products, eggs, fats, and oils, and other meat products are important sources of exposure to PBDEs. This has been found in Canada, Finland, Germany, Japan, the Netherlands, Sweden, and the United States. In terms of total intake of PBDEs, fish and shellfish are the major contributors in Europe and Japan, while meats and poultry are the major contributors in the United States and Canada (FAO/WHO JECFA, 2005). The PBDE concentration tends to be greater in fish at higher trophic levels, i.e., predatory fish (Rice, 2005). In a market basket survey conducted in Dallas, Texas (Schecter et al., 2004), the highest levels of total PBDEs were found in samples of salmon, catfish, and shark. It is notable that the congener pattern was highly variable across samples, even within types (e.g., catfish), perhaps reflecting site specificity in the magnitude and nature of the problem of PBDE contamination. Total PBDE levels were also greater in meats with relatively high fat content, such as pork sausage, hot dogs, and duck; and in dairy products with higher fat content, such as cheese and butter (Schecter et al., 2004). Similar findings were reported in a market basket survey of foods conducted in California (Luksemburg et al., 2004), in which the highest PBDE levels were found in swordfish, Alaskan halibut, and Atlantic salmon. PBDE levels were 15 times greater in Pacific farm-raised salmon than in Pacific wild salmon (Easton et al., 2002). PBDE levels are higher in salmon farmed in the United States and Europe than in Chile (Hites et al., 2004a). Limited data are available, however, on the association between seafood consumption and PBDE levels in human tissues. In a small study of 94 urban anglers in the New York–New Jersey area, greater consumption of locally caught fish was not significantly related to blood PBDE levels, suggesting that, at least at this time and in this study population, consumption of local fish is not a major route of exposure to PBDEs (Moreland et al., 2005).

Adverse Health Effects The data available on the toxicity of PBDEs are extremely limited. Experimental animal studies indicate that PBDEs affect the nervous (Viberg et al., 2003), endocrine (Stocker et al., 2004), and immune systems (Fowles et al., 1994), and that the potency of PBDEs might be comparable to that of PCBs, although considerable uncertainty remains (Kodavanti and Ward, 2005). No population-based epidemiological studies have evaluated the human health effects of environmental exposure to PBDEs. It is not known whether all PBDEs share a common mechanism of action, complicating any effort to characterize toxicity using a toxic equivalence factor approach. In light of the fact that in vitro studies with purified PBDE congeners do not show AhR activation, it is possible that the presence of trace amounts of DLCs have confounded these assessments of PBDE toxicity (FAO/WHO JECFA, 2006). The FAO/WHO Joint Expert Committee on Food Additives and Contaminants concluded that the toxicological data available on PBDEs were insufficient to establish a Provisional Tolerable Weekly Intake (FAO/WHO JECFA, 2005). The data, however, are not sufficient to identify "no observed adverse effect levels" (NOAELs) for congeners of greatest interest, and thus to draw inferences about the prevalence of exposures of concern in the US population.

Levels of POPs in Seafood

Because of their lipophilic character, persistent organic pollutants are absorbed and transported to fatty tissues in fish and marine mammals. Uptake of POPs can occur through exposure from sediments in water or via consumption of smaller fish by predatory species (Geyer et al., 2000).

Farmed fish are exposed to these contaminants to the extent that they are present in feed (Hites et al., 2004a). Recently, Hites et al. (2004a) found that, perhaps because of their higher fat levels, some farmed salmon contain significantly higher concentrations of certain organochlorine contaminants, including PCBs, than wild-caught salmon. In addition, PCB concentrations in samples of commercial salmon feed purchased in Europe were higher than those in samples purchased in North and South America, suggesting that regional differences in the composition of feed contribute to regional differences in the PCB concentrations in farmed salmon. The mean wet weight concentration of PCBs in farmed salmon was 50 ng/g or below (Hites et al., 2004a), regardless of source, and thus below the Food and Drug Administration (FDA) action level of 2 ppm for PCBs in food. Using the US EPA risk assessment for PCB and cancer risk, Hites et al. (2004a) concluded that, given the PCB levels in the fish samples, a consumer's risk will not be increased if consumption is limited to no more than 1 meal per month of farmed salmon. Given the substantial regional differences found in PCB levels, however, these analyses demonstrated the importance for the consumer of knowing whether a fish was farmed or wild-caught and also its region of origin.

In a subsequent paper, the same group of investigators reported a quantitative analysis of competing risks and benefits associated with consuming farmed Atlantic and wild-caught Pacific salmon, for both cancer and noncancer end points (Foran et al., 2005b). Sixteen organic contaminants were considered. A benefit/cancer risk ratio was calculated for cancer using cancer slope factors developed by the US EPA (assuming that a 1×10^{-5} risk is acceptable) and a benefit/noncancer risk ratio using reference doses established by the US EPA. Foran et al. (2005b) concluded that neither farmed nor wild-caught salmon can be consumed in quantities that would provide 1 g/day of EPA/DHA while still maintaining an acceptable level of carcinogenic risk (1×10^{-5}). In contrast, they determined that based on the benefit/noncarcinogenic risk ratio, wild-caught salmon could be consumed in amounts consistent with EPA/DHA intake levels recommended by the American Heart Association (see Chapter 2).

As expected, however, the results differed for farmed and wild-caught salmon. Consuming farmed salmon in amounts that provides 1 g/day of EPA/DHA would produce a cumulative cancer risk that is 24 times the acceptable cancer risk level. For wild-caught salmon, the cumulative cancer risk would be eight times the acceptable level. Both farmed and wild-caught salmon could be consumed in amounts that provide at least 1 g/day of EPA/ DHA per unit of noncarcinogenic risk (Foran et al., 2005b).

These analyses were conducted assuming salmon intake needed to provide 1 g/day of EPA/DHA. The authors interpreted the WHO intake recommendation for omega-3 fatty acids as corresponding to 2–3 g/day; this includes alpha-linolenic acid (ALA) intake, which is derived primarily from plant sources such as soy, flaxseed, and walnut oils (see Chapter 1). The analysis of Foran et al. (2005b) was based on the assumption that the 2–3 g/day of omega-3 fatty acids applied only to EPA/DHA and did not take ALA into consideration. The WHO (2003) recommendation for fish consumption is 1–2 servings per week; it assumes that this level of consumption would provide 200–500 mg of EPA/DHA, considerably less than the intake of 1 g/day EPA/DHA from fish that Foran et al. assumed. These analyses represent a "worst case" scenario in that it is assumed that consumption of salmon would be the sole source of omega-3 fatty acids. Further, it assumed that salmon would provide all omega-3 fatty acids (DHA, EPA, and ALA) and salmon is not a source of ALA. Their analysis was based on data obtained prior to the implementation of industry safety measures for the prevention of POP contamination of aquaculture products (Santerre, 2004). It is worth emphasizing that because the food supply is dynamic, benefit-risk analyses are not static (Willett, 2006).

Body Burdens of POPs

Body burden can be defined as the total amount of a chemical in the human body or in human tissue from exposure to contaminants found in the environment (DeCaprio, 1997; Mendelsohn et al., 1998; IOM, 2003). CDC monitors over 200 contaminants with the aim of identifying baseline concentrations of specific substances and determining trends in body burdens among the general population (http://www.cdc.gov/biomonitoring/overview. htm; Kamrin, 2004). CDC reports (CDC, 2004; 2005b) include data on human exposure to approximately 150 compounds, including potential seafood contaminants such as lead, mercury, and many POPs. Technological advancements now afford the ability to detect minute levels of contaminants in human tissue, although detection of such contaminants does not indicate that a hazard or risk is present. For example, individuals regularly consuming fish from the Great Lakes were reported to have higher serum dichlorodiphenyl dichloroethene (DDE) concentrations (median 10 µg/L) compared to those who did not eat fish (1 µg/L); however, they did not show impaired motor function, impaired visuospatial function, or reduced memory and learning (Schantz et al., 1999; 2001; Rogan and Chen, 2005).

Body burdens for PCBs have been reviewed in studies of fish-consuming populations by the US EPA (US EPA, 2000a,c). The review did not show any cases among the general population of PCB exposure through fish consumption that exceeded the upper limit of background exposure, although it did find that consumers who had higher consumption levels of fish with typical PCDD/PCDF profiles than the general population may receive up to five times the mean intake exposure level of the general population (Armstrong, 2002). To illustrate, sport fishers living near an industrial release site in the United States had blood PCB levels (both dioxin-like and nondioxin-like congeners) three times higher than control groups eating fish from areas that were not highly contaminated (US EPA, 2000c).

Toxicological and epidemiological data suggests that the population does not necessarily incur adverse health effects from the majority of chemicals currently detected in biomonitoring programs (US EPA, 2005). Thus, biomonitoring measures the level of the contaminant in a biological sample, which is not used to correlate such data to toxicology studies in animals; rather, biomonitoring gives a picture of a person's body burden at one particular point in time, and it can be difficult to determine when the exposure might have occurred (Paustenbach and Galbraith, 2005). Biomonitoring measurements are relevant exposure assessment tools because they indicate body burden levels from all environmental sources (e.g., air, soil, water, dust, food) combined. The purpose of the CDC national biomonitoring programs is to determine which environmental chemicals are absorbed, measure exposure levels, assess health impacts of exposure on population groups (e.g., pregnant women and children), determine exposure risks among population groups, and monitor trends over time (Source: http://www.cdc.gov/biomonitoring/overview.htm). Research investigations may be utilized to identify specific sources of the elevated exposure and action to deal with the sources (Paustenbach and Galbraith, 2005).

Summary of Evidence

Evidence for specific adverse health effects associated with exposure to POPs is inconsistent. Among confounding factors related to this class of contaminant is the uncertainty that accompanies association of specific disease outcomes with low-level exposures. An issue of particular concern is the inability to determine a threshold for an adverse effect. Thus, the determination of toxicity related to exposure to POPs is challenging and requires further research.

INTERACTIONS BETWEEN NUTRIENTS AND
CONTAMINANTS IN SEAFOOD

Selenium and Seafood Contaminants

There are several distinct ways that selenium may influence the impact of toxicants, e.g., through hepatic and extrahepatic detoxification mechanisms, effects on oxidative stress, modulating the immune response, and some novel sequestering mechanism rendering toxicants, e.g., heavy metals, inactive.

As noted previously, mercury, i.e., elemental mercury (Hg), ionic mercury (Hg^+), and organic mercury (MeHg), may exist in three different states, and each state likely governs how selenium may interact with this element. MeHg has been implicated as a neurotoxicant, a mutagen, and a teratogen in various organisms. Epidemiological studies have been conducted on the exposure of humans to mercury through consumption of fish and marine mammals in different geographical areas including Seychelles, the Canadian North, the Amazon, Faroe Islands, Papua New Guinea, and Sweden. There are inconsistencies among these studies in the toxic dose, which may be due to differences in dietary patterns between the populations studied, e.g., more whale meat is consumed in Faroe Islands and more fish in Seychelles (Chapman and Chan, 2000) (see Box 4-1). Additionally, toxicity assessments were not conducted in all of the study locations and where they were the results may not be comparable in terms of populations examined and outcomes assessed.

Coexposure to selenium may diminish the toxic effects of some forms of mercury and other heavy metals, including cadmium and silver (Whanger, 1985). The mechanisms for these interactions are only partially understood but their occurrence certainly influences the determination of safe and toxic levels of such metals for persons in the general population. Selenium was first reported to counteract acute mercuric chloride toxicity by Parizek and Ostadalova (1967). Later, Ganther et al. (1972) showed the mitigating effect of sodium selenite on the toxicity of methylmercury. When selenite and mercuric chloride are co-adminstered, these elements react in the bloodstream forming complexes at an equimolar ratio. This reaction may explain the consistent equimolar ratio of selenium and mercury in tissues of seals and other marine mammals (Koeman et al., 1973; 1975) and mercury mine workers (Kosta et al., 1975). In nearly all marine fish sampled, the stoichiometric mercury-to-selenium ratio was less than 1. In contrast, freshwater fish accumulate mercury in such a way that the stoichiometric ratio was greater than 1 (Luten et al., 1980; Whanger, 1985; Cuvin-Aralar and Furness, 1991; Ikemoto et al., 2004). Despite extremely high values for mercury and selenium, sea fish are protected against toxicity of either element. It is interesting to note that adding selenium to lakes contaminated with mercury has been shown to be an effective remediation process (Paulsson and Lundbergh, 1989).

Selenide has one of the highest known mercury binding constants and will avidly partner with mercury (Whanger, 1985). Therefore, if dietary or tissue selenium is limited, selenide will be bound by mercury resulting in a lack of selenocysteine for incorporation into vital selenoproteins. The sequestered complex of mercury-selenium is highly insoluble and can be localized in lysosomes. Such sequestered material seems to be an inconsequential accumulation, with no toxicity to the animal.

It should be noted that ocean fish, though not lake fish, are a rich source of selenium. The US Department of Agriculture (USDA) ranked fish sources as 16 of the top 25 (out of a total of 1100) selenium-containing foods (USDA, Release 18. It has been suggested that the differences in mercury toxicity found in the Faroe Islands study compared to the Seychelles study may be due to the fact that mothers in the Faroe Islands ate whale meat, which is low in selenium, while mothers in the Seychelles studies ate seafood, which is rich in selenium (Ralston, 2005). This hypothesis is likely too simplistic, however, given that the Faroese also consume large amounts of seafood other than pilot whale.

Overall, selenium in the form of selenide is pivotal with regards to forming key selenoproteins and interacting with various heavy metals, such as mercury, to form a sequestered inert complex of mercury and selenocompounds, i.e., bis(methylmercuric)selenide (BMS) (Yoneda and Suzuki, 1997; Watanabe, 2002). MeHg might be acting as a methyl donor, thereby sparing the amount of S-adenosylmethionine (SAM) required for methylation. The net effect would be demethylation of MeHg by selenide, which then could lead to other interactions between selenide molecules and newly formed ionic Hg (Gregus et al., 2001; Watanabe 2002). Evidence suggests that the two elements interact with protein through basic amino acids in the molecule and also that the protein may be one of the heparin-binding proteins (Yoneda and Suzuki, 1997).

RISKS ASSOCIATED WITH MORE ACUTE SEAFOODBORNE HAZARDS

Microbiological Hazards

The best measures of seafood safety in the United States are based on illness reports compiled by the CDC (Source: http://cdc.gov/foodnet/) and the respective epidemiology programs in each state. Complementary lists of seafoodborne illness were also compiled by the Center for Science in the Public Interest (CSPI) (DeWaal and Barlow, 2004). Although these data are compromised by limited reporting and a large portion of unidentified etiological agents or nonspecific food vehicles, they remain the best measures of causes and trends in seafoodborne illnesses.

CDC estimates during the years prior to 1980 with less informative reporting suggested approximately 11 percent of all foodborne outbreaks (an outbreak involves two or more cases from a common source) implicated fish, mollusks, or crustaceans as the food vehicle (Bryan, 1980). Compilations of CDC data from 1978–1987 indicated fish and shellfish constituted only 10.5 percent of foodborne outbreaks and 3.6 percent of total cases (IOM, 1991). Estimates from the same data indicated "both [the percentage of] people made ill from beef (4) and turkey (3.7) exceeded total illnesses from seafood (3.5), whereas pork (2.7) and chicken (2.6) were each slightly lower. When shellfish (2.3 percent) and fish (1.2 percent) were considered separately, the number of reported cases from each was lower than for any other animal meat category" (IOM, 1991). These comparisons did not adjust for per capita consumption. FAO's compilation of CDC's data indicated that the number of cases remained higher for shellfish, but that outbreaks for fish, of which 90 percent could be linked to the cause, are more common (Huss et al., 2004). The association between exposure and illness is considered higher for seafood than for other foods due to the early onset of symptoms and the particular symptoms per types of seafood. This situation reinforces reporting of seafoodborne illnesses. Table 4-4 summarizes commonly encountered hazards and risks associated with classes of seafood consumed in the United States, and systems in place to control or minimize potential exposure risks.

Estimating Frequency of Seafoodborne Illnesses

CDC estimates for foodborne illnesses (76 million/year) and related deaths (5000/year) (Mead et al., 1999) indicated that the number of cases were reduced by 6.2 and 44.4 percent, respectively, from previous estimates from Archer and Kvenberg (1985), which were based on foodborne diarrheal diseases alone. These reports did not include any specific references to seafood other than data involving various food-related *Vibrio* infections. Although *Vibrio*-related illnesses are not a CDC-reportable disease and therefore may be underreported, Mead et al. (1999) included cases and outbreaks involving *Vibrios*, which frequently implicate seafood, particularly raw molluscan shellfish, as a likely vehicle. This study accounted for underreporting of foodborne illnesses through the use of multipliers (see Table 4-5). The less serious an illness experienced by an individual, the less likely they are to seek medical attention and thus minor illnesses are less likely to be reported. A low multiplier is needed to accurately depict the actual number of cases of a serious illness, such as those associated with *Vibrio vulnificus*.

Huss et al. (2004) compiled data from CSPI indicating consumption of molluscan shellfish caused the highest percentage of seafoodborne cases (individual illnesses) during 1990–1998, but the primary causative agent was reported in the collective category for noroviruses (see Table 4-6). The general norovirus category accounted for the large majority of seafoodborne outbreaks reported by CSPI (DeWaal and Barlow, 2004) from their survey of reported illness during 1990–2003. The most recent CDC report (2005a) suggested the incidence of infections involving *Vibrio* bacteria has been increasing (Figure 4-4), using the estimated number of total incidences based on laboratory-confirmed infections divided by the population estimates. The extent of the estimated affected population was equated to 15.2 percent of the US population. This report did not distinguish the *Vibrio* species or food vehicles involved, but it did suggest some of the *Vibrio* infections may have resulted from nonfoodborne sources, e.g., previous wounds.

With the exception of concerns for *Vibrio* and Norovirus infections, in general, the CDC report (2005a) does not reflect an increase in seafoodborne illnesses, particularly of microbial origin (most commonly associated with consumption of raw molluscan shellfish). Figures reported by CDC (2005a) are imprecise due to inclusion of other nonfoodborne causes and changes in state reporting. Since 1988, CDC has maintained only a voluntary *Vibrio* surveillance system for culture-confirmed infections in the states contiguous to the Gulf of Mexico. In 1999, the Foodborne and Diarrheal Disease Branch of CDC encouraged all state epidemiology programs to improve *Vibrio* reporting and the Council for State and Territorial Epidemiologists has drafted a resolution calling for more mandatory reporting of *Vibrio*-related illnesses (Personal communication, K. Moore, Interstate Shellfish Sanitation Conference, November, 2005).

Reducing Risk of Seafoodborne Illness

Vibrio-Associated Illness The *Vibrio* family of bacteria are indigenous to most coastal environments; the particular types and amounts present are influenced by salinity and water temperature (IOM, 1991). Filter-feeding animals, e.g., oysters, will take up chemical and microbial flora, including *Vibrios*, in their immediate environment. The two species of concern are *Vibrio vulnificus* (Vv) and *Vibrio parahaemolyticus (Vp)*. Like the related *Vibrio* cholera species, Vv and Vp can live in warm seawater and have been isolated from oysters, clams, crabs, and finfish. In contrast, Vv can cause serious illness (wound infections, gastroenteritis, or a syndrome known as "primary septicemia") and death in persons with pre-existing liver disease or compromised immune systems while Vp typically causes less severe illness. Vp can infect healthy consumers yet severe disease is rare.

TABLE 4-4 Current Seafood Safety Hazards, Controls, and Risks

Hazardous Seafood[a]	Hazard[b]	Severity to Consumers	Occurrence and Trend
Raw bivalve mollusks (oysters, clams, mussels)	(1) Viruses, enteric bacteria (2) *Vibrio vulnificus* (3) *Vibrio parahaemolyticus*	(1&3) Mostly mild gastroenteritis; certain types and serotypes can be more harmful for very few consumers (2) Severe for "at-risk" consumers[c]	(1) Random by location and time; improper water classification; recreational harvests (2) Rare yet persistent; primarily warm-water products involving at-risk consumers (3) Sporadic; may be increasing
Natural toxins Finfish (1&2) Mollusk (3)	(1) Ciguatera (2) Scombroid poisoning (3) PSP, NSP, DSP, ASP	(1) Moderate to severe and reported prolonged symptoms in some cases (2) Mild and short duration (3) Mild to severe relative to toxin type	(1) Limited to certain fish species from certain areas; could increase with more imports (2) Limited but persistent for certain species subject to thermal abuse; could increase with more imports (3) Rare but can be very serious; could increase with global warming and related environmental changes
Processed seafood	(1) *Salmonella* (2) *Listeria monocytogenes* (3) *C. perfringens* (4) *C. botulinum* (5) *Shigella* (6) *Staphylococcus aureus* (7) HAV and NLV	Usually mild; can be severe to very severe for (2) and (4), respectively, yet occurrence very rare	Very limited and decreasing; more prevalent in ready-to-eat items; could increase with more and certain imports
Allergies	Host specific	Host specific; can be mild to severe	Seafood ranked in top four food allergies; could increase for pre-formulated, value-added products

NOTE: PSP = paralytic shellfish poisoning; NSP = neurotoxic poisoning; DSP = diarrhetic shellfish poisoning; ASP = amnesic shellfish poisoning; HAV = hepatitis A virus; NLV = Norwalk-like viruses (Noroviruses) spp.

[a]Fish or shellfish, the consumption of which can lead to disease. Ranked in order of concern per occurrence and risk.

Risk to Consumers	Facts Enhancing Risk	Factors Reducing Risk
High for consumers' preferred raw mollusks; particular concern for at-risk consumers	(1) Unapproved waters, improper harvest water classifications; recreational harvest disregards advice (2) Natural occurrence and host factors (3) Post-harvest temperature abuse	(1) Approved waters; revised indicator programs (2&3); cooking; rapid and continued cooling; Post Harvest Processing (PHP) methods to reduce number of organisms; thermal mapping of harvest areas; consumer education
(1) Higher in endemic areas for certain fish species; recreational harvest and illegal sales (2) High for consumption of few species; more common for certain imported species (3) High if harvest is uncontrolled or recreational interest disregards advice	(1) Commercial and recreational harvest from specific areas for certain fish, i.e., reef species; no recognized screening methods; problematic species identified (2) Temperature abuse after capture of certain fish species; no practical screening methods (3) Lack of harvest controls; recreational shellfish harvest	(1) Restrict harvest and consumption of certain fish from certain areas; designate approved fish and harvest areas; restrict recreational sales (2) Temperature controls and monitoring for histamines; harvester education; screening for imports and suspect fish (3) Regional water and product monitoring programs; consumer education
Low when adequate cooking precedes consumption	Cross-contamination; temperature abuse; processing errors; mishandling by retail sections, restaurants, and consumers	Adequate cooking; temperature controls; proper processing and food service; proper satisfaction; consumer education; use of polymerase chain reaction-based detection for viruses
Moderate without proper labeling and product identification	Formulated products with seafood ingredients; mislabeling; cross-cooking	Proper seafood identification; cleaning and sanitizing of equipment to avoid cross-contamination

[b]An organism, substance, or condition having the potential to cause disease.

[c]At-risk consumers include consumers with pre-existing health conditions, e.g., immuno-compromised, that place the consumer in a predisposed category for seafoodborne illnesses.

SOURCE: Revised from IOM, 1991.

TABLE 4-5 Multipliers Used by CDC to Estimate Total Cases for Different Foodborne Bacterial Illnesses Based on Actual Reported Cases

Agent Causing Illness	Multiplier for Estimated Cases
Campylobacteria	38
Clostridium perfringens	
Salmonella, nontyphoidal	
Staphylococcus aureus	
E. coli O157:H7	20
Shigella	
Vibrio, other spp.	
Bacillus cereus	10
Clostridium botulinum	2
Salmonella typhi	
Vibrio cholerae, toxigenic	
Vibrio vulnificus	

SOURCES: Derived from Mead et al., 1999; 2006.

TABLE 4-6 Seafoodborne Diseases Traced to "Molluscan Shellfish" in the United States from 1990 to 1998, and Outbreaks and Cases for Which the Etiological Agent Has Been Identified

Agent	Outbreaks		Cases	
	Total	Percent	Total	Percent
V. parahaemolytics	18	27	733	22
Noro-/Norwalk-like virus[a]	15	23	2175	66
PSP/toxin	14	20	92	3
Salmonella	6	9	183	6
Scombroid	2	3	4	—
Ciguatera	3	5	5	—
Shigella	2	3	17	0.5
Campylobacter	2	3	6	—
V. vulnificus	1	—	2	—
V. alginolyticus	1	—	4	—
C. perfringens	1	—	57	2
Giardia	1	—	3	—
Total	66	93	3281	100

[a]Norovirus was recently approved as the official genus name for the group of viruses provisionally described as "Norwalk-like viruses" (NLV) (http://www.cdc.gov/ncidod/dvrd/revb/gastro/norovirus.htm).

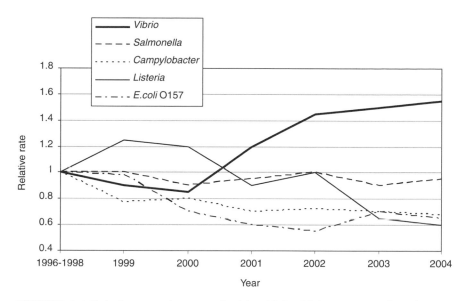

FIGURE 4-4 Relative rates (compared with 1996) of laboratory-confirmed cases of *Yersinia, Escherichia coli* O157, *Campylobacter*, and *Salmonella*, by year; from Foodborne Diseases Active Surveillance Network, United States, 1996–2004. SOURCE: CDC, 2005a.

More detailed assessment of the *Vibrio* illnesses from seafood can be found in state reports for *Vibrio vulnificus* (see Table 4-7). These reports provide more specific data for infections resulting from consumption of raw molluscan shellfish of commercial origin. With the exception of California, the majority of reported illnesses involve the oyster-producing regions about the Gulf of Mexico, due to the relative prevalence of *Vv* in warmer coastal waters. The number of *Vv* illnesses involving commercial shellfish harvests per year across all states reporting (32) during 1995–2004 averages less than one case per year (0.98 cases/year/state). The justification for the persistent concern about *Vv* stems from the potentially severe consequences for consumers in a higher risk category for infection (e.g., immunocompromised) for whom there may be as much as a 50 percent mortality rate (IOM, 1991; Hlady and Klontz, 1996).

California, Florida, Louisiana, and Texas represent "core states" designated in a *Vv* management plan designed by FDA through cooperation with the Interstate Shellfish Sanitation Conference (ISSC, 2002) to reduce *Vv* illnesses from raw oyster consumption (see Table 4-8). This plan was

TABLE 4-7 Individual Reported *Vibrio vulnificus* Cases of Illness Involving Commercial Oyster Products

State	1995	1996	1997	1998	1999	2000	2001	2002	2003	2004	Avg/Yr
CA	5	7	2	2	8	7	7	6	1		4.5
FL	8	5	6	14	12	5	11	5	12	8	8.6
LA	2	2	1	7	2	1	4	1	1	2	2.3
TX	1	8	7	2	6	9	7	5	6	3	5.4
AL	4	2	1	3		1	1		2	2	1.6
AR	1	1	1			1	1				0.5
AZ	1			2			1	1			0.5
CO										2	0.2
CT						1					0.1
GA	2	3		4	1	1	6	5	5	3	3.0
IL					1		1				0.2
IN									1		0.1
KY				1	1						0.2
MD								2		2	0.4
ME								1			0.1
MI					1					1	0.2
MO	1					1		1			0.2
MS		1	1								0.2
NC		1	2	1	1			1		1	0.7
NJ										1	0.1
NM									1	1	0.2
NV				1	1						0.2
NY		1								1	0.2
OH						1				2	0.3
OK				1				1		1	0.3
OR								1			0.1
PA					1						0.1
SC		4						3		2	0.9
TN	1							1	2		0.4
VA			1		1			1	2		0.5
VI				1		1					0.2
WI							1				0.1
Totals	26	33	21	41	36	30	40	35	33	32	
Avg/state/year											0.98

NOTE: A blank cell means no reported cases.
SOURCE: Personal communication, A.P. Rainosek, National Oceanographic and Atmospheric Administration Fisheries, National Seafood Inspection Laboratory, Pascagoula, MS, July 2005 (Data prepared for the Interstate Shellfish Sanitation Conference).

complemented with a formal risk assessment conducted for *Vv* (FAO/WHO, 2001). The plan includes specified industry performance goals for illness reduction rates and consequences if the goals are not attained.

Commercial operations have responded with post-harvest processing procedures such as high-pressure, low-temperature pasteurization and

TABLE 4-8 Abbreviated Table of Compliance for Core States as Specified in the ISSC's *Vibrio vulnificus* Management Plan

Deadline	Post-Harvest Treatments[a]	Illness Reductions[b]	Florida Example[c]
December 2004 2005–2006	25% capacity	40% (average)	9/year—baseline 5/year—goal
December 2006 2007–2008	50% capacity	60% (average)	4/year—goal
		If the 60 percent illness reduction rate is not collectively achieved by 2008, additional controls can be imposed, including harvest restrictions or closures relative to water temperatures and special labels designating product to be shucked by a certified oyster dealer.	

NOTE: Core states are California, Florida, Louisiana, and Texas.

[a]Post-harvest treatment "capacity will be based on all oysters intended for raw, half-shelled market during the months of May through September harvested from source states, to include the capacity of all operational plants and the capacity of plants under construction."

[b]Illness reductions will be based on the average illness rate for years 1995–1999 of 0.036/million persons, using data from California, Florida, Louisiana, and Texas. Adjustments in methodology can be adopted based on further review.

[c]The Florida example indicates the performance goals (total reported illnesses per year) that must be attained for compliance relative to the initial established baseline.

SOURCES: ISSC, 2001, 2002, 2003b.

"frosting" methods to kill *Vv* in the oysters as part of the illness reduction efforts. FDA (2005a) has recently approved the use of irradiation as another post-harvest processing option.

This risk management plan also includes recommendations for a public education component including programs targeting consumers of raw oysters, both those with and those without health conditions that increase their risk of *Vv* infection. In the states that were required to develop risk-management plans, Flattery and Bashin (2003) conducted a survey to elicit new information about media exposure, attitudes, and consumption behavior from consumers of raw oysters. They found that (1) generally, consumer awareness of who should avoid consuming raw oysters is limited; (2) many at-risk consumers are already taking some actions, albeit ineffective, to avoid illness; (3) one in three consumers are eating raw oysters less frequently. International Conference on Emerging Infections and Diseases (2006) also reported a decline in "risky food consumption." This survey response showed a decline of one-third in the number of individuals who reported consuming foods, including raw oysters, associated with a higher risk for foodborne disease.

Flattery and Bashin (2003) determined that to increase the effectiveness of the educational component of the plan, key messages should identify at-risk consumers; communicate effective action to prevent illness (i.e., refrain from eating raw oysters); and address popular myths about preventing illness.

It may be difficult to determine precisely the reduction in illnesses achieved because of the large standard deviation about the annual mean (the average illness rate for 1995–1999 of 0.036/million persons, based on data from California, Florida, Louisiana, and Texas) reported by ISSC (2001, 2002). At present, the number of *Vibrio* illnesses reported annually is small. For example, in Florida the 40 and 60 percent illness reduction goals represent a drop in reported illnesses from nine/year to five/year by 2006, and to four/year by 2008 (see Table 4-8 and Table 4-9). The recent increase in reporting from states that had not previously monitored *Vibrio* illnesses shows that national trends for reported illnesses are similar to those for the core states.

Management plans are also being considered to address illnesses due to *Vibrio parahaemolyticus (Vp)* from raw shellfish. Illnesses resulting from this source are less severe than for *Vv*, but occurrence is not confined to at-risk consumers. Further, international occurrence of certain *Vp* strains suggests the possibility of a pandemic infection because these strains have been identified as deriving from a known pathogenic strain of *Vp* (Chowdjury et al., 2000). *Vp* is a leading cause of seafoodborne illnesses in Japan and eastern Asian countries noted for higher consumption of raw seafood.

Infections in the United States are more sporadic and have involved crabs, shrimp, and crayfish, with cross-contamination of raw and previously cooked product as a contributing factor, although raw oysters remain the primary vehicle for *Vp* infections. *Vp* elicited little response from the National Shellfish Sanitation Program (NSSP) prior to two major outbreaks in the Gulf Coast region in 1997 and 1998, some cases of which involved a previously unreported and more virulent serotype (03:K6) from Asia (FDA, 1999). Recent outbreaks of *Vp* have also occurred in the more temperate waters of the northwest United States and Canada (Fyfe et al., 1998; CDC, 2006a,b). Infection prevention is complicated by the ability of *Vp* to grow in the oysters after harvest, particularly in the absence of adequate temperature control. Preventive measures for *Vp* are similar to those for *Vv* and include cooking, post-harvest temperature controls, and consumer and processor education and processing innovations. In the absence of regulatory mandates the FDA offers voluntary guidance indicating that no more than 10,000 bacteria per gram of raw shellfish (FDA, 2001b) should be present.

Other Bacterial Hazards

In addition to *Vibrios*, a variety of potentially pathogenic bacteria have been associated with seafood safety risks, though actual occurrence is very

TABLE 4-9 Human Pathogens Associated with Seafood

Pathogens	Isolated from Seafoods	Proven Pathogen in Seafood	Pathogen Source[a]
Organisms That Can Cause Disease in Normal, Healthy Adults			
Bacteria			
Vibrio cholerae O1	Yes	Yes	1, 2
Vibrio chloerae non-O1[b]	Yes	Yes	1
Vibrio parahaemolyticus	Yes	Yes	1
Vibrio mimicus	Yes	Yes	1
Vibrio fluvialis	Yes	Yes	1
Vibrio furnissii	Yes	Yes	1
Vibrio hollisae	Yes	Yes	1
Salmonella typhi[c]	Yes	Yes	2, 3
Salmonella (nontyphoidal)	Yes	Yes	2, 3
Campylobacter jejuni	Yes	Yes	2, 3
Escherichia coli	Yes	No	2, 3
Yersinia enterocolitica	Yes	No	2, 3
Clostridium botulinum	Yes	Yes	2, 3
Shigella	Yes	Yes	2, 3
Staphylococcus aureus	Yes	Yes	3
Hekminths			
Anisakis simplex	Yes	Yes	1
Other helminths	Yes	Yes	1
Viruses			
Poliovirus	Yes	No	2
Other picornaviruses	Yes	No	2
Norwalk/Snow Mountain/small round viruses (SRVs)	No	Yes	2
Enteral non-A, non-B, hepatitis	No	Yes	2
Hepatitis A	Yes	Yes	2, 3
Organisms That Cause Disease Most Often in Special Population Groups			
Vibrio vulnificus[d]	Yes	Yes	1
Rotavirus[e]	Yes	No	2
Listeria	Yes	No	1, 3
Organisms with Uncertain Roles as Foodborne Pathogens			
Aeromonas hydrophila[f]	Yes	Yes	1
Plesiomonas shigelloides	Yes	Yes	1
Edwardsiella tarda	Yes	No	1

[a](1) Harvest water/associated with naturally occurring aquatic bacteria; (2) harvest water/associated with fecal pollution; (3) associated with processing and preparation (cross-contamination or time/temperature abuse, infected food handlers).

[b]Causes gastroenteritis in normal, healthy hosts; can cause septicemia in persons in high-risk groups.

[c]Primarily of historical association in the United States, but remains a problem in some foreign countries and could affect imports.

[d]Illness usually confined to high-risk groups.

[e]Illness generally occurs in children under the age of 2; older persons are usually immune.

[f]Aeromonas can cause serious wound infections and septicemia; however, conclusive data on its role as a cause of gastroenteritis are lacking. Studies suggesting that it is a gastrointestinal pathogen have not implicated seafood as a risk factor for illness.

SOURCE: IOM, 1991.

rare or not reported due to lack of severity of symptoms (see Table 4-9) (IOM, 1991). The two principle pathogens of concern are *Salmonella* spp. and *Listeria monocytogenes.*

Salmonella is a bacterium of widespread occurrence in animals, especially in poultry and swine. Environmental sources of the organism include water, soil, insects, factory and kitchen surfaces, animal feces, raw meats and poultry, and raw seafoods. *S. typhi* and the paratyphoid bacteria normally cause septicemia and produce typhoid or typhoid-like fever in humans. Other forms of salmonellosis generally produce milder symptoms (Source: http://www.cfsan.fda.gov/~mow/chap1.html).

Listeria monocyotogenes is a bacterium that can cause a serious infection in humans called listeriosis. Foodborne illness caused by *L. monocytogenes* in pregnant women can result in miscarriage, fetal death, and severe illness or death of a newborn infant. Others at risk for severe illness or death are older adults and those with weakened immune systems. *L. monocytogenes* can grow at refrigerator temperatures and is found in ready-to-eat foods (Source: http://www.cfsan.fda.gov/~dms/adlister.html 2003).

Federal regulation prohibits the sale of any raw or cooked seafood products contaminated with any *Salmonella*, or cooked, ready-to-eat seafood products contaminated with any *L. monocytogenes* (CFSAN, 2001) (see Appendix Table B-4). The zero tolerance policy for *Salmonella* on any seafood product is historically based on concerns for unsanitary practices that contaminated a food after harvest. The presence of any *Salmonella* on seafood from freshwater or saltwater harvests is considered an adulterant. Inland aquacultural production can expose farmed seafood to *Salmonella* from other animal sources including neighboring wildlife. Koonse et al. (2005) evaluated both product and environments (source water and grow-out pond water) from shrimp aquaculture across six countries, and found a significant association between the concentrations of *Salmonella* and both fecal coliforms and *E. coli*. Nevertheless, the occurrence of seafoodborne salmonellosis is rare. Reported cases are usually the result of cross-contamination or unsanitary handling practices (Koonse et al., 2005). Proper sanitation that includes adherence to Hazard Analysis and Critical Control Point (HACCP) regulatory requirements for daily sanitary monitoring and records plus cooking of seafood appear to be adequately controlling *Salmonella* in seafood.

Likewise, proper sanitary practices and cooking temperature remain the primary control points to prevent potential illnesses due to contamination from particular types and amounts of *L. monocytogenes* (*Lm*) that have been found on certain seafood products (Gombas et al., 2003). The most likely vehicle of transmission is previously cooked and ready-to-eat (RTE) seafood products with prolonged refrigerated storage that could allow further growth of these more cold-tolerant pathogens. The incidence of reported illnesses for *L. monocytogenes* for all foods significantly declined by 32 percent from 1996 to 2005 (CDC, 2006a), and there are few reports involving seafood products confirmed by CDC.

Regulatory control of *C. botulinum* includes processing for canned products, reduced oxygen packaging, smoking, fermenting, and pickling (FDA, 2001a). The *C. botulinum* is destroyed by heat processing. Botulinum poisoning is rare and usually involves previously cooked and ready-to-eat (RTE) products that have not been properly heat processed. Through 2004, there have been no documented cases of botulism from any fresh seafood product regardless of packaging (Austin and Smith, 2006) with one exception. This involved a whole fresh fish including uncooked viscera, prepared and consumed in Hawaii (CDC, 1991). None of the 19 incidences of botulism cited by Bryan (1980) involved fresh fish. In addition, the CDC (2005a) reported no incidences of *C. botulinum* for foodborne illnesses cited.

The remaining bacteria with proven pathogenicity in seafood have not posed any significant risk beyond occurrences and causes recognized with other foods. The controls for these hazards are similar in terms of sanitation, proper cooking, and proper refrigeration. They currently pose no unique trend in occurrences that suggest increased exposure risk through seafood consumption.

Viruses

There are a large number of seafoodborne illnesses of unknown etiology generally classified as norovirusal. Evidence is lacking due to limitations in the methodology for culturing and enumerating viruses; further identification is difficult. Current controls rely on monitoring of harvest waters used in production of molluscan shellfish intended for raw consumption (ISSC, 2003a). Water classification or approval protocols rely on indicators associated with the presence of viruses rather than actual measures for a particular virus. Contamination of water with human fecal matter on or near oyster beds has resulted in shellfishborne "Norwalk-like" viruses (NLV) and hepatitis A (HAV) infections in consumers of raw oysters harvested from the contaminated waters (Kohn et al., 1995).

Monitoring of water for indicators associated with the presence of viruses remains the primary control for products to be consumed raw because most new post-harvesting processing methods, including irradiation, used to reduce *Vv* in raw oysters have not been proven effective for reduction of viruses. Improvements in water classification programs may include advancing methodologies using PCR-based identification and monitoring for viruses in water and seafood products.

Parasites

Consumption of raw or undercooked seafood products that had not been previously frozen has been implicated in certain human parasitic infections. Table 4-10 lists the parasites and seafood choices that have been involved in previous documented illnesses. Incidence of parasitic infection is far more common in regions of the world where raw consumption is more frequent (Table 4-11). Seafoodborne infections are more prevalent in these regions than in the United States due to agricultural practices and reliance on freshwater sources that support the life cycle of certain hazardous parasites (Rodrick and Cheng, 1989; Sakanari et al., 1995). Since their adoption, HACCP programs, which include specific controls to prevent parasite infections, suggested incidence levels were underreported and expected to increase as consumer trends favored more consumption of raw selections (Jackson, 1975; Olson, 1986; McKerrow et al., 1988). The American Gastroenterological Association (AGA) surveyed approximately 30 percent (996 members) of the active AGA practitioners located in coastal states along the Pacific, Atlantic, and Gulf of Mexico, areas prone to parasite exposure (Personal communication, G. Hoskins, FDA Office of Seafood, December 2005). Survey respondents (over 58 percent) estimated

TABLE 4-10 Parasites and Products Involved in Documented Incidences of Parasitic Infection

Fishborne parasites involved in human infections resulting from consumption[a]	Some raw and undercooked seafood dishes involved in parasitic infections for products and recipes that are not previously frozen[b]

• Tapeworms (Cestodes)
  Diphyllobothrium latum
  Diphyllobothrium pacificum
	• Cold-smoked fish (low-temperature smoked fish)
	• *Ceviche* (raw fish in lime juice or other pickling)
	• "Drunken crabs" (crabs marinated in wine and pepper)
	• Dutch green herring (light pickled herring)

• Flukes (Trematodes)
  Clonorchis sinensis
  Opisthorchis viverrini
  Heterophyes heterophyes
  Metagonimus yokogawai
	• *Gravlax* (type of cold-smoked salmon)
	• Hawaiian *lomi lomi* (chopped raw salmon with bell peppers and tomatoes)
	• Japanese "salad" (raw fish, fresh lettuce, and soy sauce)
	• Pacific Island *poisson cru* (raw fish fillet in a coconut milk recipe)

• Roundworms (Nematodes)
  Gnathostoma spinigerum
  Capillaria philippinensis
  Anisakis simplex
  Phocanema spp.
	• *Palu* (fermented fish head and viscera recipe)
	• Philippine *bagoong* (a fermented paste made from whole fish)
	• Sashimi (raw fish slices)
	• Sushi (raw seafood with rice and seaweed)
	• *Tako poki* (Japanese and Hawaiian raw squid or raw octopus dish)

SOURCES: [a]Higashi, 1985; FDA, 2001a; [b]Sakanari et al., 1995; FDA, 2001a.

TABLE 4-11 Estimated Annual Occurrence of Parasitic Infections Due to Consumption of Seafood, Based on Original Compilation by FDA

Parasite	Worldwide	USA	Source
Tapeworm	9,000,000	100,000	Bylund, 1982
Fluke	20,000,000	Relatively low	Rim, 1982
Roundworm	2000+	50	Higashi, 1985

SOURCE: As referenced in FDA, 1987.

the number of cases over 24 months during 1998–2000 at 38 parasitic infections, of which 17 were anisikiasis, 16 were diphyllobothriasis, and 5 were pseudoterranoviasis. In the final report, the AGA estimated the actual number of infections would likely be 270 cases. This survey is considered one of the most current estimates for seafoodborne parasite infections in the United States but as a single survey, it is also considered underreporting. Nevertheless, seafoodborne parasitic infections are not common in the United States.

The guidelines for seafood processing and handling that accompanied the FDA mandate for HACCP regulations introduced additional specific controls to further prevent seafoodborne parasitic infections (FDA, 2001a). The FDA identified seafood species of concern (Table 4-12) and controls for HACCP program compliance (Table 4-13). Cooking and freezing had previously been reported as effective methods to kill parasites in order to

TABLE 4-12 Seafood Identified by the FDA that Could Involve Potential Parasite Hazards If Consumed Raw and Not Previously Frozen

Bass, Sea	Herrings	Rockfish	Trevally
Caplin	Hogfish	Sablefish	Trout
Cobia	Jacks	Salmon[a]	Tuna[b]
Cod	Kahawai	Scad	Turbot
Corvina	Mackerels	Sea trout	Wolffish
Eelpout	Monkfish	Snapper	
Flounders,[a] Sole,	Mullet	Sprat	Octopus
Dab, and Fluke	Perch, Ocean	Thorny head	Squid
Grouper	Plaice	Tomcod	
Halibut	Pollock	Tongue sole	Snails

NOTES: The general market names can include numerous species from various locations. The original sources should be referenced for actual species identified.

[a]Includes wild and aquacultured sources if fresh fish or plankton used as feed.

[b]Only applies to small tuna species; excludes large tuna species such as the yellowfin, bigeye, bluefin, and albacore.

SOURCE: FDA, 2001a.

TABLE 4-13 FDA Recommended Controls to Reduce or Eliminate Potential Parasite Hazards from Seafood

Procedure	FDA Recommendation	Comment
Parasite Removal	Trimming away of suspect and identified portions and/or portions identified with candling	Not recommended as sole preventive method
Cooking	Heating of raw fish sufficient to kill bacterial pathogens	FDA Food Code (2005e) definition for cooked seafood is an internal product temperature of 145°F for 15 seconds
Freezing	Freezing and storing at –4°F or below for 7 days or freezing at –31°F or below until solid and storing at –31°F or below for 15 hours, or freezing at –31°F or below until solid and storing at –4°F or below for 24 hours	FDA's Food Code recommends these freezing conditions to retailers who provide fish intended for raw consumption

SOURCE: FDA, 2001a, International Food Safety Council (http://www.foodsafety.gov/~dms/sept/99-week1.html).

prevent infections (Bier, 1976; Deardorff and Throm, 1988; FDA, 2001a). The current HACCP program requires freezing for certain species intended for commercial use as sushi and related raw seafood products (FDA, 2001a). Given the widespread adoption of HACCP and infrequent incidence of reported infections, concern about parasitic infection may not be deterring consumers from raw seafood consumption. Consumers may still choose to consume raw seafood products that have not been frozen previously.

Naturally Occurring Toxins

Ciguatera and Scombroid

Ciguatera and scombrotoxin are the two most persistent seafoodborne toxicants (IOM, 1991). Ciguatoxins, acquired through the local environmental food chain prior to harvest, may involve a variety of toxins from certain dinoflagellates. Ciguatera arises in certain fish harvested from specific tropical to subtropical regions about South Florida, the Caribbean region, and Hawaii. Reports in Florida suggest there is no evidence for increasing incidence (Personal communication, R. Hammond, Florida Department of Health, Tallahassee, FL, December 2005) (see Table 4-14). These data do not distinguish harvest source, but they do identify the more probable species of concern. Occurrence involves recreational as well as commercial harvests. Risk of ciguatera may increase with illegal recreational sales (not subject to HACCP controls) and with increasing imports of certain fish from affected areas.

TABLE 4-14 Reported Incidences for Ciguatera and Scombroid in the United States and by Selected States

Years and Locations	Ciguatera		Scombroid Poisoning	
	Outbreaks	Cases	Outbreaks	Cases
1993–1997[a]	60 total	205 total	69 total	297 total
USA	Avg-12/year	Avg-41/year	Avg-14/year	Avg-59/year
1990–1998[b]				
Hawaii	73 total	260 total	46 total	287 total
	Avg-8/year	Avg-29/year	Avg 5/year	Avg-32/year
Florida	16 total	82 total	10 total	55 total
	Avg-2/year	Avg-9/year	Avg-1/year	Avg-6/year
Florida[c]				
1994	3	13	5	14
1995	2	4	6	55
1996	8	30	5	9
1997	9	30	4	11
1998	5	37	5	14
1999	5	21	5	19
2000	9	31	3	10
2001	5	27	8	20
2002	5	10	3	4
2003	3	5	6	35
	Avg-5 4/year	Avg-21/year	Avg-5.0/year	Avg-19/year

SOURCES: [a]Olson et al., 2000; [b]Huss et al., 2004; [c]Personal communication, R. Hammond, Florida Department of Health, Tallahassee, FL, December 2005.

Subsequent handling, storage, or cooking cannot substantially reduce the risk. The toxic dose and consumer susceptibility remain in question while regulatory controls simply call for avoidance of certain fish from suspect areas. Absence of testable material, errant recall, and consumer misnaming can confuse species identification in reported illnesses. Despite product claims for utility, there are no reliable test kits to screen for ciguatera due to limited specificity for the toxins (Hungerford, 2005). Species avoidance may be the best control to reduce the potential hazard (Lange et al., 1992; Lehane, 1999). Barracuda is a common culprit that should be avoided (Morton and Burklew, 1970). Federal regulations for controls of ciguatoxins advise against consumption of certain species, and avoidance of fish from harvest locations with prior evidence of occurrence (FDA, 2001a). This advice is compromised by lack of area designations, unpredictable changes in the local food chains, and fish migration. Future controls could involve species restrictions from designated areas.

Scombroid poisoning, also known as histamine poisoning, involves thermal abuse of certain fish resulting in elevated levels of histamine concentrations that can invoke allergic-type reactions in susceptible consumers of raw or cooked fish. Cooking does not diminish these toxins. The primary fish involved include tunas and mackerels from the *Scombridae* family of fish—thus the name—and related species mahi-mahi (*Coryphaena hippurus*), escolar (*Lepidocybium flavobrunneum*), and others. The common feature distinguishing these fish is a higher proportion of free amino acids, i.e., histidine, lysine, and ornithine, naturally occurring in the muscle tissue, which can be decarboxylated to histamine, cadaverine, and putrascine. This conversion is driven by temperatures that allow growth of certain bacteria to generate the decarboxylating enzymes. Although regulatory action levels for histamine content (<50 ppm) have been established to prevent illnesses, cadaverine and putrascine have the potential to cause illness even in the absence of histamine (FDA, 2001a). Inadequate cooling at the point of harvest is considered the primary problem, and subsequent abuse can increase the potential hazard. Temperature control from harvest until consumption is recommended by the FDA (2001a). In the United States, HACCP mandates thermal controls from harvest through processing; most illnesses which continue to appear involve recreational harvests and imports. The incidences of illness could increase as more supply of affected species is imported and the illegal sale of recreational fish is not addressed with pertinent enforcement.

Shellfish Toxins

Naturally occurring toxins that have been associated with illnesses resulting from the consumption of certain molluscan shellfish such as oysters, clams, and mussels harvested from locations with specific environmental conditions include:

- Paralytic Shellfish Poisoning (PSP)
- Neurotoxic Shellfish Poisoning (NSP)
- Diarrhetic Shellfish Poisoning (DSP)
- Amnesic Shellfish Poisoning (ASP)

The filter-feeding mollusks accumulate the toxins in their viscera from the waters harboring naturally occurring marine algae (phytoplankton) that produce the toxins. Occurrence has involved both domestic and imported marine mollusks from tropical and temperate waters, depending on the particular species of phytoplankton and water conditions. Recent international reports include a comprehensive assessment of the potential occurrences that warrant closer scrutiny of particular algal species in various locations (FAO/IOC/WHO, 2004).

Related illnesses are rare but poisoning from shellfish toxins can be severe and deadly. Cooking is not considered sufficient to control potential toxic levels in seafood (FDA, 2001a). Regulatory monitoring programs have been effective; but new toxins and plankton blooms are emerging world-wide, particularly in areas less subject to surveillance. Incidences of toxicity could increase without controls, although the likelihood for an outbreak is low. Appendix Table B-4 identifies tolerances and action levels set by federal agencies for potentially problematic products.

Chemotherapeutants

Most aquaculture operations depend on the use of various chemothera-peutants to control infectious diseases (FAO/NACA/WHO Study Group, 1999; FDA, 2001a). Aquaculture initially relied upon the same antimicro-bials employed for production of beef and poultry and other land-based farming. The resultant food safety concerns, as for land-based agriculture, include possible toxic residue in the edible portions, contributions to po-tential antibiotic-resistant diseases (for both animals and consumers), and concomitant issues involving environmental contamination. Although the volume of chemotherapeutants used in aquaculture is far less than for other medical practices and agricultural production, international aquacultural use with less scrutiny may increase. Product seizures due to the presence of chemotherapeutants in some imported farm-raised seafood have occurred. (Allshouse, 2003; http://www.fda.gov/ora/oasis/3/ora_oasis_i_16.html; http://www.fda.gov/ora/oasis/1/ora_oasis_i_16.html).

Compounds of concern have included chloramphenicol, nitrofurans, fluoroquinolone, malachite green, and others (Table 4-15). All of these an-timicrobial/antifungal agents have been used at some time for aquacultural production in the United States, prior to the implemention of restrictions by federal agencies (FDA, 2005f). The established level of controls is zero toler-

TABLE 4-15 Antimicrobial/Antifungal Agents Used at Some Time for Aquaculture Production in the United States

Illegal Antibiotic or Chemotherapeutant	Action Level Based on Detection Limit
Chloramphenicol	0.3 ppb
Nitrofurans	1.0 ppb
Malachite green	1.0 ppb
Fluoroquinolones	5.0 ppb
Quinolones (Oxolinic Acid, Flumequine)	10.0 ppb (oxolinic acid) and 20.0 ppb
Ivermectin	10.0 ppb
Oxytetracycline	2.0 ppm

NOTES: ppb = parts per billion; ppm = parts per million.
SOURCE: Personal communication, W. Jones, Food and Drug Administration, October 12, 2006.

ance, based on the most current limits for analytical detection (Hanekamp, 2003), which currently range in parts per billion (ppb) for residuals. Similar limits are in place in other developed nations that depend on seafood imports (Kulkarni, 2005).

The actual food safety risk resulting from the use of chemotherapeutants in aquaculture has been difficult to assess for lack of surveillance for the types and extent of use, and uncertainty about the hazards (FAO/NACA/WHO Study Group, 1999; Caprioli, 2000; Hanekamp, 2003). Toxic effects from the very low, ppb levels encountered in some aquacultured foods have been questioned (Hanekamp, 2003). Some studies have suggested probable transmission of antimicrobial-resistant bacteria in aquacultured food (Ervik et al., 1994; Weinstein et al., 1997; Angulo, 1999; Duran and Marshall, 2005). Yet recent reviews compiled by the Institute of Food Technologists (ITF, 2006) indicate the use of "chemical and biological antimicrobials and physical preservation systems has been remarkably successful in providing safe foods and has not been compromised by the occurrence of resistent microorganisms." The list of chemotherapeutants approved for use in aquaculture is limited and there is strict monitoring of finished products.

Analytical procedures for detecting chemotherapeutants in the ppb range are expensive and time-consuming which may deter routine sampling of aquacultured products. Prevention of illegal use of chemotherapeutants may be achieved through education and development of "best aquaculture practices" (Florida Department of Agriculture and Consumer Services, 2005). Programs are emerging to address this need in both domestic (Otwell et al., 2001; ACC, 2004) and international settings (http://www.gaalliance. org/resp.html; http://www.aquaculturecertification.org/index.html; Otwell et al., 2001). Agencies in the United States have developed programs to advance approval and use of additional chemotherapeutants, as exemplified by the recent recognition for use of florfenicol in catfish farms (FDA, 2005b).

Seafood Allergens

According to the recommended definitions for adverse food reactions (Anderson, 1986; O'Neil and Lehrer, 1995; Adverse Reactions to Food Committee, 2003), a seafood allergy involves an immunologic reaction following exposure to a seafood. The true prevalence of seafood allergies in the United States is unknown and difficult to estimate (Bush, 1995), although they remain among the most common food-induced allergies (Taylor and Bush, 1988; O'Neil et al., 1993; Hefle, 1996) (see Table 4-16). They are more commonly associated with adults (Taylor and Bush, 1988). In general, the prevalence of food allergies is overestimated (Sampson, 1992; O'Neil and Lehrer, 1995) for lack of proper diagnosis or confusion with other food sensitivities, but actual occurrence of seafood allergies is estimated

TABLE 4-16 Most Commonly Implicated Foods in Food Allergy Listed by Most Common Age Group Involved According to the Original Source

Adults	Children
Peanuts	Cow milk
Tree nuts	Eggs
Soybeans	Soybeans
Fish	Peanuts
Crustaceans	Wheat
	Tree nuts

SOURCE: Hefle, 1996.

to affect less than 2 percent of the US population (Hefle, 1996). Of this group, 280,000 to 500,000 consumers may be at risk for developing allergic reactions to seafood (Lehrer, 1993; O'Neil and Lehrer, 1995). Since exposure is the mediating factor, occurrence tends to be more prevalent near coastal regions and will likely increase as per capita seafood consumption increases (Lehrer, 1993; O'Neil et al., 1993; O'Neil and Lehrer, 1995).

Exposure can involve ingestion, inhalation (of vapors), or product handling for consumption or occupation. Likewise, potential exposure can be hidden as the presence of the particular seafood item may not be obvious or expected due to an unidentified ingredient or misidentified ingredients (i.e., fish-based surimi used in a "crab" salad). It can also result from cross-contamination of nonallergenic foods from handling either with the same improperly cleaned utensils or through subsequent cooking in the same containers or cooking media (frying oil or boiling water) as seafood (O'Neil and Lehrer, 1995; Hefle, 1996).

Similar food intolerances that are misidentified as a seafood allergy can involve an abnormal physiological or sensitive response to components accompanying the seafood (Taylor and Nordlee, 1993). Exposure to sulfiting agents is a common suspect. Sulfites are among the most widely used food additives in the food industry (IOM, 1991; Otwell et al., 2001). They are approved for use in preventing discoloration caused by indigenous enzyme activity on shrimp, lobsters, and other crustaceans (FDA, 2001a). If the sulfite residual on certain foods is excessive and not bound to the food matrix, exposure for certain asthmatic consumers could result in serious reactions. The prevalence of such reactions has been estimated at approximately 3.9 percent of asthmatic patients (Bush et al., 1986). Adverse reactions to sulfite residuals on properly treated seafood are rare, since the sulfiting agents are usually bound to the food protein matrix and are not readily released in the throat or nasal areas during consumption. Regulatory HACCP mandates also specify requirements for distinct labeling of any seafood exposed to sulfiting agents.

Consumer awareness and labeling remain the most effective measures to prevent exposure to seafood that could elicit a food sensitivity response. Commercial practices for dual processing or preparation of other foods in facilities or with utensils used for seafood must avoid potential cross-contamination that could result in unanticipated exposures. Requirements to identify seafood or any use of seafood ingredients, as well as certain food additives, have been emphasized by the HACCP mandate (FDA, 2001a) requiring appropriate hazard analysis to identify any potential food sensitivity risks controlled through proper cleaning, product segregation, or product identification in order to prevent a potential hazard.

Adverse Effects Associated with Omega-3 Supplementation

While there is extensive research suggesting health benefits from the consumption of EPA/DHA found in fish oils, there are also data that indicate that overconsumption of fish oils could have adverse consequences. Evidence suggests that EPA and DHA may increase bleeding time, specifically by reducing platelet aggregability, and prolonged bleeding times in humans whose diets were supplemented with fish oil have been observed (e.g., Jensen et al., 1988; Rodgers and Levin, 1990; Harris et al., 1991). After reviewing this literature, FDA concluded that prolonged bleeding is not a significant risk at levels of consumption of up to 3 grams per day of EPA and DHA (Source: http://www.cfsan.fda.gov/~dms/ds-ltr11.html). This conclusion was the basis for FDA's recommendation, which remains in force, that consumption of EPA and DHA combined should be limited to 3 grams per day, of which 2 might come from supplements.

Other potentially adverse effects of excessive consumption of fish oils include reduced glycemic control among diabetics, increased levels of low-density lipoprotein (LDL) cholesterol among diabetics and hyperglycemics, and immunosuppressive effects. FDA determined that limiting consumption of EPA and DHA to 3 grams per day would protect against these effects also.

Since some contaminants that may be found in seafood are lipophilic, including PCBs, DDT and its metabolites, DLCs, and polyaromatic hydrocarbons (PAHs), they may tend to concentrate in the fish oil. It is important to recognize that dietary supplements, including fish oils sold as supplements, are subject to the same regulations regarding adulteration as are conventional foods. A food is considered adulterated if it "bears or contains any poisonous or deleterious substance which may render it injurious to health" or if it "has been prepared, packed, or held under insanitary conditions whereby it may have become contaminated with filth, or whereby it may have been rendered injurious to health" (21 USC 342(a)(1) & (4)).

Fish-oil supplements are regulated by FDA under the provisions of the Dietary Supplement Health and Education Act (DSHEA). This law provides that no FDA safety notification is needed for dietary supplement ingredients that were already on the US market prior to October 15, 2004. Fish oils are "grandfathered" under this provision, and thus there are no standards of identity for commercial fish-oil dietary supplements. Further, there is no provision under any law or regulation that requires a firm to disclose to FDA or consumers the information they have about the safety or purported benefits of their fish-oil products.

FDA is, however, empowered to remove from the market any fish-oil supplement that is not of adequate purity to ensure consumer safety under normal conditions of use. Since FDA has limited resources to analyze the composition of food products, including dietary supplements, it focuses these resources first on public health emergencies and products that may have caused injury or illness. Enforcement priorities then go to products thought to be unsafe or fraudulent or in violation of the law.

Fish-oil products, as opposed to fish themselves, can be processed to remove undesirable constituents. An industry trade association, the Council for Responsible Nutrition, established voluntary standards for its members in October of 2002. These standards limit concentrations of contaminants in fish-oil products as follows:

- DLCs: ≤ 2 pg TEQ/g
- PCBs: ≤ 0.09 µg/g
- Heavy metals (lead, cadmium, mercury, arsenic): all < 1 µg/g

Data submitted to FDA by the National Fish Meal and Oil Association on pesticide and PCB analysis in fish oil, conducted under Title 21, Code of Federal Regulations, Parts 109 and 509 "Action Levels for Poisonous or Deleterious Substances in Human Food and Animal Feed," indicated that multiple samples of menhaden and fish oil (refined and crude) did not contain detectable levels of a panel of pesticides, PCBs, and dioxins (Source: http://www.fda.gov/ohrms/dockets/dailys/02/Jul02/070202/99p-5332_sup0003_01_vol1.pdf).

Summary of Evidence

In summary, while certain hazards associated with specific species (e.g., scombroid poisoning) and lack of compliance with food safety guidelines (e.g., eating raw molluscan shellfish) persist, reviews of reported seafood-borne illnesses indicate that more acute seafood safety hazards are not increasing. This trend seems to be due in part to the food safety control measures mandated since 1997 (e.g., HACCP and monitoring of sanitation control procedures); the new labeling requirements providing educational support; and specific management plans implemented by regulatory and industry partnerships to address the more serious illnesses associated with consumption of raw molluscan shellfish. However, the potential for misuse of chemotherapeutants in domestic and imported aquaculture products is a source for concern about the presence of toxins and increased antimicrobial resistance in seafood, particularly in light of increasing dependence on aquacultured products.

CHAPTER CONCLUSION

The committee's review of evidence on risks associated with consumption of seafood drew on current research reports and reviews, published reviews from stakeholder groups, invited presentations made to the committee, and correspondance with experts in areas relevant to the statement of work. One component of the committee's charge was to identify and prioritize the potential for adverse health effects from both naturally occurring and introduced toxicants in seafood. The conclusion from the committee's review of evidence is that, among chemical contaminants, methylmercury presents as a greater concern for adverse health effects, whereas the risk associated with dioxins and PCBs in seafood remains uncertain due to both the availability of evidence and the strength of the findings, and that microbial hazards, particularly those associated with handling and cooking practices, pose a more controllable yet persistent seafood-related risk from the standpoint of public health concerns.

FINDINGS

1. Levels of contaminants in seafood depend on several factors, including species, size, harvest location, age, and composition of feed. Methylmercury is the seafoodborne contaminant for which the most exposure and toxicity data are available; levels of methylmercury in seafood have not changed substantially in recent decades. Exposure to dioxins and PCBs varies by location and vulnerable subgroups (e.g., some American Indian/Alaskan Native groups living near contaminated waters) may be at increased risk. Microbial illness from seafood is acute, persistent, and a potentially serious risk, although incidence of illness has not increased in recent decades.

2. Methylmercury is the seafoodborne contaminant for which the most comprehensive exposure and toxicity data are available for the purpose of deriving quantitative estimates of the risks.

3. The evidence pertaining to the health risks associated with consumption of seafoodborne contaminants derives from observational studies, primarily cross-sectional and prospective cohort in design. The use of a randomized clinical trial to evaluate contaminant risks would be unethical.

4. The metrics used to characterize the risks associated with consumption of seafoodborne contaminants, such as the reference dose, are useful in identifying a contaminant intake level that is considered, based on available data, to be "without an appreciable risk of deleterious effects during a lifetime." Such metrics are not useful, however, in characterizing the increase in risk that is associated with intake levels that are above the reference dose. The dose-response modeling used to identify the BMD and BMDL could be used to characterize the risks although it is important to recognize that the estimates will be influenced by the assumptions made regarding, for example, the appropriate dose-response function.

5. Reference levels for the intake of contaminants, such as the RfDs for methylmercury and dioxin-like compounds, can be misinterpreted as "bright lines," i.e., that intakes above the level are "harmful" and intakes below the level are "safe."

6. With regard to trends in population exposures to chemical contaminants,

    a. On the basis of nationally representative data on the US population, the median blood mercury level was unchanged over the period 1999–2002.

    b. Exposures to PCBs and dioxin-like compounds are decreasing on a population basis, but exposures can vary greatly according to geographic region and consumption patterns so that particular subgroups of the population could be at increased risk.

7. Increased methylmercury exposure might be a risk factor for adult cardiovascular toxicity, although the data available are not extensive and uncertainties remain.

8. Considerable uncertainties are associated with estimates of the health risks to the general population from exposures to MeHg and POPs at levels present in commercially obtained seafood. The available evidence to assess risks to the US population is incomplete and useful to only a limited extent.

9. Estimates for trends in chemical contaminants in the seafood supply depend on harvest location and products of concern.

    a. Concerns regarding levels of PCBs and DLCs in certain aquacultured products can be addressed by means of further scrutiny of feed content and uses.

    b. The levels of methylmercury in marine seafood do not appear to have changed systematically in recent decades.

10. New potential chemical-associated risks continue to be identified

in seafood and other foods (e.g., polybrominated diphenyl ethers and other persistent organic pollutants), although inadequate data on exposure, toxicities, or both make it difficult to define the dimensions of the potential risks.

11. Consumers are exposed to a complex mixture of dietary and nondietary contaminants whereas most studies of the risks associated with seafood focus on a single contaminant. The extent to which such co-exposures might affect the toxicity of seafoodborne contaminants is largely unknown. Similarly, few data are available on the extent to which beneficial components of seafood, such as selenium and omega-3 fatty acids, might mitigate the risks associated with seafoodborne contaminants.

12. Reported seafoodborne illnesses indicate acute hazards are not increasing, but certain hazards associated with specific species and consumer preference (e.g., eating raw molluscan shellfish) persist.

13. Increased dependence on aquacultured and imported products is raising concerns for certain potential hazards.

　　a. Use of illegal chemotherapeutants in certain aquaculture operations.

　　b. Various microbial and chemical contaminants in products subject to limited regulatory surveillance.

RECOMMENDATIONS

Recommendation 1: Appropriate federal agencies (the National Oceanic and Atmospheric Administration [NOAA], the US Environmental Protection Agency [US EPA], and the Food and Drug Administration [FDA] of the US Department of Health and Human Services) **should increase monitoring of methylmercury and persistent organic pollutants in seafood and make the resulting information readily available to the general public.** Along with this information, these agencies should develop better recommendations to the public about levels of pollutants that may present a risk to specific population subgroups.

Recommendation 2: Changes in the seafood supply (sources and types of seafood) must be accounted for—there is inconsistency in sampling and analysis methodology used for nutrient and contaminants data that are published by state and federal agencies. Analytical data is not consistently revised, with separate data values presented for wild-caught, domestic, and imported products.

Research Recommendations

Recommendation 12: More complete data are needed on the distribution of contaminant levels among types of fish. This information should be made available in order to reduce uncertainties associated with the estimation of health risks for with specific seafoodborne contaminant exposures.

Recommendation 13: More quantitative characterization is needed of the dose-response relationships between chemical contaminants and adverse health effects in the ranges of exposure represented in the general US population. Such information will reduce uncertainties associated with recommendations for acceptable ranges of intake.

Recommendation 14: In addition, the committee recommends more research on useful biomarkers of contaminant exposures and more precise quantitative characterization of the dose-response relationships between chemical contaminants and adverse health effects in the ranges of exposure represented in the general US population, in order to reduce uncertainties associated with recommendations for acceptable ranges of intake.

REFERENCES

ACC (Aquaculture Certification Council). 2002–2006. *Aquaculture Certification.* [Online]. Available: http://www.aquaculturecertification.org [accessed March 6, 2006].

ACC. 2004. *Aquaculture Facility Certification, Guidelines for BAP Standards (Shrimp Hatcheries).* [Online]. Available: http://www.aquaculturecertification.org/ACC-PDFS/hgud1204.pdf [accessed April 3, 2006].

Adverse Reactions to Food Committee. 2003. *Academy Practice Paper: Current Approach to the Diagnosis and Management of Adverse Reactions to Foods.* Milwaukee, WI: American Academy of Allergy, Asthma, and Immunology. [Online]. Available: http://www.aaaai.org/media/resources/academy_statements/practice_papers/adverse_reactions_to_foods.asp [accessed April 3, 2006].

Allshouse J, Buzby JC, Harvey D, Zorn D. 2003. International trade and seafood safety. In: Buzby JC, ed. *International Trade and Food Safety: Economic Theory and Case Studies. Agricultural Economic Report Number 828.* Washington, DC: Economic Research Service. [Online]. Available: http://www.ers.usda.gov/publications/aer828/aer828i.pdf [accessed May 1, 2006].

Anderson JA. 1986. The establishment of common language concerning adverse reactions to food and food additives. *Journal of Allergy and Clinical Immunology* 78 (1 Part 2):140–143.

Angulo F. 1999. *Antibiotic Use in Aquaculture: Center for Disease Control Memo to the Record.* [Online]. Available: http://www.nationalaquaculture.org/pdf/CDC%20Memo%20to%20the%20Record.pdf#search=%22angulo%20and%20transmission%20of%20antimicrobial-resistant%20bacteria%20in%20aquacultured%20food%201999%22 [accessed August 26, 2006].

Archer DL, Kvenberg JE. 1985. Incidence and cost of foodborne diarrheal disease in the United States. *Journal of Food Protection* 48(10):887–894.

Armstrong SR. 2002. *Synopsis of Dietary Exposure to Dioxin-Like Compounds.* Paper prepared for the Committee on the Implications of Dioxin in the Food Supply. Washington, DC: Institute of Medicine.

ATSDR (Agency for Toxic Substances and Disease Registry). 1999. *Toxicological Profile for Mercury.* Atlanta, GA: US Department of Health and Human Services, Public Health Service. [Online]. Available: http://www.atsdr.cdc.gov/toxprofiles/tp46.html [accessed December 2, 2005].

Auger N, Kofman O, Kosatsky T, Armstron B. 2005. Low-level methylmercury exposure as a risk factor for neurologic abnormalities in adults. *Neurotoxicology* 26(2):149–157.

Austin JW, Smith JP. 2006. Botulism from fishery products: History and control. In: Otwell WS, Kristinsoon HG, Balaban MO, eds. *Modified Atmospheric Processing and Packaging of Fish.* Ames, IA: Blackwell Publishing. Pp. 193–216.

Bellanger TM, Caesar EM, Trachtman L. 2000. Blood mercury levels and fish consumption in Louisiana. *Journal of Louisiana Medical Society* 152(2):64–73.

Bertazzi PA, Zocchetti C, Guercilena S, Consonni D, Tironi A, Landi MT, Pesatori AC. 1997. Dioxin exposure and cancer risk. A 15-year mortality study after the "Seveso accident." *Epidemiology* 8(6):646–652.

Bidleman TF, Harner T. 2000. Chapter 10: Sorption to aerosols. In: Boethling RS, Mackay D, eds. 2000. *Handbook of Property Estimation Methods for Chemicals: Environmental and Health Sciences.* Boca Raton, FL: Lewis Publishers. Pp. 233–260.

Bier JW. 1976. Experimental anisakis: Cultivation and temperature tolerance determination. *Journal of Milk and Food Technology* 39(2):132–137.

Bowers WJ, Nakai JS, Chu I, Wade MG, Moir D, Yagminas A, Gill S, Pulido O, Meuller R. 2004. Early developmental neurotoxicity of a PCB/organochlorine mixture in rodents after gestational and lactational exposure. *Toxicological Sciences* 77(1):51–62.

Bryan FL. 1980. Epidemiology of foodborne diseases transmitted by fish, shellfish and marine crustaceans in the United States, 1970–1978. *Journal of Food Protection* 43:859–876.

Budtz-Jorgensen E, Keiding N, Grandjean P. 2004a. Effects of exposure imprecision on estimation of the benchmark dose. *Risk Analysis* 24(6):1689–1696.

Budtz-Jorgensen E, Grandjean P, Jorgensen P, Weihe P, Keiding N. 2004b. Association between mercury concentrations in blood and hair methylmercury-exposed subjects at different ages. *Environmental Research* 95(3):385–393.

Burge P, Evans S. 1994. Mercury contamination in Arkansas gamefish: A public health perspective. *Journal of the Arkansas Medical Society* 90(11):542–544.

Burger J, Gochfeld M. 2005. Heavy metals in commercial fish in New Jersey. *Environmental Research* 99(3):403–412.

Bush RK. 1995. Seafood allergy: Implications for industry and consumers. *Food Technology* 49(10):20.

Bush RK, Taylor SL, Holden K, Nordlee JA, Busse WW. 1986. Prevalence of sensitivity to sulfiting agents in asthmatic patients. *American Journal of Medicine* 81(5):816–820.

Bylund BG. 1982. Diphyllobothriasis. In: Jacbos L, Arambulo P. *CRC Handbook Series in Zoonoese. Section C: Parasitic Zoonoses, Volume 1.* Boca Raton, FL: CRC Press, Inc. Pp. 217–225.

Caprioli A, Busani L, Martel JL, Helmuth R. 2000. Monitoring of antibiotic resistance in bacteria of animal origin: Epidemiological and microbiological methodologies. *International Journal of Antimicrobial Agents* 14(4):295–301.

CDC (Centers for Disease Control and Prevention). 1991. Epidemiologic notes and reports fish botulism—Hawaii, 1990. *Morbidity and Mortality Weekly Report* 40(24):412–414. [Online]. Available: http://www.cdc.gov/mmwr/preview/mmwrhtml/00014498.htm [accessed April 5, 2006].

CDC. 2004. Preliminary FoodNet data on the incidence of infection with pathogens transmitted commonly through food—selected sites, United States, 2003. *Morbidity and Mortality Weekly Report* 53(16):338–343. [Online]. Available: http://www.cdc.gov/mmwr/preview/mmwrhtml/mm5316a2.htm [accessed January 12, 2006].

CDC. 2005a. *FoodNet—Foodborne Diseases Active Surveillance Network.* [Online]. Available: http://www.cdc.gov/foodnet/ [accessed October 6, 2005].

CDC. 2005b. *National Biomonitoring Program. Overview.* [Online]. Available: http://www.cdc.gov/biomonitoring/overview.htm [accessed May 11, 2006].

CDC. 2005c. Preliminary FoodNet data on the incidence of infection with pathogens transmitted commonly through food—10 Sites, United States, 2004. *Morbidity and Mortality Weekly Report* 54(14):352–356. [Online]. Available: http://www.cdc.gov/mmwr/preview/ mmwrhtml/mm5414a2.htm [accessed January 10, 2006].

CDC. 2005d. *Third National Report on Human Exposure to Environmental Chemicals.* Atlanta, GA: Centers for Disease Control and Prevention. [Online]. Available: http://www. cdc.gov/exposurereport/3rd/pdf/thirdreport.pdf [accessed March 16, 2006].

CDC. 2006a. Preliminary FoodNet data on the incidence of infection with pathogens transmitted commonly through food—10 states, United States, 2005. *Morbidity and Mortality Weekly Review* 55(14):392–395.

CDC. 2006b. *Vibrio parahaemolyticus* infections associated with consumption of raw shellfish—three states, 2006. *Morbidity and Mortality Weekly Review* 55(31):854–856. [Online]. Available: http://www.cdc.gov/mmwr/preview/mmwrhtml/mm5531a5.htm [accessed September 7, 2006].

Cernichiari E, Brewer R, Myers GJ, Marsh DO, Lapham LW, Cox C, Shamlaye CF, Berlin M, Davidson PW, Clarkson TW. 1995. Monitoring methylmercury during pregnancy: Maternal hair predicts fetal brain exposure. *Neurotoxicology* 16(4):705–710.

CFSAN (Center for Food Safety and Applied Nutrition). 2000. *Letter Regarding Dietary Supplement Health Claim for Omega-3 Fatty Acids and Coronary Heart Disease.* [Online]. Available: http://www.cfsan.fda.gov/~dms/ds-ltr11.html [accessed August 28, 2006].

CFSAN (Center for Food Safety and Applied Nutrition). 2001. *Fish and Fisheries Products Hazards and Controls Guidance: Third Edition. Appendix 5: FDA and EPA Safety Levels in Regulations and Guidance.* Washington, DC: Food and Drug Administration. [Online]. Available: http://www.cfsan.fda.gov/~comm/haccp4x5.html [accessed March 2, 2006].

CFSAN. 2003. *How to Safely Handle Refrigerated Ready-To-Eat Foods and Avoid Listeriosis.* [Online]. Available: http://www.cfsan.fda.gov/~dms/adlister.html [accessed May 11, 2006].

CFSAN. 2005. *Salmonella spp.* [Online]. Available: http://www.cfsan.fda.gov/~mow/chap1. html [accessed May 11, 2006].

CFSAN. 2006. *USDA Total Diet Study: Dioxin Analysis Results/Exposure Estimates.* [Online]. Available: http://www.cfsan.fda.gov/~lrd/dioxdata.html [accessed August 27, 2006].

Chapman L, Chan HM. 2000. The influence of nutrition on methyl mercury intoxication. *Environmental Health Perspectives* 108(Supplement 1):29–56.

Choi BH. 1989. The effects of methylmercury on the developing brain. *Progress in Neurobiology* 32(6):447–470.

Chowdhury NR, Chakraborty S, Ramamurthy T, Nishibuchi M, Yamasaki S, Takeda Y, Nair GB. 2000. Molecular evidence of clonal *Vibrio parahaemolyticus* pandemic strains. *Emerging Infectious Diseases* 6(6):631–636.

Clarkson TW, Strain JJ. 2003. Nutritional factors may modify the toxic action of methyl mercury in fish-eating populations. *Journal of Nutrition* 133(5 Supplement 1):1539S–1543S.

Cohen JT. 2004. *A Summary of the Major Studies of Prenatal Mercury Exposure and Cognitive Function.* Boston, MA: Harvard Center for Risk Analysis. [Online]. Available: http:// www.hcra.harvard.edu/Supplement_Fish_3IQ.pdf [accessed March 1, 2006].

Cole P, Trichopoulos D, Pastides H, Starr T, Mandel JS. 2003. Dioxin and cancer: A critical review. *Regulatory Toxicology and Pharmacology* 38(3):378–388.

Crump KS, Kjellstrom T, Shipp AM, Silvers A, Stewart A. 1998. Influence of prenatal mercury exposure upon scholastic and psychological test performance: Benchmark analysis of a New Zealand cohort. *Risk Analysis* 18(6):701–713.

Cuvin-Aralar ML, Furness RW. 1991. Mercury and selenium interaction: A review. *Ecotoxicology and Environmental Safety* 21(3):348–364.

Daniels JL, Longnecker MP, Rowland AS, Golding J, the ALSPAC Study Team. 2004. Fish intake during pregnancy and early cognitive development of offspring. *Epidemiology* 15(4):394–402.

Darnerud PO, Eriksen GS, Johannesson T, Larsen PB, Viluksela M. 2001. Polybrominated diphenyl ethers: Occurrence, dietary exposure, and toxicology. *Environmental Health Perspectives* 109(Supplement 1):49–68.

de Wit C, Alaee M, Muir D. 2004. Brominated flame retardants in the Arctic—An overview of spatial and temporal trends. *Organohalogen Compounds* 66:3811–3816.

Deardorff TL, Throm R. 1988. Commercial blast-freezing of third-stage Anisakis simplex larvae encapsulated in salmon and rockfish. *Journal of Parasitology* 74(4):600–603.

DeCaprio AP. 1997. Biomarkers: Coming of age for environmental health and risk assessment. *Environmental Science and Technology* 31(7):1837–1848.

DeWaal CS, Barlow K. 2004. *Outbreak Alert! Closing the Gaps in Our Federal Food-Safety Net*. Washington, DC: Center for Science in the Public Interest. [Online]. Available: http://www.cspinet.org/new/pdf/outbreakalert2004.pdf [accessed October 6, 2005].

Dorea JG, de Souza JR, Rodrigues P, Ferrari I, Barbosa AC. 2005. Hair mercury (signature of fish consumption) and cardiovascular risk in Munuruku and Kayabi Indians of Amazonia. *Environmental Research* 97(2):209–219.

Duran GM, Marshall DL. 2005. Ready-to-eat shrimp as an international vehicle of antibiotic-resistant bacteria. *Journal of Food Protection* 68(11):2395–2401.

Easton MD, Luszniak D, Von der GE. 2002. Preliminary examination of contaminant loadings in farmed salmon, wild salmon and commercial salmon feed. *Chemosphere* 46(7):1053–1074.

Erickson MD. 1997. *Analytical Chemistry of PCBs, Second Edition*. Boca Raton: CRC/Lewis. P. 667.

Ervik A, Thorsen B, Eriksen V, Lunestad BT, Samuelsen OB. 1994. Impact of administering antibacterial agents on wild fish and blue mussels Mytilus edulis in the vicinity of fish farms. *Diseases of Aquatic Organisms* 18(1):45–51.

Evans MS, Noguchi GE, Rice CP. 1991. The biomagnification of polychlorinated biphenyls, toxaphene, and DDT compounds in a Lake Michigan offshore food web. *Archives of Environmental Contamination and Toxicology* 20(1):87–93.

FAO/IOC/WHO (Food and Agriculture Organization/Intergovernmental Oceanographic Commission of UNESCO/World Health Organization). 2004. *Report of the Joint FAO/IOC/WHO Ad Hoc Expert Consultation on Biotoxins in Bivalve Molluscs. Oslo, Norway, September 26–30, 2004*. [Online]. Available: ftp://ftp.fao.org/es/esn/food/biotoxin_report_en.pdf [accessed May 1, 2006].

FAO/NACA/WHO Study Group. 1999. *Food Safety Issues Associated with Products from Aquaculture*. Technical Report Series, No. 883. Geneva, Switzerland: World Health Organization. [Online]. Available: http://www.who.int/foodsafety/publications/fs_management/en/aquaculture.pdf [accessed April 3, 2006].

FAO/WHO JECFA (Food and Agriculture Organization/World Health Organization Joint Expert Committee on Food Additives). 2003. *Summary and Conclusions, 61st Meeting, Rome, Italy, 10–19 June, 2003*. [Online]. Available: http://www.who.int/ipcs/food/jecfa/summaries/en/summary_61.pdf [accessed March 9, 2006].

FAO/WHO JECFA. 2005. *Summary and Conclusions, 64th Meeting, Rome, Italy, 8–17 February 2005*. [Online]. Available: http://www.who.int/ipcs/food/jecfa/summaries/summary_report_64_final.pdf [accessed March 22, 2006].

FAO/WHO JECFA. 2006. *Evaluation of Certain Food Contaminants (Sixty-fourth report of the Joint FAO/WHO Expert Committee on Food Additives)*. WHO Technical Report Series, No. 930. Geneva, Switzerland: World Health Organization. [Online]. Available: http://whqlibdoc.who.int/trs/WHO_TRS_930_eng.pdf [accessed August 26, 2006].

FAO/WHO. 2001. *Hazard Identification, Exposure Assessment and Hazard Characterization of Campylobacter spp. in Broiler Chickens and Vibrio spp. in Seafood.* Geneva, Switzerland: World Health Organization. [Online]. Available: http://www.who.int/foodsafety/publications/micro/en/july2001_en.pdf [accessed March 2, 2006].

Faroon O, Jones D, de Rosa C. 2001. Effects of polychlorinated biphenyls on the nervous system. *Toxicology and Industrial Health* 16(7–8):305–333.

FDA (Food and Drug Administration). 1987. *Food Preparation—Raw, Marinated or Partially Cooked Fishery Products. Retail Food Protection Program Information Manual. Part 6—Inspection.* Washington, DC: Center for Food Safety and Applied Nutrition.

FDA. 2001a. *Fish and Fishery Products Hazards Controls Guidance: Third Edition.* Washington, DC: Center for Food Safety and Applied Nutrition. [Online]. Available: http://www.cfsan.fda.gov/~comm/haccp4.html [accessed January 11, 2006].

FDA. 2001b. *Draft Risk Assessment on the Public Health Impact of Vibrio parahaemolyticus in Raw Molluscan Shellfish.* Washington, DC: Center for Food Safety and Applied Nutrition. [Online]. Available: http://www.cfsan.fda.gov/~dms/vprisk.html [accessed April 5, 2006].

FDA. 2005a. 21 Code of Federal Regulations, Part 179. Irradiation in the Production, Processing, and Handling of Food. *Federal Register* 70(157):48057–48073. [Online]. Available: http://frwebgate.access.gpo.gov/cgi-bin/getpage.cgi [accessed March 6, 2006].

FDA. 2005b. 21 Code of Federal Regulations, Parts 556 and 558. New Animal Drugs: Florfenicol. *Federal Register* 70(223):70046–70047. [Online]. Available: http://a257.g.akamaitech.net/7/257/2422/01jan20051800/edocket.access.gpo.gov/2005/05-22935.htm [accessed April 3, 2006].

FDA. 2005c. *21 Code of Federal Regulations, Part 510—New Animal Drugs, Volume 6.* [Online]. Available: http://www.accessdata.fda.gov/scripts/cdrh/cfdocs/cfcfr/CFRSearch.cfm?CFRPart=510&showFR=1[accessed April 3, 2006].

FDA. *Refusal Actions by FDA as Recorded in OASIS.* [Online]. Available: http://www.fda.gov/ora/oasis/3/ora_oasis_i_16.html and http://www.fda.gov/ora/oasis/1/ora_oasis_i_16.html [accessed May 11, 2006].

Fein GG, Jacobson JL, Jacobson SW, Schwartz PM, Dowler JK. 1984. Prenatal exposure to polychlorinated biphenyls: Effects on birth size and gestational age. *Journal of Pediatrics* 105(2):315–320.

Flattery J, Bashin M. 2003. *A Baseline Survey of Raw Oyster Consumers in Four States.* Columbia, SC: Interstates Shellfish Sanitation Conference. [Online]. Available: http://www.cpa.gov/gmpo/pubinfo/pdf/accomp-app-d.pdf [accessed April 11, 2006].

Florida Department of Agriculture and Consumer Services. 2005. *Aquaculture Best Management Practices Rule.* Tallahassee, FL: Florida Department of Agriculture and Consumer Services. [Online]. Available: http://www.floridaaquaculture.com/publications/BMP%20Rule-Manual112805.pdf [accessed April 10, 2006].

Foran JA, Hites RA, Carpenter DO, Hamilton MC, Mathews-Amos A, Schwager SJ. 2004. A survey of metals in tissues of farmed Atlantic and wild Pacific salmon. *Environmental Toxicology and Chemistry* 23(9):2108–2110.

Foran JA, Carpenter DO, Hamilton MC, Knuth BA, Schwager SJ. 2005a. Risk-based consumption advice for farmed Atlantic and wild Pacific salmon contaminated with dioxins and dioxin-like compounds. *Environmental Health Perspectives* 113(5):552–556.

Foran JA, Good DH, Carpenter DO, Hamilton MC, Knuth BA, Schwager SJ. 2005b. Quantitative analysis of the benefits and risks of consuming farmed and wild salmon. *Journal of Nutrition* 135(11):2639–2643.

Fowles JR, Fairbrother A, Baecher-Steppan L, Kerkvliet NI. 1994. Immunologic and endocrine effects of the flame-retardant pentabromodiphenyl ether (DE-71) in C57BL/6J mice. *Toxicology* 86(1–2):49–61.

Fries GF. 1995a. A review of the significance of animal food products as potential pathways of human exposures to dioxins. *Journal of Animal Science* 73(6):1639–1650.

Fries GF. 1995b. Transport of organic environmental contaminants to animal products. *Reviews of Environmental Contamination and Toxicology* 141:71–109.

Fyfe M, Kelly MT, Yeung ST, Daly P, Schallie K, Buchanan S, Waller P, Kobayashi J, Therien N, Guichard M, Lankford S, Stehr-Green P, Harsch R, DeBess E, Cassidy M, McGivern T, Mauvais S, Fleming D, Lippmann M, Pong L, McKay RW, Cannon DE, Werner SB, Abbott S, Hernandez M, Wojee C, Waddell J, Waterman S, Middaugh J, Sasaki D, Effler P, Groves C, Curtis N, Dwyer D, Dowdle G, Nichols C. 1998. Outbreak of vibrio parahaemolyticus infections associated with eating raw oysters—Pacific Northwest, 1997. *Morbidity and Mortality Weekly Report* 47(22):457–462. [Online]. Available: http://www.cdc.gov/mmwr/preview/mmwrhtml/00053377.htm [accessed April 11, 2006].

Ganther HE, Goudie C, Sunde ML, Kopecky MJ, Wagner P, Oh S-H, Hoekstra WG. 1972. Selenium: Relation to decreased toxicity of methylmercury added to diets containing tuna. *Science* 175(26):1122–1124.

Geyer HJ, Rimkus GG, Scheunert I, Kaune A, Schramm K-W, Kettrup A, Zeeman M, Muir DCG, Hansen LG, Mackay D. 2000. Bioaccumulation and occurrence of endocrine-disrupting chemicals (EDC), persistent organic pollutants (POPs), and other organic compounds in fish and other organisms including humans. In: Hutzinger O, Beek B, eds. *Bioaccumulation, New Aspects and Developments. The Handbook of Environmental Chemistry, Vol. 2, Part J*. Berlin, Germany: Springer Verlag. Pp. 1–166.

Global Aquaculture Alliance. 2004. *Responsible Aquaculture Program*. [Online]. Available: http://www.gaalliance.org/resp.html [accessed April 3, 2006].

Gombas DE, Chen Y, Clavero RS, Scott VN. 2003. Survey of Listeria monocytogenes in Ready-to-Eat Foods. *Journal of Food Protection* 66(4):559–569.

Grandjean P, Weihe P, White RF, Debes F, Araki S, Yokoyama K, Murata K, Sorensen N, Dahl R, Jorgensen PJ. 1997. Cognitive deficit in 7-year-old children with prenatal exposure to methylmercury. *Neurotoxicology and Teratology* 19(6):417–428.

Grandjean P, Weihe P, Burse VW, Needham LL, Storr-Hansen E, Heinzow B, Debes F, Murata K, Simonsen H, Ellefsen P, Budtz-Jorgensen E, Keiding N, White RF. 2001. Neurobehavioral deficits associated with PCB in 7-year-old children prenatally exposed to seafood neurotoxicants. *Neurotoxicology and Teratology* 23(4):305–317.

Gregus Z, Gyurasics A, Csanaky I, Pinter Z. 2001. Effects of methylmercury and organic acid mercurials on the disposition of exogenous selenium in rats. *Toxicology and Applied Pharmacology* 174(2):177–187.

Guallar E, Sanz-Gallardo I, Veer PV, Bode P, Aro A, Gomez-Aracena J, Kark JD, Riemersma RA, Martin-Moreno JM, Kok FJ. 2002. Mercury, fish oils, and the risk of myocardial infarction. *New England Journal of Medicine* 347(22):1747–1754.

Hanekamp JC, Frapporti G, Olieman K. 2003. Chloramphenicol, food safety and precautionary thinking in Europe. *Environmental Liability* 11:209–221. [Online]. Available: http://www.richel.org/theodoc/pdf/Chloramphenicol.pdf [accessed May 1, 2006].

Harris WS, Windson SL, Dujovne CA. 1991. Effects of four doses of n-3 fatty acids given to hyperlipidemic patients for six months. *Journal of the American College of Nutrition* 10(3):220–227.

Hefle SL. 1996. The chemistry and biology of food allergens. *Food Technology* 50(3):86–92.

Higashi GJ. 1985. Foodborne parasites transmitted to man from and other aquatic foods. *Food Technology* 39(3):69–74.

Hightower JM, Moore D. 2003. Mercury levels in high-end consumers of fish. *Environmental Health Perspectives* 111(4):604–608.

Hites RA. 2004. Polybrominated diphenyl ethers in the environment and in people: A meta-analysis of concentrations. *Environmental Science and Technology* 38(4):945–956.

Hites RA, Foran JA, Carpenter DO, Hamilton MC, Knuth BA, Schwager SJ. 2004. Global assessment of organic contaminants in farmed salmon. *Science* 303(5655):226–229.

Hlady W, Klontz K. 1996. The epidemiology of Vibrio infections in Florida, 1981–1993. *Journal of Infectious Diseases* 173(5):1176–1183.

Huisman M, Koopman-Esseboom C, Lanting CI, van der Paauw CG, Tuinstra LG, Fidler V, Weisglas-Kuperus N, Sauer PJ, Boersma ER, Touwen BC. 1995. Neurological condition in 18-month-old children perinatally exposed to polychlorinated biphenyls and dioxins. *Early Human Development* 43(2):165–176.

Humphrey H. 1988. Human exposure to persistent aquatic contaminants. In: Schmidtke NW, ed. *Toxic Contamination in Large Lakes.* Chelsea, MI: Lewis Publishers. Pp. 227–238.

Hungerford JM. 2005. Committee on Natural Toxins and Food Allergens: Marine and freshwater toxins. *Journal of the Association of Official Analytical Chemists International* 88(1):299–324.

Huss HH, Ababouch L, Gram L. 2004. *Assessment and Management of Seafood Safety and Quality.* Technical Paper No. 444. Rome, Italy: Food and Agricultural Organization. [Online]. Available: http://www.fao.org/DOCREP/006/Y4743E/y4743e06.htm [accessed March 30, 2006].

ICEID (International Conference on Emerging Infectious Diseases). 2006. *Consumption of Risky Foods Declines.* Atlanta, GA: International Conference on Emerging Infectious Diseases. [Online]. Available: http://www.asm.org/ASM/files/LeftMarginHeaderList/DOWNLOADFILENAME/000000002017/risky%20foods.pdf [accessed April 11, 2006].

IFT (Institute of Food Technologists). 2006. *Antimicrobial Resistance: Implications for the Food System, Summary.* IFT Expert Report. [Online]. Available: http://members.ift.org/NR/rdonlyres/17A8181C-143C-4D94-8885-9093C4AFC533/0/OnePagerSummary.pdf [accessed August 26, 2006].

IISD (International Institute for Sustainable Development). 1998. Report of the first session of the INC for an international legally binding instrument for implementing international action on center persistent organic pollutants (POPS): 29 June–3 July 1998. *Earth Negotiations Bulletin* 15(10):1. [Online]. Available: http://www.iisd.ca/download/pdf/enb1510e.pdf [accessed March 13, 2006].

Ikemoto T, Kunito T, Tanaka H, Baba N, Miyazaki N, Tanabe S. 2004. Detoxification mechanism of heavy metals in marine mammals and seabirds: Interaction of selenium with mercury, silver, copper, zinc, and cadmium in liver. *Archives of Environmental Contamination and Toxicology* 47(3):402–413.

Ikonomou MG, Rayne S, Addison RF. 2002. Exponential increases of the brominated flame retardants, polybrominated diphenyl ethers, in the Canadian Arctic from 1981 to 2000. *Environmental Science and Technology* 36(9):1886–1892.

IOM (Institute of Medicine). 1991. *Seafood Safety.* Washington, DC: National Academy Press.

IOM. 2003. *Dioxins and Dioxin-Like Compounds in the Food Supply: Strategies to Decrease Exposure.* Washington, DC: The National Academies Press.

ISSC (Interstate Shellfish Sanitation Conference). 2001. *Vibrio Management Committee Meeting, Biloxi, MS, November 8–9, 2001.* [Online]. Available: http://issc.org/Archives/old-newsletters/Nov-2002/VMCNOV.htm [accessed April 28, 2006].

ISSC. 2002. *Vibrio vulnificus Risk Management Plan for Oysters.* [Online]. Available: http://www.issc.org/Vibrio_vulnificus_Education/1/II%20A%20Vibrio%20vulnificus%20Risk%20Management%20Plan.doc [accessed March 2, 2006].

ISSC. 2003a. *Guide for the Control of Molluscan Shellfish 2003.* National Shellfish Sanitation Program, Interstate Shellfish Sanitation Conference. [Online]. Available: http://www.cfsan.fda.gov/~ear/nss2-toc.html [accessed April 20, 2006].

ISSC. 2003b. *Florida Vibrio vulnificus Risk Reduction Plan for Oysters.* [Online]. Available: http://www.issc.org/Vibrio_vulnificus_Education/1/II%20B%20a%20Florida%20Vib rio%20Vulnificus%20Risk%20Reduction%20Plan%20for%20Oy.rtf [accessed April 28, 2006].

Jackson GJ. 1975. The new disease status of human anisakiasis and North American cases: A review. *Journal of Milk and Food Technology* 38(12):769–773.

Jacobson JL, Jacobson SW. 1996. Dose-response in perinatal exposure to polychlorinated biphenyls (PCBs): The Michigan and North Carolina cohort studies. *Toxicology and Industrial Health* 12(3–4):435–445.

Jacobson JL, Jacobson SW. 2003. Prenatal exposure to polychlorinated biphenyls and attention at school age. *Journal of Pediatrics* 143(6):780–788.

Jacobson JL, Jacobson SW, Humphrey HE. 1990. Effects of in utero exposure to polychlorinated biphenyls and related contaminants on cognitive functioning in young children. *Journal of Pediatrics* 116(1):38–45.

Jensen CD, Spiler GA, Wookey VJ, Wong LG, Whitman JH, Scala J. 1988. Plasma lipids on three levels of fish oil intake in healthy human subjects. *Nutrition Reports International* 38:165–171.

Jensen TK, Grandjean P, Jorgensen EB, White RF, Debes F, Weihe P. 2005. Effects of breast feeding on neuropsychological development in a community with methylmercury exposure from seafood. *Journal of Exposure Analysis and Environmental Epidemiology* 15(5):423–430.

Johansson N, Basun H, Winblad B, Nordberg M. 2002. Relationship between mercury concentration in blood, cognitive performance, and blood pressure, in an elderly urban population. *BioMetals* 15(2):189–195.

Kamrin MA. 2004. Bisphenol A: A scientific evaluation. *Medscape General Medicine* 6(3):7.

Kimbrough RD. 1987. Human health effects of polychlorinated biphenyls (PCBs) and polybrominated biphenyls (PBBs). *Annual Review of Pharmacology and Toxicology* 27: 87–111.

Kimbrough RD, Squire RA, Linder RE, Strandberg JD, Montalli RJ, Burse VW. 1975. Induction of liver tumor in Sherman strain female rats by polychlorinated biphenyl aroclor 1260. *Journal of the National Cancer Institute* 55(6):1453–1459.

Kingman A, Albertini T, Brown LJ. 1998. Mercury concentrations in urine and whole blood associated with amalgam exposure in a US military population. *Journal of Dental Research* 77(3):461–471.

Kjellstrom T, Kennedy S, Wallis S, Mantell C. 1986. *Physical and Mental Development of Children with Prenatal Exposure to Mercury from Fish. Stage I: Preliminary Tests at Age 4.* Solna, Sweden: National Swedish Environmental Protection Board.

Kjellstrom T, Kennedy S, Wallis S, Stewart A, Friberg L, Lind B, Wutherspoon T, Mantell C. 1989. *Physical and Mental Development of Children with Prenatal Exposure to Mercury from Fish. Stage II: Interviews and Psychological Tests at Age 6.* Solna, Sweden: National Swedish Environmental Protection Board.

Kodavanti PR, Ward TR. 2005. Differential effects of commercial polybrominated diphenyl ether and polychlorinated biphenyl mixtures on intracellular signaling in rat brain in vitro. *Toxicological Sciences* 85(2):952–962.

Koeman JH, Peeters WH, Koudstaal-Hol CH, Tjioe PS, de Goeij JJ. 1973. Mercury-selenium correlations in marine mammals. *Nature* 245(5425):385–386.

Koeman JH, van de Ven WS, de Goeij JJ, Tjioe PS, van Haaften JL. 1975. Mercury and selenium in marine mammals and birds. *Science of the Total Environment* 3(3):279–287.

Kohn MA, Farley TA, Ando T, Curtis M, Wilson SA, Jin Q, Monroe SS, Baron RC, McFarland LM, Glass RI. 1995. An outbreak of Norwalk virus gastroenteritis associated with eating raw oysters. Implications for maintaining safe oyster beds. *Journal of the American Medical Association* 273(6):466–471.

Kong KY, Cheung KC, Wong CK, Wong MH. 2005. Residues of DDTs, PAHs and some heavy metals in fish (Tilapia) collected from Hong Kong and mainland China. *Journal of Environmental Science and Health. Part A: Toxic/Hazardous Substances and Environmental Engineering* 40(11):2105–2115.

Koonse B, Burkhardt W, Chirtel S, Hoskins GP. 2005. Salmonella and the sanitary quality of aquacultured shrimp. *Journal of Food Protection* 68(12):2527–2532.

Kosta L, Byrne AR, Zelenko V. 1975. Correlation between selenium and mercury in man following exposure to inorganic mercury. *Nature* 254(5497):238–239.

Kraepiel AM, Keller K, Chin HB, Malcolm EG, Morel FM. 2003. Sources and variations of mercury in tuna. *Environmental Science and Technology* 37(24):5551–5558.

Kulkarni P. 2005. *The Marine Seafood Export Supply Chain in India: Current State and Influence of Import Requirements*. Winnipeg, Manitoba, Canada: International Institute for Sustainable Development. [Online]. Available: http://www.tradeknowledgenetwork. net/pdf/tkn_marine_export_india.pdf [accessed May 2, 2006].

Lange WR, Snyder FR, Fudala PJ. 1992. Travel and ciguatera fish poisoning. *Archives of Internal Medicine* 152(10):2049–2053.

Law RJ, Alaee M, Allchin CR, Boon JP, Lebeuf M, Lepom P, Stern GA. 2003. Levels and trends of polybrominated diphenylethers and other brominated flame retardants in wildlife. *Environment International* 29(6):757–779.

Lehane L. 1999. *Ciguatera Fish Poisoning: A Review in a Risk-Assessment Framework*. Canberra, Australia: National Office Animal and Plant Health, Agriculture, Fisheries and Forestry. [Online]. Available: http://www.affa.gov.au/corporate_docs/publications/pdf/ animalplanthealth/chief_vet/ciguatera.pdf [accessed April 3, 2006].

Lehrer SB. 1993. Seafood allergy. Introduction. *Clinical Reviews in Allergy* 11(2):155–157.

Longnecker MP, Wolff MS, Gladen BC, Brock JW, Grandjean P, Jacobson JL, Korrick SA, Rogan WJ, Weisglas-Kuperus N, Hertz-Picciotto I, Ayotte P, Stewart P, Winneke G, Charles MJ, Jacobson SW, Dewailly E, Boersma ER, Altshul LM, Heinzow B, Pagano JJ, Jensen AA. 2003. Comparison of polychlorinated biphenyl levels across studies of human neurodevelopment. *Environmental Health Perspectives* 111(1):65–70.

Luksemburg W, Wenning R, Maier M, Patterson A, Braithwaite S. 2004. Polybrominated diphenyl ethers (PBDE) and polychlorinated dibenzo-p-dioxins (PCDD/F) and biphenyls (PCB) in fish, beef, and fowl purchased in food markets in northern California U.S.A. *Organohalogen Compounds* 66:3982–3987.

Lunder S, Sharp R. 2003. *Tainted Catch: Toxic Fire Retardants Are Building Up Rapidly in San Francisco Bay Fish—And People*. Washington, DC: Environmental Working Group. [Online]. Available: http://www.ewg.org/reports_content/taintedcatch/pdf/PBDEs_final. pdf [accessed September 12, 2005].

Luten JB, Ruiter A, Ritskes TM, Rauchbaar AB, Riekwel-Booy G. 1980. Mercury and selenium in marine- and freshwater fish. *Journal of Food Science* 45:416–419.

Mahaffey KR, Clickner RP, Bodurow CC. 2004. Blood organic mercury and dietary mercury intake: National Health and Nutrition Examination Survey, 1999 and 2000. *Environmental Health Perspective* 112(5):562–570.

McDowell MA, Dillon CF, Osterloh J, Bolger PM, Pellizzari E, Fernando R, Montes de Oca R, Schober SE, Sinks T, Jones RL, Mahaffey KR. 2004. Hair mercury levels in US children and women of child-bearing age: Reference range data from NHANES 1999–2000. *Environmental Health Perspectives* 112(11):1165–1171.

McKerrow JH, Sakanari J, Deardorff TL. 1988. Anisakiasis: Revenge of the sushi parasite. *New England Journal of Medicine* 319(18):1228–1229.

Mead PS, Slutsker L, Dietz V, McCaig LF, Bresee JS, Shapiro C, Griffine PM, Tauxe RV. 1999. Food-related illness and death in the United States. *Emerging Infectious Diseases* 5(5):607–625. [Online]. Available: http://www.cdc.gov/ncidod/eid/vol5no5/mead.htm [accessed January 12, 2006].

Mead PS, Slutsker L, Dietz V, McCaig LF, Bresee JS, Shapiro C, Griffine PM, Tauxe RV. 2006. Food-related illness and death in the United States. *Emerging Infectious Diseases* 5(5):607–625.

Meironyté D, Norén K, Bergman A. 1999. Analysis of polybrominated diphenyl ethers in Swedish human milk: A time-related trend study, 1972–1997. *Journal of Toxicology and Environmental Health, Part A* 58(6):329–341.

Mendelsohn ML, Mohr LC, Peeters JP. 1998. *Biomarkers: Medical and Workplace Applications.* Washington, DC: Joseph Henry Press.

Mocarelli P, Gerthoux PM, Brambilla P, Marocchi A, Beretta C, Bertona M, Cazzaniga M, Colombo L, Crespi C, Ferrari E, Limonta G, Sarto C, Signorini, Tramacere PL. 1999. Dioxin health effects on humans twenty years after Seveso: A summary. In: Ballarin-Denti A, Bertazzi PA, Facchetti S, Mocarelli P, eds. *Chemistry, Man, and Environment: The Seveso Accident 20 Years On: Monitoring, Epidemiology and Remediation.* Pp. 41–52.

Moreland KB, Landrigan PJ, Sjödin A, Gobeille AK, Jones RS, McGahee EE, Needham LL, Patterson DG. 2005. Body burdens of polybrominated diphenyl ethers among urban anglers. *Environmental Health Perspectives* 113(12):1689–1692.

Morton RA, Burklew MA. 1970. Incidence of ciguatera in barracuda from the west coast of Florida. *Toxicon* 8(4):317–318.

Myers GJ, Davidson PW, Cox C, Shamlaye CF, Palumbo D, Cernichiari E, Sloane-Reeves J, Wilding GE, Kost J, Huang LS, Clarkson TW. 2003. Prenatal methylmercury exposure from ocean fish consumption in the Seychelles child development study. *Lancet* 361 (9370):1686–1692.

National Fish Meal and Oil Association. 2002. *Certificate of Analysis and Pesticide Scans.* Provided to the FDA by Thionville Laboratories, Inc. [Online]. Available: http://www.fda.gov/ohrms/dockets/dailys/02/Jul02/070202/99p-5332_sup0003_01_vol1.pdf [accessed August 28, 2006].

Nguon K, Baxter MG, Sajdel-Sulkowska EM. 2005. Perinatal exposure to polychlorinated biphenyls differentially affects cerebellar development and motor functions in male and female rat neonates. *Cerebellum* 4(2):112–122.

NRC (National Research Council). 1999. *Hormonally Active Agents in the Environment.* Washington, DC: National Academy Press.

NRC. 2000. *Toxicological Effects of Methylmercury.* Washington, DC: National Academy Press.

NRC. 2006. *Health Risks from Dioxin and Related Compounds: Evaluation of the EPA Reassessment.* Washington, DC: The National Academies Press.

Ocean Nutrition Canada. 2004. *Manufacturing: MEG-3.* [Online]. Available: http://www.ocean-nutrition.com/inside.asp?cmPageID=158/ [accessed May 11, 2006].

O'Neil CE, Lehrer SB. 1995. Seafood allergy and allergens: A review. *Food Technology* 49(10):103–116.

O'Neil C, Helbling AA, Lehrer SB. 1993. Allergic reactions to fish. *Clinical Reviews in Allergy* 11(2):183–200.

Oken E, Wright RO, Kleinman KP, Bellinger D, Hu H, Rich-Edwards JW, Gillman MW. 2005. Maternal fish consumption, hair mercury, and infant cognition in a US cohort. *Environmental Health Perspectives* 113(10):1376–1380.

Olsen SJ, MacKinon LC, Goulding JS, Bean NH, Slutsker L. 2000. Surveillance for foodborne disease outbreaks—United States, 1993–1997. *Morbidity and Mortality Weekly Report* 49(Surveillance Summary 1):1–51. [Online]. Available: http://www.cdc.gov/mmwr/preview/mmwrhtml/ss4901a1.htm [accessed March 31, 2006].

Olson RE. 1986. Marine fish parasites of public health importance. In: Kramer DE, Liston J, eds. *Seafood Quality Determination*. Amsterdam, the Netherlands: Elsevier Science Publishers. Pp. 339–355.

Ortiz-Roque C, Lopez-Rivera Y. 2004. Mercury contamination in reproductive age women in a Caribbean island: Vieques. *Journal of Epidemiology and Community Health* 58(9):756–757.

Otwell S, Garrido L, Garrido V, Benner R. 2001. *Farm-raised Shrimp: Good Aquacultural Practices for Product Quality and Safety*. Florida Sea Grant Publication SGEB-53. Gainesville, FL: Florida Sea Grant University. [Online]. Available: http://www.uhh.hawaii.edu/~pacrc/Mexico/files/manual/08_shrimp_farming_methods.pdf [accessed May 3, 2006].

Parizek J, Ostadalova I. 1967. The protective effect of small amounts of selenite in sublimate intoxication. *Experientia* 23(2):142–143.

Passos CJ, Mergler D, Gaspar E, Morais S, Lucotte M, Larribe F, Davidson R, de Grosbois S. 2003. Eating tropical fruit reduces mercury exposure from fish consumption in the Brazilian Amazon. *Environmental Research* 93(2):123–130.

Patandin S, Lanting CI, Mulder PG, Boersma ER, Sauer PJ, Weisglas-Kuperus N. 1999. Effects of environmental exposure to polychlorinated biphenyls and dioxins on cognitive abilities in Dutch children at 42 months of age. *Journal of Pediatrics* 134(1):33–41.

Paulsson K, Lundbergh K. 1989. The selenium method for treatment of lakes for elevated levels of mercury in fish. *Science of the Total Environment* 87–88:495–507.

Paustenbach D, Galbraith D. 2005. *Biomonitoring: Measuring Levels of Chemicals in People—and What the Results Mean*. New York, NY: American Council on Science and Health. [Online]. Available: http://www.acsh.org/docLib/20050721_biomonitoring.pdf [accessed March 28, 2006].

Peele C. 2004. *Washington State Polybrominated Diphenyl Ether (PBDE) Chemical Action Plan: Interim Plan*. Olympia, WA: Washington State Department of Ecology, Department of Health. [Online]. Available: http://www.ecy.wa.gov/pubs/0403056.pdf [accessed March 22, 2006].

Ralston NVC. 2005 (April 11). *Selenium Modulation of Toxicants in Seafood*. Presented to the Committee on Nutrient Relationships in Seafood: Selections to Balance the Benefits and Risks, Washington, DC, Institute of Medicine.

Rayne S, Ikonomou MG, Antcliffe B. 2003. Rapidly increasing polybrominated diphenyl ether concentrations in the Columbia River system from 1992 to 2000. *Environmental Science and Toxicology* 37(13):2847–2854.

Rice DC. 2000. Identification of functional domains affected by developmental exposure to methylmercury: Faroe Islands and related studies. *Neurotoxicology* 21(6):1039–1044.

Rice DC. 2004. The US EPA reference dose for methylmercury: Sources of uncertainty. *Environmental Research* 95(3):406–413.

Rice, DC. 2005 (February). *Brominated Flame Retardants: A Report to the Joint Standing Committee on Natural Resources, 122nd Maine Legislature*. Prepared by the Bureau of Health and Department of Environmental Protection. [Online]. Available: http://mainegov-images.informe.org/dep/rwm/publications/legislativereports/pdf/bromfeb2005.pdf#search=%22rice%20brominated%20flame%20retardants%3A%20a%20report%20to%20the%20joint%20standing%20committee%20on%20natural%20resources%22 [accessed August 26, 2006].

Rim H. 1982. Clonorchiasis. In: Hillyer G, Hopla C, eds. *CRC Handbook Series in Zoonoses, Volume II*. Boca Raton, FL: CRC Press Inc. Pp. 17–32.

Rissanen T, Voutilainen S, Nyyssonen K, Lakka TA, Salonen JT. 2000. Fish oil-derived fatty acids, docosahexenoic acid and docosapentaenoic acid, and the risk of acute coronary events—The Kuopio Ischaemic Heart Disease Risk Factor Study. *Circulation* 102(22):2677–2679.

Robson MG, Hamilton GC. 2005. Pest control and pesticides. In: Frumkin H, ed. *Environmental Health: From Global to Local*. San Fransisco: John Wiley and Sons, Inc. Pp. 544–580.

Rodgers RPC, Levin J. 1990. A critical reappraisal of the bleeding time. *Seminars in Thrombosis and Hemostasis* 16(1):1–20.

Rodrick GE, Cheng TG. 1989. Parasites: Occurrence and significance in marine animals. *Food Technology* 43(11):98–102.

Roegge CS, Schantz SL. 2006. Motor function following developmental exposure to PCBS and/or MEHG. *Neurotoxicology and Teratology* 28(2):260–277.

Roegge CS, Wang VC, Powers BE, Klintsova AY, Villareal S, Greenough WT, Schantz SL. 2004. Motor impairment in rats exposed to PCBs and methylmercury during early development. *Toxicological Sciences* 77(2):315–324.

Rogan WJ, Chen A. 2005. Health risks and benefits of bis(4-chlorophenyl)-1,1,1-trichloroethane (DDT). *Lancet* 366(9487):763–773.

Ross G. 2004. The public health implications of polychlorinated biphenyls (PCBs) in the environment. *Ecotoxicology and Environmental Safety* 59:275–291.

Ryan LM. 2005. *Effects of Prenatal Mercury Exposure on Childhood IQ: A Synthesis of Three Studies*. Report to the US Environmental Protection Agency.

Ryan JJ, Patry B, Mills P, Beaudoin NG. 2002. Recent trends in levels of brominated diphenyl ethers (BDEs) in human milks from Canada. *Organohalogen Compounds* 58:173–176.

SACN (Scientific Advisory Committee on Nutrition). 2004. *Advice on Fish Consumption: Benefits and Risks*. London, England: The Stationery Office.

Saint-Phard D, Gonzalez P, Sherman P. 2004. Unsuspected mercury toxicity linked to neurologic symptoms: A case series. *Archives of Physical and Medical Rehabilitation* 85:E25 (abstract).

Sakanari JA, Moser M, Deardorff TL. 1995. *Fish Parasites and Human Health: Epidemiology of Human Helminthic Infections*. California Sea Grant College, University of California.

Salonen JT, Seppanen K, Nyyssonen K, Korpela H, Kauhanen J, Kantola M, Tuomilehto J, Esterbauer H, Tatzber F, Salonen R. 1995. Intake of mercury from fish, lipid peroxidation, and the risk of myocardial infarction and coronary, cardiovascular, and any death in eastern Finnish men. *Circulation* 91(3):645–655.

Salonen JT, Seppanen K, Lakka TA, Salonen R, Kaplan GA. 2000. Mercury accumulation and accelerated progression of carotid atherosclerosis: A population-based prospective 4-year follow-up study in men in eastern Finland. *Atherosclerosis* 148(2):265–273.

Sampson HA. 1992. Food hypersensitivity: Manifestations, diagnosis, and natural history. *Food Technology* 46:141–156.

Santerre CR. 2004. Farmed salmon: Caught in a numbers game. *Journal of Food Technology* 58(2):108. [Online]. Available: http://seafood.ucdavis.edu/organize/santerresalmon.pdf [accessed April 27, 2006].

Schantz SL, Gardiner JC, Gasior DM, Sweeney AM, Humphrey HE, McCaffrey RJ. 1999. Motor function in aging Great Lakes fisheaters. *Environmental Research* 80(2 Part 2): S46–S56.

Schantz SL, Gasior DM, Polverejan E, McCaffrey RJ, Sweeney AM, Humphrey HE, Gardiner JC. 2001. Impairments of memory and learning in older adults exposed to polychlorinated biphenyls via consumption of Great Lakes fish. *Environmental Health Perspectives* 109(6):605–611.

Schantz SL, Widholm JJ, Rice DC. 2003. Effects of PCB exposure on neuropsychological function in children. *Environmental Health Perspectives* 111(3):1–27.

Schecter A, Päpke O, Tung K-C, Staskal D, Birnbaum L. 2004. Polybrominated diphenyl ethers contamination of United States food. *Environmental Science and Technology* 38(20):5306–5311.

Schecter A, Papke O, Tung KC, Joseph J, Harris TR, Dahlgren J. 2005. Polybrominated diphenyl ether flame retardants in the U.S. population: Current levels, temporal trends, and comparison with dioxins, dibenzofurans, and polychlorinated biphenyls. *Journal of Occupational and Environmental Medicine* 47(3):199–211.

Seychelles Medical and Dental Journal. 2004. Special Issue: Volume 7, Number 1. [Online]. Available: http://www.seychelles.net/smdj/ [accessed January 12, 2006].

Shamlaye C, Davidson PW, Myers GJ. 2004. The Seychelles Child Development Study: Two decades of collaboration. *Seychelles Medical and Dental Journal,* Special Issue 7(1):92–99. [Online]. Available: http://www.seychelles.net/smdj/SECIVB.pdf [accessed March 9, 2006].

Sjödin A, Jones RS, Focan J-F, Lapcza C, Wang RY, McGahee EE III, Zhang Y, Turner WE, Slazyk B, Needham L, Patterson DG Jr. 2004a. Retrospective time-trend study of polybrominated diphenyl ether and polybrominated and polychlorinated biphenyl levels in human serum from the United States. *Environmental Health Perspectives* 112(6):654–658.

Sjödin A, Päpke O, McGahee E III, Jones R, Focant J-F, Pless-Mulloli T, Toms L-M, Wang R, Zhang Y, Needham L, Herrmann T, Patterson D Jr. 2004b. Concentration of polybrominated diphenyl ethers (PBDEs) in house hold dust from various countries—inhalation a potential route of human exposure. *Organohalogen Compounds* 66:3817–3822.

Smith AG, Gangolli SD. 2002. Organochlorine and chemicals in seafood: Occurrence and health concerns. *Food and Chemical Toxicology* 40:767–779.

Stern AH, Smith AE. 2003. An assessment of the cord:maternal blood methylmercury ratio: Implications for risk assessment. *Environmental Health Perspectives* 111(12):1465–1470.

Stewart PW, Reihman J, Lonky EI, Darvill TJ, Pagano J. 2003. Cognitive development in preschool children prenatally exposed to PCBs and MeHg. *Neurotoxicology and Teratology* 25(1):11–22.

Stoker TE, Laws SC, Crofton KM, Hedge JM, Ferrell JM, Cooper RL. 2004. Assessment of DE-71, a commercial polybrominated diphenyl ether (PBDE) mixture, in the EDSP male and female pubertal protocols. *Toxicological Sciences* 78(1):144–155.

Taylor SL, Bush RK. 1988. Allergy by ingestion of seafood. In: Tu AT, ed. *Handbook of Natural Toxins, Volume 3, Marine Toxins and Venoms.* New York: Marcel Dekker. Pp. 149–183.

Taylor SL, Nordlee JA. 1993. Chemical additives in seafood products. *Clinical Reviews in Allergy* 11(2):261–291.

Ulbrich B, Stahlmann R. 2004. Developmental toxicity of polychlorinated biphenyls (PCBs): A systematic review of experimental data. *Archives in Toxicology* 78(5):252–268.

UNEP (United Nations Environment Programme). 2002. *Global Mercury Assessment.* Geneva, Switzerland: UNEP Chemicals. [Online]. Available: http://www.chem.unep.ch/mercury/Report/GMA-report-TOC.htm [accessed March 1, 2006].

UNEP Global Environmental Facility. 2003. *Regionally Based Assessment of Persistent Toxic Substances. Global Report 2003.* Geneva, Switzerland: United Nations. [Online]. Available: http://www.chem.unep.ch/pts/gr/Global_Report.pdf [accessed April 26, 2006].

US EPA (United States Environmental Protection Agency). 1987. *National Dioxin Study. Tiers 3, 5, 6, and 7.* EPA-440/4-87-003. Washington, DC: Office of Water Regulations and Standards.

US EPA. 1991. Guidelines for developmental toxicity risk assessment. *Federal Register* 56: 63798-63826. [Online]. Available: http://www.epa.gov/ncea/raf/pdfs/devtox.pdf [accessed April 26, 2006].

US EPA. 1994. *Exposure and Human Health Reassessment of 2,3,7,8-tetrachlorodibenzo-p-dioxin ((TCDD) and Related Compounds.* National Academy of Sciences (NAS) Review Draft. Washington, DC: National Center for Environmental Assessment.

US EPA. 1995. *The Use of the Benchmark Dose Approach in Health Risk Assessment.* EPA/630/R-94-007, Washington, DC: Office of Research and Development.

US EPA. 1997. *Mercury Report for Congress. Volume 1. Executive Summary.* EPA-452/R-97-003. Washington, DC: Office of Air Quality Planning and Standards and Office of Research and Development. [Online]. Available: http://www.epa.gov/ttn/oarpg/t3/reports/volume1.pdf [accessed January 12, 2006].

US EPA. 2000a. *Exposure and Human Health Reassessment of 2,3,7,8-tetrachlorodibenso-p-dioxin (TCDD) and Related Compounds.* Draft Final Report. Washington, DC: US EPA. [Online]. Available: http://cfpub.epa.gov/ncea/cfm/part1and2.cfm?ActType=default [accessed March 2, 2006].

US EPA. 2000b. *Guidance for Assessing Chemical Contaminant Data for Use in Fish Advisories. Volume II: Risk Assessments and Consumption Limits. Third Edition.* Washington, DC: Environmental Protection Agency. [Online]. Available: http://www.epa.gov/ost/fishadvice/volume2/index.html [accessed March 2, 2006].

US EPA. 2000c. *Exposure and Human Health Reassessment of 2,3,7,8-tetrachlorodibenso-p-dioxin (TCDD) and Related Compounds. Part III: Dioxin: Draft Integrated Summary and Risk Characterization for 2,3,7,8-Tetrachlorodibenzo-p-Dioxin (TCDD) and Related Compounds.* [Online]. Availabe: http://cfpub.epa.gov/ncea/cfm/part1and2.cfm?ActType=default [accessed August 26, 2006].

US EPA. 2001. *Water Quality Criterion for the Protection of Human Health: Methylmercury. Chapter 4: Risk Assessment for Methylmercury.* Washington, DC: Office of Sciences and Technology, Office of Water, EPA. [Online]. Available: http://www.epa.gov/waterscience/criteria/methylmercury/merc45.pdf [accessed September 12, 2005].

US EPA. 2003. *2001 Toxics Release Inventory Data Release Questions and Answers.* [Online]. Available: http://www.epa.gov/tri/tridata/tri01/external_qanda_for_revision.pdf [accessed March 13, 2006].

US EPA. 2005. *The Inventory of Sources and Environmental Releases of Dioxin-Like Compounds in the United States: The Year 2000 Update.* [Online]. Available: http://www.epa.gov/ncea/pdfs/dioxin/2k-update/ [accessed March 13, 2006].

US EPA. 2006. *Health Effects of PCBs.* [Online]. Available: http://www.epa.gov/pcb/pubs/effects.html [accessed March 2, 2006].

USDA (United States Department of Agriculture). 2005. *National Nutrient Database for Standard Release 18.* [Online]. Available: http://www.nal.usda.gov/fnic/foodcomp/Data/SR18/sr18.html) [accessed May 11, 2006].

Van den Berg M, Birnbaum L, Bosveld AT, Brunstrom B, Cook P, Feeley M, Giesy JP, Hanberg A, Hasegawa R, Kennedy SW, Kubiak T, Larsen JC, van Leeuwen FX, Liem AK, Nolt C, Peterson RE, Poellinger L, Safe S, Schrenk D, Tillitt D, Tysklind M, Younes M, Waern F, Zacharewski T. 1998. Toxic equivalency factors (TEFs) for PCBs, PCDDs, PCDFs for humans and wildlife. *Environmental Health Perspectives* 106(12):775–792.

Van Wijngaarden E, Beck C, Shamlaye CF, Cernichiari E, Davidson PW, Myers GJ, Clarkson TW. 2006. Benchmark concentrations for methyl mercury obtained from the 9-year follow-up of the Seychelles Child Development Study. *Neurotoxicology* 27(5):702–709.

Verity MA. 1997. Pathogenesis of methyl mercury neurotoxicity. In: Yasui M, Strong MJ, Ota K, Verity MA, eds. *Mineral and Metal Neurotoxicology.* Boca Raton, FL: CRC Press. Pp. 159–167.

Viberg H, Fredriksson A, Eriksson P. 2003. Neonatal exposure to polybrominated diphenyl ether (PBDE 153) disrupts spontaneous behaviour, impairs learning and memory and decreases hippocampal cholinergic receptors in adult mice. *Toxicology and Applied Pharmacology* 192(2):95–106.

Virtanen, JK, Voutilainen S, Rissanen TH, Mursu J, Tuomainen TP, Korhonen MJ, Valkonen VP, Seppanen K, Laukkanen JA, Salonen JT. 2005. Mercury, fish oils, and risk of acute coronary events and cardiovascular disease, coronary heart disease, and all-cause mortality in men in eastern Finland. *Arteriosclerosis, Thrombosis and Vascular Biology* 25(1):228–233.

Vreugdenhil HJ, Lanting CI, Mulder PG, Boersma ER, Weisglas-Kuperus N. 2002a. Effects of prenatal PCB and dioxin background exposure on cognitive and motor abilities in Dutch children at school age. *Journal of Pediatrics* 40(1):48–56.

Vreugdenhil HJ, Slijper FM, Mulder PG, Weisglas-Kuperus N. 2002b. Effects of perinatal exposure to PCBs and dioxins on play behavior in Dutch children at school age. *Environmental Health Perspectives* 110(10):A593–A598.

Vreugdenhil HJ, Mulder PG, Emmen HH, Weisglas-Kuperus N. 2004. Effects of perinatal exposure to PCBs on neuropsychological functions in the Rotterdam cohort at 9 years of age. *Neuropsychology* 18(1):185–193.

Vupputuri S, Longnecker MP, Daniels JL, Guo X, Sandler DP. 2005. Blood mercury level and blood pressure among US women: Results from the National Health and Nutrition Examination Survey, 1999–2000. *Environmental Research* 97(2):195–200.

Walkowiak J, Wiener JA, Fastabend A, Heinzow B, Kramer U, Schmidt E, Steingruber HJ, Wundram S, Winneke G. 2001. Environmental exposure to polychlorinated biphenyls and quality of the home environment: Effects on psychodevelopment in early childhood. *Lancet* 358(9293):1602–1607.

Watanabe C. 2002. Modification of mercury toxicity by selenium: Practical importance? *Tohoku Journal of Experimental Medicine* 196(2):71–77.

Weil M, Bressler J, Parsons P, Bolla K, Glass T, Schwartz B. 2005. Blood mercury levels and neurobehavioral function. *Journal of the American Medical Association* 293(15):1875–1882.

Weinstein MR, Litt M, Kertesz DA, Wyper P, Ross D, Coulter M, McGreer A, Facklam R, Ostach C, Willey BM Borczyk A, Low DE, and the Investigative Team. 1997. Invasive infection due to a fish pathogen: Streptococcus iniae. *New England Journal of Medicine* 337(9):589–594.

Whanger PD. 1985. Metabolic interactions of selenium with cadmium, mercury, and silver. *Advances in Nutritional Research* 7:221–250.

WHO (World Health Organization). 1990. *Environmental Health Criteria 101: Methylmercury.* Geneva, Switzerland: WHO. [Online]. Available http://www.inchem.org/documents/ehc/ehc/ehc101.htm [accessed March 9, 2006].

WHO. 2001. Consultation on Risk Assessment of Non-Dioxin-Like PCBs. 2001 (September 3–4). Presented at the Federal Institute for Health Protection of Consumers and Veterinary Medicine (BgVV), Berlin, Germany. [Online]. Available: http://www.who.int//pcs/docs/consultation_%20pcb.htm [accessed March 17, 2006].

WHO. 2003. *Diet, Nutrition, and the Prevention of Chronic Diseases.* Geneva, Switzerland: WHO. [Online]. Available: http://www.who.int/hpr/NPH/docs/who_fao_expert_report.pdf [accessed March 2, 2006].

Willett, WC. 2006. Fish: Balancing health risks and benefits. *American Journal of Preventive Medicine* 29(4):320–321.

Winneke G, Walkowiak J, Lilienthal H. 2002. PCB-induced neurodevelopmental toxicity in human infants and its potential mediation by endocrine dysfunction. *Toxicology* 181–182:161–165.

Yokoo EM, Valente JG, Grattan L, Schmidt SL, Platt I, Silbergeld EK. 2003. Low level methylmercury exposure affects neuropsychological function in adults. *Environmental Health* 2(1):8.

Yoneda S, Suzuki KT. 1997. Detoxification of mercury by selenium by binding of equimolar Hg-Se complex to a specific plasma protein. *Toxicology and Applied Pharmacology* 143(2):274–280.

Yoshizawa K, Rimm EB, Morris JS, Spate VL, Hsieh C-C, Spiegelman D, Stampfer MJ, Willett WC. 2002. Mercury and the risk of coronary heart disease in men. *New England Journal of Medicine* 347(22):1755–1760.

5

Analysis of the Balancing of Benefits and Risks of Seafood Consumption

The committee's task included a charge to develop a decision path appropriate to the needs of US consumers for selecting seafood in ways that balance nutritional benefits against exposure risks. In the committee's judgment, there are three distinct steps in the process of designing consumer guidance about balancing benefits and risks in making seafood consumption decisions (see Box 5-1). After a brief overview, this chapter addresses the first step in the process: the scientific assessment and balancing of the benefits and risks of seafood consumption. Subsequent chapters address the second and third steps in the process.

The scientific assessment and balancing of the benefits and risks of seafood consumption contained in this chapter is based on the evidence presented in Chapters 3 and 4. The committee found that its ability to quantify benefit-risk trade-offs was limited from the benefit side (e.g., the quantitative link between eicosapentaenoic acid/docosahexaenoic acid [EPA/DHA] consumption and health benefits), the risk side (e.g., the quantitative risk of methylmercury [MeHg] exposure for adult men), and in terms of benefit-risk interactions. Because of this uncertainty, the committee concluded that it was not feasible to present a quantitative benefit-risk assessment and balancing. Thus it relied on its expert judgement to produce a qualitative scientific benefit-risk analysis and balancing of the benefits and risks of seafood consumption.

INTRODUCTION

Advice to consumers about balancing the benefits and risks of seafood consumption must be based on the best available scientific information. The

---

BOX 5-1
A Three-Step Process to Design Consumer Guidance on Balancing Benefits and Risks Associated with Seafood Consumption

Step 1: Scientific benefit-risk analysis and balancing of the benefits and risks (including attention to characteristics [e.g., age, sex] that distinguish target populations and the effects of potential food substitutions made by consumers).

Step 2: Empirical analysis of consumer perceptions and decision-making (understanding decision contexts and their variability; eliciting input from consumers regarding how they perceive and make choices) (see Chapter 6).

Step 3: Design and evaluation of the guidance program itself (including the format of guidance, program structure and media [e.g., brochures, websites, public meetings or programs, radio spots, point-of-purchase displays, hotlines], and the combination of communication products and processes) (see Chapter 7).

---

scientific assessment and balancing of the benefits and risks associated with seafood consumption is a complex task. Diverse evidence, of varying levels of completeness and uncertainty, on different types of benefits and risks must be combined to carry out the balancing required in the first step in designing consumer guidance. To produce coordinated benefit-risk advice requires combining expertise from several disciplines, as this committee has done.

In other settings, balancing benefits and risks has been approached through a variety of summary metrics. These include: Quality Adjusted Life Years (QALYs), which combine the quantity and quality of life; Disability Adjusted Life Years (DALYs), which are the sum of years of potential life lost due to premature mortality and the years of productive life lost due to disability (Gold et al., 2002); monetary measures; utility measures (estimates from multi-attribute utility analyses); and deliberative decision-making exercises. These decision-making exercises focus on trade-offs as a means to inform policymakers about, first, decision attributes of different choices and, second, development of means-ends objectives networks that illustrate values people want to achieve and how they think those can best be achieved (Gregory and Wellman, 2001; Gregory et al., 2001). However, in the case where benefits and risks have an outcome on the same endpoint, such as MeHg and EPA/DHA impacts on neurologic development, it is not necessary to artificially link the benefit and risk through a separate construct such as QALYs.

In light of uncertainty in the scientific information associated with both nutrient intake and contaminant exposure from seafood, it is the committee's judgment that no summary metric adequately captures the complexity of seafood benefit-risk trade-offs. The committee outlined an approach to balance benefits against risks, conducted an analysis of the trade-offs, and considered additional factors that informed each in order to produce a decision framework that incorporates benefit and risk analysis. Over time, the process of balancing benefits and risks must be iterative, with systematic, objective reviews following strict profiles, and updates and reinterpretation as new evidence is developed. This can be accomplished through the convening of an expert group such as this committee or through the organization of expertise within federal agencies to provide comprehensive benefit-risk analysis rather than piecemeal benefit-by-benefit and risk-by-risk analysis.

APPROACH TO BALANCING BENEFITS AND RISKS

In developing its approach to balancing benefits and risks, the committee considered previous approaches developed to analyze scientific evidence and balance benefits and risks: two of these approaches are risk-risk or risk-trade-off analysis and risk relationship analysis.

"Risk-risk" or "risk-trade-off" analysis was developed as a means of further evaluating regulatory and other actions targeted at reducing a specific risk (Gray and Hammitt, 2000; Hammitt, 2000; IOM, 2003). This approach emphasizes that in reducing a targeted risk, it is possible that other risks would be created or increased. This approach also provides a means for considering multiple countervailing risks that may indicate whether it is either riskier to remediate a problem or take no action.

"Risk-relationship" analysis goes a step further, recognizing the possible existence of ancillary benefits as well as countervailing risks that may result from adopting a particular risk-management option (IOM, 2003). For example, efforts to reduce a contaminant in a specific food product may pose a countervailing risk if the efforts make a nutrient-rich food too expensive for some consumers to afford. In addition, the higher price of the product could cause consumers to switch to alternative products that pose similar or higher risk from the same or other contaminants. However, if the product is high in a food component that is unhealthful, then a switch away from it may generate ancillary benefits such as reduced risk for chronic disease.

The committee concluded that its charge goes an important additional step beyond risk-relationship analysis. Risk-relationship analysis starts with a targeted risk reduction and attempts to identify significant potential ancillary benefits and countervailing risks that may affect the risk reduction actually achieved through a risk management option. In the case of designing guidance to consumers on selecting seafood, there is a suite of benefits and risks that needs to be simultaneously targeted and considered. The target of analysis is the overall effect of seafood selection and consumption decisions, and not reduction of a specific risk or enhancement of a specific benefit. For this reason, the construct of ancillary benefits and countervailing risks is not applicable.

For Step 1 of the three-step process, the committee developed the approach of *benefit-risk analysis* to design consumer guidance on balancing benefits and risks associated with seafood consumption, shown in Box 5-1. The approach points to the types of information needed to improve benefit-risk decisions. An expert judgment technique is one approach to this task, given the uncertainty in the data that supports the evidence on benefits and risks. In its deliberations, the commmittee adapted a four-part protocol based on previous work (IOM, 2003) to complete Step 1, scientific benefit-risk analysis, in the process of designing seafood guidance.

Part A. Identify and determine the magnitude of the benefits and risks associated with different types of consumption for the population as a whole and, if appropriate, for specific target populations.

Part B. Identify the benefits and risks that evidence suggests are important enough to be included in the balancing process used to develop consumption guidance for the population as a whole and, if appropriate, for specific target populations.

Part C. Evaluate changes in benefits and risks associated with changes in consumption patterns. The magnitude of the changes depends on the magnitude of exposure to specific agents, either nutrients or contaminants, and how the magnitude of the response varies in relation to changes in intake or exposure.

Part D. Balance the benefits and risks to arrive at specific guidance for healthy consumption for the population as a whole and, if appropriate, for specific target populations.

SCIENTIFIC BENEFIT-RISK ANALYSIS FOR SEAFOOD CONSUMPTION

Part A. Identify and Determine the Magnitude of the Benefits and Risks

The committee identified the range of benefits and risks that the evidence suggests are important to balance in developing seafood choice guidance. The nutritional benefits of seafood include: it is a source of protein that is low in saturated fat, and contains several essential micronutrients, especially selenium. Seafood also is a primary source of the omega-3 fatty acids EPA and DHA. The evidence detailed in Chapter 3 indicates that consumption of seafood and/or EPA/DHA by pregnant females may provide benefits to their developing fetuses. Infants receiving EPA/DHA either from breast milk or supplemented formula may benefit in terms of neurological and visual development. Similarly, there is evidence that consumption of fish is associated with cardiovascular benefits in the general population.

These benefits must be balanced against risks to health, as reviewed in Chapter 4, from exposure to chemical and/or microbial contamination that may be present in some seafood available to US consumers. The best-characterized risk from chemical contamination of seafood is from methylmercury, a potent neurotoxin. Thus, the population groups at greatest risk from exposure to contaminants in seafood are the developing fetus, infants, and young children. As discussed in Chapter 4, a Reference Dose (RfD) has been established for methylmercury on the basis of developmental tests in children born to mothers from populations where seafood is a major part of their diets. At the same time, evidence suggests the fetus and infant may be among the principal beneficiaries from certain nutrients in seafood. Evidence available on levels of MeHg that may be detrimental to nonpregnant adults has not allowed the formulation of a similar reference dose based on risks to these population segments.

In establishing their joint advisory targeted at pregnant women and children, the US Environmental Protection Agency (US EPA) and Food and Drug Administration (FDA) examined potential intakes of MeHg that would occur in pregnant women given consumption patterns using various available commercial sources of seafood. If predatory fish high in mercury were avoided completely, they concluded that up to 12 ounces of fish (four 3-ounce servings per week) could be consumed without exceeding the RfD dose that has been established with studies in populations of women consuming substantial amounts of seafood (US EPA/FDA, 2004) (see Chapter 4). Though the committee recognized that the RfD was not a "bright line" that established a firm cutoff for risk, the FDA/EPA fish advisory provides reasonable guidelines for pregnant women to consume seafood in amounts that may confer benefit without significantly increasing risk. There is little evidence available about levels of methylmercury that may be detrimental to other segments of the population.

Risks from other contaminants in seafood are, comparatively, less well-characterized than methylmercury. Contamination from persistant organic pollutants (POPs) has been characterized at exposure levels that result from industrial releases or occupational exposure, and for fish-consumers in geographic areas where contaminants are more concentrated. However, at lower levels of exposure there is less information available on adverse health effects. In addition, levels of dioxin-like compounds (DLCs) and polychlorinated biphenyls (PCBs) vary considerably among different types of seafood, with relatively higher levels found in fatty compared to lean fish. There is limited available data on levels of DLCs and PCBs in seafood and terrestrial animal products, but levels in seafood may on average be comparable to or higher than those in red meat and full-fat dairy products (IOM, 2003). Risks from microbiological hazards will vary, largely according to handling and preparation methods (e.g., consuming raw rather than cooked seafood).

Part B. Identify Important Benefits and Risks in the Balancing Process

Although some guidance applies to all groups, e.g., general nutritional benefits and microbial risks, a key conclusion of the committee's deliberations is that the evidence in regard to the benefits and risks associated with seafood consumption varies in important ways across target populations. Thus, guidance should be tailored to these populations. Equally important is that everyone in the population be covered by specific guidance.

Given the current evidence reviewed in this report, decisions about seafood consumption for the general population consuming commercially available seafood fall into four target populations: (1) females who are or may become pregnant, and those who are breastfeeding; (2) infants and children up to age 12; (3) adolescent males, adult males, and females who will not become pregnant; and (4) adult males and females at risk for coronary heart disease. During the committee's initial deliberations, adult males and females with a *history* of coronary heart disease were considered as a separate target population. However, recent evidence suggests that the guidance for these persons is not different from that for adult males and females at risk of coronary heart disease.

The committee recognizes that there are additional groups of consumers for whom guidance must be further tailored, such as subsistence and recreational fishers. However, designing guidance for these groups requires further separate, specific analyses of benefit and risk impacts. As noted in Chapter 4, to date there is little known about the impact of high seafood consumption, beyond that previously reported on neurological development in fetuses and young children. The committee decided there was insufficient evidence to set an upper limit on the amount of seafood consumed each week by the general public, except where research supports such recommendations.

Part C: Evaluating Changes in Benefits and Risks Associated with Changes in Consumption Patterns

The committee conducted several analyses to evaluate and understand changes in benefits and risks that may be associated with changes in consumption patterns that could occur due to the type of guidance provided to consumers. The extent of these changes depends on the magnitude of exposure to a specific agent—either nutrients or contaminants—and how the change of the response varies in relation to changes in intake or exposure. These analyses and their implications for the design of consumer guidance are discussed below.

Substitution Impact on Selected Nutrients

The committee reviewed the impact of substitution in two ways. First, it considered the quantity of various foods that would need to be eaten to provide approximately 100 mg of EPA/DHA. Next, the committee reviewed the differences in selected nutrients contributed by 3-ounce portions of various meat, poultry, and seafood sources. While recognizing that there are many species of seafood, those chosen for this analysis represent the most frequently eaten types in the United States (e.g., shrimp, tuna, and salmon). The committee further considered the contribution of specific nutrient levels (e.g., EPA/DHA in species of salmon) in developing consumer guidance (see Figures 7-5 through 7-8b). The committee looked at the specific impact of food choice trade-offs involving calories, saturated fat, EPA/DHA, selenium, and iron. The committee did not consider potential impacts of seafood choices on other vitamins and minerals because it relied on the conclusions already drawn by the Dietary Guidelines Advisory Committee (DGAC) that the substitution of two servings of seafood for two servings of animal protein foods would not substantially impact the vitamin and mineral content of the diet of the average American consumer (DGAC, 2005).

Figure 5-1 compares the number of portions (servings) from various animal foods that an individual would need to select to consume 100 mg EPA/DHA. The graph shows that to achieve a similar EPA/DHA intake level, a smaller amount of a high-EPA/DHA seafood, e.g., salmon, is needed compared to other food sources. This difference (consuming higher quantities of food to achieve an equivalent intake of EPA/DHA) is significant because of the corollary increase in total caloric and saturated fat intake from most other foods (see Table 5-1). Nonanimal sources of omega-3 fatty acids are not included in this comparison.

Weighing benefits against risks from consuming seafood needs to be considered in the context of the total diet. Table 5-1 highlights nutritional factors that may influence the assessment of the benefits and risks associated with seafood consumption by comparing nutrient levels from one 3-ounce serving of different animal protein foods commonly consumed by Americans. The foods selected as examples include lean (10 percent fat) and fatty (20 percent fat) beef, chicken (< 5 percent fat), shrimp, and canned tuna, both light and white (albacore). Preparation methods chosen were the low-

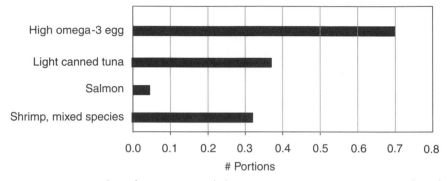

FIGURE 5-1 Number of portions* needed to consume 100 mg EPA/DHA in selected animal protein foods.
*Portion size = 100 g uncooked for all foods except eggs (~85 g = 1 egg).
SOURCE: US Department of Agriculture [USDA] *Nutrient Database, Release 18.* [Online]. Available: http://www.nal.usda.gov/fnic/foodcomp/Data/SR18/sr18.html; Sindelar et al., 2004.

est in fat (e.g., baked). It should be noted that any adjustments to the total diet to accommodate the addition of one food choice can be balanced by decreases in other choices (e.g., higher and lower energy foods). Benefits associated with selecting a specific food may be counterbalanced by risks associated with food preparation methods, e.g., the introduction of more calories and saturated fat by frying fish.

Although most seafood choices are lower in fat than animal meats, poultry, and eggs, the impact on energy and saturated fat intake depends on the particular substitution being made. For example, although salmon provides less energy and saturated fat than either of the beef choices shown in Table 5-1, it is higher in both these nutrients than chicken or eggs. Nonetheless, the substitution of salmon for all other animal protein sources results in increases in EPA/DHA intake levels (from 0.0 to 1.8 g). In fact, the substitution of any of the seafood choices listed in Table 5-1 for any of the beef, chicken, or egg choices results in more EPA/DHA and selenium. Finally, it can be seen that salmon and tuna are generally lower in iron than beef, which may be a consideration for pregnant females, other females of childbearing age, and individuals at risk for iron deficiency anemia.

Substitution Impact on Selected Contaminants

There are limited available data from which to construct scenarios of the risk impacts of substituting seafood for other animal protein sources. Contaminants for which there are reported values are methylmercury and dioxins and DLCs. Food choices are compared in Table 5-1. For a 57 kg reference female to make a weekly selection of two 3-ounce servings of seafood and not exceed the RfD level for methylmercury (5.7 µg MeHg per day) requires that no more than one of those selections be white (albacore) tuna. In contrast, levels of DLCs in two 3-ounce servings of white (albacore) or light canned tuna or salmon do not exceed target exposure limits. Making a trade-off of 20 percent fat beef for salmon will not decrease the exposure levels to DLCs, although it will for MeHg. Selecting light canned tuna in place of white (albacore) tuna will decrease exposure levels to both MeHg and DLCs, but will also significantly decrease intake levels of EPA/DHA.

Uncertainties in Substitution Analysis

The substitution analyses presented above are based on nutrient and contaminant values. However, there are several sources of uncertainty in the estimates of these nutrient and contaminant values. Mean estimates of nutrients represent best estimates of the value one would expect to find in any specific case. A common indication of how much one can expect individual values to vary from the mean is a confidence band, the calculation of which is based on the individual sample values observed. The committee did not have access to individual sample values or estimates of the variability in those for the estimates reported in Table 5-1.

Table 5-2 characterizes some of what is known about the data from which the estimates in Table 5-1 were derived (i.e., their provenance). As Table 5-2 illustrates, sample sizes and ages vary tremendously. While it is difficult to determine just how significant it is, variability in sample sizes and approaches, together with changes over time in analytical methods (Igarashi et al., 2000; Siddiqui et al., 2003) and in feed (e.g., reductions in the use of fishmeal in poultry feed) are noteworthy sources of uncertainties (Barlow, 2001). The EPA/DHA levels in chicken provide a case in point.

Comparison of the estimates in Table 5-1 with those from other sources also suggests considerable variability and uncertainty. Hamilton et al. (2005) illustrate that levels of omega-3 fatty acids in salmon vary by source. Using samples of farmed, wild, and store-purchased salmon from a large number of locations, they estimated that omega-3 fatty acid levels in farmed Atlantic salmon are more than twice as high as in salmon from other sources. Further, their estimate of omega-3 fatty acid levels in farmed Atlantic salmon is almost twice as high as that shown in Table 5-1.

Importantly, specific population subgroups, e.g., Native Alaskans who previously relied on seafood and marine mammal consumption and followed advice to decrease their intake of these foods to reduce the risks associated with exposure to contaminants, suffered negative consequences in overall nutrition (Wheately and Wheately, 1981; Murphy et al., 1995;

TABLE 5-1 Estimated Levels of Selected Nutrients and Contaminants per 3-ounce Cooked Serving of Seafood and Animal Food Choices

Food Choice	Energy # Data points	kcal/3 oz[a,*]	Saturated Fat # Data points	g/3 oz[a,*]	Cholesterol # Data points	mg/3 oz[a,*]	EPA/DHA # Data points	g/3 oz[a,*]
Salmon	N/A	175	N/A	2.1	2	54	2	1.8
White (albacore) tuna	N/A	109	N/A	0.7	N/A	36	N/A	0.7
Light tuna	N/A	99	N/A	0.2	3	26	5	0.2
Shrimp	N/A	84	N/A	0.2	0	166	11	0.3
Beef, 20% fat	N/A	230	35	5.8	36	77	N/A	0
Beef, 10% fat	N/A	184	35	4	36	72	N/A	0
Chicken[j]	N/A	140	N/A	0.9	0	72	N/A	0.03
Egg[i]	N/A	132	N/A	2.8	7	360	37	0.04
Point of Reference	EER[1,d] Men ≈ 2700 kcal/day Women ≈ 2100 kcal/day Pregnant ≈ +300 kcal/day Lactating ≈ +500 kcal/day		As low as possible while consuming a nutritionally adequate diet[1]		As low as possible while consuming a nutritionally adequate diet[1]		AI of total omega-3[1,e] Men = 1.6 g/day Women = 1.1 g/day Pregnant = 1.4 g/day Lactating = 1.3 g/day *Assume that 10% of total omega-3 fatty acids come from EPA/DHA*	

Food Choice	Selenium # Data points	µg/3 oz[a,*]	Iron # Data points	mg/3 oz[a,*]	Methylmercury # Data points	µg/3 oz[b,**]	Dioxin/Dioxin-like Compounds # Data points	TEQ/3 oz[c,***]
Salmon	N/A	35.2	2	0.3	N/A	1	N/A	21
White (albacore) tuna	2	55.8	5	0.8	N/A	29	N/A	No data
Light tuna	45	68.3	30	1.3	N/A	10	N/A	1

Shrimp	58	33.7	N/A	2.6	4	N/A	4
Beef, 20% fat	72	18.3	36	2.1	0	N/A	20
Beef, 10% fat	72	18.4	36	2.3	0	N/A	10
Chicken[i]	20	23.5	16	0.9	0	N/A	2
Egg[i]	69	26.2	14	1	0	N/A	2
Point of Reference	RDA[2,f] Men and women = 55 µg/day Pregnant = 60 µg/day Lactating = 70 µg/day		RDA[3,f] Men = 8 mg/day Women = 18 mg/day Pregnant = 27 mg/day Lactating = 9 mg/day		Rfd[4,g] Men and women = 0.1 µg/kg/day		TDI[5,h] Men and women = 1–4 TEQ/kg/day

NOTE: N/A means that the values are not available.

[a]For nutrient data: Salmon = Salmon, Atlantic, farmed, cooked; White tuna = Tuna, white, canned in water, drained; Light tuna = Tuna, light, canned in water, drained; Shrimp = Shrimp, cooked, moist heat; Beef, 20% fat = Beef, ground, 80% lean/20% fat, broiled; Beef 10% fat = Beef, ground, 90% lean/10% fat, broiled; Chicken = Chicken, breast, meat only, cooked, roasted; Egg = Egg, whole, cooked, hard-boiled.

[b]For methylmercury data: White tuna = Tuna (canned, albacore); Light tuna = Tuna (canned, light); Beef = Beef w/vegetables in sauce, from Chinese restaurant; Chicken = Chicken breast, roasted; Egg = Egg, boiled.

[c]TEQ = Toxicity Equivalency (see Chapter 4 for explanation); Because of different analytical methods, the dioxin/DLC data are averaged from 2001, 2002, and 2003. Ground beef represents lower-fat beef, chuck roast represents higher-fat beef, roasted chicken breast data was used for "chicken," and boiled egg data was used for "egg."

[d]EER = Estimated Energy Requirements. EER for men aged 19 years and older = 662 − (9.53 × age in years) + PA(15.91 × weight in kilograms + 539.6 × height in meters); reference man is 70 kg in weight, 1.77 m in height, PA of 1.11 (low active). EER for women aged 19 years and older = 354 − (6.91 × age in years) + PA(9.36 × weight in kilograms + 726 × height in meters); reference women is 57 kg in weight, 1.63 m in height, PA of 1.12 (low active).

[e]AI = Adequate Intake; the recommended average daily intake level that is assumed to be adequate for a group (or groups) of apparently healthy people, used when an RDA cannot be determined.

[f]RDA = Recommended Dietary Allowances; the average daily dietary nutrient intake level sufficient to meet the nutrient requirement of 97 to 98 percent of healthy individuals in a particular life stage and gender group.

[g]Rfd = Reference Dose; an estimate (with uncertainty spanning perhaps an order of magnitude) of daily exposure to the human population (including sensitive subgroups) that is likely to be without an appreciable risk of deleterious effects during a lifetime; for a 70 kg reference man the Rfd is 7 µg/day; for a 57 kg reference women the Rfd is 5.7 µg/day.

continued

TABLE 5-1 Continued

[b]TDI = Tolerable Daily Intake; represents an index for a contaminant similar to the Adequate Daily Intake, used for food additives. These limits are based on the assumption of an experimental threshold dose level below which no toxic effect is found in animal models and includes an additional uncertainty factor for extrapolation to humans. TEQ = Toxicity Equivalency.

[i]EPA/DHA levels in chicken and egg are based on existing published data; changes in the use of fishmeal in feed sources may have an impact on levels detected in the future.

SOURCES:
*USDA, 2005.
**Adapted from http://www.cfsan.fda.gov/~frf/sea-mehg.html; Carrington et al., 2004; Mahaffey, 2004; CFSAN, 2005b.
***Adapted from CFSAN, 2005a.
[1] IOM, 2002/2005.
[2] IOM, 2000.
[3] IOM, 2001.
[4] NRC, 2000.
[5] IOM, 2003.

TABLE 5-2 Data Available on Sampling of Selenium, EPA/DHA, and Mercury in Food

Food	Selenium[a]	EPA/DHA[a]	Methylmercury[b]
Salmon (Atlantic, farmed, cooked)	N/A*	2 samples	5 samples: 4 from 1992, 1 from 1993
Tuna (light, canned in water, drained)	45 samples	5 samples	2 samples from 1991–1992 (plus 131 samples for methylmercury from 2003–2004)
Shrimp	58 samples	11 samples	19 samples from 1991–1992, 1993, 1996 (plus 2 samples for methylmercury from 1993 and 1995)
Chicken[c]	20 samples (data over 20 years old); New data forthcoming show most nutrient levels comparable to earlier samples, but EPA/DHA levels as undetectable.		44 samples from 1990–1993 through 2003–2004

*N/A means that the values are not available.

SOURCES:
[a]Data from USDA Agriculture Handbook 8 (1976–1992) and its four supplements (1990–1993) as listed in USDA, 2005.
[b]CFSAN, 2006a.
[c]Personal communication, J.M. Holden, USDA-ARS-BHNRC-NDL, Beltsville, MD, March 30, 2006.

Nobmann and Lanier, 2001). Native Alaskans who switched from their traditional diet high in seafood products had few affordable healthful substitution foods from which to choose. When they decreased their seafood intake, they purchased more processed foods that were less nutrient-dense (such as manufactured snack products) and actually decreased the overall quality of their diets (see discussion Chapter 2, *American Indian/Alaska Native and First Nations Populations*).

Table 5-2 illustrates the available sampling data on nutrients and contaminants in food. The Agricultural Research Service (ARS) of the US Department of Agriculture (USDA) has begun updating its nutrient database through its National Food and Nutrient Analysis Program in collaboration with the National Institutes of Health (NIH). This ambitious project, which began in 1997, includes instituting a monitoring program for key foods and critical nutrients; conducting a thorough analysis of selected poultry products, restaurant foods, and items on FDA's list of the most commonly consumed fruits, vegetables, and seafood; and developing databases of foods of importance to ethnic subpopulations (Source: http://www.ars.usda.gov/ Research/docs.htm?docid=9446).

In the committee's judgment, it is important to conduct substitution analyses of the potential impacts of changes in consumption despite the uncertainties about the underlying nutrient and contamination levels. These analyses are incorporated into the balancing of benefits and risks in the following discussion.

Part D: Balancing the Benefits and Risks to Arrive at Specific Guidance for Healthy Consumption

To complete the scientific analysis considering benefits and risks together, the committee developed the following consumption guidance for each of the four target population groups:

1. Females who are or may become pregnant or who are breast-feeding:
    a. May benefit from consuming seafood, especially those with relatively higher concentrations of EPA and DHA;
    b. A reasonable intake would be two 3-ounce (cooked) servings but can safely consume 12 ounces per week;
    c. Can consume up to 6 ounces of white (albacore) tuna per week;
    d. Should avoid large predatory fish such as shark, swordfish, tilefish, or king mackerel.
2. Children up to age 12:
    a. May benefit from consuming seafood, especially those with relatively higher concentrations of EPA and DHA;

b. A reasonable intake would be two 3-ounce (cooked), or age-appropriate, servings but can safely consume 12 ounces per week;

c. Can consume up to 6 ounces (or age-appropriate servings) of white (albacore) tuna per week;

d. Should avoid large predatory fish such as shark, swordfish, tilefish, or king mackerel.

3. Adolescent males, adult males, and females who will not become pregnant:

a. May reduce their risk for cardiovascular disease by consuming seafood regularly, e.g., two 3-ounce servings per week;

b. Who consume more than two servings a week should choose a variety of types of seafood to reduce the risk for exposure to contaminants from a single source;

4. Adult males and females who are at risk of cardiovascular disease:

a. May reduce their risk of cardiovascular disease by consuming seafood regularly, e.g., two 3-ounce servings per week;

b. Although supporting evidence is limited, there may be additional benefits from including high-EPA/DHA seafood selections;

c. Who consume more than two servings a week should choose a variety of types of seafood to reduce the risk for exposure to contaminants from a single source.

This information differs from the dietary guidance and advisories available from federal agencies and private organizations (see Chapter 2) in three important ways. First, the information combines benefit and risk information to yield coordinated statements. Second, the information comprehensively covers everyone in the population so that population groups are not left with uncertainties about which information applies to them. Third, while previous guidance has had tailored messages for people with a risk for cardiovascular disease (and to those with a history of such disease), the committee concludes that current scientific evidence suggests that the guidance for them is not materially different from that for the more general "adolescent males, adult males, and females who will not become pregnant" reflected above. For this reason the decision pathway that follows focuses on target populations 1–3 identified above. This suggested guidance should be reconsidered periodically as new data on risks and benefits associated with seafood consumption emerge.

The suggested guidance presented above is the endpoint of judgements about the important benefits and risks, as well as how they balance. The process of forming such guidance can be made more transparent with the use of tables that present the key considerations. Table 5-3 illustrates this

TABLE 5-3 Potential for Benefits and Risks Associated with Seafood Choices by Population Group

Seafood Choices for Females Who Are or May Become Pregnant and Those Who Are Breastfeeding

Choice	Consume locally caught freshwater fish (commercial and recreational catches) only after checking state advisories.
Potential for Benefit	Might reduce food costs; continues family traditions.
Potential for Risk	Potential for increased MeHg, dioxin, and PCB exposure compared to other seafood selections. Risk for bacterial contamination will increase if consumed raw. Intake levels of iron will be lower than meat selections.
Choice	**May benefit from consuming seafood, especially those with relatively higher concentrations of EPA and DHA. A reasonable intake would be two 3-ounce (cooked) servings but can safely consume 12 ounces per week; should avoid large predatory fish such as shark, swordfish, tilefish, or king mackerel.**
Potential for Benefit	Seafood is a high-quality low-fat protein source. Intake levels of saturated fat will likely decrease compared to meat selections. Intake levels of EPA/DHA will increase compared to meat and "nonfatty" seafood selections. Intake of selenium may increase compared with beef, pork, and poultry selections.
Potential for Risk	Available data suggest levels of MeHg are not associated with adverse health effects if consumption is limited to no more than four 3-ounce servings per week. Potential risk from exposure to dioxins and PCBs is similar to meat selections. Risk for bacterial contamination will increase if raw seafood is consumed. Intake levels of iron will be lower than meat selections.
Choice	**Can consume up to 6 ounces of white (albacore) tuna per week.**
Potential for Benefit	Seafood is a high-quality low-fat protein source. Intake levels of saturated fat will likely decrease compared to meat selections. Intake levels of EPA/DHA will increase compared to meat and leaner seafood selections. Intake of selenium may increase compared with beef, pork, and poultry selections.
Potential for Risk	Available data suggest levels of MeHg are not associated with adverse health effects if consumption is limited to 6 ounces per week. Potential risk from exposure to dioxins and PCBs is similar to meat selections. Risk for bacterial contamination will increase if raw seafood is consumed. Intake levels of iron will be lower than meat selections.

Seafood Choices for Children up to Age 12

Choice	**May benefit from consuming seafood, especially those with relatively higher concentrations of EPA and DHA.**
Potential for Benefit	Decreased caloric intake from total and saturated fats and increased intake of selenium compared with beef, pork, and poultry selections. Intake levels of EPA/DHA will increase compared to meat and lean seafood selections.
Potential for Risk	Available data suggests levels of MeHg in high-EPA and -DHA seafood are not associated with adverse health effects at recommended consumption levels. Potential risk from exposure to dioxins and PCBs is similar to meat selections. Decreased intake of iron compared to meat selections. Risk for bacterial contamination will increase if raw seafood is consumed.

continued

TABLE 5-3 Continued

Choice	A reasonable intake would be two 3-ounce (cooked) or age-appropriate servings but they can safely consume 12 ounces per week.
Potential for Benefit	Intake levels of EPA/DHA will increase compared to meat and lean seafood selections. Decreased caloric intake from total and saturated fats compared with beef, pork, and poultry selections, but increased compared to lean seafood selections. Increased intake of selenium compared to meat selections.
Potential for Risk	Potential for greater exposure to dioxins and PCBs compared with lean seafood. Decreased intake of iron compared to meat selections.
Choice	Should avoid large predatory fish such as shark, swordfish, tilefish, or king mackerel.
Potential for Benefit	Available data suggests reduced exposure to MeHg. No anticipated impact on exposure to POPs.
Potential for Risk	Intake levels of EPA/DHA and selenium will be lower if meat is selected as a substitute.
Choice	Can consume up to 6 ounces of white (albacore) tuna per week.
Potential for Benefit	Seafood is a high-quality low-fat protein source. Intake levels of saturated fat will likely decrease compared to meat selections. Intake levels of EPA/DHA will increase compared to meat and leaner seafood selections. Intake of selenium may increase compared with beef, pork, and poultry selections.
Potential for Risk	Available data suggest levels of MeHg are not associated with adverse health effects if consumption is limited to two 3-ounce servings per week. Potential risk from exposure to dioxins and PCBs is similar to meat selections. Risk for bacterial contamination will increase if raw seafood is consumed. Intake levels of iron will be lower than meat selections.

Seafood Choices for Adolescent Males, Adult Males, and Females Who Will Not Become Pregnant

Choice	Consume seafood regularly, e.g., two 3-ounce servings per week; if more are consumed, then insure a variety of choices are made to reduce exposure to contaminants.
Potential for Benefit	Decreased caloric intake from total and saturated fats and increased intake of selenium compared with beef, pork, and poultry selections. Intake levels of EPA/DHA will increase compared to meat selections if high EPA/DHA seafood is selected.
Potential for Risk	Available data suggest levels of MeHg, dioxins, and PCB exposure will likely be within exposure guidelines regardless of type of seafood selected. The potential for exposure to contaminants is increased if locally caught seafood is consumed without regard to local advisories. Increased risk for exposure to infectious microorganisms if raw seafood is consumed. Decreased intake of iron compared to meat selections.

more detailed background approach to the design of guidance intended for the four target populations.

A decision tree or other decision representation is another way of depicting the consumption guidance listed above. This kind of diagram highlights the variables that group consumers into specific target populations who face different benefits and risks and who should receive tailored advice. In the committee's judgment, the variables that distinguish between target populations facing different benefit-risk balances, based on existing evidence, are age, gender, and pregnant or could become pregnant, or breastfeeding. A fourth distinguishing variable explored by the committee was risk of cardiovascular disease. However, as noted above, the committee believes the evidence is insufficient to warrant separate guidance to this group beyond that which would be offered based on age, gender, and pregnancy or breastfeeding status. These three variables, as they apply to the target population groups, are arrayed in a decision pathway, shown in Figure 5-2, that illustrates the committee's final analysis of the balance between benefits and risks associated with seafood consumption.

Acknowledging Limitations of the Benefit-Risk Analysis

The committee believes that it is fundamentally important to acknowledge that benefit-risk analysis as conducted here will always have limitations related to the availability of data on and evaluation of benefits and risks. For example, here the committee relied on data that contain a variety of uncertainties. In the case of seafood consumption, the potential for an adverse health effect from exposure to a contaminant is presumed to depend upon, among other things, differences in prior exposure levels as well as differences in sensitivity to toxicants among individuals. Likewise, persons may receive variable benefits, including no benefit, from nutrients that are found in higher concentrations in seafood than in most other foods, i.e., EPA/DHA and selenium. Those already at low risk for cardiovascular disease, for example, may see little cardiovascular benefit from seafood consumption. Furthermore, it is difficult to obtain information regarding when sampling occurred, the number of samples taken, and the methodology used to identify and quantitate specific nutrients over time, resulting in uncertainty about the variability of nutrient levels in seafood. Finally, no two samples of seafood, either from the same species or from different tissues in the same seafood will contain the same level of either nutrients or contaminants.

In the committee's judgment, these uncertainties may reduce the applicability of the guidance to a specific person, but the general guidance for safe seafood consumption applies to most persons in a category. The

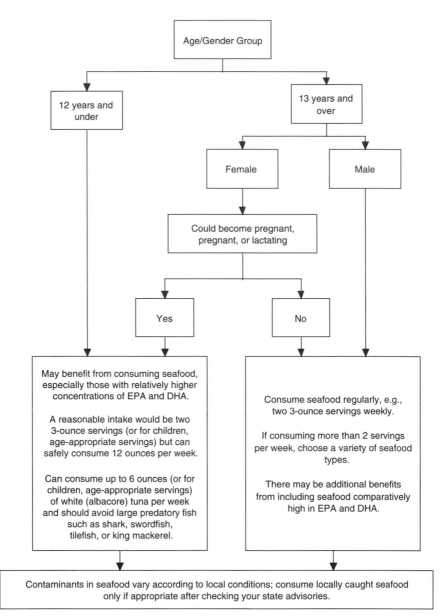

FIGURE 5-2 A decision pathway or representation of the balance between benefits and risks associated with seafood consumption. This diagram highlights the variables that group consumers into specific target populations who should receive tailored advice. Specific details about consumer advice are discussed in Chapter 7.

following points illustrate the variables that influence what can be generally applicable:

• Concentrations of contaminants in seafood are known to be influenced by factors such as location of harvest, seasonal variations, size, and species. General guidance to consumers must be based on available data for average levels of potential contaminants in type or species of seafood. Sparse data on adverse health effects associated with some contaminants make it difficult to estimate the variability of specific contaminant levels in seafood, as well as levels of EPA and DHA.

• Levels of EPA and DHA in seafood depend upon the fatty acid content of the type of seafood consumed, the source of fat in feed for farmed fish, and serving size. Sparse data make it difficult to determine variability in the EPA and DHA content. As more seafood is produced by aquaculture rather than wild-caught, EPA and DHA levels within species could change.

• There is considerable uncertainty about the concentration of contaminants that present a health risk. Methylmercury exposure levels that pose a risk were established for the most vulnerable members of the population, i.e., the fetus, infant, and young child. However, methylmercury exposure levels that pose a risk for adverse health effects for other population categories listed above are unknown. Similarly, exposure limitations for persistant organic pollutants, dioxins and dioxin like compounds, and PCBs are unclear.

• Methylmercury intake exposures that are used to indicate a potential for risk for the fetus, infant, and young child are adjusted (as noted in Chapter 4) to make them more conservative than levels of observed risk.

These uncertainties mean that guidance to individual consumers can, at best, present the broad trade-offs of benefits and risks associated with seafood selections and consumption patterns, and inform consumers of the inherent uncertainties therein. The committee is aware that considerations other than health benefits or risks also may influence consumers' choice of seafood. These include environmental concerns about aquaculture and the sustainability of wild seafood stocks. These considerations are beyond the charge to the committee and are not included in the decision pathway.

FINDINGS

1. Relatively few studies have attempted to simultaneously assess both the health benefits and the risks associated with seafood consumption. However, there is emerging evidence of the trade-offs between the benefits

and risks associated with seafood consumption for health endpoints such as infant development and cardiovascular disease.

2. Given the uncertainty in the underlying exposure data and evolving health impacts, there is no summary metric that can adequately capture the complexity of seafood choices to balance benefits and risks for purposes of providing guidance to consumers. An expert judgement technique can be used to consider benefits and risks together, to yield specific suggested consumption advice.

3. Developing guidance on seafood consumption requires the development of a benefit-risk analysis that identifies the magnitude of benefits and risks associated with different types of consumption, identifies which are important enough to be included in the balancing process, evaluates changes in benefits and risks associated with changes in consumption patterns, and balances the benefits and risks to arrive at specific guidance for healthy consumption for the population as a whole or, if appropriate, for specific target populations.

4. Current evidence suggests that important benefits and risks to be considered in benefit-risk analysis vary across the following target populations: (1) females who are or may become pregnant and those who are breastfeeding; (2) children up to age 12; and (3) adolescent and adult males, and females who will not become pregnant. The committee did not find evidence that adult males and females who are at risk of cardiovascular disease differ from group 3 in terms of potential benefits and risks.

5. The impact of substituting selected species of seafood for other animal protein sources can result in increased consumption of EPA/DHA and selenium; however, impacts on saturated fats and energy intakes vary depending on the seafood selected.

6. The impact of substituting selected species of seafood for other animal protein sources on exposure to environmental toxicants other than methylmercury is uncertain due to inadequate supporting evidence.

7. Considering benefits and risks together yields specific suggested consumption guidance for the three targeted populations enumerated in Finding 4 above.

8. Guidance should be reconsidered periodically, and on an ongoing basis, as new data on both risks and benefits associated with seafood consumption emerge.

CONCLUSIONS

Combining expertise from the disparate relevant disciplines to consider benefits and risks simultaneously is an essential step to producing a comprehensive benefit-risk balancing analysis. An organization of experts is needed among appropriate federal agencies to oversee and manage coordinated benefit-risk judgments and to implement a coordinated research effort to generate the data needed by agencies to issue timely, accurate, and continuously updated advice to consumers, including target populations.

REFERENCES

ARS (Agriculture Research Service). 2006. *National Food and Nutrient Analysis Program.* [Online]. Available: http://www.ars.usda.gov/Research/docs.htm?docid=9446 [accessed May 11, 2006].

Barlow S. 2001 (October). *Fishmeal and Oil—Supplies and Markets.* A presentation to Group Fish Forum, St. Albans, UK, International Fishmeal and Fish Oil Organization. [Online]. Available: http://www.iffo.org.uk/Supplies.pdf#search=%22Fishmeal%20and%20oil%3A%20resources%20and%20markets%22 [accessed August 24, 2006].

Carrington CD, Montwill B, Bolger PM. 2004. An intervention analysis for the reduction of exposure to methylmercury from the consumption of seafood by women of child-bearing age. *Regulatory Toxicology and Pharmacology* 40(3):272–280.

CFSAN (Center for Food Safety and Applied Nutrition). 2005a. *Dioxin Analysis Results/ Exposure Estimates.* [Online]. Available: http://www.cfsan.fda.gov/~lrd/dioxdata.html [accessed April 17, 2006].

CFSAN. 2005b. *Total Diet Study Statistics on Element Results.* College Park, MD: US Food and Drug Administration. [Online]. Available: http://www.cfsan.fda.gov/~acrobat/tds1byel.pdf [accessed April 17, 2006].

CFSAN. 2006a. *CFSAN Mercury Concentrations in Fish: FDA Monitoring Program (1990–2004).* [Online]. Available: http://www.cfsan.fda.gov/~frf/seamehg2.html [accessed April 19, 2006].

CFSAN. 2006b. *Mercury Levels in Commercial Fish and Shellfish.* [Online]. Available: http://www.cfsan.fda.gov/~frf/sea-mchg.html [accessed April 17, 2006].

DGAC (Dietary Guidelines Advisory Committee). 2005. *Dietary Guidelines Advisory Committee Report.* Washington, DC: Department of Health and Human Services and the Department of Agriculture. [Online]. Available: http://www.health.gov/dietaryguidelines/dga2005/report/ [accessed November 29, 2005].

Gold MR, Stevenson D, Fryback DG. 2002. HALYS and QALYS and DALYS, oh my: Similarities and differences in summary measures of population health. *Annual Review of Public Health* 23(1):115–134.

Gray GM, Hammitt JK. 2000. Risk/risk trade-offs in pesticide regulation: An exploratory analysis of the public health effects of a ban on organophosphate and carbamate pesticides. *Risk Analysis* 20(5):665–680.

Gregory R, Wellman K. 2001. Bringing stakeholder values into environmental policy choices: A community-based estuary case study. *Ecological Economics* 39(1):37–52.

Gregory R, McDaniels T, Fields D. 2001. Decision aiding, not disputing resolution: Creating insights through structured environmental decisions. *Journal of Policy Analysis and Management* 20(3):415–432.

Hamilton MC, Hites RA, Schwager SJ, Foran JA, Knuth BA, Carpenter DO. 2005. Lipid composition and contaminants in farmed and wild salmon. *Environmental Science and Technology* 39(22):8600–8629.

Hammitt JK. 2000. Analytic methods for environmental regulations in the United States: Promises, pitfalls and politics. *International Journal for Risk Assessment and Management* 1(1/2):105–124.

Igarashi T, Aursand M, Hirata Y, Gribbestad IS, Wada S, Nonaka M. 2000. Nondestructive quantitative determination of docosahexaenoic acid and n-3 fatty acids in fish oils by resonance spectroscopy. *Journal of the American Oil Chemists' Society* 77:737–748.

IOM (Institute of Medicine). 2000. *Dietary Reference Intakes for Vitamin C, Vitamin E, Selenium, and Carotenoids.* Washington, DC: National Academy Press.

IOM. 2001. *Dietary Reference Intakes for Vitamin A, Vitamin K, Arsenic, Boron, Chromium, Copper, Iodine, Iron, Manganese, Molybdenum, Nickel, Silicon, Vanadium and Zinc.* Washington, DC: National Academy Press.

IOM. 2002/2005. *Dietary Reference Intakes for Energy, Carbohydrate, Fiber, Fat, Fatty Acids, Cholesterol, Protein, and Amino Acids.* Washington, DC: The National Academies Press.

IOM. 2003. *Dioxins and Dioxin-Like Compounds.* Washington, DC: The National Academies Press.

Mahaffey KR. 2004. Fish and shellfish as dietary sources of methylmercury and the omega-3 fatty acids, eicosahexaenoic acid and docosahexaenoic acid: Risks and benefits. *Environmental Research* 95(3):414–428.

Murphy NJ, Schraer CD, Thiele MC, Boyko EJ, Bulkow LR, Doty BJ, Lanier AP. 1995. Dietary change and obesity associated with glucose intolerance in Alaska Natives. *Journal of the American Dietetic Association* 95(6):676–682.

Nobmann ED, Lanier AP. 2001. Dietary intake among Alaska native women resident of Anchorage, Alaska. *International Journal of Circumpolar Health* 60(2):123–137.

NRC (National Research Council). 2000. *Toxicological Effects of Methylmercury.* Washington, DC: National Academy Press.

Siddiqui N, Sim J, Silwood CJL, Toms H, Iles RA, Grootveld M. 2003. Multicomponent analysis of encapsulated marine oil supplements using high-resolution ^{1}H and ^{13}C NMR techniques. *Journal of Lipid Research* 44(12):2406–2427.

Sindelar CA, Scheerger SB, Plugge SL, Eskridge KM, Wander RC, Lewis NM. 2004. Serum lipids of physically active adults consuming omega-3 fatty acid-enriched eggs or conventional eggs. *Nutrition Research* 24(9):731–739.

US EPA/FDA. 2004. *What You Need to Know About Mercury in Fish and Shellfish.* [Online]. Available: http://www.epa.gov/waterscience/fishadvice/advice.html or http://www.cfsan.fda.gov/~dms/admehg3.html [accessed August 27, 2006].

USDA. 2005. *USDA National Nutrient Database for Standard Reference Release 18.* [Online]. Available: http://www.nal.usda.gov/fnic/foodcomp/Data/SR18/sr18.html [accessed October 10, 2005].

Wheatley MA, Wheatley B. 1981. The effect of eating habits on mercury levels among Inuit residents of Sugluk, P.Q. *Etudes/Inuit/Studies* 5(1):27–43.

6

Understanding Consumer Decision Making as the Basis for the Design of Consumer Guidance

Chapter 5 outlined the three steps the committee deemed necessary to designing guidance to consumers about balancing benefits and risks in making seafood consumption decisions (see Box 5-1): scientific assessment and analysis of the benefits and risks; analysis of the consumer's decision making context; and production and evaluation of the guidance. Chapter 5 then detailed Step One: the evidence base for the information to include in the guidance (or what the consumer needs to know to make an informed decision). This chapter presents an approach to Step Two: developing an understanding of how consumers make seafood choices and the informational environment in which they do so. This environment includes both what information the consumer has access to and what the consumer needs or wants to know. Included in this chapter is an overview of the types of information that are currently available and evidence of the degree to which consumer choice has been influenced by it. The chapter then discusses reasons why consumer guidance may have weak or unintended impacts on consumer choice and what must be understood about the consumer decision-making context in order to design effective guidance.

INTRODUCTION

As noted in the previous chapters, there is a wide variety of guidance on seafood consumption currently available to consumers. Based on their analysis of nutritional benefits, some governmental agencies and nongovernmental organizations (NGOs) have recommended that most Americans consume two 3-ounce (cooked) servings of seafood weekly, with one of these being a fatty fish (see Chapter 1). Other guidance cautions some consumers against specific types of seafood due to health risks. As shown in preceding chapters, different populations have different benefit-risk profiles, and guidance to consumers should be tailored to reflect this.

Receiving new information, such as dietary guidance, does not automatically lead consumers to change their food consumption patterns. Food choice is influenced by a complex informational environment that also includes labeling, point-of-purchase information, commercial advertising and promotion, and Web-based health information. Specific guidance may have a limited impact, although evidence suggests that this varies significantly and in general is not well measured or understood; current advice may create unintended consequences in consumer choices. A better understanding of the sociocultural, environmental, economic, and other individual factors that influence consumer choice is necessary for the design of effective consumer guidance, especially where the intent is to communicate balancing of benefits and risks associated with its consumption.

FOOD CHOICE BEHAVIOR

Food Consumption Decisions

Identification of Factors Influencing Food Consumption Decisions

Studies of food choice behavior have identified both individual and environmental factors that influence the complex process of decision making (Lutz et al., 1995; Galef, 1996; Drewnowski, 1997; Nestle et al., 1998; Booth et al., 2001; Wetter et al., 2001; Bisogni et al., 2002; Devine, 2005; Raine, 2005; Shepard, 2005). Factors influencing seafood consumption choices are similar to those for other foods (e.g., taste, convenience, or ease of preparation) (Gempesaw et al., 1995).

Individual Influences When consumers are asked what is most important when choosing food, taste is the most likely response (Drewnowski, 1997). However, a variety of other individual factors (e.g., habit) (Honkanen et al., 2005) also influence consumer decisions about consumption or avoidance of specific foods (Lutz et al., 1995; Galef, 1996; Drewnowski, 1997; Nestle et al., 1998; Booth et al., 2001; Bisogni et al., 2002; Devine, 2005). For example, some people will override taste to select foods to benefit their health (Stewart-Knox et al., 2005). The choice for healthfulness is further affected by choice of preparation method and food consumption outside the home (Blisard et al., 2002). For other consumers, issues of convenience, availability, and cost may play greater roles than concerns about health. What is unknown is the degree to which these factors determine final food selection.

Environmental Influences Taste is influenced by genetics (Birch, 1999; Mennella et al., 2005a) and exposure throughout life (Birch, 1998; Birch and Fisher, 1998; Mennella et al., 2005b). Other environmental factors that influence seafood choices include accessibility of seafood as a subsistence food (Burger et al., 1999b), cultural tradition (Willows, 2005), price of seafood and of seafood substitutes (Hanson et al., 1995), and health and nutrition concerns (Gempesaw et al., 1995; Trondsen et al., 2003). For example, some consumers make seafood choices based on concerns about environmental impact (see Monterey Bay Aquarium's Seafood Watch [http://www.mbayaq.org/cr/seafoodwatch.asp], production methods, or geographical origin (Figure 6-1).

An individual's food choices are made based on their history but are influenced by a changing environment over time (Devine, 2005; Wethington, 2005). While most patterns of choice (trajectories) are stable throughout life, significant societal and personal events, as well as relationships, influence these patterns. The timing of these events may greatly influence subsequent food choices. In response to these external events and internal changes, individuals may or may not choose to adopt strategies to improve their health and change their lifestyle behaviors. Using the pregnant woman as an example (see Appendix C-1), one can examine the complexity of food choice using the Life Course Perspective framework (see Appendix C-2).

Economic Considerations Associated with Food Choice Behavior

Economic considerations may also influence consumer food choice behavior. Evidence suggests that seafood is a good substitute for other protein foods (Salvanes and DeVoretz, 1997; Huang and Lin, 2000). US consumers have the lowest income elasticity of demand (the percentage change in demand for a 1 percent change in income) for the overall category of "food, beverages, and tobacco" of 114 countries, based on an analysis of 1996 data (Seale et al., 2003). This indicates that, on average, their food expenditures are not very sensitive to income changes. For the subcategory of fish, Seale et al. also found the US expenditure elasticity (the percentage change in demand for a 1 percent change in expenditures on a category) lowest among the 114 countries studied. Similarly, US consumers had the lowest own-price elasticities of demand (the percentage change in demand for a one percent change in price) for fish among the countries studied.

More detailed analysis within the United States suggests further income and price considerations that may influence how consumers implement guidance on seafood choices. For example, Huang and Lin (2000) used 1987–1988 National Food Consumption Survey data to estimate expenditure and own-price elasticities adjusting for changes in the quality of the foods consumed across different income groups. Expenditure and own-

220

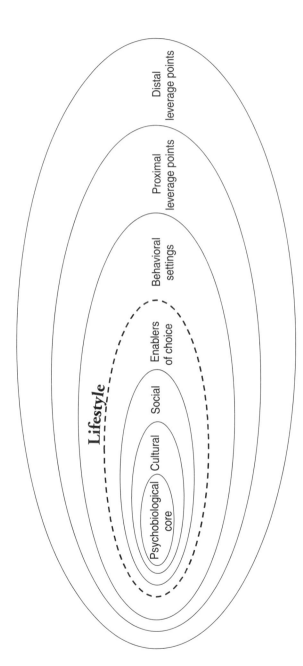

FIGURE 6-1 Framework for factors influencing healthy eating and physical activity behaviors. The schema depicts a psychobiological core composed of genetic, psychological (e.g., self-esteem, body image, disagreement with personal vulnerability or gain from choices), and physiological influences (e.g., gender, age, health status, responses to specific components in food, hunger, and satiety). This core is embedded within a social-cultural context (e.g., families and friends, religion and tradition, economic and other resources, awareness and knowledge of the implications of choice), and impact of consumer advertising and information that can either enhance or inhibit healthful food choices and other lifestyle behaviors. In addition to these individual characteristics, the larger environment (e.g., neighborhoods, communities, schools, worksites) along with policy decisions (e.g., health advisories and guidance; economic and political priorities) greatly influence the individual's food decisions (Wetter et al., 2001; Raine, 2005). Food availability, convenience, cost considerations, and food subsidies also are included in the environmental layers of influence. SOURCE: Adapted, with permission, from Booth et al. (2001). Copyright 2001 by International Life Sciences Institute.

price elasticities vary between low-, medium-, and high-income consumers, although the extent differs between food products (Yen and Huang, 1996; Huang and Lin, 2000). They also conclude that the quality of items chosen by consumers (e.g., different cuts of beef within the beef subcategory) is clearly linked to income level. Similarly, an analysis of household expenditures on fruits and vegetables shows significant differences in expenditure per capita between low-income and higher-income households, as well as differences in the income elasticity of demand (Blisard et al., 2004). These results suggest that population averages may conceal significant differences between income groups in terms of their demand responses to income, expenditure, and price changes.

Impact of Factors Influencing Food Consumption Decisions

In general, when consumers are presented with new information, e.g., balancing health benefits with risks of seafood choices, food choice behavior theories suggest that they will interpret and respond to this information in light of their existing beliefs, attitudes, and habits, and will be influenced by situational factors as much as or more than by the content of the information.

For example, in a long-term, randomized controlled study involving advice to men with angina to eat more fish and vegetables, small increases in fish consumption were observed (Ness et al., 2004), but this did not appear to improve survival (Ness et al., 2002). Even with carefully planned prospective studies of the consequences of giving advice, it can be difficult to discern the effect of advice, due to potentially confounding influences (see also *Impact of State Advisories* below). Advice provided publicly may be focused on by the media, reinforced or contradicted by other policy measures, or obscured by other news (Kasperson et al., 2003).

As Ness et al. (2004) illustrated, knowledge does not necessarily lead to the intended changes in consumption patterns. In addition, once a decision is made, many processes are involved in implementing and sustaining a change (Appendix C-3). Among the many theories used to explain both food choice behavior (and its subsequent impact on health) and behavior change (Achterberg and Trenker, 1990), a few are highlighted in Appendix C-2.

The Current Information Environment Influencing Seafood Choices

Consumers have access to several different types of communication that form a complex information environment in which they make decisions. Each of these plays a role in their decisions, either as a source of information or as a facilitator of choice.

A striking aspect of the information available to consumers is that it is not systematically coordinated. This lack of coordination would not be unexpected between public agencies and private organizations, or between groups who may have different interpretations of the evidence about what is a healthful eating pattern as well as different goals in giving advice. However, even within the federal government, guidance to consumers has not been systematically coordinated, either on a benefit-by-benefit or risk-by-risk basis, as illustrated by the differences between recommendations on portion sizes and frequency of consumption (see Table 1-2 and Appendix Table B-3).

Elements of the information environment which government agencies can control include labels, other point-of-purchase information in the retail environment, and restaurant and fast-food outlet menus.

Labels and Other Point-of-Purchase Information

Ingredient and Nutrition Labeling Ingredient labeling gives consumers content information about packaged seafood products. In some cases, regulation also restricts use of terms in identifying products. For example, only albacore tuna can be labeled as "white tuna," while "chunk light tuna" may include several species of tuna.

Nutrition labeling in the form of the Nutrition Facts panel is mandatory in the United States for packaged products, while the use of voluntary nutrient content and health claims is also regulated. Fresh foods are exempt from mandatory labeling. In 1992, the US Food and Drug Administration (FDA) issued guidelines for a voluntary point-of-purchase nutrition information program for fresh produce and raw fish. The guidelines are scheduled to be revised in 2006 to make them more consistent with mandatory nutrition labeling requirements (Personal communication, K. Carson, Food and Drug Administration, April 1, 2006). To meet the guidelines, a retailer must include the following nutrition information on the point-of-purchase label for seafood that is among the 20 types most commonly eaten in the US: seafood type; serving size; calories per serving; protein, carbohydrate, total fat, cholesterol, and sodium content per serving; and percent of the US Recommended Dietary Allowances (RDA) for iron, calcium, and vitamins A and C per serving (FDA, 2004a). A serving is defined as 3 ounces or 85 grams cooked weight, without added fat or seasoning.

Qualified Health Claims Labeling While the standard Nutrition Facts format informs consumers about several nutrition characteristics of seafood products, it does not list omega-3 fatty acid content. In 2004, the FDA announced the availability of a qualified health claim for reduced risk of coronary heart disease on conventional foods that contain eicosapentaenoic acid (EPA) and docosahexaenoic acid (DHA). Qualified health claims on foods must be supported by scientific evidence as outlined in the guidance document, *Guidance for Industry and FDA: Interim Procedures for Qualified Health Claims in the Labeling of Conventional Human Food and Human Dietary Supplements* (CFSAN, 2003). In addition, the FDA is conducting further consumer studies to make sure the language used in claims is well understood by consumers (FDA, 2004b).

In the interim period, the FDA will prioritize health claims for review based on the potential significance of the product's health impact on a serious or life-threatening illness, and the strength of evidence in support of the claim. The health claims that will be evaluated first include the benefits of eating foods high in omega-3 fatty acids, including certain fatty fish like ocean salmon, tuna, and mackerel, for reducing the risk of heart disease.

Country of Origin and Other Labeling   The 2002 Supplemental Appropriations Act amended the Agricultural Marketing Act of 1946 to require retailers to inform consumers of the country of origin of wild and farm-raised fish and shellfish. This information can be conveyed by label, stamp, mark, placard, or other clear and visible sign on the product, package, display, holding unit, or bin containing the seafood at the final point of consumption. Food service establishments are exempt, as are processed products.

Box 6-1 describes an unresolved issue over which governmental sector has the authority to control the consumer's access to certain information

---

BOX 6-1
Challenge to California's Proposition 65

In 2005, the Food and Drug Administration claimed that California's action was a violation of federal law. On March 8, 2006, the House passed HR 4167, the *National Uniformity for Food Act,* which amends the Federal Food, Drug, and Cosmetic Act to "provide for uniform food safety warning notification requirements" and to supersede state legislation and practices on food-warning labels, including Proposition 65. At the writing of this report, the Act had not passed the Senate. An amendment to the Act included a clause to exclude mercury warnings: "Nothing in this Act or the amendments made by this Act shall have any effect upon a State law, regulation, proposition or other action that establishes a notification requirement regarding the presence or potential effects of mercury in fish and shellfish."

SOURCE: http://www.govtrack.us/data/us/bills.text/109/h/h4167.pdf.

regarding food. In 2004, the Attorney General of California joined a lawsuit filed by the Public Media Center, a nonprofit media and consumer advocacy agency in San Francisco, against the nation's three largest canned tuna companies to enforce Proposition 65, California's 1986 law requiring warnings about exposure to contaminants, such as methylmercury.

Restaurant and Fast-Food Menu Information The away-from-home sector is exempt from nutritional and country of origin labeling requirements. Further, many restaurants do not identify seafood products such as breaded fish sandwiches by species. Some of this information is provided voluntarily, and this may increase with consumer demand for specific types of seafood.

In April 2003, the Attorney General of California filed suit against major restaurant chains in the state for violating Proposition 65 requirements to inform consumers of potential exposure to "substances known by the state to cause cancer or reproductive toxicity" by failing to post "clear and reasonable" consumer warnings about exposure to mercury in seafood (i.e., shark, swordfish, and tuna). The suit was settled in early 2005, when most of the restaurants agreed to put up warnings about the risks from mercury in seafood near the front door, hostess desk or reception area, or entry or waiting area (California Office of the Attorney General, [http://ag.ca.gov/newsalerts/2005/05-011.htm]). The information provided in this sector remains largely unregulated. The outcome of the lawsuit concluded that labeling under Proposition 65 was preempted for mercury in tuna, although the decision was specific to the circumstances in the case. All applications of Proposition 65 to food were not preempted by the decision. Moreover, this decision was by a state judge and specific to Proposition 65 and California—not other laws or other states.

Regulated Point-of-Purchase Information Retailers may place nutrition information on individual food wrappers or on stickers affixed to the outside of the food. Compliance with point-of-purchase guidelines is checked by biennial surveys of 2,000 food stores that sell raw produce or fish and the results are reported to Congress. Additionally, every 2 years the FDA publishes, in the Federal Register, revised nutrition labeling data for the 20 most frequently consumed raw fruits, vegetables, and fish.

Recent research suggests that the amount of information available on fresh seafood products in retail settings varies markedly, with counter staff frequently unable to provide additional information (Burger et al., 2004). In addition to the quantity and types of information available to consumers, the accuracy of information should also be considered. Limited tests indicate that seafood products may be misrepresented—for example, sold as wild when they are in fact farmed (Is Our Fish Fit to Eat, 1992; Burros, 2005).

Advertising and Promotion

Advertising and promotion may include nonregulated point-of-purchase information, which can be displayed on placards, shelf tags, or in pamphlets or brochures. In addition to regulated labeling and point-of-purchase information, several types of retail information are available to consumers making food choices. For processed foods, packaging information includes the brand, product name, and unregulated product claims and other information. It is estimated that $7.3 billion was spent on advertising food in 1999 (Story and French, 2004).

As well, several other forms of point-of-purchase (e.g., signage, brochures) and other forms of information (e.g., websites) may be provided. Other means to convey this information to consumers may include live demonstrations, computer booths, or recorded presentations as adjuncts to the printed information.

Web-Based Health Information

Interactive Health Communication Much of the rapidly rising use of the Internet is devoted to seeking health information: four out of five Internet users (95 million Americans) have Internet access to look for health-related information; 59 percent of female users have used the Internet to look for information on nutrition (Fox, 2005). The promise of eHealth and, in particular, interactive health communication (IHC) (Eng et al., 1999; Eng and Gustafson, 1999; Wyatt and Sullivan, 2005), has captured the attention of health communicators, in part due to the ability to target and tailor communications, disseminate them rapidly, and engage the audience in an exchange of information, rather than a one-way message delivery (Gustafson et al., 1999); compared with Griffiths et al., 2006. Evaluation of IHC, which falls under the category of eHealth, remains challenging (Eysenbach and Kummervold, 2005). While ethical issues such as unequal access to the Internet and maintaining confidentiality of information pose challenges, IHC has become an important tool for health communicators.

Online Seafood Information and Advocacy There are currently several examples of online seafood consumption information and advocacy available, as illustrated in Table 6-1. For example, Oceans Alive, a nongovernmental organization (Environmental Defense Network), offers "Buying Guide: Becoming a Smarter Seafood Shopper," on its website (http://www.oceansalive.org/eat.cfm). Other sites offer nutrition information about seafood; however, a cursory glance suggests that some sites may not be updated frequently, and so may provide out-of-date nutritional and other guidance. Updating is likely to be a challenge for any interactive guidance

TABLE 6-1 A Sampling of Online Consumer Information and Advocacy Sites Which Include Mercury Calculators

Website	Organization	Type of Organization/Project	Input
http://www. ewg.org/issues/ mercury/20031209/ calculator.php	Environmental Working Group (EWG)	Public health and environmental action organization	Consumer's weight (lbs) Consumer's gender
http://www. fishscam.com/ mercuryCalculator. cfm	FishScam.com	A project of the Center for Consumer Freedom A nonprofit organization supported by restaurants, food companies, and individuals, created by Berman & Co., a public affairs firm which has represented various animal production industries	Consumer's weight (lbs) Fish of choice (dropdown menu provided)
http://gotmercury. org/english/ advanced.htm	Got Mercury?	A project of Turtle Island Restoration Network Public education and campaign to reduce exposure to methylmercury from seafood	Consumer's weight (lbs) Type of fish consumer has eaten in a week Amount (oz) of up to three different fish consumer has eaten in a week (dropdown menu provided)

Output	Notes/Quoted Extracts
Amount of canned albacore and canned light tuna you can safely eat (g/kg of weight/day) Based on FDA's health standard (i.e., safe dose)	Assumes that you do not eat any other seafood. Assumes that every can of tuna has an average amount of mercury. The FDA recommends up to 12 ounces a week of a variety of fish. If you eat other seafood, the amount of tuna that you can eat safely will be less than calculated here. EWG recommends that women of childbearing age and children under 5 not eat albacore tuna at all, because a significant portion of albacore tuna has very high mercury levels. People eating this tuna will exceed safe exposure levels by a wide margin.
Amount (oz) of each fish you can eat weekly without introducing new health risks from mercury Based on the US EPA's Reference Dose Links the US EPA's "Reference Dose" and the theoretical harm threshold (a number ten times greater, called the "Benchmark Dose lower limit") to the Glossary section of this website	The EPA knows the level of exposure that represents a hypothetical risk, but it adjusts it by a factor of 10 in order to arrive at its "Reference Dose." It's this smaller, hyper-cautionary number that environmental groups use to scare Americans into thinking that tiny amounts of mercury in fish represent a real health hazard. According to fishy math from EWG and SeaWeb, for instance, your health is in grave danger if you consume just 12 ounces of tuna (canned chunk light) in a given week. This trickery is responsible for a great deal of needless fear. And food-scare groups ignore the fact that health risks from mercury take an entire lifetime to accumulate. It's simply not possible to get mercury poisoning from eating a week's worth of any commercially available fish.
Mercury exposure (% of EPA limit) Based on the US EPA's reference dose	Please be aware that these values are averages. The concentration of mercury in seafood can be significantly higher or lower than what is represented here. As a precautionary approach, we recommend that women (especially of childbearing age) avoid seafood species that contain higher average levels of mercury. Mercury information for many shellfish species is currently unavailable. Data source: FDA website (http://www.cfsan.fda.gov/~frf/sea-mehg.html). Two exceptions are the troll-caught albacore data which come from an Oregon State University study and canned albacore data, which come from an FDA dataset that is not yet published on its site.

continued

TABLE 6-1 Continued

Website	Organization	Type of Organization/Project	Input
http://www.nrdc. org/health/effects/ mercury/index.asp	Natural Resources Defense Council (NRDC)	An environmental action organization	Consumer's weight (lbs) Types of fish consumer has eaten in the last month Number of portions consumer has eaten of each fish Portion sizes for each fish meal
http://www. oceanconservancy. org/site/PageServer? pagename=mercury Calculator	The Ocean Conservancy	A research, education, advocacy organization advocating for the oceans	Consumer's weight (lbs) Average number of 6 oz servings/week of different seafood types (list provided)

tool. Information on the nutrient content of foods, including seafood, can be obtained through the USDA nutrient database (USDA, 2005b; Source: http://www.nal.usda.gov/fnic/foodcomp/Data/SR18/sr18.html) (see also Chapter 5, Table 5-2 and discussion).

Currently, much of the interactive seafood consumption information available on the Web consists of mercury intake calculators that may include tailoring by the decision-maker's weight, sometimes gender, and the type and amount of seafood consumed (Table 6-1). In addition, the computerized nutritional information approach has been successful and shown some promise in other domains (Lancaster and Stead, 2002; Eng et al., 1999). Computerized nutrition information in the form of menu planning has been ongoing since the mid-1960s (Balintfy, 1964; Eckstein, 1967) and is still being developed (Bouwman et al., 2005).

Northern Contaminants Program

The Northern Contaminants Program (NCP) is funded by a commitment of one million dollars a year from the Canadian government and managed by aboriginal communities. The aim of the program is to reduce

Output	Notes/Quoted Extracts
Estimated level of blood mercury (µg/L), level of blood mercury that the US EPA considers safe Based on the US EPA's Reference Dose Link to FDA's 2003 data on levels of mercury in 17 types of fish	Because the numbers used in the mercury calculator are averages, the fish you eat may contain mercury at levels significantly higher or lower than the numbers used in this calculator. The results of the calculator are only an estimate of the possible level of mercury in your blood and should not be considered definitive. The estimate does not predict any risk to you or your family. If you are concerned about the calculator's results or wish to get a more accurate reading through a blood mercury test, you should talk to your doctor.
Total mg/kg mercury per week Based on the US EPA's Reference Dose	If your results are less than 0.7 below, your mercury levels are likely within EPA's recommended range. If your results exceed 0.7, your levels may be higher than EPA recommends. Data source: "Mercury Levels in Commercial Fish & Shellfish," by FDA and EPA (http://vm.cfsan.fda.gov/~frf/sea-mehg.html)

and eliminate some of the contaminants reaching the Arctic, and to inform and educate Northerners about the issue of contaminants. Relevant to this report is the work that is being done to inform and educate Northerner Dwellers about the issue and how to manage their diet around existing and emerging contaminant issues.

The initial response of Northern aboriginal communities to information on contaminants in aquatic food was a dramatic switch away from eating "country foods." In a region where there are few readily available and affordable nutritional alternatives and 56 percent of the population is "food insecure," this exposed the population to a greater risk from poor nutrition than that posed by the contaminants. Communication about contaminants also affected the social structure of the region as it had a negative impact on the practice of sharing food, due to concerns that hunters might be poisoning friends and family. There was also a negative impact on the efforts of health workers to encourage breastfeeding in the region.

Under the NCP, any contaminant information has to be filtered through a community committee made up of representatives from the aboriginal and Inuit organizations, and health and wildlife workers. This committee is responsible for taking the messages that scientists may develop, and turning them into something that can be presented to and discussed with the communities. This communication process has enabled the scientific assessments to be merged into different communication practices that result in better public perception and understanding.

In the Inuit culture, each community has its own particular system of knowledge and way of understanding, and the NCP has adapted communication activities to these systems. Among the targeted and tailored communications activities are school curriculums for children, posters, little newsletters, and fact sheets. Radio, video shows, and a whole myriad of different technologies are used to communicate these messages.

Most of these communications relate to benefits—country foods are good for you and important for good nutrition. Little is said about contaminants because the community had established that people really do not care about bioaccumulation or PCBs. They want to know if their food is good to eat. The community has told the scientists that contaminant messages cannot just be "dumped" on communities. Information has to be put into a context of an overall health and nutrition message. The NCP is delivering these tailored health and nutrition messages, targeted to specific audiences such as youth and pregnant or nursing women through a community-based stakeholder program (Personal communication, E. Loring, Inuit Tapiriit Kanatami, August 3, 2006; http://www.ainc-inac.gc.ca/ncp/).

Summary

In summary, guidance to consumers regarding the benefits and risks of seafood consumption may inform individual choices about which types of seafood and how much to consume. The design of guidance should consider the context of other product information, particularly labeling, available to consumers to facilitate choice. These other information sources affect choice as well as influence how effectively consumers can implement their decisions once they are made. This distinction is important. For example, labels provide information that consumers use to decide which products to buy just as consumer guidance does. But they also facilitate choices that have already been made. If, following guidance, consumers decide to add a particular type of seafood from a specific region to their diets, will they be able to effectively identify this product in a retail store? Do restaurant and fast-food outlet menus give sufficient information for consumers to implement their choices made on the basis of guidance?

IMPACT OF INFORMATION ON CONSUMER DECISION MAKING

Although it is difficult to attribute observed behavior changes to specific advice, like national and local fish advisories, awareness of advisories suggests that they contribute to avoidance. For example, shifts away from traditional (country) foods, much of which is seafood, due to concerns that include mercury and other pollutants, have resulted in striking increases in anemia, dental caries, obesity, heart disease, and diabetes among the native populations of Northern Canada (Willows, 2005). Another example of an unanticipated effect of risk information is the Alar controversy of 1989 (Marshall, 1991), which effectively stigmatized apple consumption until Alar was pulled from the market later that year.

As these examples show, reactions to risk information can prevail over, and change, preferences and markets; consumer information may appear to have little direct influence, but it can have substantial unanticipated consequences. The combination of responses to and changing understanding of food consumption choice consequences can amplify the effects of risk information, which can be further amplified by the media, government, and other parties (Kasperson et al., 2003). Providing information about risks in the absence of benefit information is likely to produce negative responses (Finucane et al., 2003; Slovic et al., 2004), compounding the tendency to omit consideration of factors that are not mentioned explicitly (Fischhoff et al., 1978).

Seafood choices, like all consumption choices, may entail value trade-offs (see Chapter 7). Well-designed guidance and information can simplify making such trade-offs for consumers by:

- Taking into account consumers' own decision objectives;
- Understanding consumers' decision contexts and prior beliefs;
- Providing adequate, comprehensible measures for the full range of consequences;
- Recognizing that value trade-offs are dependent on individual preferences and tastes; and
- Supporting consistency checks, to help people make decisions consistent with their preferences (Keeney, 2002).

Interpretation of new messages—including labels, warnings, and risk communications—depends on prior knowledge and beliefs (Sattler et al., 1997; Argo and Main, 2004), ethnic and cultural background (Burger et al., 1999a,b; Bostrom and Löfstedt, 2003; Knuth et al., 2003), and other characteristics of individual message recipients, as well as attributes of the messages. In addition to specific content (Bostrom et al., 1994) and attributes such as format, structure, graphics, and wording choices (Schriver, 1989; Atman et al., 1994; Wogalter et al., 1996; Sattler et al., 1997; Schriver, 1997), how messages are processed depends also on the reader's attributes and motivation, and the salience and importance of the topic to the reader (Wogalter et al., 1996; Zuckerman and Chaiken, 1998).

Knowing how consumers make such decisions is also critical to assessing the likelihood of success of different communication strategies. Hence the design of consumer information about benefits and risks associated with seafood consumption requires assessing the decision goals and decision processes of consumers through formative analyses involving interviews or focus groups, and observational studies, as well as quantitative survey analyses and experimental testing of presentation formats and dissemination outlets. The following discussion summarizes the evidence to date regarding the effects of seafood advisories, labels, point-of-purchase information, and other consumer communications.

Evaluating the Effects of Previous Seafood Consumption Guidance

Evaluating the impact of previous guidance on seafood purchasing behavior can be done either qualitatively or quantitatively. Focus groups have been the traditional qualitative method; responses to surveys provide the quantitative information (Source: http://www.cfsan.fda.gov/~dms/adme-hg3g.html). Simulations, predictions, and scenarios also can be employed.

Impact of Federal Fish Advisories

In a report to the Interagency Working Group on Mercury Communications, Levy and Derby (2000) described the results of eight focus groups conducted prior to the 2001 US EPA fish advisory. They characterize prior concerns about mercury in fish as low, with the perception that mercury in fish is primarily a pollution problem. Reactions to statements about hazards of mercury in fish and fish consumption advice were interpreted as demonstrating two kinds of spillover effects. The first was a failure to narrow the perception of the at-risk group to be pregnant women who eat a lot of fish; focus group participants concluded that the general public must be at risk for consuming mercury from fish. The second was a general tendency to categorize fish as safe or not without paying much attention to quantitative consumption advice. Also noted was the fact that participants wanted information on fish that were safe to eat as well as on those that were not safe to eat.

Oken et al. (2003) and Shimshack et al. (2005) conducted post hoc analyses of the effects of the 2001 US EPA fish advisory on seafood consumption. Oken et al. (2003) found that issuance of the advisory was correlated with decreased consumption of "dark meat" fish, canned tuna, and "white meat" fish in a study of pregnant women. However, it is unclear whether the decrease is attributable to the advisory because the study lacks controls for other known possible influences on consumption. Shimshack et al. (2005) find evidence suggestive of a decrease in canned fish consumption after the advisory among those who regularly read newspapers or magazines. Overall, they conclude that the advisory had an effect in that over the period studied the mean expenditure share for canned fish fell for some targeted consumers compared to nontargeted consumers. Again, the study does not control for other factors that may have an important influence on changes in consumption. In addition, neither study controls for actual awareness of the advisory, which makes any attribution of the observed changes difficult. The business press refers to a drop in demand after the joint 2004 US EPA/FDA fish advisory (e.g., Warner, 2005). The committee cannot evaluate these claims due to the lack of any statistical information and controls for other factors that affect sales beyond the effects of the advisories. To the best of the committee's knowledge there have been, to date, no studies done by government, industry, academia, consumer, or environmental groups that offer a credible measure of market impacts of the 2004 US EPA/FDA fish advisory.

Cohen et al. (2005) carried out simulations of consumer behavior under what they call optimistic, moderate, and pessimistic scenarios for responses to the 2001 advisory. Their optimistic scenario assumes that only women of childbearing age respond to the advisory, and do so by substituting low-mercury seafood for higher mercury seafood. Their moderate scenario assumes that women of childbearing age reduce their seafood consumption by 17 percent in response to the 2001 advisory, with no change in types of seafood consumed. Their pessimistic scenario assumes that all adults decrease seafood consumption by 17 percent. In both the moderate and pessimistic scenarios, an overall decrease in benefits results (estimated changes in Quality Adjusted Life Years from a benefit-risk analysis). The optimistic scenario estimates an increase in net benefits if there is compliance with the 2001 advisory, with no spillover effects. The greatest benefit is derived from eating one fish meal a week, as opposed to none. In summary, the analysis by Cohen et al. suggests that the advisory was appropriate, in theory; but the study is not an empirical evaluation of the effects of the advisories. Further, the study assumed some coronary and stroke risk-reduction benefits that recent reviews suggest may not be empirically substantiated.

The US EPA and FDA carried out two sets of focus group studies prior to issuing their joint 2004 US EPA/FDA fish advisory, for a total of 16 focus groups in seven locations (SOURCE: http://www.epa.gov/waterscience/fishadvice/factsheet.html). In a public presentation, an FDA spokesperson summarized findings from the first eight focus groups in four main points: (1) most participants preferred a simple message conveying that consuming high amounts of methylmercury may harm a child's development, and what to do to avoid high amounts; (2) some participants wanted more information about how methylmercury would affect health, and more data on particular species of fish; (3) some participants think of fish consumption as a whole, and do not distinguish between commercially and sport- or recreationally caught fish; (4) almost all participants reported that they and their children would avoid species designated "do not eat," regardless of whether or not they were in the targeted audience (Davidson, 2004).

Detailed reports from these focus group studies are not available, although information shows that the focus groups included pregnant or lactating women and racially diverse groups of both sexes, and were conducted in coastal as well as noncoastal locations (Davidson, 2004).

Impact of State Fish Advisories

Survey evaluations suggest that awareness of state fish advisories is low overall. Between one-half and two-thirds of sports fishers reported awareness of state or local advisories in studies of advisory effectiveness (Burger and Waishwell, 2001; Anderson et al., 2004). Tilden et al. (1997), Anderson et al. (2004), and Knobeloch et al. (2005) found that awareness was higher among males than females, with less than half of the women who consume recreationally caught fish aware of advisories.

Risk information of the type found in fish advisories appears to increase reluctance to consume seafood proportionately to benefits when the risks are low, and without regard to benefits when the risks are high (Knuth et al., 2003). Further, there is preliminary evidence suggesting that risk-risk information (comparing the risks of seafood with risks of other foods) may influence risk perceptions more than benefit-risk information (for risks and benefits of seafood) (Knuth et al., 2003).

As is shown in Table 1-2 and Appendix Table B-3, seafood advisories and guidance have been issued by federal, state, and local authorities with conflicting objectives and differing assumptions, even to the point of inconsistent serving sizes. Even an expert reader would find it challenging to integrate these different pieces of advice with one another.

In general, it requires careful experimental design to be able to attribute the effects of specific communications (Golding et al.,1992; Johnson et al., 1992). Experimental evidence shows that warnings can change perceptions and beliefs (Wolgater and Laughrey, 1996; Sattler et al., 1997; Burger and Waishwell, 2001; Riley et al., 2001; Argo and Main, 2004; Knobeloch et al., 2005), but unintended effects, such as overreactions, may occur (Wheatley and Wheatley, 1981; Levy and Derby, 2000; Shimshack et al., 2005).

Labeling Effectiveness and Effects of Health Claims

While there is little evidence pertaining to seafood labels per se, there is considerable evidence on labeling effectiveness in general. In their systematic review of 129 studies, Cowburn and Stockley (2003) concluded that most consumers claim to look at nutrition labels at least sometimes, but actual use is not widespread. Evidence on consumer understanding of nutrition labels is mixed; while nutrition labels appear to enable simple comparisons, consumers have difficulty using them for more complex tasks, like placing food into consumers' overall dietary context. The review summarizes findings on label formatting as well, and recommends using boxes for the information; standard, familiar, consistent formatting; and thin alignment lines. Other formatting information reviewed suggested that pie charts are difficult for consumers to understand and should not be used, and that consumers using bar charts tended to compare the length of the bars without taking note of the scales (Cowburn and Stockley, 2003). Recent formative research on more graphic presentation of nutritional information suggests that "traffic light" formats (Food Standards Agency, 2005) may be effective. These rely on the familiarity of the traffic light metaphor, and the ease with which people interpret their colors.

Research on Qualified Health Claims as Applied to Functional Foods In their survey of consumers in Finland, Denmark, and the United States (n=1533, stratified by country), Bech-Larsen and Grunert (2003) found that perceived healthiness of functional foods was primarily determined by the perceived healthiness of the base foods (orange juice, yogurt and non-butter spread) used in their experiment regardless of the additional functional component. Health claims on the label increased the perceived healthiness of functional foods (Bech-Larsen and Grunert, 2003; Williams, 2005).

The optimal presentation of health claims may be a short health claim on the package front, with a longer panel on the back (Wansink et al., 2004). While health claims can change attitudes toward foods, qualifying such claims appropriately based on the quality of the underlying science is a challenging communications task. In tests of several formats, including adjectives embedded in statements and various report card formats (Derby and Levy, 2005), strength-of-science disclaimers did not have the intended effects.

Table 6-2 summarizes the current seafood consumption information environment. Information from the table can be used to identify opportunities for improving this environment with existing information. As illustrated in the table, the most salient gap is insufficient evaluation of the current consumer seafood information environment (e.g., marketing research) and a lack of emphasis on benefits of seafood consumption. Most information available focuses on risks alone. Other shortfalls include the limited reach of state advisories, lack of or potentially misleading (out of date, or inappropriate use of Reference Dose [RfD]) use of quantitative benefit and risk information in interactive online consumer guidance, and limited provision

TABLE 6-2 Summary of Current Seafood Consumption Information Environment

	Benefit/Risk Message	Source	Medium/Channel	Intended Audience(s)	Available Evaluation Evidence
Federal Advisories	Mercury risks	FDA, US EPA	Mass media, broadcast	Females of childbearing age, infants, and children	Insufficient evaluation of market impact Suggestion of spillover effects, including possible stigmatization of seafood (Levy and Derby, 2000; Davidson, 2004)
State Advisories	Risks: 30 percent on mercury	State health and environmental agencies	Brochures, government websites, signs	Various	Evaluations suggest limited effectiveness One-fifth to one-half of sports fishers are aware of state or local advisories in studies of advisory effectiveness (Burger and Waishwell, 2001; Anderson et al., 2004)
Regulated Point-of-Purchase Information	Nutritional information, country of origin, risk	Safeway, Albertson's, Wal-Mart, Whole Foods, etc.	Point-of-purchase placards, shelf tags, pamphlets/ brochures; individual food wrappers and stickers on the outside of food	All consumers	Suggestion that these displays can increase market share of product by 1–2 percent over 2 years (Cowburn and Stockley, 2003) No specific evaluations of point-of-purchase displays of mercury in seafood; evaluations of point-of-purchase displays for seafood source suggest false claims are made regarding origin (Burger et al., 2004)
Labeling	Types of seafood and how much to consume; nutritional information and risks	Retailers	Point-of-purchase placards, shelf tags, pamphlets/ brochures; individual food wrappers and stickers on the outside of food	All consumers	Most consumers claim to look at nutrition labels at least sometimes, but actual use is less widespread (Cowburn and Stockley, 2003) No specific evaluation of seafood labels— limited labeling requirements

Qualified Health Claims	Eating foods high in omega-3 fatty acids to decrease risk of heart disease	Producers	On products/menus	All consumers	These claims increase the perceived healthfulness of functional foods (Bech-Larsen and Grunert, 2003; Williams, 2005)
Web-based Health Information	Nutrition information (although often not updated), risk, mercury, Dioxin-like Compounds, ecological	Environmental Non-govenmental Organizations	Internet, interactive	Internet users, environmentally concerned	Committee unaware of any evaluations. Advice is given in a limited number of categories; limited quantitative information; very limited info on benefits of seafood consumption
Mercury Intake Calculators	Risk focus: mercury	Various organizations (public health, environmental action, nonprofit, education/campaign, research advocacy)	Internet, interactive	Internet users, concerned consumers (inferred)	Misuse of RfD, committee unaware of any evaluations
Northern Contaminants Program	Benefits, balancing choices	Health Canada	Mixed media, participative program	Northern communities	Program limited to Northern Canada (Kuhnlein et al., 2000; Mos et al., 2004; Willows, 2005), evaluations suggest program effectively prevents substituting low nutrition foods for seafood; questions about costs

of point-of-purchase information. Notably, federal and state government agencies are not currently providing interactive online guidance.

SETTING THE STAGE FOR DESIGNING CONSUMER GUIDANCE

Seafood is a complex commodity, with a very wide range of individual products with varying price levels, and nutrient and contaminant profiles. The availability and affordability of seafood products is changing (see Chapter 2); this is likely to influence the ability of consumers to implement the seafood choices that they want to make to balance benefits and risks. The market context in which consumers make choices should be kept in mind when designing guidance. For example, information accompanying the guidance could point to lower-cost alternatives for increasing intake of seafood rich in EPA and DHA.

Seafood choices, like all consumption choices, entail value trade-offs; for example, seafood higher in EPA and DHA may cost more than seafood that is lower. Other seafood may be more economical but contain higher levels of contaminants. Some individuals will accept high risks to achieve what they value as high benefits (e.g., consume raw seafood because of its pleasurable taste), while others may prefer to "play it safe."

Individual differences in tastes, preferences, beliefs and attitudes, and situations complicate the task of informing and supporting benefit-risk trade-off decisions. Food choices may be predicated on different objectives—a healthy baby for the pregnant woman, or weight loss for someone who is overweight. Audience segmentation and targeting is essential for effective communication (see above), not only because decision objectives and risk attitudes vary, but because people's knowledge and interest varies.

Tailored communications are more effective than general advice (de Vries and Brug, 1999; Rimer and Glassman, 1999). For example, access to appropriate, science-based information on both the benefits and risks of seafood consumption is particularly critical for pregnant women to enable them to adhere to health guidance messages (Athearn et al., 2004). Therefore, constructing information on balancing the benefits and risks of seafood consumption during pregnancy must address pregnant women separately from other consumers.

A recent multi-state focus group study (Athearn et al., 2004) revealed that most but not all women were aware of and followed the recommendation to avoid undercooked or raw seafood during pregnancy. In contrast, the recommendation not to serve smoked fish cold without heating was less familiar, which was reflected in higher reported consumption levels (25.8 percent for smoked fish vs. 14.5 percent for undercooked or raw seafood consumption). This appeared to be related to lack of exposure to this recommendation (especially from participants' doctors) and lack of publicized evidence of risk (in terms of outbreaks, case studies, or risk assessment measures). It was also related to the lack of clarity as to whether "smoked" fish included lox and hot-smoked and/or cold-smoked fish. The authors concluded that it is critical for pregnant women to understand why the information is being targeted to them, and to make certain to entitle food safety information as "applicable to pregnant women" specifically.

Consumer messages about diet and nutrition need to be understandable, achievable, and consistent across information sources. They must also "address sources of discomfort about dietary choices; they must engender a sense of empowerment; and they should motivate both by providing clear information that propels toward taking action and appeals to the need to make personal choices" (Borra et al., 2001). Consumers need access to information that is in a clear and easy-to-understand format, that is structured to support decision-making, and that allows consumers access to additional layers of information when they want them (Morgan et al., 2001).

It is important for those designing consumer guidance to conduct an empirical analysis of the decision-making process. Part of this assessment is understanding consumers' decision context when they are presented with guidance suggesting changes in food choice behavior. One way to gain such understanding is to construct an empirically based scenario reflective of the consumers' world, rather than that of the scientist, as described in the Family Seafood Selection Scenario shown in Appendix C-4. This should be based on the best available evidence from consumer research.

Pre-implementation and post hoc evaluation of the impact of consumer guidance must control for differences, as well as changes in factors including incomes and prices, that occur during the period studied in order to isolate the effect of the guidance itself. Otherwise, the effect of the guidance on changes in consumption may be over- or underestimated. These types of controls have been lacking in previous evaluations, making the effect of the guidance unclear.

FINDINGS

1. Consumers are faced with a multitude of enablers and barriers when making and implementing food choices. Dietary advice is just one component in making food choices.

2. Advice to consumers from the federal government and private organizations on seafood choices to promote human health has been fragmented. Benefits have been addressed separately from risks; portion sizes differ from one piece of advice to another. Some benefits and some risks have been addressed separately from others for different physiological systems and age groups. As a result, multiple pieces of guidance—sometimes conflicting—exist simultaneously for seafood.

3. The existence of multiple pieces of advice, without a balancing of benefits and risks, may lead to consumer misunderstanding. As a result, individuals may under- or overconsume foods relative to their own health situations.

4. There is inconsistency between current consumer advice in relation to portion sizes. For example, the FDA/US EPA fish advisory uses a 6-ounce serving size whereas nutritional advice from some government agencies uses a 3-ounce serving size.

5. Evidence is insufficient to document changes in general seafood consumption in response to the 2001 or 2004 methylmercury advisories.

6. It is apparent that messages about consumption often have to be individualized for different groups such as pregnant females, children, the general population, subsistence fishermen, and native populations.

7. Involving representatives of targeted subpopulations (e.g., Arctic Circle campaign) in both the design and evaluation of communications intended to reach those subpopulations can improve the effectiveness of those communications.

8. There are models for designing guidance, e.g., using full programs, that some individual communities (e.g., Arctic Circle campaign) have contributed to understanding the effects of different modes of health communication and modifying messages to achieve the desired community and/or individual response.

RECOMMENDATIONS

Recommendation 1: Appropriate federal agencies should develop tools for consumers, such as computer-based, interactive decision support and visual representations of benefits and risks that are easy to use and to interpret. An example of this kind of tool is the health risk appraisal (HRA), which allows individuals to enter their own specific information and returns appropriate recommendations to guide their health actions. The model developed here provides this kind of evidence-based recommendation regarding seafood consumption. Agencies should also develop alternative tools for populations with limited access to computer-based information.

Recommendation 2: New tools apart from traditional safety assessments should be developed, such as consumer-based benefit-risk analyses. A better way is needed to characterize the risks combined with benefit analysis.

Recommendation 3: A consumer-directed decision path needs to be properly designed, tested, and evaluated. The resulting product must undergo methodological review and update on a continuing basis. Responsible agencies will need to work with specialists in risk communication and evaluation, and tailor advice to specific groups as appropriate.

Recommendation 4: Consolidated advice is needed that brings together different benefit and risk considerations, and is tailored to individual circumstances, to better inform consumer choices. Effort should be made to improve coordination of federal guidance with that provided through partnerships at the state and local level.

Recommendation 5: Consumer messages should be tested to determine if there are spillover effects for segments of the population not targeted by the message. There is suggestive evidence that risk-avoidance advice for sensitive subpopulations may be construed by other groups or the general population as appropriate precautionary action for themselves. While emphasizing trade-offs may reduce the risk of spillover effects, consumer testing of messages should address the potential for spillover effects explicitly.

RESEARCH RECOMMENDATIONS

Recommendation 1: Research is needed to develop and evaluate more effective communication tools for use when conveying the health benefits and risks of seafood consumption as well as current and emerging information to the public. These tools should be tested among different communities and subgroups within the population and evaluated with pre- and post-test activities.

Recommendation 2: Among federal agencies there is a need to design and distribute better consumer advice to understand and acknowledge the context in which the information will be used by consumers. Understanding consumer decision making is a prerequisite. The information provided to consumers should be developed with recognition of the individual, environmental, social, and economic consequences of the advice. In addition, it is important that consistency between agencies be maintained, particularly with regard to communication information using serving sizes.

SUMMARY

Mass communication has inarguably changed the world, using a one-size-fits-all model. There are health messages that everyone of a certain generation has heard ("Just Say No"). But like shoes, advice is more helpful if it is sized appropriately and designed appropriately for the intended use. As communications technologies have advanced, the communicator's ability to tailor communications to reach large audiences rapidly, and interact with them, has also advanced.

REFERENCES

Achterberg C, Trenkner LL. 1990. Developing a working philosophy of nutrition education. *Journal of Nutrition Education* 22(4):189–193.

Anderson HA, Hanrahan LP, Smith A, Draheim L, Kanarek M, Olsen J. 2004. The role of sport-fish consumption advisories in mercury risk communication: A 1998–1999 12-state survey of women age 18–45. *Environmental Research* 95(3):315–24.

Argo JJ, Main KJ. 2004. Meta-analyses of the effectiveness of warning labels. *Journal of Public Policy and Marketing* 23(2):193–208.

Athearn PN, Kendall PA, Hillers VV, Schroeder M, Bergmann V, Chen G, Medeiros LC. 2004. Awareness and acceptance of current food safety recommendations during pregnancy. *Maternal and Child Health Journal* 8(3):149–162.

Atman CJ, Bostrom A, Fischhoff B, Morgan MG. 1994. Designing risk communication: Completing and correcting mental models of hazardous processes, Part I. *Risk Analysis* 14(5):779–788.

Balintfy JL. 1964. Menu planning by computer. *Communications of the ACM* 7(4):255–259.

Bech-Larsen T, Grunert KG. 2003. The perceived wholesomeness of functional foods: A conjoint study of Danish, Finnish, and American consumers' perception of functional foods. *Appetite* 40:9–14.

Birch LL. 1998. Development of food acceptance patterns in the first years of life. *Proceedings of the Nutrition Society* 57(4):617–624.

Birch LL. 1999. Development of food preferences. *Annual Review of Nutrition* 19(1): 41–62.

Birch LL, Fisher JO. 1998. Development of eating behaviors among children and adolescents. *Pediatrics* 101(3 Part 2):539–549.

Bisogni CA, Connors M, Devine CM, Sobal J. 2002. Who we are and how we eat: A qualitative study of identities in food choice. *Journal of Nutrition and Education Behavior* 34(3):128–139.

Blisard N, Lin B-H, Cromartie J, Ballenger N. 2002. America's changing appetite: Food consumption and spending to 2020. *FoodReview* 25(1):2–9.

Blisard, Noel, Hayden Stewart, and Dean Jolliffe. 2004 (May). *Low-Income Households' Expenditures on Fruits and Vegetables*. US Department of Agriculture, Economic Research Service. Agricultural Economic Report Number 833.

Booth SL, Sallis JF, Ritenbaugh C, Hill JO, Birch LL, Frank LD, Glanz K, Himmelgreen DA, Mudd M, Popkin BM, Rickard KA, St Jeor S, Hays NP. 2001. Environmental and societal factors affect food choice and physical activity: Rationale, influences, and leverage points. *Nutrition Reviews* 59(3 Part 2):S21–S39.

Borra S, Kelly L, Tuttle M, Neville K. 2001. Developing actionable dietary guidance messages: Dietary fat as a case study. *Journal of the American Dietetic Association* 101(6):678–684.

Bostrom A, Lofstedt RE. 2003. Communicating risk: Wireless and hardwired. *Risk Analysis* 23(2):241–248.

Bostrom A, Atman CJ, Fischhoff B, Morgan MG. 1994. Evaluating risk communication: completing and correcting mental models of hazardous processes, Part II. *Risk Analysis* 14(5):789–798.

Bouwman LI, Hiddink GJ, Koelen MA, Korthals M, van't Veer P, van Woerkum C. 2005. Personalized nutrition communication through ICT application: How to overcome the gap between potential effectiveness and reality. *European Journal of Clinical Nutrition* 59(Suppl 1):S108–S115.

Burger J, Waishwell L. 2001. Are we reaching the target audience? Evaluation of a fish fact sheet. *Science of the Total Environment* 277(1–3):77–86.

Burger J, Pflugh KK, Lurig L, Von Hagen LA, Von Hagen S. 1999a. Fishing in urban New Jersey: Ethnicity affects information sources, perception, and compliance. *Risk Analysis* 19(2):217–229.
Burger J, Stephens WL Jr, Boring CS, Kuklinski M, Gibbons JW, Gochfeld M. 1999b. Factors in exposure assessment: Ethnic and socioeconomic differences in fishing and consumption of fish caught along the Savannah River. *Risk Analysis* 19(3):427–438.
Burger J, Stern AH, Dixon C, Jeitner C, Shukla S, Burke S, Gochfeld M. 2004. Fish availability in supermarket and fish markets in New Jersey. *Science of the Total Environment* 333(1):89–97.
Burros M. 2005 (April 10). Stores say wild salmon but tests say farm bred. *New York Times.* [Online]. Available: http://www.rawfoodinfo.com/articles/art_wildsalmonfraud.html [accessed October 17, 2005].
CFSAN (Center for Food Safety and Applied Nutrition). 2003. *Guidance for Industry and FDA: Interim Procedures for Qualified Health Claims in the Labeling of Conventional Human Food and Human Dietary Supplements.* Rockville, MD: Food and Drug Administration. [Online]. Available: http://www.cfsan.fda.gov/~dms/hclmgui3.html [accessed October 17, 2005].
CFSAN. 2005. *Methylmercury in Fish—Summary of Key Findings from Focus Groups about the Methylmercury Advisory.* [Online]. Available: http://www.cfsan.fda.gov/~dms/admehg3g.html [accessed August 28, 2006].
CFSAN. 2006a. *Mercury Levels in Commercial Fish and Shellfish.* [Online]. Available: http://vm.cfsan.fda.gov/~frf/sea-mehg.html [accessed August 28, 2006].
CFSAN (Center for Food Safety and Applied Nutrition). 2006. *Mercury Levels in Commercial Fish and Shellfish.* [Online]. Available: http://www.cfsan.fda.gov/~frf/sea-mehg.html [accessed August 28, 2006].
Cohen et al. 2005. A quantitative risk-benefit analysis of changes in population fish consumption. *American Journal of Preventive Medicine* 29(4):325–334.
Cowburn G, Stockley L. 2003. *A Systematic Review of the Research on Consumer Understanding of Nutrition Labelling.* Brussels, Belgium: European Heart Network.
Davidson M. 2004 (January 25–28). *Presentation for the National Forum on Contaminants in Fish.* San Diego, CA. [Online]. Available: http://www.epa.gov/waterscience/fish/forum/2004/presentations/monday/davidson.pdf [accessed May 11, 2006].
de Vries H, Brug J. 1999. Computer-tailored interventions motivating people to adopt health promoting behaviours: Introduction to a new approach. *Patient Education Counseling* 36(2):99–105.
Derby BM, Levy AS. 2005. *Working Paper: Effects of Strength of Science Disclaimers on the Communication Impacts of Health Claims.* [Online]. Available: http://www.fda.gov/OHRMS/dockets/dockets/03N0496/03N-0496-rpt0001.pdf [accessed August 29, 2006].
Devine CM. 2005. A life course perspective: Understanding food choices in time, social location, and history. *Journal of Nutrition Education and Behavior* 37(3):121–128.
Drewnowski A. 1997. Taste preferences and food intake. *Annual Review of Nutrition* 17:237–253.
Eckstein EF. 1967. Menu planning by computer: The random approach. *Journal of the American Dietetic Association* 51(6):529–533.
Eng TR, Gustafson DH, Henderson J, Jimison H, Patrick K. 1999. Introduction to evaluation of interactive health communication applications. *American Journal of Preventive Medicine* 16(1):10–15.
EWG (Environmental Working Group). 2006. *EWG Tuna Calculator.* [Online]. Available: http://www.ewg.org/issues/mercury/20031209/calculator.php [accessed August 28, 2006].

Eysenbach G, Kummervold PE. 2005. Is cybermedicine killing you? The story of a cochrane disaster. *Journal of Medical Internet Research* 7(2):e21. [Online]. Available: http://www.jmir.org/2005/2/e21/ [accessed September 7, 2006].

FDA. 2004a. Food Labeling, Title 21. *Federal Register 2:20–52*. [Online]. Available: http://a257.g.akamaitech.net/7/257/2422/12feb20041500/edocket.access.gpo.gov/cfr_2004/aprqtr/21cfr101.9.htm [accessed March 22, 2006].

FDA. 2004b. *FDA Implements Enhanced Regulatory Process to Encourage Science-Based Labeling and Competition for Healthier Dietary Choices*. [Online]. Available: http://www.cfsan.fda.gov/~dms/nuttfbg.html [accessed March 22, 2006].

Finucane ML, Peters E, Slovic P. 2003. Chapter 10: Judgment and decision making: The dance of affect and reason. In: Schneider SL, Shanteau J, eds. *Emerging Perspectives on Judgment and Decision Research*. Cambridge, UK: Cambridge University Press. Pp. 327–364.

Fischhoff B, Slovic P, Lichtenstein S. (1978). Fault trees: Sensitivity of assessed failure probabilities to problem representation. *Journal of Experimental Psychology: Human Perception and Performance* 4:330–344.

FishScam.com. *Mercury Calculator*. [Online]. Available: http://www.fishscam.com/mercury-Calculator.cfm [accessed August 28, 2006].

Focus Groups about the Methylmercury Advisory. [Online]. Available: http://0-www.cfsan.fda.gov.lilac.une.edu/~dms/admehg3g.html [accessed May 11, 2006].

Fox S. 2005. *Health Information Online*. Pew Internet and American Life Project, Washington DC, May 17, 2005. [Online]. Available: http://www.pewInternet.org/pdfs/PIP_Healthtopics_May05.pdf [accessed April 10, 2006].

FSA (Food Standards Agency). 2005. *Signpost Labelling: Creative Development of Concepts Research Report*. UK: Food Standards Agency. [Online]. Available: http://www.food.gov.uk/multimedia/pdfs/signpostingnavigatorreport.pdf [accessed April 13, 2006].

Galef BG Jr. 1996. Food selection: Problems in understanding how we choose foods to eat. *Neuroscience and Biobehavioral Reviews* 20(1):67–73.

Gempesaw CM, Bacon JR, Wessels CR, Manalo A. 1995. Consumer perceptions of aquaculture products. *American Journal of Agriculture Economics* 77:1306–1312.

Golding D, Krimsky S, Plough A. 1992. Evaluationg risk communication: Narrative versus technical presentations of information about radon. *Risk Analysis* 12(1):27–35.

Got Mercury? Eating Lots of Seafood? Use This Advanced Mercury Calculator to See Your Exposure. [Online]. Available: http://gotmercury.org/english/advanced.htm [accessed August 28, 2006].

Griffiths F, Lindenmeyer A, Powell J, Lowe P, Thorogood M. 2006. Why are health care interventions delivered other the Internet? A systematic review of the public literature. *Journal of Medical Internet Research* 8(2):e10. [Online]. Available: http://www.jmir.org/2006/2/e10/ [accessed September 7, 2006].

Gustafson DH, Hawkins R, Boberg E, Pingree S, Serlin RE, Granziano F, Chan CL. 1999. Impact of a patient-centered, computer-based health information/support system. *American Journal of Preventive Medicine* 16(1):1–9.

Hanson GD, Herrmann RO, Dunn JW. 1995. Determinants of seafood purchase behavior: Consumers, restaurants, and grocery stores. *American Journal of Agricultural Economics* 77(5):1301–1305.

Honkanen P, Olsen SO, Verplanken B. 2005. Intention to consume seafood—the importance of habit. *Appetite* 45(2):161–168.

Huang KS, Lin B-H. 2000. *Estimation of Food Demand and Nutrient Elasticities from Household Survey Data*. Economic Research Service Technical Bulletin No. 1887. Washington, DC: US Department of Agriculture.

Indian and Northern Affairs Canada. *Northern Contaminants Program*. [Online]. Available: http://www.ainc-inac.gc.ca/ncp/ [accessed September 7, 2006].

Is Our Fish Fit to Eat. 1992. *Consumer Reports* 57(2):103.

Johnson BB, Sandman PM, Miller P. 1992. *Testing the Role of Technical Information in Public Risk Preception.* [Online]. Available: http://www.piercelaw.edu/risk/vol3/fall/johnson.htm [accessed August 27, 2006].

Kasperson JX, Kasperson RE, Pidgeon N, Slovic P. 2003. Chapter 1: The social amplification of risk: Assessing fifteen years of research and theory. In: Pidgeon N, Kasperson RE, Slovic P, eds. *The Social Amplification of Risk.* Cambridge, UK: Cambridge University Press. Pp. 13–46.

Keeney RL. 2002. Common mistakes in making value trade-offs. *Operations Research* 50(6):935–945.

Knobeloch L, Anderson HA, Imm P, Peters D, Smith A. 2005. Fish consumption, advisory awareness, and hair mercury levels among women of childbearing age. *Environmental Research* 97(2):220–227.

Knuth BA, A Connelly N, Sheeshka J, Patterson J. 2003. Weighing health benefit and health risk information when consuming sport-caught fish. *Risk Analysis* 23(6):1185–1197.

Kuhnlein HV, Receveur O, Chan HM, Loring E. 2000. *Centre for Indigenous People's Nutrition and Environment (CINE).* Ste-Anne-de-Bellevue, QC: CINE.

Lancaster T, Stead L. 2005. Self-help interventions for smoking cessation. *Cochrane Database of Systematic Reviews* (3):CD001118.

Levy AS, Derby B. 2000. *Report Submitted to Interagency Working Group on Mercury Communications.* Findings from focus group testing of mercury-in-fish messages. [Online]. Available: http://www.cfsan.fda.gov/~acrobat/hgfoc10.pdf [accessed May 11, 2006].

Lutz SM, Smallwood DM, Blaylock JR. 1995. Limited financial resources constrain food choices. *FoodReview* 18(1):13–17.

Marshall E. 1991. A is for apple, Alar, and—alarmist. *Science* 254(5028):20–22.

Mennella JA, Pepino MY, Reed DR. 2005a. Genetic and environmental determinants of bitter perception and sweet preferences. *Pediatrics* 115(2):e216–e222.

Mennella JA, Turnbull B, Ziegler PJ, Martinez H. 2005b. Infant feeding practices and early flavor experiences in Mexican infants: An intra-cultural study. *Journal of the American Dietetic Association* 105(6):908–915.

Monterey Bay Aquarium. 1999–2006. *Seafood Watch: Make Choices for Healthy Oceans.* [Online]. Available: http://www.mbayaq.org/cr/seafoodwatch.asp [accessed August 28, 2006].

Morgan MG, Fischhoff B, Bostrom A, Atman CJ. 2001. *Risk Communication: A Mental Models Approach.* Cambridge, UK: Cambridge University Press.

Mos L, Jack J, Cullon D, Montour L, Alleyne C, Ross PS. 2004. The importance of imarine foods to a near-urban first nation community in coastal British Columbia, Canada: Toward a benefit-risk assessment. *Journal of Toxicology and Environmental Health, Part A* 67(8–10):791–808.

Ness AR, Hughes J, Elwood PC, Whitley E, Smith GD, Burr ML. 2002. The long-term effect of dietary advice in men with coronary disease: Follow-up of the Diet and Reinfarction trial (DART). *European Journal of Clinical Nutrition* 56(6):512–518.

Ness AR, Ashfield-Watt PA, Whiting JM, Smith GD, Hughes J, Burr ML. 2004. The long-term effect of dietary advice on the diet of men with angina: The diet and angina randomized trial. *Journal of Human Nutrition and Diet* 17(2):117–119.

Nestle M, Wing R, Birch L, DiSogra L, Drewnowski A, Middleton S, Sigman-Grant M, Sobal J, Winston M, Economos C. 1998. Behavioral and social influences on food choice. *Nutrition Review* 56(5 Pt 2):S50–S64; discussion S64–S74.

NRDC (Natural Resources Defense Council). 2006. *Mercury Contamination in Fish. A Guide to Staying Healthy and Fighting Back.* [Online]. Available: http://www.nrdc.org/health/effects/mercury/index.asp [accessed December 8, 2006].

The Ocean Conservancy. 2001–2006. *Mercury Calculator.* [Online]. Available: http://www.oceanconservancy.org/site/PageServer?pagename=mercuryCalculator [accessed August 28, 2006].

Oceans Alive. 2005. *Buying Guide: Becoming a Smarter Seafood Shopper.* [Online]. Available: www.oceansalive.org/eat.cfm?subnav=buy [accessed October 17, 2005].

Office of the Attorney General. 2001. *Attorney General Lockyer Announces Court Approval of Settlement Requiring Major Restaurant Chains to Post Warnings About Mercury in Fish.* [Online]. Available: http://ag.ca.gov/newsalerts/2005/05-011.htm [accessed May 11, 2006].

Oken E, Kleinman KP, Berland WE, Simon SR, Rich-Edwards JW, Gillman MW. 2003. Decline in fish consumption among pregnant women after a national mercury advisory. *Obstetrics and Gynecology* 102(2):346–351.

109th Congress, 2D Session. 2006. H.R. 4167: An Act. [Online]. Available: http://www.govtrack.us/data/us/bills.text/109/h/h4167.pdf [accessed August 28, 2006].

Park H, Thurman WN, Easley JE Jr. 2004. Modeling inverse demands for fish: Empirical welfare measurement in Gulf and South Atlantic Fisheries. *Marine Resource Economics* 19:333–351.

Raine K. 2005. Determinants of healthy eating in Canada. *Canadian Journal of Public Health* 96(Supplement 3):S8–S14.

Riley DM, Fischhoff B, Small M, Fischbeck P. 2001. Evaluating the effectiveness of risk-reduction strategies for consumer chemical products. *Risk Analysis* 21(2):357–369.

Rimer, BK, Glassman B. 1999. Is there a use for tailored print communications in cancer risk communication? *Journal of the National Cancer Institute, Monographs* 25:140–148.

Salvanes KG, DeVoretz DJ. 1997. Household demand for fish and meat products: Separability and demographic effects. *Marine Resource Economics* 12(1):37–55.

Sattler B, Lippy B, Jordan TG. 1997. *Hazard Communication: A Review of the Science Underpinning the Art of Communication for Health and Safety.* Washington, DC: US Department of Labor.

Schriver K. 1989. Evaluating text quality: The continuum from text-focused to reader-focused methods. *IEEE Transactions on Professional Communication* 32(4):238–255.

Schriver KA. 1997. *Dynamics in Document Design: Creating Text for Readers.* New York: John Wiley and Sons, Inc.

Science Panel on Interactive Communication and Health. 1999. *Wired for Health and Well-Being: The Emergence of Interactive Health Communication.* Washington, DC: US Department of Health and Human Services. [Online]. Available: http://www.health.gov/scipich/pubs/finalreport.htm [accessed September 6, 2006].

Seale J Jr, Regmi A, Bernstein J. 2003 (October). *International Evidence on Food Consumption Patterns.* US Department of Agriculture, Economic Research Service, Technical Bulletin Number 1904.

Shepard R. 2005. Influences on food choice and dietary behavior. Elmadfa I editor. *Diet Diversifications and Health Promotion.* Basel, Switzerland: S. Karger AG. Pp. 36–43.

Shimshack JP, Ward MB, Beatty TKM. 2005. Working paper: Are mercury advisories effective? Information, education, and fish consumption.

Slovic P, Finucane ML, Peters E, MacGregor DG. 2004. Risk as analysis and risk as feeling: Some thoughts about affect, reason, risk, and rationality. *Risk Analysis* 24(2):311–322.

Stewart-Knox B, Hamilton J, Parr H, Bunting B. 2005. Dietary strategies and uptake of reduced fat foods. *Journal of Human Nutrition and Diet* 18(2):121–128.

Story M, French S. 2004. Food advertising and marketing directed at children and adolescents in the US. *International Journal of Behavior, Nutrition, and Physical Activity.* Published online February 10 at http://www.pubmedcentral.nih.gov/articlerender.fcgi?artid=416565.

Tilden J, Hanrahan LP, Anderson H, Palit C, Olson J, Kenzie WM. 1997. Health advisories for consumers of Great Lakes sport fish: Is the message being received? *Environmental Health Perspectives* 105(12):1360–1365.

Trondsen T, Scholderer J, Lund E, Eggen AE. 2003. Perceived barriers to consumption of fish among Norwegian women. *Appetite* 41(3):301–314.

USDA. 2005a. Briefing Rooms: Food CPI, Prices and Expenditures: Food Expenditure Tables. [Online]. Available: http://www.ers.usda.gov/Briefing/CPIFoodAndExpenditures/Data/ [accessed May 11, 2006].

USDA. 2005b. *USDA National Nutrient Database for Standard Reference Release 18.* [Online]. Available: www.nal.usda.gov/fnic/foodcomp/Data/SR18/sr18.html [accessed October 17, 2005].

US EPA (US Environmental Protection Agency). 2006. *Joint Federal Advisory for Mercury in Fish.* [Online]. Available: http://www.epa.gov/waterscience/fishadvice/factsheet.html [accessed August 28, 2006].

Wansink B, Sonka ST, Hasler CM. 2004. Front-label health claims: When less is more. *Food Policy* 29:659–667.

Warner M. 2005 (August 19). With sales plummeting, tuna strikes back. *New York Times— Late Edition.* C. P. 3.

Wellman KF. 1992. The United States retail demand for fish products: An application of the almost ideal demand System. *Applied Economics* 24(4):445–457.

Wethington E. 2005. An overview of the life course perspective: Implications for health and nutrition. *Journal of Nutrition and Education Behavior* 37(3):115–120.

Wetter AC, Goldberg JP, King AC, Sigman-Grant M, Baer R, Crayton E, Devine C, Drewnowski A, Dunn A, Johnson G, Pronk N, Saelens B, Snyder D, Walsh K, Warland R. 2001. How and why do individuals make food and physical activity choices? *Nutrition Reviews* 59(3 Part 2):S11–S21.

Wheatley MA, Wheatley B. 1981. The effect of eating habits on mercury levels among Inuit residents of Sugluk, P.Q. *Etudes/Inuit/Studies* 5(1):27–43.

Williams P. 2005. Consumer understanding and use of health claims for foods. *Nutrition Review* 63(7):256–264.

Willows ND. 2005. Determinants of healthy eating in Aboriginal peoples in Canada: The current state of knowledge and research gaps. *Canadian Journal of Public Health* 96 (Suppl. 3):S32–S36, S36–S41.

Wogalter MS, Laughery KR. 1996. WARNING! Sign and label effectiveness. *Current Directions in Psychological Science* 5(2):33–37.

Wyatt JC, Sullivan F. 2005. eHealth and the future: Promise or peril? *British Medical Journal* 331(7529):1391–1392.

Yen ST, Huang CL. 1996. Household demand for finfish: A generalized double-hurdle model. *Journal of Agriculture and Resources Economics* 21(2):220–234.

Zuckerman A, Chaiken S. 1998. A heuristic-systematic processing analysis of the effectiveness of warning labels. *Psychology and Marketing* 15(7):621–642.

7

Balancing Choices:
Supporting Consumer Seafood
Consumption Decisions

This chapter presents Step 3 (see Box 5-1) of the process for designing consumer guidance on balancing benefits and risks associated with seafood consumption. This step focuses on the design and evaluation of the guidance program itself, including the format of the guidance; its communication through media, health care partners, and other channels; and mock-up examples of ways to integrate the benefit and risk considerations from previous chapters into consumer guidance. The chapter also discusses other communication and decision-support design considerations.

INTRODUCTION

The goal of this chapter is to advise agencies on how to develop a consumer seafood information program to support consumers who are trying to balance benefits and risks in their seafood consumption decisions. Such advice necessarily builds on an assessment of the benefits and risks, as well as an assessment of what decisions consumers actually face, and how they currently approach those decisions. A related and essential element of the process is use of the best available social and behavioral science research on the design of effective communications programs and messages to inform consumer benefit-risk decisions. In addition, we present several specific options for informing seafood consumption decisions, in order to highlight the features of alternative formats for informing consumers' seafood consumption decisions for themselves and their families.

While there is a role for simple slogans and overall guidance to the general population, the committee believes that it cannot be emphasized too much that communications tailored for specific audiences are likely to be more effective and thus are an important element in communications programs. This is especially important for benefit-risk choices where target population groups differ in their risk susceptibility, and in the degree to which they are likely to benefit. For both education and marketing, understanding the audience and targeting it appropriately are critical.

A successful communications program starts with clear objectives and measurable goals, and includes the steps outlined in the two preceding chapters followed by implementation and evaluation, as discussed below. The development strategy should be iterative, such that program evaluation is built into the program from the outset and used to refine it over time. One widely used health communications program planning document, the National Institutes of Health "Pink Book" (SOURCE: http://www.cancer. gov/pinkbook), suggests these components for a health communications program plan: a general description of the program, including intended audiences, goals, and objectives; a market research plan (i.e., for researching the consumer context and choice process); message and materials development and pretesting plans; materials production, distribution, and promotion plans; partnership plans; a process evaluation plan; an outcome evaluation plan; a task and timetable; and a budget.

For demonstration purposes, the committee takes as a working objective the facilitation of consumer use of information for decision making and balancing choices, for a wide variety of consumers. Corresponding measurable end points would be increased awareness of both benefits and risks of seafood consumption, and increased ease of access and usability of seafood benefit-risk information.

Table 6-2 in Chapter 6 provides a summary of the current seafood consumption information environment. Opportunities for improving the current information environment include: (1) providing more comprehensive and systematic evaluation of current consumer seafood information and information environments for target populations ("marketing research"); (2) increasing the emphasis on benefits of seafood consumption; (3) assessing the overall role of state advisories in consumer seafood consumption decisions, taking into account their limited reach; (4) increasing the availability of quantitative benefit and risk data for seafood consumption, and addressing any errors in how quantitative benefit and risk information is used in interactive online consumer guidance; (5) increasing the use and usefulness of point-of-purchase displays; and (6) developing partnership programs.

Notably, while US federal and state agencies provide websites for consumers (e.g., http://www.foodsafety.gov/~fsg/fsgadvic.html; http://health. nih.gov), these do not currently provide interactive online guidance; other parties are now providing quantitative risk information, as discussed in Chapter 6. Much has been written about program evaluation (CDC, 1999;

Mark et al., 2000; Ryan and DeStefano, 2000) and the evaluation of communications (Schriver, 1990; Spyridakis, 2000); the paucity of information available regarding both formative (e.g., the Food and Drug Administration focus groups) and summative (e.g., overall effects on attitudes or consumption) evaluation of national seafood consumption advisories suggests that agencies should devote additional attention and resources to evaluation. The committee touches on the importance of evaluation in the context of partnerships, to assess whether communications are appropriate and effective for target populations.

STEP 3: DESIGNING COMMUNICATIONS TO SUPPORT INFORMED DECISION-MAKING

Interactive Health Communication

In seafood consumption, "one size does not fit all," and messages about consumption often have to be individualized for different groups. There is a need to consider developing tools for consumers such as web-based, interactive programs that provide easy-to-use seafood consumption decision tools. Real-time, interactive decision support that is easily available to the public has the potential to increase informed actions for some portion of the population. In the absence of federal investment in such tools, some organizations have invested in online mercury calculators or consumption guides (Table 6-1). Many of these focus solely on risks from seafood consumption, and while well-intentioned, may be providing misleading information, for example, by interpreting the Reference Dose (RfD) as a "bright line" to determine whether consuming seafood puts a consumer at risk.

One model for developing comprehensive consumer tools is a health risk appraisal (HRA) that would allow individuals to enter their own specific information and would provide feedback in the form of appropriate information or advice to guide the user's health actions, such as seafood consumption. There are a myriad of health risk appraisal tools commercially available; of those in the public domain the Centers for Disease Control and Prevention (CDC) has extensive experience in the development and use of HRAs (SOURCE: http://www.cdc.gov). In order to be most useful and appropriately directed, tools such as the HRA must be based on a body of knowledge that substantiates both benefits and risks. This kind of approach can be seen in the *Clinical Guide to Preventive Services* from the Agency for Healthcare Research and Quality (AHRQ), which adopted recommendations based on medical evidence and the strength of that evidence in practice (USPSTF, 2001–2004).

The *Clinical Guide to Preventive Services* is an example of an interactive health communication approach to providing one-on-one guidance, along with the degree of evidence for that guidance, which is used to categorize a spectrum of recommendations. These tools are generally not set up to provide information to individuals, but rather to public health practitioners and individual care providers. Their recommendations are evidence-based but not easily translatable to the lay community. Although the *Clinical Guide to Preventive Services* is aimed toward practitioners, AHRQ has tried to make it understandable to the general public—e.g., if you are over 50, and have a risk factor, then get a mammogram.

A more coordinated approach is needed for developing and disseminating evidence-based recommendations to health care practioners that can then be provided to consumers. Such recommendations should be updated on a continuous, rotating basis, to allow for more rapid translation of science to practice. Where HRA tools are targeted for intermediaries who are experts in their own right, guidance or additional tools are necessary to help them translate and target information for consumers. The *Clinical Guide to Preventive Services* has a handbook that attempts to provide user-friendly tools to help providers translate and target information to consumers. If the goal is to guide consumption decisions that balance benefits and risks, there needs to be a similar translation mechanism because of the limited and continuously evolving knowledge base concerning seafood benefits and safety. Currently, consumers are receiving piecemeal information about methylmercury and persistent organic pollutants such as dioxins and polychlorinated biphenyls (PCBs); for the most part, that information is not pulled together sufficiently to facilitate consumers' understanding it in context and thus being able to use it to inform their choices (see Table 6-2). (Also see Chapter 6 for discussion of the effectiveness of online nutrition information.)

A general framework for developing this kind of communication is a consumer checklist that engages the user in interactive identification of his or her benefit-risk factors, and uses that information to produce a tailored benefit-risk estimation and associated recommended actions. Determining how to communicate the resulting estimates and actions requires a series of judgements, including whether and how to represent this information as text, numbers, or graphics. Empirical testing of the effects of the final tool is essential, given the difficulties of predicting the effects of communications on individual consumers, or even specific target populations.

Decision Support for Consumers

The committee's balancing of the benefits and risks of different patterns of seafood consumption for different target populations resulted in the analysis presented in Chapter 5. This type of expert identification of the characteristics that distinguish target populations who face substantially different consequences from seafood consumption is an important component of audience segmentation and targeting.

If a target population believes they are exempt from general advice because of some specific condition, they may either ignore the available advice or interpret it in unanticipated ways. The spillover effects discussed in Chapter 6 illustrate the kinds of problems that may arise. While expert recommendations such as those summarized in Chapter 5 could, in theory, be used directly by federal agencies as advice to consumers on seafood consumption, such advice is unlikely to be effective if it ignores consumers' contexts and information needs.

As discussed in Chapter 6, there are multiple reasons why expert benefit-risk analyses alone comprise an insufficient communication design strategy. Examples include when consumers distrust experts, when there are widespread misconceptions about a risk or benefit, or when experts use technical jargon that makes their reasoning opaque to nonexperts. Some consumers may want more information, and some will want to be able to independently verify experts' advice.

One previously tested consumer-centered approach to providing information is the development of decision support focused on the decisions and decision contexts faced by consumers, as discussed in Chapter 6. Through a brief set of questions, a decision pathway can segment and channel consumers into relevant target populations in order to provide benefit and risk information that is tailored to each group, as illustrated in Figures 7-1 and 7-2.

Figure 7-2 includes a separate question about cardiovascular health, which differentiates it from Figure 5-2. This question is included because the committee anticipates that the many recommendations and guidelines specially targeting higher eicosapentaenoic acid/docosahexaenoic acid (EPA/DHA) consumption for those with cardiovascular health concerns may have created a belief in that target population that they would benefit more than others from high EPA/DHA consumption. As is evident from the recommendations in both Figure 5-2 and 7-2, the committee's analysis does not support this distinction. This assumption about cardiovascular patients' beliefs would need to be verified empirically before it was included as part of a communications program.

Alternative formats for presenting information can serve the interests of consumers who desire different levels of information as inputs to their decision-making, and provide those most interested with additional insight regarding the quality of information, including uncertainties. Alternative guidance structures might be relevant for consumers focused on different goals and decisions, such as the estimated benefits and risks of eating a specific seafood meal, as illustrated in Figure 7-3. Figure 7-3 uses consumption of one 3-ounce serving of Atlantic farmed salmon as an example of the type of information that could be presented with this tool. The committee notes

1. What is your age?

    ☐ 2-19

    ☐ 20-39

    ☐ 40+

2. What is your sex?

    ☐ Male

    ☐ Female

    If female, could you become pregnant or are you currently pregnant or lactating?

    ☐ Yes

    ☐ No

3. Are you at risk of cardiovascular disease?

    ☐ Yes

    ☐ No

4. Do you eat fish caught in local waters, as opposed to commercially available fish?

    ☐ Yes

    ☐ No

FIGURE 7-1 Example of set of questions to identify benefit-risk target populations for seafood consumption.

that the eocological effects of increasing salmon aquaculture are highly debated (e.g., Naylor et al., 2001). Further consideration would have to be given to this debate if the decision tool were to also incorporate a weighing of the ecological impacts of food choices.

Another alternative format structure might be a comparison of two meal options, as illustrated in Figures 7-4a and 7-4b for the example of consuming a serving of salmon vs. a serving of chicken. Full development of this comparison approach would require information, such as that shown in Table 5-1, on a full range of seafood and other food products that consumers may substitute for each other.

Decision analyses can be presented in several formats (e.g., Figures 7-3, 7-4a, and 7-4b) or used to lead consumers through a decision pathway, for example, via an interactive Web-based program that graphically provides tailored information. In a Web-based format, the consumer could proceed by answering a set of questions such as those shown in Figure 7-1.

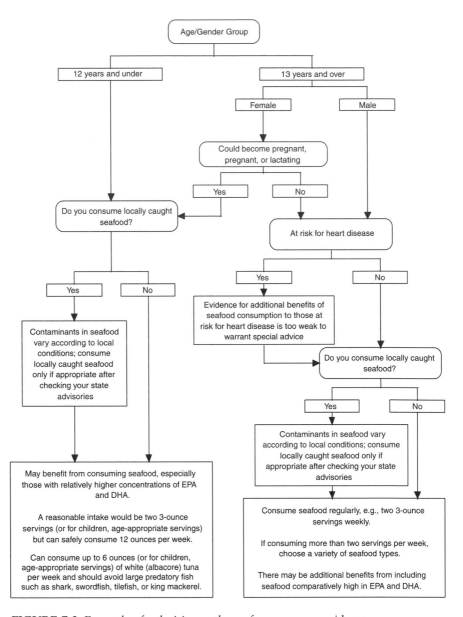

FIGURE 7-2 Example of a decision pathway for consumer guidance.
NOTE: The wording in this figure has not been tested among consumers. Designers will need to test the effects of presenting information on seafood choices in alternative formats.

This week I am planning on eating:

Meal 1: **(number entered by consumer)** ounces of
(type of seafood, entered by consumer from dropdown menu), and

Meal 2: **(number entered by consumer)** ounces of
(type of seafood, entered by consumer from dropdown menu).

(If you plan on eating additional seafood meals, click here).

Is this a good idea?
Enter your age (**from menu)** and gender (**from menu**), then
click here for **advice**, here for **analysis**.

Example:
This week I am planning on eating

Meal 1: **3 ounces** of **Atlantic farmed salmon**
(no additional meals)
What will I be getting from this seafood?

ADVICE:

Eating **3 ounces** of **Atlantic farmed salmon** a week is good for everyone. Including children and women of childbearing age.

Evidence suggests that you could benefit from eating more seafood than this every week.

Serving size check: **3 ounces** is about the size of a pack of cards.

Click here for more details on nutrients and contaminants* in your seafood meals.
Click here for more general seafood consumption advice.

link to Nutrients and Contaminants

ANALYSIS of nutrients and contaminants in your seafood meals:

3 ounces of **Atlantic farmed salmon** has:

Nutrients:*
Calories...............175
Saturated fat........ 2.1 grams
Selenium.............. 35.2 micrograms
Iron......................0.3 micrograms
EPA/DHA..............1.8 grams

Contaminants:*
Methylmercury......1 microgram
Dioxin/DLC........... 21 toxicity equivalents

*Hotlink the nutrients and contaminants to explanations, definitions, and relevant standards, similar to the Notes at the bottom of Table 5-1. Include links from these to data sources.

FIGURE 7-3 Example of seafood meal analysis decision tool—Would I receive a benefit or risk from eating this seafood meal? Questions: portion size (3 or 6 ounces), kind of seafood (all of the most commonly eaten kinds), specific species/type (where applicable and data available—e.g., for salmon).

What happens if I eat 3 ounces of salmon instead of 3 ounces of chicken?

Tabular Comparison[a]

		Salmon (3 oz)	Chicken[c] (3 oz)
Nutrients	Energy (kcal)[b]	175	140
	EPA/DHA (g)[b]	1.8	0.03
Contaminants	Methylmercury (μg)[b]	1	0
	Dioxin/DLC (TEQ)[b]	21	2

FIGURE 7-4a Example of a substitution question approach with tabular presentation of information—What happens if I eat seafood X (e.g., salmon) instead of food Y (e.g., chicken)?

[a]Continue the table with other nutrients/contaminants/other factors of interest.

[b]Hot link the units to explanations and definition (for example, TEQ = sum of toxicity equivalency factors (TEF); where TEF is a numerical index that is used to compare the toxicity of different congeners and substances, in this case dioxin congeners.

[c]Note that EPA/DHA levels in chicken and eggs are based on existing published data; changes in the use of fishmeal in feed sources may have an impact on levels detected in the future.

The example decision pathway shown in Figure 7-2 distinguishes between consumer target populations in order to tailor consumption advice based on current evidence regarding the benefits and risks of seafood consumption. It also assumes that consumers agree with and accept the health goals and risk assessments implicit in federal nutritional guidelines and risk advisories.

Additional information can be added to explain branching in the decision pathway and the reasons for it. Designers will need to test the effects of presenting information on seafood choices in alternative formats. The first set of hypertext explanations would link the questions asked in the decision pathway to the research used to create the pathway, to explain the questions' relevance to assessment of benefits and risks, and to provide consumers with links to more detailed information on the personal benefits and risks associated with seafood consumption. Table 7-1 shows examples of the types of explanations that might be used as added information in the

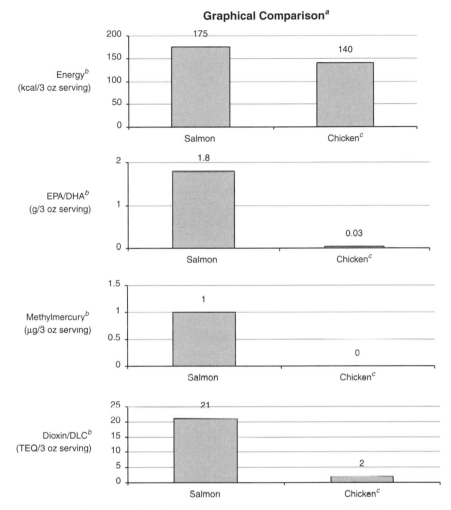

What happens if I eat 3 ounces of salmon instead of 3 ounces of chicken?

Graphical Comparison[a]

FIGURE 7-4b Example of a substitution question approach with graphical presentation of information—What happens if I eat seafood X (e.g., salmon) instead of food Y (e.g., chicken)?

[a]Continue the graphs with other nutrients/contaminants/other factors of interest.

[b]Hot link the units to explanations and definitions (for example, TEQ = sum of toxicity equivalency factors (TEF); where TEF is a numerical index that is used to compare the toxicity of different *congeners* and substances, in this case dioxin congeners.

[c]Note that EPA/DHA levels in chicken and eggs are based on existing published data; changes in the use of fishmeal in feed sources may have an impact on levels detected in the future.

TABLE 7-1 Examples of Possible Additional Layers of Information to Provide to Interested Consumers

	Possible Content of "Click Here for More Background Information"
Age	Children should eat age-appropriate portions. (hypertext link to table or pictures of age-appropriate portions)
Gender	Mercury accumulates in the body, and so can pose a risk to a nursing infant or future baby. This is why gender is important.
Pregnant, could become pregnant, lactating	Mercury accumulates in the body, and so can pose a risk to a nursing infant or future baby
Prior cardiovascular event	The evidence that suggests that those who have had heart attacks may reduce their risk by consuming EPA and DHA is weaker than previously thought. (link to additional data, source)
Seafood type, source, and preparation method	Explanatory paragraphs could summarize benefit and risk data for various species, by geographical origin (where data exist to distinguish in this way), and whether commercially available or self-caught fish. They could also discuss preparation methods—risks of raw fish (see Chapter 4) and cooking methods (e.g., frying, breading) that can abbrogate nutritional benefits. Current data do not support distinctions between seafood types beyond those made in the Food and Drug Administration/US Environmental Protection Agency 2004 advisory.
Alternative sources of nutrients; benefits, risks, and costs of alternatives	As addressed in Chapters 3, 4, and 5, other foods and fish-oil supplements are also sources of EPA and DHA. Other trade-offs identified in Chapter 5 could also be summarized for consumers. Regular updating would be necessary, given that changes in the use of fishmeal and other content in feed has changed and will change the nutritional value of animal products.

formats. Designers will need to test the effects of presenting information on seafood choices in alternative formats.

Presenting Quantitative Benefit-Risk Information: The Promise and Peril of Visual Information

Both anecdotal and experimental evidence support the use of visual information as superior to either text or numbers in many contexts. The inclusion of alternative presentations of benefit-risk information in the design of consumer advice recognizes that while some consumers prefer to follow the advice given them by experts, others want to decide on the benefit-risk trade-offs for themselves. Consumers differ in their ability to interpret specific benefit or risk metrics. As discussed in Chapter 6, effectively informing decision-making requires the use of metrics that consumers can evaluate and use. A consumer-centered information design and evaluation approach is needed that makes information "easily available, accurate, and timely" (Hibbard and Peters, 2003). One approach is to present numerical information graphically (Hibbard et al., 2002). Consumers should be familiar with rating systems that represent benefits and risks in a small number of categories (often five), as is done for crash test ratings (TRB, 2002). The UK Food Standards Agency (FSA) has proposed "red-amber-green" multiple traffic light labeling for foods (FSA, 2005, 2006; http://www.food.gov. uk/foodlabelling/signposting/signpostlabelresearch/).

Graph comprehension depends on experience and expectations, as well as on the design of the graph in question (Shah and Hoeffner, 2002). Familiarity with an analog, as in the multiple traffic light system proposed by the FSA, can aid comprehension. Consumer testing carried out by Navigator for FSA (FSA, 2005) suggests that the multiple traffic light system helps consumers choose more nutritious foods, although the system has been criticized for its simplicity (Fletcher, 2006). Other common graphical approaches to presenting benefits or risks include "thermometers," rank-ordered bar charts, or a more complex graphic embedded in a matrix of benefit and risk information, as is done by *Consumer Reports*.

While some of these approaches have been tested empirically, an agency developing consumer guidance should test prototypes on representative consumers. A potential problem in presenting benefit and risk metrics together is that the consumer may misinterpret the relationship between benefit and risk. For example, consumers are likely to infer that side-by-side thermometers or bars are directly comparable, even if they are labeled with different numerical scales.

Formats such as those presented by the committee in Figures 7-2 through 7-4b can serve as suitable advice for consumers who want general guidance on seafood consumption. However, other consumers may want specific information for different seafood products. In Navigator's testing, consumers preferred additional text to be informational rather than advisory (FSA, 2005). For these consumers, there is a large family of graphics that could be used to present choices across a broad range of seafood products. The committee developed several examples of graphical presentations of guidance to illustrate possible approaches. In presenting such graphics, the committee emphasizes its finding that it is not possible to have a single metric that captures complex benefit-risk relationships. Any sort of score system is unlikely to capture the inherent uncertainties in what is known about the underlying benefit-risk trade-offs. Graphical formats should be carefully and empirically tested to insure that they effectively communicate with consumers.

Multiple design decisions are required to produce graphical guidance; all could influence the impression the consumer takes away. These decisions include the selection of the seafood types to show; the colors, order, and formatting of bars to use; and whether to employ error bars to communicate uncertainty about point estimates. The graphical examples presented in Figures 7-5 through 7-8b below focus on information on EPA/DHA and methylmercury in seafood selections. A particularly important design choice here is the inclusion/exclusion and relative size of the scale of EPA/DHA bars as compared to the scale of methylmercury bars. Similar decisions would need to be made in presenting other benefit (e.g., low-fat profiles) and risk (e.g., other contaminants) information in these types of formats. In the figures presented here, the relative lengths of the EPA/DHA and methylmercury scales have been chosen arbitrarily, as the committee has not determined quantitatively the relative values of benefits from EPA/DHA and risks from methylmercury. The graphics present information that the consumer would use in conjunction with specific guidance that is appropriate for them (e.g., consumption of EPA/DHA, avoidance of methylmercury).

Figures 7-5 through 7-7 are examples of formats that could be tested with consumers. In the discussion here, the committee highlights considerations in the alternative approaches. All of these graphics relate to the benefit-risk tradeoff between EPA/DHA consumption and methylmercury intake. The use of this example reflects the fact that information is more complete here than for other nutrient and toxicant effects, not that these are the only benefit-risk tradeoffs that are relevant to consumers. However, the effect of graphics like these is likely to be to draw consumers' attention to this information, and to ignore other possibly relevant information.

Figure 7-5 emphasizes the EPA/DHA content of different fish in grams per 3-ounce serving. This monochromatic graph is intended to emphasize benefits and provide guidance on seafood choices to enhance EPA/DHA consumption. This figure may be appropriate by itself for the guidance of adolescent males, adult males, and females who will not become pregant. For females who could become pregnant, are pregnant, or are lactating, and for infants and young children, the graph might include colored bars (red and yellow) to indicate fish (e.g., tilefish) containing levels of methylmercury that increase the potential for adverse health effects for these groups.

Figures 7-6a and 7-6b combine the presentation of information on EPA/DHA and methylmercury levels in a 3-ounce serving for different types of seafood. Two versions of this graph are presented in order to emphasize the design issues involved. These issues arise from the fact that the committee could not use a single scale, quantitative metric (e.g., Quality Adjusted Life Year, Disability Adjusted Life Year) for the combined benefit-risk profile of different seafoods. Thus, the information for methylmercury and EPA/DHA must be presented in separate metric scales that are not directly comparable.

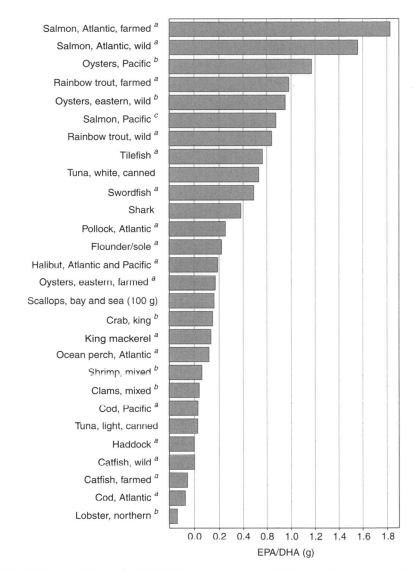

FIGURE 7-5 Estimated EPA/DHA amount (grams [g]) in one 3-ounce portion of seafood.
NOTES: The scale used in this figure for EPA/DHA content is arbitrary. Designers will need to carefully test the effect of the scale used for the bars on the message received by consumers.

[a]Cooked, dry heat.
[b]Cooked, moist heat.
[c]The EPA and DHA content in Pacific salmon is a composite from chum, coho, and sockeye.

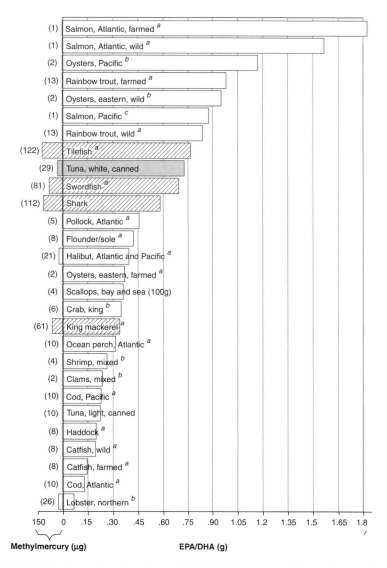

FIGURE 7-6a Example of estimated EPA/DHA (grams [g]) and methylmercury (microgram [µg]) amounts in one 3-ounce portion of seafood.
NOTES: The scales used in this figure for EPA/DHA and methylmercury content are arbitrary. Designers will need to carefully test the effect of the scales used for the bars on the message received by consumers.

[a]Cooked, dry heat.
[b]Cooked, moist heat.
[c]The EPA and DHA content in Pacific salmon is a composite from chum, coho, and sockeye.

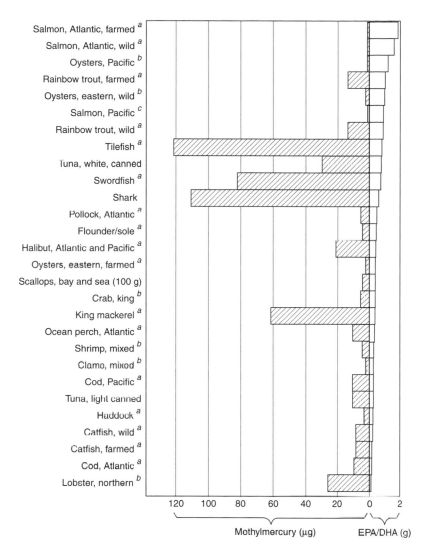

FIGURE 7-6b Example of estimated EPA/DHA (grams [g]) and methylmercury (microgram [µg]) amounts in one 3-ounce portion of seafood, with emphasis on methylmercury.

NOTES: The scales used in this figure for EPA/DHA and methylmercury content are arbitrary. Designers will need to carefully test the effect of the scales used for the bars on the message received by consumers.

[a]Cooked, dry heat.

[b]Cooked, moist heat.

[c]The EPA and DHA content in Pacific salmon is a composite from chum, coho, and sockeye.

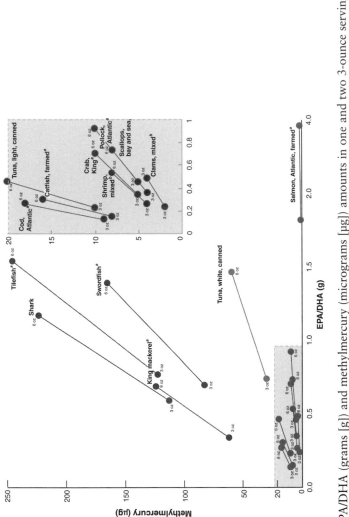

FIGURE 7-7 Estimated EPA/DHA (grams [g]) and methylmercury (micrograms [µg]) amounts in one and two 3-ounce servings per week amounts.

NOTES: The scales used in this figure for EPA/DHA and methylmercury content are arbitrary. Designers will need to carefully test the effect of the scales used for the bars on the message received by consumers.

[a]Cooked, dry heat.
[b]Cooked, moist heat.

Figures 7-6a and 7-6b illustrate that the choice of scales to use for each can greatly affect the graph's appearance. Testing with consumers is required to assess the impression made by alternative formats.

The scales used in Figure 7-6a have the effect of emphasizing information on EPA/DHA content and illustrate that there are a number of seafood choices, with varying levels of EPA and DHA, available with low exposure to methylmercury. The figure does not provide information about levels of lipophilic contaminants such as dioxins and PCBs because of the limited availability of data for various types of seafood. However, evidence presented in Chapter 4 suggests that levels of these contaminants in commercially obtained seafood do not pose a risk of adverse health effects even among the most at-risk groups, i.e., females who could become pregnant, are pregnant, or are lactating, and infants and young children, when consumed in the amount of two 3-ounce servings per week. As shown, Figure 7-6a may be appropriate for guidance to females who could become pregnant, are pregnant, or are lactating, and for infants and young children, as the shaded bars indicate types of seafood that should be avoided or consumed in limited amounts by individuals in these target populations. For adolescent males, adult males, and females who will not become pregnant, Figure 7-6a could be used for guidance without any specially shaded bars.

Figure 7-6b uses alternative scales to show the methylmercury and EPA/DHA content in 3-ounce servings of different seafoods. The design tends to emphasize the methylmercury and deemphasize the EPA/DHA information. A side-by-side comparison of Figures 7-6a and 7-6b illustrates the impact of design choices on how consumer guidance information is presented. The committee again emphasizes that the scales used in Figures 7-6a and 7-6b for EPA/DHA and methylmercury content are arbitrary. Designers will need to carefully test the effect of the scales used for the bars on the message received by consumers.

Figure 7-7 also provides information on both EPA/DHA and methylmercury content, although for a smaller number of seafood choices to make the figure easier to read. The figure's advantage is that it combines information on one and two 3-ounce servings per week. The corresponding disadvantage is that it may be harder for consumers to grasp. Graphs like this can be helpful in identifying product consumption patterns that provide benefits with little risk to most consumers as compared to those that raise risk concerns for some consumers. Figure 7-7 may be useful guidance for females who could become pregnant, are pregnant, or are lactating, and for infants and young children. If the EPA/DHA-methylmercury tradeoff is less important, for example, for adolescent males, adult males, and females who will not become pregant, then Figure 7-5, which focuses solely on EPA/DHA content, may provide more useful guidance. Here, the committee again notes that the choice of scale on the horizontal and vertical axes may have an important effect on the message received by consumers. This effect should be carefully tested in the design phase.

Finally, Figures 7-8a and 7-8b illustrate the use of color to highlight information that is important to specific target populations. Figure 7-8a is a color version of Figure 7-6a. Seafood choices containing levels of methylmercury that exceed recommended safe intakes for females who could become pregnant, are pregnant, or are lactating, and for infants and young children and that should be avoided by these groups are shown in red. White (albacore) tuna is shown in yellow to indicate that consumption should be limited to 6 ounces per week for these at-risk population groups. Figure 7-8b, a color version of Figure 7-7, uses the same color scheme to emphasize choices for these groups.

The sample graphics presented here do not include a representation of uncertainty. Uncertainty can be represented with additional symbols (e.g., adding error bars), text or numbers, or with variations on the original graphic (e.g., by fading out the ends of the bars in a bar chart to indicate uncertain values or quantities. A consumer right-to-know perspective suggests that agencies are obligated to report or reveal uncertainties to interested consumers, and should strive to do so as transparently as possible. Representing uncertainty explicitly has the potential to improve decision-making (Roulston, 2006); failure to communicate uncertainty can increase public distrust (Frewer, 2004). However, testing is essential, as explicit representation of uncertainty can have unanticipated effects (Johnson and Slovic, 1995, 1998).

Given the weaknesses in the data underlying current conclusions on benefits and risks, strengthened collaboration between federal agencies appears to be an important goal for development of improved seafood consumption guidance. A federal advisory committee is one mechanism that could be used to coordinate across agencies.

In addition to collaboration between agencies, collaborating with non-traditional partners can assist federal agencies not only with dissemination of guidance, but with design and formative evaluation by engaging relevant target populations and providing a privileged relationship with them through the partnering organization. There are large networks of health care providers including but not limited to federal agencies that dispense daily advice on health and wellness and recommendations for medical care to broad segments of the population, including groups at high risk for poor health outcomes (SOURCE: http://www.healthfinder.gov). There are many opportunities to communicate benefit and risk information to at-risk population groups; a dramatic increase in immunization rates for children achieved in the mid-1990s illustrates one successful effort (CDC, 1996). A coordinated and tailored approach to individual consumer decision-making would have utility in working with federal agencies and other public health providers.

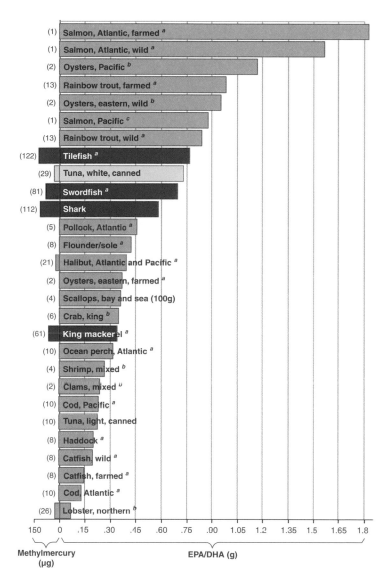

FIGURE 7-8a Color version of Figure 7-6a.
NOTES: The scales used in this figure for EPA/DHA and methylmercury content are arbitrary. Designers will need to carefully test the effect of the scales used for the bars on the message received by consumers.

[a]Cooked, dry heat.
[b]Cooked, moist heat.
[c]The EPA and DHA content in Pacific salmon is a composite from chum, coho, and sockeye.

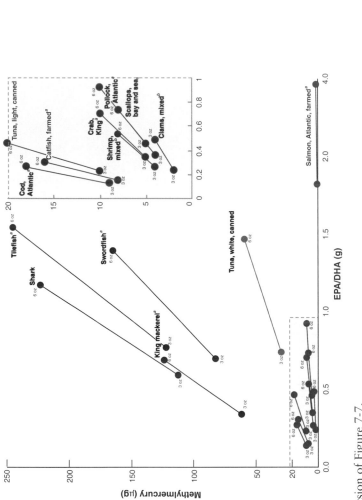

FIGURE 7-8b Color version of Figure 7-7.

NOTES: The scales used in this figure for EPA/DHA and methylmercury content are arbitrary. Designers will need to carefully test the effect of the scales used for the bars on the message received by consumers.

[a]Cooked, dry heat.
[b]Cooked, moist heat.

Communicating this information to these groups would often entail little or no increased cost. The limiting factor may be education of the providers (e.g., public health nurses) themselves. National associations could be an easy point of access for communicating information and networking (e.g., http://www.naccho.org).

Most state public health agencies, as well as many city and county agencies, have some statutory responsibility for seafood safety (advisories and posting regulatory actions, e.g., based on bacterial testing of oyster beds). Most of these agencies have health education programs including nutrition staff who provide individual counseling as well as health education to the general public. These agencies touch virtually every community and citizen in this country—there are more than 3000 local public health departments, not including county and state departments (SOURCE: http://www.naccho. org).

Community and migrant primary health care centers are funded through section 330 of the US Public Health Service Act and are charged with providing primary care and disease prevention services to low-income and other at-risk groups. Growth of their network has been a priority of the federal government, and the number of local sites exceeds 400, reaching millions of people daily (SOURCE: http://www.hrsa.gov). These centers are more often than not placed in communities at-risk. The community migrant health centers have also shown that when emphasis and training on disease prevention issues have been made a priority, disease (e.g., breast and cervical cancers) prevention interventions can actually exceed those provided to members of the general population who are not regarded as at risk. Community migrant health could be an important vehicle in helping consumers make informed seafood choices.

Collaborative Approaches: Federal Coordination and Communicating Health Messages Through Nontraditional Partners

There are a variety of federally funded but locally administered consumer education (e.g., Cooperative Extension System, see Box 7-1) and maternal-child health agencies (e.g., Title 5, Women, Infants, and Children Program [WIC], Head Start) that provide guidance and care to the general public, and to mothers and children. Although located in different agencies (e.g., WIC is administered through the US Department of Agriculture, Head Start is administered through the Administration for Children and Families [ACF]), these programs frequently serve either similar or the same populations. As with health partners in community health centers, they have a similar emphasis on health education and communication, and present significant opportunities for influencing consumer decision making.

BOX 7-1
Cooperative Extension

The Cooperative Extension is another nationwide educational network that delivers information to people in their homes, workplaces, and communities. Each US state and territory has a state office at its land-grant university and a network of local or regional offices. Extension links the resources and expertise of nearly 3150 county extension offices, 107 land-grant colleges and universities, and the federal government. County offices are staffed by one or more experts who provide useful, practical, and research-based information through printed and media-based materials, Web-based information sites, the telephone, community programs, and not-for-credit classes. This system is an excellent resource for disseminating health information and correcting misinformation.

The Need for Pretest and Post Hoc Evaluation

One of the challenges in supporting informed consumer choice is how governmental agencies communicate health benefits and risks to both the general population and to target populations. Previous attempts at communicating benefits and risks may have resulted in misinterpretation or misuse, including a reduction or total elimination of seafood consumption, by the intended audiences (Willows, 2005). Federal agencies should develop new and consumer-friendly tools to disseminate current and emerging information to the public. Developing effective tools requires formative evaluation, as well as an iterative approach to design.

Some individual communities have made substantial progress in understanding the effects of different modes of health communication and modifying the message to achieve the desired community and/or individual response. One such example is the Inuit community in Alaska, where communication of health risks from fish consumption previously resulted in changing patterns of food consumption from traditional foods to highly processed and often unhealthy alternative foods. Through the use of tailored messages and the involvement of the community throughout the entire process, a more effective message is now being provided to local communities.

Implementation: Embedding Consumer Advice Within a Larger Consumer Information Program

Consumers face challenging choices about seafood. Both the seafood supply and the information about benefits and risks of consuming that sea-food are changing rapidly. Fortunately, rapid advances in information and communication technologies now make it possible for agencies to distribute more up-to-date and detailed information, more widely, than ever before. Over 80 percent of US adults under age 40 use the Internet (Fox, 2005). This, however, does not negate the role of point-of-purchase information and the broader information context.

Further, there are communication structures in place within various federal agencies that are often duplicative and not effectively utilized. There is no functional mechanism in place for planning and implementing a new or evolving communication system that is synergistic and not duplicative. The committee is not aware of any significant efforts in place that would coordinate access to various programs within and between agencies and departments. There is potential for implementation of an effective system for communicating benefits and risks associated with consumption of seafood, but the means for implementation are not apparent. Achieving a coordinated and consistent approach that gives consumers information they can use and understand is likely to require some kind of coordinating mechanism, such as oversight by an interagency task force.

RECOMMENDATIONS

The committee offers the following general recommendations relevant to the design of seafood consumption advice.

Recommendation 1: The decision pathway the committee recommends, which illustrates its analysis of the current balance between benefits and risks associated with seafood consumption, should be used as a basis for developing consumer guidance tools for selecting seafood to obtain nutritional benefits balanced against exposure risks. Real-time, interactive decision tools, easily available to the public, could increase informed actions for a significant portion of the population, and help to inform important intermediaries, such as physicians.

Recommendation 2: The sponsor should work together with appropriate federal and state agencies concerned with public health to develop an interagency task force to coordinate data and communications on seafood consumption benefits, risks, and related issues such as fish stocks and seafood sources, and begin development of a communication program to help consumers make informed seafood consumption decisions. Empirical evaluation of consumers' needs and the effectiveness of communications should be an integral part of the program.

Recommendation 3: Partnerships should be formed between federal agencies and community organizations. This effort should include targeting and involvement of intermediaries, such as physicians, and use of interactive Internet communications, which have the potential to increase the usefulness and accuracy of seafood consumption communications.

REFERENCES

CDC (Centers for Disease Control and Prevention). 1996. National, state and urban area vaccination average levels among children ages 19–35 months—United States, April 1994–March 1995. *Morbidity and Mortality Weekly Report* 45(7):145–150. [Online]. Available: http://www.cdc.gov/mmwr/PDF/wk/mm4507.pdf [accessed May 12, 2006].

CDC. 1999. Framework for program evaluation in public health. *Morbidity and Mortality Weekly Report: Recommendations and Reports* 48(11):1–40. [Online]. Available: http://www.phppo.cdc.gov/dls/pdf/mmwr/rr4811.pdf [accessed April 21, 2006].

CDC. [Online]. Available: http://www.cdc.gov [accessed May 12, 2006].

Fletcher A. 2006. Academic slams food labelling plans as 'too simplistic.' *FoodNavigator.com, Europe*. [Online]. Available: http://www.foodnavigator.com/news/ng.asp?id=66287-kellogg-weetabix-pepsico [accessed August 27, 2006].

FoodSafety.gov. 2005. *Consumer Advice*. [Online]. Available: http://www.foodsafety.gov/~fsg/fsgadvic.html [accessed April 21, 2006].

Fox S. 2005. *Data Memo*. Generations online. PEW/Internet. [Online]. Available: http://www.pewInternet.org/pdfs/PIP_Generations_Memo.pdf [accessed April 21, 2006].

Frewer L. 2004. The public and effective risk communication. *Toxicology Letters* 149(1–3):391–397.

FSA (Food Standards Agency). 2005. *Signpost Labelling: Creative Development of Concepts Research Report*. UK: Food Standards Agency. [Online]. Available: http://www.food.gov.uk/multimedia/pdfs/signpostingnavigatorreport.pdf [accessed April 13, 2006].

FSA. 2006. *Board Agrees Principles for Front of Pack Labelling. Press Release, March 9, 2006*. Food Standards Agency. [Online]. Available: http://www.food.gov.uk/news/news-archive/2006/mar/signpostnewsmarch/ [accessed April 21, 2006].

Hibbard J, Peters E. 2003. Supporting informed consumer health care decisions: Data presentation approaches that facilitate the use of information in choice. *Annual Review of Public Health* 24:413–433.

Hibbard JH, Slovic P, Peters E, Finucane ML. 2002. Strategies for reporting health plan performance information to consumers: Evidence from controlled studies. *Health Services Research* 37(2):291–313.

HRSA (Health Resources and Services Administration). [Online]. Available: http://www.hrsa.gov [accessed May 12, 2006].

Johnson BB, Slovic P. 1995. Presenting uncertainty in health risk assessment: Initial studies of its effects on risk perception and trust. *Risk Analysis* 15(4):485–494.

Johnson BB, Slovic P. 1998. Lay views on uncertainty in environmental health risk assessments. *Journal of Risk Research* 1(4):261–279.

Mark MM, Henry GT, Julnes G, eds. 2000. *Evaluation: An Integrated Framework for Understanding, Guiding, and Improving Policies and Programs*. San Francisco, CA: Jossey-Bass, Inc.

NACCHO (National Association of County and City Health Officials). [Online]. Available: http://www.naccho.org [accessed May 12, 2006].

Naylor RL, Goldburg RJ, Primavera J, Kautsky N, Beveridge MCM, Clay J, Folke C, Lubchenco J, Mooney H, Troell M. 2001. Effects of aquaculture on world fish supplies. *Issues in Ecology* 8:1–12.

NCI (National Cancer Institute). 2003. *Pink Book—Making Health Communication Programs Work*. [Online]. Available: http://www.cancer.gov/pinkbook/ [accessed April 21, 2006].

NIH (National Institutes of Health). 2006. *Health Information.* [Online]. Available: http://health.nih.gov/ [accessed April 21, 2006].

Roulston MS. 2006. A laboratory study of the benefits of including uncertainty information in weather forecasts. *Weather and Forecasting* 21(1):116–122.

Ryan KE, DeStefano, eds. 2000. *Evaluation as a Democratic Process: Promoting Inclusion, Dialogue, and Deliberation: New Directions for Evaluation.* San Francisco, CA: Jossey-Bass, Inc.

Schriver KA. 1990. *Evaluation Text Quality: The Continuum from Text-Focused to Reader-Focused Methods.* Technical Report No. 41. Berkley, CA: National Center for the Study of Writing. [Online]. Available: http://www.writingproject.org/cs/nwpp/download/nwp_file/136/TR41.pdf?x-r=pcfile_d [accessed April 21, 2006].

Shah P, Hoeffner J. 2002. Review of graph comprehension research: Implications for instruction. *Educational Psychology Review* 14(1):47–69.

Spyridakis JH. 2000. Guidelines for authoring comprehensible web pages and evaluating their success. *Technical Communication* 47(3):301–310. [Online]. Available: http://www.uwtc.washington.edu/research/pubs/jspyridakis/Authoring_Comprehensible_Web_Pages.pdf [accessed April 21, 2006].

TRB (Transportation Research Board). 2002. *An Assessment of the National Highway Traffic Safety Administration's Rating System for Rollover Resistance.* Washington, DC: The National Academies Press.

USDA. *Healthfinder.* [Online]. Available: http://www.healthfinder.gov [accessed May 12, 2006].

USPSTF (US Preventive Services Task Force). 2001–2004. *Guide to Clinical Preventive Services, 2001–2004.* Rockville, MD: Agency for Healthcare Research and Quality. [Online]. Available: http://www.ahrq.gov/clinic/gcpspu.htm [accessed April 21, 2006].

Willows ND. 2005. Determinants of healthy eating in Aboriginal peoples in Canada: The current state of knowledge and research gaps. *Canadian Journal of Public Health* 96(Supplement 3):S32–S36; S36–S41.

A

Glossary and Supplementary Information

GLOSSARY

Abbreviations/Acronyms

5-HT	*In vivo* synaptic serotonin
AA	Arachidonic acid
ADHD	Attention Deficit Hyperactivity Disorder
AEDS	Atopic eczema/dermatitis syndrome
AHA	American Heart Association
AHR	Airway hyperresponsiveness
AHRQ	Agency for Healthcare Research and Quality
AI	Adequate Intake
ALA	Alpha-linolenic acid
ALSPAC	Avon Longitudinal Study of Parents and Children
AMI	Acute myocardial infarction
ANOVA	Analysis of variance
AOCS	American Oil Chemists Society
APC	Aerobic bacterial counts
APGAR	Activity, Pulse, Grimace, Appearance, and Respiration
APO	Apolipoprotein
APTT	Activated partial thromboplastin time
ARS	Agricultural Research Society
AUC	Area under the curve
BDI	Beck Depression Inventory

BMD   Benchmark dose
BMDLs   Benchmark dose lower bound
BMI   Body Mass Index

CAD   Coronary artery disease
CAPS   Childhood Asthma Prevention Study
CAT   Clinical Adaptive Test
CD   Cluster of differentiation (molecule)
CDC   Centers for Disease Control and Prevention
CDDs   Chlorinated dibenzo-p-dioxins
CDFs   Chlorinated dibenzofurans
CFR   Code of Federal Regulations
CGOST   Combined Cow and Gate Premium and Osterfeed formulae
CHD   Coronary heart disease
CI   Confidence interval
CLAMS DQ   Clinical Linguistic and Auditory Milestone Scale—
                  Development Quotient
CNPase   2′,3′-cyclic nucleotide 3′-phosphodiesterase
CNS   Central nervous system
COPD   Chronic obstructive pulmonary disease
COT   Committee on Toxicity
CRP   C-reactive protein
CSFII   Continuing Survey of Food Intake by Individuals
CSPI   Center for Science in the Public Interest
CVD   Cardiovascular disease

DART   Diet and Reinfarction Trial; Diet and Angina Randomized
                  Trial
DALY   Disability adjusted life years
DBD   Disruptive Behavior Disorders
DBP   Diastolic blood pressure
DDE   Dichlorodiphenyldichloroethane
DDST   Denver Developmental Screening Test
DDT   Dichlorodiphenyltrichloroethane
DGA   *Dietary Guidelines for Americans*
DGAC   Dietary Guidelines Advisory Committee
DGLA   Dihomo-gamma-linolenic acid
DHA   Docosahexaenoic acid
DHHS   Department of Health and Human Services
DNA   Deoxyribonucleic acid
DPA   Docosapentaenoic acid
DQ   Developmental quotient
DRI   Dietary Reference Intake

DSM	Diagnostic and Statistical Manual of Mental Disorders
DTA	Docosatetraenoic acid
ECG	Electrocardiogram
EFA	Essential fatty acids
EFSA	European Food Safety Authority
EPA	Eicosapentaenoic acid
EPDS	Edinburgh Postpartum Depression Scale
EPIC	European Prospective Investigation into Cancer and Nutrition
ETA	Eicosatrienoic acid
FAO	Food and Agriculture Organization of the United Nations
FDA	Food and Drug Administration
FDCA	Federal Food, Drug, and Cosmetic Act
FFQ	Food Frequency Questionnaire
FSA	Food Standards Agency (UK)
FVEP	Flash-visual evoked potential
GLA	Gamma-linolenic acid
GRAS	Generally recognized as safe
GSH-Px	Glutathione peroxidase
HACCP	Hazard Analysis and Critical Control Point
Hb	Hemoglobin
HDL-C	High-density lipoprotein cholesterol
HHS	Health and Human Services
HIV	Human immunodeficiency virus
HR	Hazard ratio
HRA	Health risk appraisal
HRT	Hormone replacement therapy
HSCL	Hopkins Symptom Checklist
HUFA	Highly unsaturated fatty acid
HVA	Homovanillic acid
IFN-γ	Interferon-gamma
IgG	Immunoglobin G
IgM	Immunoglobin M
IHC	Interactive Health Communication
IHD	Ischemic heart disease
IL	Interleukin
IMT	Intima-media thickness
IOM	Institute of Medicine

IQ	Intelligence quotient
IRR	Incidence rate ratio
ISAAC	International Study of Asthma and Allergy in Childhood
ISSC	Interstate Shellfish Sanitation Conference
JECFA	Joint FAO/WHO Expert Committee on Food Additives and Contaminants
K-ABC	Kaufman Assessment Battery for Children
KPS	Knobloch, Passamanik, and Sherrad's Developmental Screening Inventory
LA	Linoleic acid
LCPUFA	Long-chain polyunsaturated fatty acids
LDL-C	Low-density lipoprotein cholesterol
LNA	Linolenic acid
LOAEL	Lowest observed adverse effect level
MCDI	MacArthur Communicative Development Inventory
MDI	Bayley Scales of Infant Development Mental Index
MEC	Multiethnic Cohort Study
MFFT	Matching Familiar Figures Test
MI	Myocardial infarction
MPCOMP	Mental Processing Composite
MPN	Most probable number
NCP	Northern Contaminants Program
NHANES	National Health and Nutrition Examination Survey
NIH	National Institutes of Health
NLV	Norwalk-like viruses
NMFS	National Marine Fisheries Service
NOAA	National Oceanic and Atmospheric Administration
NOAEL	No observed adverse effect level
NONVERB	Nonverbal abilities
NRC	National Research Council
NYHA	New York Heart Association
OA	Oleic acid
OR	Odds ratio
OVA	Ovalbumin
PC	Phosphatidylcholine
PCB	Polychlorinated biphenyls

PCDD	Polychlorinated di-benzo-*p*-dioxin
PCDF	Polychlorinated di-benzo-*p*-furan
PCR	Polymerase chain reaction
PDI	Psychomotor Developmental Index
PE	Phosphatidylethanolamine
PGF2α	Prostaglandin $F_{2\alpha}$
PHP	Post-harvest processing
PL	Phospholipid
Ppm	Parts per million
PT	Prothrombin time
PUFA	Polyunsaturated fatty acids
QALYs	Quality Adjusted Life Years
RBC	Red blood cell
RCT	Randomized clinical trial or randomized controlled trial
RDA	Recommended Dietary Allowance
RR	Relative risk
RRR	Relative risk reduction
RTE	Ready-to-eat
SACN	Scientific Advisory Committee on Nutrition (UK)
SBP	Systolic blood pressure
SCDS	Seychelles Child Development Study
SCID-CV	Statistical Manual of Mental Disorders, Fourth Edition, Axis I Disorders—Clinical Version
SE	Standard error
SEQPROC	Sequential processing
SIMPROC	Simultaneous processing
TCDD	Tetrachlorodibenzo-*p*-dioxin
TDE	Tetrachlorodiphenylethane
TDI	Tolerable Daily Intake
TEF	Toxicity Equivalency Factor
TEQ	Toxicity Equivalency
TF	Total fatty acids
TG	Triglycerides
TNF-α	Tumor necrosis factor alpha
TOVA	Test of Variables of Attention
UNEP	United Nations Environmental Programme
USDA	US Department of Agriculture
US EPA	US Environmental Protection Agency

VEP   Visual evoked potential
VLDL   Very low-density lipoprotein
VRM   Visual recognition memory

WHO   World Health Organization
WIC   Special Supplemental Nutrition Program for Women, Infants,
               and Children

Definitions

24-hour recall   A method of collecting food consumption data; an interviewer solicits detailed information regarding what a study participant ate and drank in the previous 24 hours or on the previous day

Adipose tissue   Fat tissue

Aflatoxin   Any of a group of toxic compounds produced by certain molds that contaminate stored food supplies such as animal feed and peanuts

Analysis of variance (ANOVA)   To identify sources of variability; to describe the relationship between a continuous dependent variable and one or more nominal independent variables

Anglers   Those who crab and/or fish

Anthropogenic   Of human origin

Aquaculture   Rearing or cultivating marine or freshwater fish or shellfish under controlled conditions for food

Arrhythmia   An irregular heartbeat

Assay   The evaluation of a substance for impurities, toxicity, etc.

Atherosclerosis   A condition in which plaques containing cholesterol and lipids are deposited on the innermost layer of the walls of large and medium-sized arteries

Atopic   Of, relating to, or caused by a hereditary predisposition toward developing certain hypersensitivity reactions, such as hay fever, asthma, or chronic urticaria, upon exposure to specific antigens

Axonal   The usually long process of a nerve fiber that generally conducts impulses away from the body of the nerve cell

Bayesian hierarchical model   A statistical method to make inferences about an unknown parameter in a multi-level model

Benchmark dose modeling   A technique for quantitative assessment of noncancer health effects; based on the level at which the prevalence of a defined health abnormality exceeds the background prevalence of the abnormality by a specified amount

Benefit-risk analysis   Comparison of the benefits of a situation to its related risks

Best practices   A technique or methodology that, through experience and research, has reliably proven to lead to a desired result

Bioaccumulative pollutants   Substances that increase in concentration in living organisms as they take in contaminated air, water, or food because they are very slowly metabolized or excreted

Biomagnification   The process by which the concentration of toxic substances increases in each successive link in the food chain

Body burden   The total amount of a chemical in the human body or in human tissue from exposure to contaminants in the environment

Boston naming test   A type of picture-naming vocabulary test used in the examination of children with learning disabilities and the evaluation of brain-injured adults

Calcarine fissure   A narrow groove in the mesial surface of the occipital lobe of the cerebrum

Case-control study   An epidemiological and observational study in which persons are selected because they have a specific disease or other outcome (cases) and are compared to a control (referent comparison) group without the disease to evaluate whether there is a difference in the frequency of exposure to possible disease risk factors; also termed a retrospective study or case referent study

Cerebellum   A region of the brain that plays an important role in the integration of sensory perception and motor output

Chloracne   A severe skin condition with acne-like lesions that occur mainly on the face and upper body after exposure to high doses of dioxin and dioxin-like compounds

Cholesterol   The chief sterol in all animal tissues, especially brain, nerve, adrenal cortex, and liver; it functions as a constituent of bile and as a precursor of vitamin D; cholesterol circulates in the blood as lipoprotein, in combination with protein and other blood lipids

Ciguatera   A natural toxin occurring sporadically in certain fish harvested from specific tropical to subtropical regions (i.e., South Florida, the Caribbean, and Hawaii)

***Clostridium botulinum* (*C. botulinum*)**   A specific microorganism that, under anaerobic conditions and thermal abuse, can produce an extremely potent toxin (destroyed by sufficient heating); produces spores that can be hazardous to babies, individuals on antibiotic therapy, or immunocompromised individuals

Cochrane review   Systematic literature reviews based on the best available information about health care interventions. They explore the evidence for and against the effectiveness and appropriateness of treatments (medications, surgery, education, etc.) in specific circumstances

Complex mixture   A mixture that is a combination of many chemicals, has a commonly known generic name, and is naturally occurring; a fraction of a naturally occurring mixture that results from a separation process; or a modification of a naturally occurring mixture or a modification of a fraction of a naturally occurring mixture that results from a chemical modification process

Confounder A factor that is associated with both the exposure and outcome of interest and can distort the apparent magnitude or direction of the studied effect

Congener One of two or more compounds of the same kind with respect to classification

Correlation coefficient A measure of the extent to which two variables are related

Cortical Relating to the outer portion of an organ

Crustaceans Aquatic arthropods characteristically having a segmented body, a chitinous exoskeleton, and paired, jointed limbs; includes lobsters, crabs, shrimps, and barnacles

Cytokines Hormone-like proteins which regulate the intensity and duration of immune responses and are involved in cell-to-cell communication

De novo Anew; often applied to particular biochemical pathways in which metabolites are newly biosynthesized

Dioxins and dioxin-like compounds Unintentional contaminants that are released into the environment from combustion processes and accumulate, through the food chain, in the lipid component of animal foods

Disappearance model The total supply of imported and landed food converted to edible weight, subtracting exports, nonfood uses, and other decreases in supply, adding imports, and then dividing by the total population to estimate per capita consumption

Dose-response relationship A relationship between the amount of an agent (either administered, absorbed, or believed to be effective) and changes in certain aspects of the biological system, apparently in response to the agent

Dysarthria A disturbance of speech and language

Effect modifier Variation(s) in the association between an exposure and outcome occurring across different strata of a third variable (e.g., the association between oral contraceptive use and myocardial infarction differs between smokers and nonsmokers)

Efficacy measurement endpoint Measure of an intervention's influence on a disease or health condition

Epidemiology The study of the distribution and determinants of health-related states and events in populations and the control of health problems

Erythrocyte A mature red blood cell

Essential fatty acids Fatty acids that cannot be synthesized by the body and therefore must be included in the diet (e.g., ALA)

Etiology Cause and origin of a disease

Experimental trials A type of study in which human or animal exposure to a substance occurs in a controlled environment for the purpose of studying its effects; in humans, experimental trials are only ethical when there is equipoise between the two arms of the trial

Fate and transport Models used by risk assessors to estimate the movement and chemical alteration of contaminants as they move through the environment (e.g., air, soil, water, groundwater)

Fibrinogen A protein in blood plasma that is essential for the coagulation of blood

Filter-feeding animal An aquatic animal, such as a clam, barnacle, or sponge, that feeds by filtering particulate organic material from water

First Nation An organized aboriginal group or community, especially any of the bands officially recognized by the Canadian government

Flora The microorganisms that normally inhabit a bodily organ or part

Food frequency questionnaire (FFQ) A method of collecting food consumption data; a self-administered questionnaire that asks a study participant how often he/she consumed, on average, a list of specific foods in the past weeks, months, or years to determine a usual long-term diet

Functional foods Foods or dietary components that may provide a health benefit beyond basic nutrition

Genotoxin A toxin (poisonous substance) that harms the body by damaging DNA molecules

Geometric mean A measure of central tendency by which all N terms are multiplied together and the Nth root extracted; useful for summarizing highly skewed data and ratios

Global (in the sense of study) Involving the whole population

Grating stimuli A geometric pattern used as a substitute for letters or symbols in tests of visual acuity in infants

Half-life The time required for the elimination of half a total dose from the body

Hazard ratio (HR) Broadly equivalent to relative risk (RR); applying information collected at different times, it is useful when the risk is not constant with respect to time; the term is typically used in the context of survival over time; if the HR is 0.5, then the relative risk of death for one group is half the risk of death in the other group

Health Professionals Follow-up Study A study initiated in 1986 and conducted by researchers at the Harvard School of Public Health; enrolled 51,529 male health professionals (dentists, pharmacists, optometrists, osteopath physicians, podiatrists, and veterinarians), aged 40–75, to evaluate the relationship between nutritional factors and the incidence of serious illnesses such as cancer, heart disease, and other vascular diseases in men; follow-up questionnaires were mailed out every two years to update exposure information and identify cases; designed to complement the all-female Nurses' Health Study (see below)

Health risk appraisal (HRA)   An instrument commonly used in worksite preventive health care to identify the likelihood that an individual will develop a preventable or chronic disease, based on personal, medical, and lifestyle indications; comprises a questionnaire, risk estimation, and educational information

Histamine   A hormone/chemical transmitter involved in local immune responses, regulating stomach acid production, and in allergic reactions as a mediator of immediate hypersensitivity; has been implicated in seafood toxicants from certain species of fish exposed to thermal abuse

Homeostasis   The state of equilibrium in the body with respect to various functions and to the chemical compositions of the fluids and tissues

Hot spots   Localized areas with high pollutant concentrations

Immunoglobulin A (IgA)   The class of antibodies produced predominantly against ingested antigens, found in body secretions such as saliva, sweat, or tears, and functioning to prevent attachment of viruses and bacteria to epithelial surfaces

In vitro   In an artificial environment outside the living organism

Intima-media thickness   A unique diagnostic and monitoring service to determine the presence of coronary atherosclerosis in its early stages; refers to a measurement of the first two layers of the artery (intima and media)

Intrauterine growth retardation   A condition resulting in a fetal weight less than the 10th percentile of predicted weight for gestational age

Inuit   A general term for a group of culturally similar indigenous peoples inhabiting the Arctic coasts of Siberia, Alaska, the Northwest Territories, Nunavut, Québec, Labrador, and Greenland

Lean meat equivalent   Amounts of meat alternatives that count as equivalent to 1 ounce of cooked lean meat, e.g., 1/2 cup of cooked dry beans or peas, 1/2 cup tofu, 2 tablespoons of peanut butter, 1/3 cup of nuts, or 1/4 cup of seeds

Leukocyte   White blood cell; blood cells that engulf and digest bacteria and fungi; an important part of the body's defense system

Linear model   Fitting a straight line to the data to help describe a pattern in the data; the term "linear" refers to the fitted straight line, and the term "model" refers to the equation that summarizes the fitted line

Lipids   Members of a large group of organic compounds insoluble in water and soluble in fat solvents; lipids of nutritional importance include essential fatty acids, triglycerides, and sterols

Lipophilic compounds   Substances capable of dissolving, of being dissolved in, or of absorbing lipids; lipid soluble

Lipoprotein   A compound protein consisting of protein and lipid; has the solubility characteristics of protein and hence is involved in lipid transport

High-density lipoprotein (HDL)   A complex of lipids and proteins in approximately equal amounts that functions as a transporter of cholesterol in the blood; high levels are associated with a decreased risk of atherosclerosis and coronary heart disease

Low-density lipoprotein (LDL)   A lipoprotein that transports cholesterol in the blood; composed of a moderate amount of protein and a large amount of lipid; high levels are thought to be associated with increased risk of atherosclerosis and coronary heart disease

Listeria monocytogenes   A principal pathogenic bacterium that has been associated with safety risk from a large variety of foods, including seafoods

Lipoprotein (a) [Lp(a)]   An LDL-like particle that is produced in the liver; numerous studies have found that concentrations of plasma Lp(a) above 0.3 g/L (note reference ranges may vary between laboratories) are associated with an increased risk of coronary heart disease

Maximum likelihood   A popular statistical method used to make inferences about parameters of the underlying probability distribution of a given dataset

Mechanistic   Of or relating to the philosophy of mechanism, especially tending to explain phenomena only by reference to physical or biological causes

Meta-analysis   Combined results of several studies that address a set of related research hypotheses

Metaphase   A stage of mitosis; condensed chromosomes, carrying genetic information, align in the middle of the cell before being separated into each of the two daughter cells

Methylmercury   The form of mercury of greatest concern with regard to seafood consumption; results when mercury from other forms is deposited in bodies of water and biotransformed through the process of methylation by microorganisms; it bioaccumulates through the food chain, and thus its highest concentrations are in large long-lived predatory species

Minimal risk level   An estimate of the daily human exposure to a hazardous substance that is likely to be without appreciable risk of adverse noncancer health effects over a specified duration of exposure

Mitotic   Of or relating to mitosis, the process by which a cell separates its duplicated genome into two identical halves

Molar   A unit of concentration for solutions

Molluscan   Of or relating to numerous chiefly marine invertebrates, typically having a soft unsegmented body, a mantle, and a protective calcareous shell; includes edible shellfish and snails

Monte Carlo analysis   Randomly generates values for uncertain variables over and over to simulate a model

Muktuk   The skin and underlying fat (blubber) layer of a whale

Multicenter   A single study conducted in more than one location

Multipliers   Quantifies the additional effects of an exposure/intervention beyond those that are immediately attributable to the intervention alone

Multivariate analysis   A method in which several dependent variables can be considered simultaneously; not to be confused with multivariable analysis that involves several variables, even if only one dependent variable is considered at a time

Myocardial infarction   Sudden insufficiency of arterial or venous blood supply involving the middle layer of the heart usually as a result of a closed, or closing, coronary artery

Myometrium   The muscular wall of the uterus

MyPyramid   Released in 2005 by the US Department of Agriculture (USDA) to help consumers make choices from every food group, find their balance between food intake and physical activity, and get the most nutrition out of their calories; replaced the Food Guide Pyramid; can be found at http://www.mypyramid.gov

Norovirus   A group of related, single-stranded RNA, nonenveloped viruses that cause acute gastroenteritis in humans; transmitted primarily through the fecal-oral route, either by consumption of fecally contaminated food or water, or by direct person-to-person spread

Northern dwellers   Native people living in the far north

Nunavik   The arctic region of Québec, Canada; an Inuit homeland

Nurses' Health Study   A study initiated in 1976 and conducted by researchers at the Channing Lab, Harvard Medical School and the Departments of Epidemiology and Nutrition, Harvard School of Public Health; enrolled 121,700 female registered nurses aged 30–55 living in 11 states to assess risk factors for cardiovascular disease and cancer; follow-up questionnaires were mailed out every two years to update exposure information and identify cases and, as of 1980, included a diet assessment

Observational studies   Study types that follow a population (either prospectively or retrospectively) to examine how exposure to risk factors influences one's probability of developing a disease in the absence of intervention; includes cross-sectional studies, cohort studies, and case-control studies

Occipital cortex   The part of the brain used to process visual information

Odds ratio (OR)   In a case-control study (see above), the exposure odds among cases compared to the exposure odds among controls, where the exposure odds are the number of individuals with the exposure relative to the number of individuals without the exposure (e.g., if 3 out of 10 people are exposed, then the exposure odds are 3:7)

Omega-3 fatty acids (n-3 fatty acids)   Polyunsaturated fatty acids found in oil from fatty fish as well as plant sources; characterized by the presence of a double bond 3 carbons from the methyl end in the carbon chain; includes alpha-linolenic acid (ALA), eicosapentaenoic acid (EPA), and docosahexaenoic acid (DHA)

Omega-6 fatty acids (n-6 fatty acids)   Polyunsaturated fatty acids found in animal and vegetable sources of fat; characterized by the presence of a double bond 6 carbons from the methyl end in the carbon chain; includes linoleic acid (LA) and arachidonic acid (AA)

One component pharmacokinetic model   Assumes that the drug in question is evenly distributed throughout the body into a single compartment and that the rate of elimination is proportional to the amount of drug in the body; only appropriate for drugs which rapidly and readily distribute between the plasma and other body tissues

P-value   As in hypothesis testing; the probability of getting a value of the test statistics as extreme as, or more extreme than, the value observed, if the null hypothesis (i.e., no association, no effect of treatment) were true; the alternative hypothesis determines the direction of "extreme"; usually p<0.05 means that the null hypothesis is rejected and the association between the exposure and outcome is statistically significant

Parenteral   The introduction of substances into an organism by intravenous, subcutaneous, intramuscular, or intramedullary injection

Paresthesia   A skin sensation, such as burning, prickling, itching, or tingling, with no apparent physical cause

Pathogenic bacteria   Bacteria that cause disease or abnormality

Pelagic fish   Fish living in open oceans or seas rather than waters adjacent to land or inland waters

Persistent organic pollutants (POPs)   Organic chemicals that remain intact in the environment for long periods, become widely distributed geographically, bioaccumulate up the food chain by accumulating in fatty tissues of animals, and pose a risk of causing adverse effects to human health and to the environment

Plasma lipids   Lipids in the fluid portion of anticoagulated blood

Platelet   A type of blood cell that helps prevent bleeding by causing blood clots

Population attributable risk   The proportion of disease in a population that would be prevented if the risk factor were removed from the entire population

Post hoc   Formulated after the fact; for example, a post hoc analysis is designed and applied to data already collected for another study

Precentral gyrus   The convolution of the frontal lobe of the brain that is bounded in back by the central sulcus and that contains the motor area

Preeclampsia   A toxic condition developing in late pregnancy characterized by a sudden rise in blood pressure

Prophylactic   Preventing disease

Prospective cohort study   An epidemiological and observational study in which a defined group of persons known to be exposed to a potential disease risk factor is followed over time and compared to a group of persons who were not known to be exposed to the potential risk factor, to evaluate the differences in rates of the outcome; also termed a prospective observational study, follow-up study, incidence study

Prostaglandins   Lipid-based membrane-associated chemical messengers synthesized by most tissue cells; act locally as a hormone-like substance; may be synthesized from both omega-3 and omega-6 fatty acids

Provisional tolerable weekly intake   Exposure limit presented in micrograms of contaminant per week and per 1 kg body mass

Public Health Service Act   Defines the federal agencies and their personnel who are are part of the federal Public Health Service

Reference Dose (RfD)   An estimate (with uncertainty spanning perhaps an order of magnitude) of daily exposure to the human population (including sensitive subgroups) that is likely to be without an appreciable risk of deleterious effects during a lifetime

Regression coefficient   The slope of the straight line that most closely relates two correlated variables; the number of units that a dependent variable changes for each one unit increase in an independent variable

Relative risk (RR)   Rate of the outcome of interest in a population compared with the rate in the reference population

Risk assessment   An organized process used to describe and estimate the likelihood of adverse health outcomes from environmental exposures to chemicals; the four steps are hazard identification, dose-response assessment, exposure assessment, and risk characterization

Salmonella **spp.**   A genus of bacteria including several pathogenic species that have been associated with risk from contaminated foods, including seafoods

Saturated fat   Fatty acids with no double bonds; fats that are solid enough to hold their shape at room temperature (about 70°F)

Science-based knowledge   Conclusions (findings and recommendations) based on clear and consistent evidence from both observational and experimental study designs

Scombroid poisoning   Intoxication by foods that contain high levels of histamine caused by bacterial contamination

Serum lipids   Lipids in the fluid portion of coagulated blood

Shellfish   Common terminology used to identify crustacean and/or molluscan seafoods

Standard deviation   A statistic that shows how tightly all the various data points are clustered around the mean in a set of data

Tertile   A contiguous grouping (low, middle, high) of one-third of a sample or population

Thermal abuse   Improper refrigeration or heat exposure during preparation, storage, or transfer

Toxicant   Any substance or material that can injure living organisms through physicochemical interactions

Toxicity equivalency factor   A numerical index that is used to compare the toxicity of different congeners and substances

Toxicokinetic   The processes of absorption, distribution, metabolism, and excretion that occur between the time a toxic chemical enters the body and when it leaves

Toxin   A poisonous substance (of animal, mineral, vegetable, or microbial origin) that can cause damage to living tissues

Trophic   Of or relating to nutrition

Triglycerides (TG)   A naturally occurring ester of three fatty acids and glycerol that is the chief constituent of fats and oils

Uncertainty factor (UF)   One of several (generally 10-fold factors) used in operationally deriving the Reference Dose (RfD) from experimental data. UFs are intended to account for (1) the variation in sensitivity among members of the human population; (2) the uncertainty in extrapolating animal data to the case of humans; (3) the uncertainty in extrapolating from data obtained in a study that is of less-than-lifetime exposure; and (4) the uncertainty in using Lowest Observed Adverse Effect Level data rather than No Observed Adverse Effect Level data

Value trade-off   The willingness to pay a higher price for something with a higher value rating attached

Vibrio vulnificus   A bacterium usually associated with raw molluscan shellfish

Voluntary Seafood Inspection Program   A program for inspection and certification of seafood processing plants, designed to ensure quality more than product safety; conducted by the National Marine Fisheries Service

SUPPLEMENTARY INFORMATION ON NUTRIENTS OF SPECIAL INTEREST IN SEAFOOD

Omega-3 Fatty Acids

Omega-3 fatty acids occur widely throughout the plant and animal kingdoms. Algae, fungi, bacteria, insects, and some vertebrates possess the array of enzymes needed for de novo synthesis of these fatty acids (Gill and Valivety, 1997a). Genetically complex plants, though they may be good sources of alpha-linolenic acid (ALA), rarely produce polyunsaturated fatty acids longer than 18 carbons and thus are not sources of eicosapentaenoic acid (EPA) and docosahexaenoic acid (DHA). Though more genetically complex animals can synthesize EPA and DHA from ALA (Qiu, 2003), the rate of synthesis in most species is low. Fish are good sources of EPA and DHA primarily because their natural diets contain these fatty acids, not because they are able to synthesize them de novo. Organisms low on the food chain consume the algal and microbial sources of EPA and DHA, which become concentrated in the lipid stores of those species higher up in the food chain.

Derivation of the Omega-3 Fatty Acids

Omega-3 fatty acids are long-chain polyunsaturated fatty acids that are characterized by the presence of a double bond at the omega position (3 carbon atoms from the methyl end) in the carbon chain. This position is what identifies them as omega-3 fatty acids. EPA and DHA are not endogenously synthesized from saturated, monounsaturated, or omega-6 fatty acids; they can only be made from the precursor omega-3 fatty acid, ALA. Figure A-1 shows the synthesis pathways for omega-3 fatty acids.

The omega-3 fatty acids include:

• Alpha-linolenic acid, 18:3 n-3, a plant-derived source of fatty acid. ALA can be converted to the omega-3 fatty acids EPA and DHA through a series of desaturation and chain elongation events, but the conversion in humans is inefficient and varies with the content of other fatty acids in the diet (see discussion below for more information about conversion efficiency);

• Eicosapentaenoic acid, 20:5 n-3, a fatty acid synthesized from ALA and found primarily in fatty fish. EPA is a precursor molecule in the human synthesis of one family of eicosanoids, including prostaglandins, thromboxane, leukotrienes, hydroxy fatty acids, and lipoxins. These compounds serve as modulators of cardiovascular, pulmonary, immune, reproductive, and secretory functions at the cellular level;

• Docosahexaenoic acid, 22:6 n-3, a fatty acid synthesized from ALA and found primarily in fatty fish. It is a component of all membrane structural lipids in neural and retinal tissues and spermatozoa. The developing brain accumulates large amounts of DHA late in fetal life. This accumulation continues through at least the first 2 postnatal years.

Selenium

Selenium is an element classified within Group VIA in the periodic table following oxygen and sulfur but preceding tellurium and polonium.

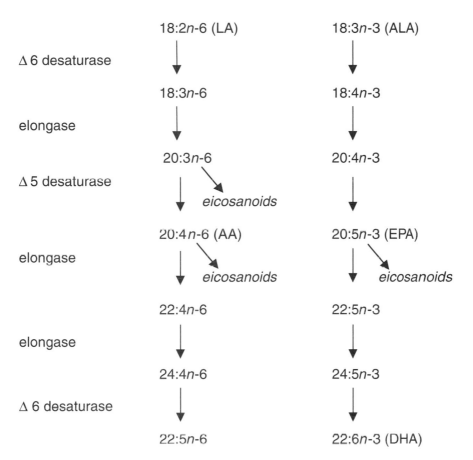

FIGURE A-1 Biosynthesis of long-chain fatty acids.
NOTES: LA = Linoleic acid; AA = Arachidonic acid; ALA = Alpha-linolenic acid;
EPA = Eicosapentaenoic acid; DPA = Docosapentaenoic acid; DHA = Docosahexaenoic
acid.
SOURCE: Derived from IOM, 2002/2005.

This position in the periodic table leads to the classification of selenium as
a metalloid element with unique chemistry and biochemistry, i.e., exhibiting
both metallic and nonmetallic properties. Selenium can form bonds with
other selenium atoms, a characteristic referred to as catenation and shared
with other elements like carbon, silicon, and sulfur. Elemental selenium is
found in three forms: the gray-black form or metallic hexagonal selenium,
an amorphous white form, and a monoclinic red form. Selenium has six
electrons in the 4s and 4p, orbital and the empty $d\pi p\pi$ bonds of selenium,
like sulfur, can be filled by $p\pi$ electrons of oxygen. Selenium and sulfur have

similar radii Δ, 1.03 and 1.07 (covalent radii), and similar electronegativities of 2.44 and 2.48, respectively. Thus, the chemical reactivity of selenium and sulfur are similar. However, the reduction potential of selenous and selenic acids are much greater than those of the analogous sulfur acids so that when both are in the same mixture, selenite will be reduced to elemental selenium but sulfite will be oxidized to sulfate.

Selenium Essentiality

Selenium occurs in all the cells and tissues of mammalian species and reflects the level of dietary selenium over a wide range of intakes. Selenium was recognized as an essential nutrient when Schwarz and Foltz (1957) showed that a form of liver necrosis developed in rats if either vitamin E or selenium was excluded from their diet. It is now recognized that both selenium and vitamin E have important roles in the detoxification of hydro-peroxides and free radical byproducts (Sunde, 2001).

Selenium deficiency has been demonstrated in premature infants and patients utilizing long-term selenium-free enteral or parenteral solutions. Deficiency symptoms include red blood cell hemolysis, cardiomyopathy, growth retardation, cataract formation, abnormal placenta retention, lack of spermatogenesis, and skeletal muscle degeneration. There is a decline of selenoproteins, particularly glutathione peroxidase activity. Selenium deficiency has been found to be endemic in regions of China, where it is called Keshan disease. Children are particularly susceptible, and the disease is characterized by cardiomyopathy. Selenite-enriched salt has been shown to assist in the reversal of this deficiency, but it is likely that selenium is only one factor. Coxsackie virus has been isolated from persons with Keshan disease, and recent animal research has provided evidence that viral infections may be influenced by selenium status. The Institute of Medicine has recommended an intake of no less than 55 and no more than 400 μg of selenium per day as sufficient to meet the needs of the average adult (IOM, 2000).

Selenium is an essential element in a group of proteins, i.e., selenoproteins. Sulfur amino acids and selenium are involved in the synthesis of these selenoproteins via selenophosphate to form selenocysteine, catalyzed by the enzyme selenophosphate synthetase. Approximately 25 selenoproteins have been identified, with half characterized with respect to their function (Kryukov et al., 2003). Of those characterized for function, over half perform free radical detoxification. The list of established selenoproteins and their respective biological functions are listed in Table A-1 (Sunde, 2000). The selenium is incorporated into the peptide backbone of selenium-containing proteins as selenocysteine. Novel metabolic pathways are necessary to convert various dietary forms of selenium into the selenocysteine entity. Dietary selenate and selenite are reductively converted to selenide,

TABLE A-1 Selenoproteins and Biological Functions

Selenoproteins	Function
Cytosolic glutathione peroxidase, GPX1	Major form of selenium, protects against hydroperoxides
Phospholipid hydroperoxide glutathione peroxidase, GPX4	Lipophilic, works within membranes to destroy peroxides
Gastrointestinal glutathione peroxidase, GPX2	Protect intestine against external peroxides
Extracellular glutathione peroxidase, plasma GPX, GPX3	Secreted GPX, major form of selenium in milk
Selenoprotein W, SELW	Small 9.8 kDa selenoprotein found in muscle, postulated to have antioxidant function
Selenoprotein P, SELP	Major plasma selenoprotein, postulated to protect the cardiovascular system against oxidant damage
Thioredoxin reductase, TRRs	Reduce small intracellular molecules, regulate intracellular redox state, and may have important roles in antioxidant defense
Iodothyronine deiodinase	Activation and metabolism of thyroid hormone
Sperm capsule selenoprotein	

SOURCE: Derived from Sunde, 2001.

usually in the intestinal or erythrocyte cells. Selenium released from seleno-methionine breakdown will also enter this pool as selenide. Subsequently, synthesis of selenocysteine involves several unique intermediates but it is the selenide that serves as the precursor to selenocysteine.

Selenium Food Sources

Plant and animal levels of selenium vary widely, reflecting the wide range of selenium content of soils (Sunde, 2001). Corn, rice, and soybeans grown in a selenium-poor region of China contain 0.0005, 0.007, and 0.010 µg/g, respectively, while those grown in seleniferous areas of China can have a selenium content as high as 8.1, 4.0, and 11.9 µg/g, respectively. Organ meats and seafood are usually good sources for this element (USDA, 2005), with levels ranging from 0.4 to 1.5 µg/g, whereas levels in muscle meats range from 0.1 to 0.4 µg/g, and in dairy products, less than 0.1 to 0.3 µg/g. Drinking water usually has a negligible selenium content, unless it comes from well waters in seleniferous areas (Sunde, 2001).

Selenium Toxicity

Berzelius first reported the existence of selenium as a metal in 1817. In nature, selenium is often found in combination with lead, copper, mercury, and silver as selenides, similar to sulfur counterparts. Localized seleniferous areas can be found in various parts of the Great Plains in North America. Seleniferous areas also have been identified in Ireland, Israel, Australia, Russia, and South Africa. In grazing livestock of North America, the disease associated with excess selenium intake is known as alkali disease or blind staggers. Selenium accumulator plants ingested by livestock are often the source of selenosis or selenium poisoning. Selenium poisoning can be a mild chronic condition, or severely acute, resulting in death. Acute selenium poisoning resulting in death is often preceded by blindness, abdominal pain, salivation, grinding of the teeth, and paralysis. Death is usually due to respiratory failure, which is often complicated by starvation resulting from loss of appetite, marked restriction of food intake, anemia, and severe pathological changes in the liver (Hogberg and Alexander, 1986). Dullness and lack of vitality, emaciation and roughness of coat, loss of hair, erosion of the joints, atrophy of the heart and cirrhosis of the liver, and anemia characterize chronic selenium poisoning. Chronic selenium poisoning can occur in rats and dogs given diets containing 5–10 ppm selenium. It is likely that the minimum toxic level is 4–5 ppm selenium. Acute toxicity in humans occurs when selenium intake is in excess of 750 µg/day. Usually toxicity occurs when individuals are exposed to high dietary intake and industrial conditions (smelters) that increase the body burden of selenium.

The precise ways in which selenium at toxic intakes exerts toxicity are not completely understood. Inhibition of oxygen consumption by tissues appears to be mediated through a poisoning of succinic dehydrogenase.

When selenium intake is high, it can be methylated through S-adenosyl-methione by either microsomal or cytosolic methyltransferases, forming the products methyl, dimethyl, trimethyl derivatives. Dimethyl selenide is the volatile seleno derivative giving the garlic-like odor (Sunde, 2001).

References

Gill I, Valivety R. 1997. Polyunsaturated fatty acids, part 1: Occurrence, biological activities and applications. *Trends in Biotechnology* 15:401–409.
Hogberg J, Alexander J. 1986. *Selenium.* In: Friberg, L, Norberg, G, Vouk VB, eds. *Handbook on the Toxicology of Metals.* Vol 2. Amsterdam, Netherlands: Elsevier. Pp. 482–512.

IOM (Institute of Medicine). 2000. *Dietary Reference Intakes for Vitamin C, Vitamin E, Selenium, and Carotenoids.* Washington, DC: National Academy Press. Pp. 284–324.

IOM. 2002/2005. *Dietary Reference Intakes for Energy, Carbohydrate, Fiber, Fat, Fatty Acids, Cholesterol, Protein, and Amino Acids.* Washington, DC: The National Academies Press.

Kryukov GV, Castellano S, Novoselov SV, Lobanov AV, Zehtab O, Guigo R, Gladyshev VN. 2003. Characterization of mammalian selenoproteins. *Science* 300:1439–1443.

Qui X. 2003. Biosynthesis of docosahexaenoic acid (DHA, 22:6–4, 7, 10, 13, 16, 19): Two distinct pathways. *Prostaglandins, Leukotrienes and Essential Fatty Acids* 68:181–186.

Schwartz K, Foltz CM. 1957. Selenium as an integral part of factor 3 against dietary necrotic liver degeneration. *Journal of the American Chemical Society* 79(12):3292–3293.

Sunde RA. 2001. Selenium. In: Bowman BA, Russel RM, eds. *Present Knowledge in Nutrition.* Washington, DC: International Life Sciences Institute Press. Pp. 352–365.

USDA (US Department of Agriculture). 2005. *National Database for Standard Release 18.* [Online]. Available: http://www.nal.usda.gov/fnic/foodcomp/Data/SR18/sr18.html) [accessed December 4, 2006].

B

Data Tables

Note: Abbreviations/acronyms included in the following data tables are included in the Glossary (see Appendix A).

Studies on Women, Infants, and Children

TABLE B-1a Studies on Preeclampsia: Effects on Women Who Increase Seafood and/or Omega-3 Fatty Acid Intake

Author	Study Type	Subjects	Exposure	Timing of Exposure
Sibai, 1998	Review	3 randomized controlled trials	Fish-oil supplement	
Sindelar et al., 2004	Randomized Controlled Trial	Men (n=8) Women (n=4) Mean age of 33 years Lincoln, NE Non-Hispanic White Recruited at YMCA marathon and triathlon training group meetings and word of mouth Exercising regularly as members of a running training group sponsored by the local YMCA No being treated with eating disorders or depression, or those unable to eat eggs, or those using medications known to affect serum lipids	n-3 PUFA-enriched eggs	2 weeks baseline period, 4 weeks treatment period (crossover design), 4 weeks washout period between treatments
Haugen and Helland, 2001	Randomized Controlled Trial	Pregnant women (n=37) Mean age about 27-31 years Oslo, Norway Normotensive without proteinuria, had uncomplicated term pregnancies, randomly taken from another study investigating the influence of omega-3 fatty acids on fetal, neonatal, and child development Another group had moderate preeclampsia	Cod-liver oil supplement	16-20 weeks gestation through pregnancy

Amount	Results	Conclusion*
	"The beneficial effects of fish oil on the incidence of preeclampsia are supported by observational studies and 1 large, uncontrolled early trial."	N
	Three randomized trials "reveal no reduction in the incidence of preeclampsia in the fish oil group."	
n-3 PUFA-enriched eggs: flaxseed added to hens' diet 350 mg n-3 PUFA/60 g egg 0.25 g LA, 0.10 g DHA/60 g egg 1 egg/day for 6 days and no eggs on day 7	LA, DHA, and total n-3 dietary intake of those randomized to n-3 PUFA-enriched egg treatment were significantly higher than at baseline and compared to the conventional egg treatment (p<0.05).	N/A
Conventional eggs: 60 mg of n-3 PUFA/60 g egg 0.04 g LA, 0.02 g DHA/60 g egg 1 egg/day for 6 days and no eggs on day 7	There were no significant differences in serum total cholesterol, LDL C and HDL C in physically active adults from baseline to end of treatment or between groups. Serum triglycerides were significantly higher with n-3 PUFA-enriched egg treatment than those from baseline and compared to the conventional egg treatment (p<0.05).	
Cod-liver oil group: 10 mL/day	"The pressure increase was significant in both groups, but no significant differences in the constrictory response or in the proportions of preparations displaying dilatatory responses were observed when compared to appropriate control groups."	N
Corn oil group: 10 mL/day	"Neither preeclampsia nor dietary supplementation with cod-liver oil had any significant effect on the vasoactive response to PGF2α in umbilical cord arteries."	

continued

TABLE B-1a Continued

Author	Study Type	Subjects	Exposure	Timing of Exposure
Salvig et al., 1996	Randomized Controlled Trial	Pregnant women (n=533) Aged 18-44 years Aarhus, Denmark No history of placental abruption in an earlier pregnancy or a serious bleeding episode in the present pregnancy, no prostaglandin inhibitors regularly, no allergy to fish and regular intake of fish oil	Fish-oil supplement	30th week gestation through pregnancy
Onwude et al., 1995	Randomized Controlled Trial	Pregnant women (n=233) Aged 18-39 years for fish oil group Aged 16-40 for placebo group Leeds, UK Multigravida with a history of one or more small babies, a history of proteinuric or nonproteinuric pregnancy-induced hypertension, or a history of unexplained stillbirth Primigravida with abnormal uterine arcuate artery Doppler blood flow at 24 weeks gestation	EPA/DHA supplement	Until 38th week gestation; enrollment time unspecified
Bulstra-Ramakers, 1995	Randomized Controlled Trial	Pregnant women (n=63) Groningen, Netherlands Birth weight below the 10th percentile in association with pregnancy-induced hypertension or chronic renal disease, or with placenta abnormalities	EPA supplement	12-14 weeks gestation until delivery

Amount	Results	Conclusion*
Fish oil group: 2.7 g/day (4 capsules/day, each capsule contains 32% EPA, 23% DHA, 2 mg tocopherol/ml) Olive oil group: 1 g; 72% oleic acid and 12% LA/capsule 4 capsules/day Control = no capsule	"Mean blood pressure increased during the course of the 3rd trimester," but this change was not statistically different among the three groups. "No differences were seen between the groups in proportions of women with a systolic blood pressure above 140 mmHg or a systolic blood pressure above 90 mmHg, although the proportion of women with diastolic above 90 mmHg tended to be lower in the fish oil group compared to the olive oil group (RR=0.48, p=0.07)."	N
2.7 g/day (1.62 g/day of EPA) (1.08 g/day of DHA)	There were no significant differences between the two groups for proteinuric pregnancy-induced hypertension, nonproteinuric pregnancy-induced hypertension, birth weight, gestation length, perinatal death, duration of labor, onset of labor (spontaneous, induced, or prelabor section), or mode of delivery.	N
4 capsules 3 times/day (each capsule contains 0.25 mg EPA) vs. placebo	"Addition of 3 g/day of EPA to the diet did not result in either a lowering of the incidence of pregnancy induced hypertension or intrauterine growth retardation." "Birth weight centiles were slightly lower and the recurrence rate of pregnancy-induced hypertension was slightly higher in the EPA group," compared to the control group, although these differences were not significant.	N

continued

TABLE B-1a Continued

Author	Study Type	Subjects	Exposure	Timing of Exposure
Schiff et al., 1993	Controlled Trial	Pregnant women (n=16) Aged 25-34 years Nulliparous Nonsmokers, no history of hyper- tension, coagulation disorders, thrombocytopenia, or chronic vascular, renal, or other disease	Fish-oil supplement	32-34 weeks through the next 21 days
Olsen and Secher, 1990	Randomized Controlled Trial	Pregnant women (n=5022) Aged 15-44 years London People's League of Health, 1946 Attending antenatal clinics of 10 hospitals No disease or physical abnormality	EPA/DHA supplement	Enrolled at <24 weeks gestation; treatment lasts for <15 weeks (n=288), 16-19 weeks (n=411), 20-23 weeks (n=414), or 24+ weeks (n=417)

Amount	Results	Conclusion*
6 capsules/day (each capsule contains 1000 mg of concentrated fish oil, 26% of which is n-3 fatty acids)	"Mean excretion of 11-dehydro-thromboxane B_2 before and after 21 days of fish oil consumption was reduced among the fish oil-treated women from 1606±411 pg/mg of creatinine to 779±299 pg/mg after treatment ($p<0.0001$, paired t test). In all 11 patients the decreased excretion of this metabolite was considerable, ranging from 32% to 71%." No significant change was detected among the control women.	B
0.1 g/day of EPA+DHA from halibut oil in supplement vs. no supplement Supplement includes 0.26 g ferrous iron; 0.26 g calcium; minute quantities of iodine, manganese and copper; 0.60 g thiamin/g; 0.10 g vitamin C; 0.36 g halibut liver oil	In primiparae, the OR for preeclampsia was significant when comparing the treatment to the control group (OR=0.689, 95% CI 0.50-0.95). In primiparae, the OR for albuminuria was statistically significant when comparing the treatment to the control group (OR=0.717, 95% CI 0.54-0.96). In primiparae, the OR for hypertension was not significant when comparing the treatment to the control group (OR=0.862, 95% CI 0.73-1.02). In multiparae, these statistics were OR=0.677 (95% CI 0.43-1.07), OR=0.675 (95% CI 0.44-1.04), and OR=1.121 (95% CI 0.89-1.42). There were no significant effects on the occurrences of stillbirths, early neonatal deaths (before 8 days), perinatal deaths, sepsis, or the duration of labor.	B

continued

TABLE B-1a Continued

Author	Study Type	Subjects	Exposure	Timing of Exposure
Clausen et al., 2001	Cohort	Pregnant women (n=3133) Mean age 29.8 years 51.8% nulliparous Representing all socioeconomic classes Aker University Hospital, Oslo, Norway No pregestational diabetes or twin/triplet pregnancies	Fatty acids from food	17-19 weeks gestation until after delivery

Amount	Results	Conclusion*
Tertiles of saturated fatty acids (%energy) Mean = ≤12.0, 12.0-15.0, >15.0	After adjusting for energy, age, smoking, BMI, systolic blood pressure for 20 weeks' gestation, nullipara and energy:	N
Tertiles of monounsaturated fatty acids (%energy) Mean = ≤10.5, 10.5-13.0, >13.0	Statistically significant ORs for preeclampsia, comparing the highest group to the lowest group of fatty acid intakes, were observed for polyunsaturated fatty acids (p=0.01) and omega-6 fatty acids (p=0.05); and	
Tertiles of polyunsaturated fatty acids (%energy) Mean = ≤5.2, 5.2-7.5, >7.5	Statistically nonsignificant ORs for preeclampsia, comparing the highest group to the lowest group of fatty acid intakes, were	
Tertiles of omega-3 fatty acids (%energy) Mean = ≤0.9, 0.9-1.6, >1.6	observed for saturated fat (p=0.10), monounsaturated fat (p=0.59), and omega-3 fatty acids (p=0.06).	
Tertiles of omega-6 fatty acids (%energy) Mean = ≤3.8, 3.8-5.8, >5.8		

continued

TABLE B-1a Continued

Author	Study Type	Subjects	Exposure	Timing of Exposure
Velzing-Aarts et al., 1999	Case-control	Cases (n=27) = preeclamptic women Controls (n=24) = normotensive, nonproteinuric women Pregnant women Mean age about 27 years Curacao	Fatty acid composition in maternal and umbilical platelets and umbilical arteries and veins	During delivery or within 2 hours after birth

Amount	Results	Conclusion*
Mean fatty acid composition in maternal platelets (in mol%): Controls = 9.66±2.75 LA; 0.27±0.10 ALA; 0.29±0.14 EPA; 2.03±0.62 DHA Cases = 7.02±1.91 LA; 0.22±0.11 ALA; 0.21±0.07 EPA; 2.16±0.93 DHA	"Newborns of preeclamptic women had significantly lower birth weights and gestational ages at delivery," compared to newborns of non-preeclamptic women. Preeclamptic women had significantly lower maternal platelet levels of LA (p<0.001) and EPA (p<0.05) compared to normotensive women.	B
Mean fatty acid composition in umbilical cord platelets (in mol%): Controls = 3.73±0.76 LA; 0.14±0.10 ALA; 0.16±0.07 EPA; 2.33±0.58 DHA Cases = 4.16±1.51 LA; 0.21±0.11 ALA; 0.17±0.07 EPA; 1.97±0.30 DHA	Preeclamptic women had significantly lower umbilical arteries levels of EPA (p<0.01) and DHA (p<0.001) compared to normotensive women. No other significant differences were found for LA, ALA, EPA, or DHA.	
Mean fatty acid composition in umbilical veins (in mol%): Controls = 2.69±0.44 LA; 0.10±0.05 ALA; 0.09±0.04 EPA; 4.26±0.85 DHA Cases = 2.89±0.56 LA; 0.11±0.05 ALA; 0.07±0.02 EPA; 3.35±0.96 DHA		
Mean fatty acid composition in umbilical arteries (in mol%): Controls = 1.87±0.39 LA; 0.10±0.04 ALA; 0.09±0.03 EPA; 4.83±0.76 DHA Cases = 1.74±0.75 LA; 0.10±0.06 ALA; 0.06±0.03 EPA; 3.73±1.03 DHA		

continued

TABLE B-1a Continued

Author	Study Type	Subjects	Exposure	Timing of Exposure
Kesmodel et al., 1997	Nested case-control	Cases = women with preeclampsia (n=43), pregnancy-induced hypertension (n=179), intrauterine growth retardation (n=182), delivering preterm (n=153), delivering postterm (n=189) Control = sample from whole cohort (n=256) Pregnant women Aarhus, Denmark	Seafood and fish-oil supplement	Between 6 months and 3 1/2 years after delivery
Williams et al., 1995	Case-control	Cases (n=22) = preeclamptic Controls (n=40) = normotensive Pregnant women Mean age 28.6-31.2 years White (n=17 in preeclamptic group, n=23 in non-preeclamptic group) Seattle, Washington About 21% Medicaid recipient	Maternal erythrocytes fatty acid profiles	Day after delivery

Amount	Results	Conclusion*

Low intake =
  Maximum of 1 fish snack/
  week and 1 fish meal/month
  and no fish oil
	After adjusting for maternal smoking habits,
	maternal height, maternal weight before
	pregnancy, parity, maternal social status, and
	average daily calcium intake:
		N

High intake =
  Minimum of 4 fish snacks/
  week or 4 fish meals/month
  or intake of fish oil during
  pregnancy
	There were no significant ORs of pregnancy-
	induced hypertension, preeclampsia, intra-
	uterine growth retardation, preterm delivery
	or postterm delivery for the middle-intake
	group or the high-intake group compared to
	the low-intake group.	

Middle intake = Everyone else		
Tertiles of EPA: Median = 0.20, 0.26, 0.36	After adjusting for parity and pre-pregnancy BMI, the OR of preeclampsia for the lowest tertile of EPA, compared to the highest ter- tile of EPA was 5.54 (95% CI 1.06-28.79).	B
Tertiles of DPA: Median = 1.54, 1.75, 2.02	After adjusting for parity and pre-pregnancy BMI, the OR of preeclampsia for the lowest tertile of DPA, compared to the highest ter- tile of DPA was 3.33 (95% CI 0.65-16.99).	
Tertiles of DHA: Median = 4.38, 5.14, 6.40	After adjusting for parity and pre-pregnancy BMI, the OR of preeclampsia for the lowest tertile of DHA, compared to the highest ter- tile of DHA was 7.54 (95% CI 1.23-46.22).	
Tertiles of total long-chain n-3 fatty acids: Median = 6.23, 7.09, 8.50	After adjusting for parity and pre-pregnancy BMI, the OR of preeclampsia for the lowest tertile of the sum of long-chain omega-3 fatty acids, compared to the highest tertile of long-chain omega-3 fatty acids was 7.63 (95% CI 1.43-40.63).	

continued

TABLE B-1a Continued

Author	Study Type	Subjects	Exposure	Timing of Exposure
Wang et al., 1991	Case-control	Cases (n=9) = preeclamptic women ControlsA (n=11) = normal pregnant women ControlsB (n=10) = nonpregnant women Aged 20-40 years Term (pregnant women) Not on oral contraceptives (nonpregnant women)	Plasma fatty acid analysis	During pregnancy

*N = Evidence of no association or no clear association; B = Evidence of a benefit; N/A = A conclusion is not available; these data are presented for background information only.

Amount	Results	Conclusion*
Nonpregnant women (mg/L±SE): 79.51±3.47 total PUFA, 60.79±2.28 LA, 10.99±1.01 AA, 1.88±0.17 ALA, 0.26±0.04 EPA, 5.58±0.60 DHA	Plasma total polyunsaturated fatty acid levels, LA, ALA, and EPA were all significantly higher in the normal pregnant women than in the preeclamptic women ($p<0.05$, $p<0.01$, $p<0.05$, $p<0.05$, respectively).	B
Normal pregnant women (mg/L±SE): 90.60±6.68 total PUFA, 62.93±4.69 LA, 12.81±0.87 AA, 3.68±0.99 ALA, 1.08±0.33 EPA, 10.40±0.94 DHA	EPA and DHA were significantly lower in the nonpregnant women compared to the pregnant women ($p<0.05$ and $p<0.01$, respectively). No other significant differences between the plasma polyunsaturated fatty acid levels in the three groups were found.	
Preeclamptic women (mg/L±SE): 67.42±3.88 total PUFA, 45.98±2.80 LA, 11.44±1.00 AA, 1.11±0.25±ALA, 0.11±0.11 EPA, 8.94±0.69 DHA	"No statistical differences were noted in the five polyunsaturated fatty acid levels between fasting and non fasting states in both non-pregnant and normal pregnant subjects."	

TABLE B-1b Studies on Postpartum Depression: Effects on Women Who Increase Seafood and/or Omega-3 Fatty Acid Intake

Author	Study Type	Subjects	Exposure	Timing of Exposure
Marangell et al., 2004	Open trial	Pregnant women (n=7) Aged 31-42 years Married, Caucasian (except for one married, Hispanic) Baylor College of Medicine History of a depressive episode in the postpartum period, not suffering from a current depressive episode No psychotropic medications within 2 weeks of baseline, history of nonreponse to two or more antidepressants, serious comorbid medical or psychiatric illness, or significant risk of dangerousness to self or others	Fish-oil supplement	34-36 weeks gestation until 12 weeks postpartum
Llorente et al., 2003	Randomized Controlled Trial	Pregnant women (n=89) Aged 18-42 years No chronic medical condition, no dietary supplements other than vitamins, no smoking, who had not been pregnant >5 times Planned to breastfeed infants exclusively for at least 4 months Part of a larger cohort study on effects of DHA on breastfeeding mothers and their infants	Algae-derived triglyceride supplement	Within a week of delivery to 4 months after delivery
Hibbeln and Salem, 1995	Review	Summary of three cohorts	DHA depletion	

Amount	Results	Conclusion*
Fish oil group: 2960 mg fish oil/day 173 mg EPA and 123 mg DHA per day 10 capsules/day	Trial was terminated because of a high relapse rate observed after enrolling only seven participants.	N
Algae-derived triglyceride capsule (about 200 mg DHA/day) vs. placebo	"Repeated measures analysis of variance, with the use of data only from the women who completed the questionnaires at both baseline and 4 months, showed no difference between the two groups at any time" with regards to postpartum depression.	N
	"There were no significant differences between groups in the EPDS and SCID-CV scores, particularly in current or past episodes of depression, as detected by the SCID-CV."	
	"There were no significant correlations between plasma phospholipid DHA content and BDI, EPDS, or SCID-CV scores."	
	"The relative maternal depletion of DHA may be one of the complex factors leading to increased risk of depression in women of childbearing age and in postpartum periods."	B

continued

TABLE B-1b Continued

Author	Study Type	Subjects	Exposure	Timing of Exposure
Timonen et al., 2004	Cohort	Live female births (n=2968) Live male births (n=2721) Unselected, genetically homogeneous Northern Finland 1966 Birth Cohort	Seafood	Previous 6 months (during pregnancy) until 31 years of age

Amount	Results	Conclusion*

Rare eaters: ≤1 time/month
 	
Regular eaters: ≥1 time/week
 	
Serving size unspecified
	After adjusting for body mass index, serum total cholesterol level, and socioeconomic situation, women who ate fish rarely had a higher OR for depression, compared to women who ate fish regularly. This statistic was observed by various measurements:
	    Doctor-diagnosis:
	      OR=1.3 (95% CI 0.9-1.9);
	    HSCL-25 <2.01:
	      OR=1.4 (95% CI 1.1-1.9);
	    HSCL-25 <2.01 and doctor-diagnosis:
	      OR=2.6 (95% CI 1.4-5.1).
	
	After adjusting for alcohol intake, smoking, physical inactivity, and marital status, women who ate fish rarely had a higher OR for depression, compared to women who ate fish regularly. This statistic was observed by various measurements:
	    Doctor-diagnosis:
	      OR=1.2 (95% CI 0.9-1.6);
	    HSCL-25 <2.01:
	      OR=1.4 (95% CI 1.1-1.8);
	    HSCL-25 <2.01 and doctor-diagnosis:
	      OR=2.4 (95% CI 1.4-4.2).
	
	Among men, none of these ORs were significant.
		B

continued

TABLE B-1b Continued

Author	Study Type	Subjects	Exposure	Timing of Exposure
Otto et al., 2003	Cohort	Participated in 2 earlier studies Pregnant women (n=112) Mean age around 30 years Caucasian Southern Limburg, Netherlands Fish intake <2 times/week No metabolic, cardiovascular, neurologic, renal, or psychiatric disorders No medications, except for multi-vitamins and iron supplements Singleton pregnancy Term delivery No blood transfusions in the perinatal period Gestational age <14 weeks at entry, Caucasian, fish consumption <2 times a week (for Study 2 only)	Venous (plasma) blood fatty acid composition	36 weeks gestation, at delivery, and 32 weeks postpartum
Otto et al., 2001	Cohort	Pregnant women (n=57) Mean age around 30 years Southern Limburg, Netherlands No metabolic, cardiovascular, neurologic, or renal disorders No medications, except multivitamins and iron supplements Singleton pregnancy Term delivery No blood transfusions in the perinatal period	Diet and venous blood fatty acid profiles	36-37 weeks gestation; 2-5 days after delivery; 1, 2, 4, 8, 16, 32, 64 weeks postpartum

Amount	Results	Conclusion*
Absolute amount not specified	No significant relationship was observed between DHA, n-6DPA, or their ratio and the EPDS scores at delivery or at 32 weeks postpartum.	N
	No statistically significant relationships between depression and fatty acid status were observed with DHA or n-6DPA, neither for the levels at delivery, nor for their postpartum changes.	
	"The improvement of the DHA status during the postpartum period, as reflected by the increase of the DHA/n-6DPA ratio during this period, was higher in the non-depressed than in the depressed women (OR=0.90, p=0.04)."	
	Similar results remained after adjusting for Study 1 or 2, parity, education level, maternal age at test moment, breastfeeding, smoking, and alcohol use (OR=0.88, p=0.03).	
Absolute amount not specified	"After delivery, total fatty acids in plasma phospholipids decreased significantly over time in the lactating and nonlactating women (p<0.0001)."	N/A
	"The amounts of ALA, DHA, and total n-3 fatty acids showed significant downward trends postpartum in both groups, whereas the amounts of EPA and DPA increased significantly after delivery."	

continued

TABLE B-1b Continued

Author	Study Type	Subjects	Exposure	Timing of Exposure
Al et al., 1995	Cohort	Pregnant women (n=110) Aged 19-43 years Maastricht, Netherlands Caucasian Singleton pregnancy DBP <90 mmHg No metabolic, cardiovascular, neurological or renal disorder	Maternal venous and umbilical vein fatty acid profiles	10, 14, 18, 22, 26, 30, 32, 34, 36, 38, 40 weeks gestation; after delivery; 6 months after delivery
Holman, 1991	Cohort	Pregnant women (n=19) Aged 24-36 years Caucasian Normotensive, normal singleton pregnancies Mayo Clinic, Minnesota Controls (n=59) = staff and students from the University of Minnesota, aged 19-48 years	Blood fatty acid composition	36 weeks gestation, during labor, 6 weeks postpartum

Amount	Results	Conclusion*
Absolute amount not specified	"The average total amount of fatty acid (TF) in maternal venous plasma PL increased significantly (p<0.0001) during pregnancy, but the rise in TF became less pronounced towards the end of gestation (p<0.0001)."	N/A
	"Total fatty acids increased from 1238.11 mg/L at week 10 to 1867.84 mg/L at week 40 of gestation, and all of the fatty acid families showed a similar course."	
	"The mean amount of total fatty acids in umbilical plasma phospholipids was substantially lower (p<0.0001) than all maternal values" for all fatty acid families.	
	"In contrast to the absolute amounts of AA and DHA, the mean relative amounts of AA and DHA in umbilical plasma phospholipids were significantly (p<0.0001) higher than all maternal values."	
Normal controls of non-pregnant women of child-bearing age All in mol%±SEM: 24.1±0.39 LA, 12.5±0.24 AA, 0.22±0.01 ALA, 0.53±0.03 EPA, 1.04±0.04 DPA, 3.71±0.14 DHA	All individual PUFA were less than normal in pregnant women at 36 weeks of pregnancy than in the nonpregnant women, where EPA was 42% of normal values.	N/A
	"The fatty acid profile of plasma phospholipids during labor was similar to that at 36 weeks except for the subnormal LA and ALA values became significant at p<0.01 and p<0.05, respectively, and the elevated 22:5n-6 became significant at 0.001."	
	The fatty acid profile of plasma phospholipids for lactating women 6 weeks postpartum was similar to those during pregnancy and labor except that AA status improved, diminished ALA, and increased EPA and DPA toward normal.	
	The fatty acid profile of plasma phospholipids for nonlactating women 6 weeks postpartum was similar to that of the lactating women, expect that abnormalities were less severe or of lower significance.	

continued

TABLE B-1b Continued

Author	Study Type	Subjects	Exposure	Timing of Exposure
Hibbeln, 2002	Cross-sectional	Pregnancy women (n=14,532) 23 countries 41 different studies	Seafood	During pregnancy, unspecified

*N = Evidence of no association or no clear association; B = Evidence of a benefit; N/A = A conclusion is not available; these data are presented for background information only.

Amount	Results	Conclusion*
Absolute amount not specified	"Greater apparent seafood consumption predicted DHA content of mothers' milk ($p<0.006$)" and "higher DHA content in mothers' milk predicted a lower prevalence rate of postpartum depression ($p<0.0001$)." "Higher national seafood consumption predicted lower prevalence rates of postpartum depression ($p<0.0001$)."	B

TABLE B-1c Studies on Gestation and Birth Weight: Effects on Infants of Mothers Who Increase Seafood and/or Omega-3 Fatty Acid Intake

Author	Study Type	Subjects	Exposure	Timing of Exposure
de Groot et al., 2004	Randomized Controlled Trial	Pregnant women (n=79) Mean age of 29-30 years Maternal education about 4 (on an 8-point scale) Maastricht, Heerlen, Sittard, southeastern Netherlands White origin, gestational age <14 weeks, normal health, fish consumption <2 times/week No hypertensive, metabolic, cardiovascular, renal, psychiatric, or neurologic disorder	ALA-supplemented margarine	14 weeks gestation until delivery
Smuts et al., 2003a	Randomized Controlled Trial	Pregnant women (n=73) Mainly African-American Aged 16-35 years Reachable by telephone Planned to deliver at the Regional Medical Center in Memphis, TN No more than four pregnancies	DHA-enriched egg	24-28 weeks gestation until delivery
Smuts et al., 2003b	Randomized Controlled Trial	Pregnant women (n=291) Aged 16-36 years Mainly African-descent Plan to deliver at Truman Medical Center in Kansas City, MO Able and willing to consume eggs, access to refrigeration Singleton gestation No weight >240 pounds at baseline, cancer, lupus, hepatitis, infectious disease, diabetes, gestational diabetes, elevated blood pressure at baseline	DHA-enriched egg	24-28 weeks gestation until delivery

Amount	Results	Conclusion*
Experimental group (% total fatty acids): ALA-enriched high-LA margarine 25 g margarine 45.36 LA, 14.18 ALA Control group (% total fatty acids): No ALA high-LA margarine 25 g margarine/day 55.02 LA, 0.17 ALA	Newborns in the experimental group had a significantly higher mean birth weight than those in the control group (p=0.043). No significant differences in gestational age, APGAR score, or umbilical plasma DHA concentrations in phospholipids were found between the two groups.	B (birth weight only)
High-DHA egg group: mean = 183.9±71.4 mg DHA/day ranged from 27.6 to 264.9 mg/day Ordinary egg group: mean = 35.1±13.2 mg DHA/day ranged from 0 to 36 mg/day Low egg intake group: mean = 10.8±4.0 mg DHA/day ranged from 0 to 36 mg/day	"Mean weight, length, and head circumference of infants in the high-DHA egg group were greater than in the ordinary egg group, and gestation was 5.6 days longer."	B
High-DHA egg group: mean = 133±15 mg DHA/egg ranged from 108 to 165 mg/egg Ordinary egg group: mean = 33±11 mg DHA/egg ranged from 22 to 51 mg/egg	After controlling for maternal BMI at enrollment and number of prior pregnancies, the mean difference in gestational age between the two groups was 6.0±2.3 days (p=0.009). After controlling for maternal BMI at enrollment and maternal race, the mean difference in birth weight between the two groups was not significant.	B (gestation only)

continued

TABLE B-1c Continued

Author	Study Type	Subjects	Exposure	Timing of Exposure
Haugen and Helland, 2001	Randomized Controlled Trial	Pregnant women (n=37) Mean age about 27-31 years Oslo, Norway Normotensive without protein-uria, had uncomplicated term pregnancies, randomly taken from another study investi-gating the influence of omega-3 fatty acids on fetal, neona-tal, and child development Another group had moderate preeclampsia	Cod-liver oil supplement	16-20 weeks gestation through pregnancy
Helland et al., 2001	Randomized Controlled Trial	Pregnant women (n=590) Aged 19-35 years Oslo, Norway Single pregnancies, Nulli- or primipara Intention to breastfeed No supplement of n-3 LCPUFA earlier during the pregnancy No premature births, birth asphyxia, infections, and anomalies in the infants that required special attention	Cod-liver oil supplement	17-19 weeks gestation until 3 months after delivery

Amount	Results	Conclusion*
Cod-liver oil group: 10 mL/day Corn-oil group: 10 mL/day	There were no significant differences in gestational age between the four groups (cod-liver oil group, corn oil group, preeclamptic group, and the normotensive group). Birth weight was significantly higher in the corn oil group compared to the cod-liver oil group ($p<0.05$) and significantly higher in the normotensive group compared to the preeclamptic group ($p<0.0001$).	A (birth weight only)
10 mL/day cod-liver oil vs. corn oil Cod-liver oil group: 803 mg of EPA/10 mL; 1183 mg DHA/10 mL Corn-oil group: 0 mg of EPA/10 mL; 8.3 mg DHA/10 mL	"There were no significant differences in gestational length or birth weight between the two supplement groups. Birth length, head circumference, and placental weight were also similar in the 2 supplement groups."	N

continued

TABLE B-1c Continued

Author	Study Type	Subjects	Exposure	Timing of Exposure
Olsen et al., 2000	Randomized Controlled Trial	Pregnant women (n=1619) 19 hospitals in Denmark, Scotland, Sweden, England, Italy, Netherlands, Norway, Belgium, and Russia Participated in one of six previous trials (four prophylactic trials and two therapeutic trials)	Fish-oil supplement	20 weeks (prophylactic) or 33 weeks (therapeutic) gestation, delivery
Olsen et al., 1992	Randomized Controlled Trial	Pregnant women (n=533) Mean age 29 years Aarhus, Denmark Main midwife clinic, covers a well-defined geographic area No placental abruption in previous pregnancy or serious bleeding in current pregnancy; no prostaglandin inhibitors regularly No multiple pregnancy, allergy to fish, and regular intake of fish oil	Fish-oil supplement	Enrolled at 30 weeks gestation; end time not specified

Amount	Results	Conclusion*
2.7 g/day fish oil vs. olive oil in the prophylactic trials 6.1 g/day fish oil vs. olive oil in the therapeutic trials	In the trial of women who experienced preterm delivery in an earlier pregnancy, those randomized to fish oil had statistically significant longer gestation duration (difference = 8.5 days) compared to those randomized to olive oil (p=0.01). In the trial of women who experienced preterm delivery in an earlier pregnancy, those randomized to fish oil had children with a significantly higher mean birth weight (difference = 208.7 g) compared to those randomized to olive oil (p=0.02). In the trial of women with threatening preeclampsia in the current pregnancy, the mean difference of duration until delivery was 8.8 days less for those randomized to fish oil compared to those randomized to olive oil (p=0.19). In the trial of women with suspected intrauterine growth retardation in the current pregnancy, the mean difference of weight for gestational age was 29 g higher in those randomized to fish oil compared to those randomized to olive oil (p=0.75).	B
2.7 g/day fish oil vs. olive oil	The average gestational length for those in the fish-oil group was 4 days longer (95% CI 1.5-6.4, p<0.005) than those in the olive oil group. The average gestational length for those in the fish-oil group was 2.8 days longer (95% CI 0.8-4.8, p<0.01)) than those in the olive-oil and control groups. Birth weight (p=0.07) and length (p=0.1) trended higher in the fish-oil group than in the olive-oil group (3 way ANOVA between fish oil, olive oil, no oil).	B

continued

TABLE B-1c Continued

Author	Study Type	Subjects	Exposure	Timing of Exposure
Olsen and Secher, 1990	Randomized Controlled Trial	Pregnant women (n=5022) Aged 15-44 years London People's League of Health, 1946 Attending antenatal clinics of 10 hospitals No disease or physical abnormality	EPA/DHA supplement from halibut oil	Enrolled at <24 weeks gestation; treatment lasts for <15 weeks (n=288), 16-19 weeks (n=411), 20-23 weeks (n=414), or 24+ weeks (n=417)
People's League of Health, 1946	Randomized Controlled Trial	Pregnant women (n=5022) London Not beyond the 24th week of pregnancy No physical disease or abnormality	n-3 supplement	
People's League of Health, 1942	Randomized Controlled Trial	Pregnant women (n=5022) London	Additional diet, which includes halibut liver oil	Enrolled if due date more than 16 weeks away; until delivery

Amount	Results	Conclusion*
0.1 g/day of EPA+DHA from halibut oil in supplement vs. no supplement Supplement includes 0.26 g ferrous iron; 0.26 g calcium; minute quantities of iodine, manganese, and copper; 0.6 g thiamin/g; 0.1 g vitamin C; 0.36 g halibut liver oil	"In primiparae, a 19.9% (p=0.012) reduction in the odds of delivering earlier than 40 weeks was seen in the treatment group, whereas in multiparae a reduction of 21.2% (p=0.028) was seen," compared to the control group. "No significant effects were seen on the odds of delivering after 40 weeks of gestation." "No significant effects were seen on average birth weight."	B (gestation only)
	"A smaller incidence of prematurely was revealed among the treated women, and this is particularly significant since about 50% of infant deaths under 1 month are due to prematurely."	B
Weekly intake score for consumption of "the more important foodstuffs" such as milk, butter, wholemeal bread, fresh vegetables, fatty fish, fruit, eggs, etc. Additional diet: 0.26 g ferrous iron; 0.26 g calcium; minute quantities of iodine, manganese, and copper; 1 g adsorbate of vitamin B1; 100 mg vitamin C; 0.36 g halibut liver oil (vitamins A and D)	Among primigravida women, 20.1±1.10% of those who received additional diet experienced a preterm delivery compared to 23.9±1.10% of those who did not receive additional diet. This difference was statistically significant. Among multiparae women, 20.1±1.33% of those who received additional diet experienced a preterm delivery compared to 24.2±1.33% of those who did not receive additional diet. This difference was statistically significant.	B

continued

TABLE B-1c Continued

Author	Study Type	Subjects	Exposure	Timing of Exposure
Lucas et al., 2004	Cohort	Postpartum women (n=491) and their infants Mean age of 23.7 years Inuit 14 coastal villages of Nunavik and southern Quebec Delivered at Tulattavik Health Center (Ungava Bay) or Inuulitsivik Health Center (Hudson Bay)	Cord venous sample	At delivery

Amount	Results	Conclusion*
Tertiles of EPA (% of total fatty acids): Tertile 1 = <0.21 Tertile 2 = 0.21-0.39 Tertile 3 = >0.39 Tertiles of DHA (% of total fatty acids): Tertile 1 = <2.99 Tertile 2 = 2.99-4.03 Tertile 3 = >4.03 Tertiles of %n-3 HUFA (% of total HUFA): Tertile 1 = <18.60 Tertile 2 = 18.60-22.96 Tertile 3 = >22.96	After adjusting for weight gain during pregnancy, gestational diabetes, cord blood mercury, lead, and PCB congener 153, those in the third tertile of n-3 HUFA (% of total HUFA) had significantly longer gestation (278.4 days) compared to those in the first tertile (273.0 days) ($p<0.05$). After adjusting for pre-pregnancy weight, weight gain during pregnancy, parity, smoking status during pregnancy, gestational diabetes, age, cord blood mercury, and PCB congener 153, those in the third tertile of n-3 HUFA (% of total HUFA) had babies with a higher birth weight (3551 g) compared to those in the first tertile (3475 g), but this difference was not significant. There were no significant differences in birth weight or gestation based on the tertiles of EPA and DHA in the cord blood.	B

continued

TABLE B-1c Continued

Author	Study Type	Subjects	Exposure	Timing of Exposure

Oken et al., 2004	Cohort	Pregnant women (n=2109)
		Aged 14-44 years
		16% Black,
		  7% Hispanic-American,
		  6% Asian-American
		Massachusetts
		Project Viva
			Seafood	Last menstrual period until enrollment, 3 months prior to 26-28 weeks of gestation, the month prior to delivery

Olsen and Secher, 2002	Cohort	Pregnant women (n=8729)
		Aarhus, Denmark
		Gave birth to singleton, live-
		  born babies without detected
		  malformations
		Had not consumed fish-oil
		  supplements
			Seafood	From when first knew of pregnancy until completion of questionnaires at 16 and 30 weeks gestation

Amount	Results	Conclusion*
Seafood tertiles: None or <1 serving/month, the remaining subjects were divided into tertiles with the highest intake group used as the referent	After adjusting for enrollment site, infant sex, and maternal age, height, intrapartum weight gain, pre-pregnancy BMI, race/ethnicity, smoking during pregnancy, education, and gravidity:	B
First trimester quartiles of EPA+DHA: Quartile 1 = 0.00-0.05 Quartile 2 = 0.06-0.12 Quartile 3 = 0.12 0.24 Quartile 4 = 0.24-2.53	Significant negative trends based on EPA+DHA intake were found for the first trimester [birth weight (p=0.01) and fetal growth (p=0.001)], the second trimester [fetal growth (p=0.03)], and the third trimester [birth weight (p=0.001) and fetal growth (p=0.003)];	
Second trimester quartiles of EPA+DHA: Quartile 1 = 0.00-0.05 Quartile 2 = 0.06-0.12 Quartile 3 = 0.12-0.23 Quartile 4 = 0.24-2.71	No other significant trends were observed for change in birth weight, fetal growth or length of gestation with EPA+DHA intake during the three trimesters;	
Third trimester quartiles of EPA+DHA: Quartile 1 and 2 = 0.00-0.06 Quartile 3 = 0.60-0.11 Quartile 4 = 0.11-1.72	Significant negative trends were observed for change in birth weight and fetal growth with seafood consumption, but only during the first trimester (p=0.05 and p=0.08, respectively); and No other significant trends were observed for change in birth weight, fetal growth, or length of gestation with seafood intake during the first two trimesters.	
0.0, 0.5, 2.0, 4.0, 20.0, 28.0 serving/28 days Hot fish meal: 144 g fish/serving 1627 µg n-3 fatty acids/serving	"Low birth weight, preterm birth, and intrauterine growth retardation all tended to decrease with increasing fish consumption, and mean birth weight, duration of gestation, and birth weight adjusted for gestational age tended to increase with increasing fish consumption."	B
Fish sandwich: 29 g fish/serving 431 µg n-3 fatty acids/serving Fish salad: 50 g fish/serving 149 µg n-3 fatty acids/serving	Low consumption of seafood was a strong risk factor for preterm delivery and low birth weight. The associations were strongest below a daily intake of 0.15 g long change n-3 fatty acids or 15 g fish.	

continued

TABLE B-1c Continued

Author	Study Type	Subjects	Exposure	Timing of Exposure
Grandjean et al., 2001	Cohort	Singleton term births (n=182) Faroe Islands Delivered at the National Hospital in Torshavn Birth at >36 weeks of gestation; no congenital neurological disease	Maternal and cord serum and seafood intake	Maternal blood taken at week 34, cord blood taken at delivery, questionnaire administered 2 weeks after parturition
Olsen et al., 1991	Cohort	Mothers of live-born singleton infants (n=99) Mean age about 27 years Faroese (n=62) and Danish women (n=37) Delivered at the Landss-jukrahusid and Aarhus Kommenehospital No preeclampsia, rhesus immu-nization, insulin-dependent diabetes mellitus, or twin pregnancies	Peripheral venous blood sample	5-48 hours after delivery

Amount	Results	Conclusion*
Information on fish species or portion sizes was not collected	Gestational length showed a significant positive association with cord serum DHA concentration (p<0.001) and DTA (p=0.004).	B
Fish dinners/week: 0, 1, 2, ≥3	After adjusting for nonsmoking, average-height and nulliparous mother with term birth of male baby, birth weight showed a significant positive association with cord serum ETA (p=0.001), EPA (p=0.015), and DPA (p=0.002).	
Whale meat dinners/month: 0, 1, ≥2		
Whale blubber dinners/month: 0, 1-2, >2	After adjusting for gender, parity, gestational length, smoking, and maternal height, birth weight decreases by 246 g for every one unit increase in cord serum EPA concentration (%) (p=0.037).	
Faroese women: Mean of 0.83±0.039% EPA Mean of 2.08±0.059% DPA Mean of 5.87±0.12% DHA Mean of 12.07±0.15% AA	There were no significant differences in gestational age (p=0.3) and birth weight (p=0.1) between the two groups.	N
Danish women: Mean of 0.61±0.051% EPA Mean of 2.08±0.076% DPA Mean of 4.65±0.159% DHA Mean of 12.07±0.19% AA	After controlling for maternal pre-pregnant weight, height, age, parity, marital status, smoking, and employment during pregnancy a significant association was found between the (3/6) ratio from blood and gestational age in the Danish women (p=0.02) but not in the Faroese women (p=0.6).	

continued

TABLE B-1c Continued

Author	Study Type	Subjects	Exposure	Timing of Exposure
Harper et al., 1991	Case-control	Cases = born to Orkney Island residents, delivered in Orkney Islands (n=899) or Aberdeen (n=116) Controls = born to Aberdeen City district residents (n=2997) Singleton live births Scotland	Resident of Orkney (a proxy for eating more seafood)	

*B = Evidence of a benefit; A = Evidence of an adverse effect; N = Evidence of no association or no clear association.

Amount	Results	Conclusion*
The Orcandians eat 30% more fish than the Aberdonians, but absolute amount undetermined	Mean birth weight of the infants born to residents of Orkney Islands was 3521 g and for residents of Aberdeen was 3287 g (p=0.01).	B
	Gestational age was 0.36 weeks longer in the Orkney women than in the Aberdeen women (p=0.01).	
	18.3% of infants born to Orkney women and 10.0% of infants born to Aberdeen women were over the 90th percentile for birth weight (corrected for gestational age and parity) (p=0.01).	
	4.8% of infants born to Orkney women and 12.2% of infants born to Aberdeen women were below the 10th percentile for birth weight (corrected for gestational age and parity) (p=0.01).	
	Being a resident of Orkney explains a significant proportion of the difference in birth weights between Orkney and Aberdeen women ($R^2 = 0.489$).	

TABLE B-1d Studies on Development (Anthropometry, Visual Acuity, and Cognition): Effects on Infants of Mothers Who Increase Seafood and/or Omega-3 Fatty Acid Intake

Author	Study Type	Subjects	Exposure	Timing of Exposure
Cohen et al., 2005	Review	Aggregated 8 random-ized controlled trials (one study of maternal dietary supplementation and seven studies of for-mula supplementation)	DHA supplement	
Jensen et al., 2005	Randomized Controlled Trial	Pregnant women (n=114 in DHA group; n=113 in control group) Aged 18-40 years Houston, TX White (75% DHA group; 79% control group) African American (19% DHA group; 13% control group) Gestational age >37 weeks Infant birth weight 2500-4200 g No chronic maternal dis-orders as well as major congenital anomalies and obvious gastroin-testinal or metabolic disorders of the infant	DHA supplement	Day 5 after delivery until 4 months postpartum

Amount	Results	Conclusion*
	An increase in maternal intake of DHA during pregnancy of 1 g/day will increase child IQ by 0.8-1.8 points.	B
	"Prenatal maternal DHA intake increasing the child plasma (RBC) DHA phospholipid fraction by 1% has the same impact on cognitive development as formula DHA supplementation that increases the child's plasma (RBC) DHA phospholipid fraction by 1%."	
	"Because typical DHA intake associated with fish consumption is well under 1 g/day, changes in fish consumption will result in IQ effects amounting to a fraction of a point," but they are not clinically detectable.	
DHA capsule: Algal triacylglycerol 200 mg DHA/day Control capsule: Soy and corn oil	There were no significant differences in visual acuity (from either the Teller Acuity Card or Sweep VEP) at 4 or 8 months of age between the two groups. There were no significant differences in mean transient VEP latency at 4 and 8 months of age between the two groups; but the transient VEP amplitude was significantly lower in the infants of the DHA group compared to the infants of the control group. There were no significant differences in Gesell Gross Motor Inventory, CAT, CLAMS DQ, or Bayley MDI between the two groups at 12 or 30 months of age; but Bayley PDI at 30 months of age was 8.4 points higher (p=0.005) in infants of the DHA group compared to infants of the control group.	N

continued

TABLE B-1d Continued

Author	Study Type	Subjects	Exposure	Timing of Exposure
Dunstan et al., 2004	Randomized Controlled Trial	Pregnant women (n=83) Atopic pregnancies Western Australia History of doctor diagnosed allergic rhinitis and/or asthma One or more positive skin prick test to house mites; grass pollens; molds; cat, dog, or cockroach extracts Nonsmokers No other medical problems, complicated pregnancies, seafood allergy, or >2 fish meals/week Term, healthy infants considered at high risk of allergic disease	Fish-oil supplement	20 weeks gestation until delivery
Jensen et al., 2004	Randomized Controlled Trial	Breast-feeding mothers (n=89 in treatment group; n=85 in placebo group)	DHA supplement	Delivery until 4 months postpartum

Amount	Results	Conclusion*
Fish-oil group: 3.7 g/day fish oil 56% DHA and 27.7% EPA 4 capsules/day	Breast milk concentrations of DHA, DPA, and EPA were significantly higher (p<0.001) and AA was significantly lower (p=0.045) in fish-oil supplemented mothers compared with controls.	N/A
Olive-oil group: 66.6% n-9 oleic acid and <1% n-3 PUFA 4 capsules/day	"There were no significant differences in the detection or level of free cytokines or IgA between the 2 groups."	
200 mg/day of DHA vs. placebo	There were no significant differences between the two groups in visual function or neurodevelopment until 30 months of age.	B
	At age 30 months, the Bayley PDI of infants whose mothers were randomized to DHA was 0.55 standard deviations higher (p<0.01) than that of infants whose mothers were randomized to the placebo.	
	There were no significant differences between the two groups in visual function; transient VEP; sweep VEP; stereoacuity; and gross and fine motor, executive, perceptual/visual or verbal domains at age 5.	
	At age 5, infants whose mothers were randomized to DHA had significantly higher Sustained Attention Subtest of the Leiter International Performance Scale than those whose mothers were randomized to the placebo (p<0.008).	

continued

TABLE B-1d Continued

Author	Study Type	Subjects	Exposure	Timing of Exposure
Helland et al., 2003	Randomized Controlled Trial	Pregnant women (n=48 in cod-liver oil group; n=36 in corn oil group) Aged 19-35 years Oslo, Norway Healthy women with, singleton pregnancy, nulli- or primiparous, intention to breastfeed No supplement of n-3 LCPUFA earlier during pregnancy, premature births, birth asphyxia, general infections, or anomalies in the infants that required special attention	Cod-liver oil supplement	From 18 weeks of pregnancy until 3 months after delivery

Amount	Results	Conclusion*

Cod-liver oil:
10 mL/day
1183 mg DHA,
   803 mg EPA
 	
Corn oil:
10 mL/day
4747 mg LA,
   92 mg ALA
	K-ABC scores were significantly higher for the sub-set MPCOMP among children from the cod-liver oil group compared to the corn oil group (p=0.049). The scores for the other subtests (SEQPROC, SIMPROC, NONVERB) were also higher in the cod-liver oil group compared to the corn oil group, but they were not significant.	B

continued

TABLE B-1d Continued

Author	Study Type	Subjects	Exposure	Timing of Exposure
Auestad et al., 2001	Randomized Controlled Trial	Infants (n=294 formula fed; n=165 breastfed) Kansas City, MO; Little Rock, AR; Pittsburgh, PA; Tucson, AZ Good health, term status, either ≤9 days of age (formula group) or ≤11 days of age and currently breastfeeding (breastfeeding group), birth weight ≥2500 g, 5-minute APGAR score ≥7, ability to tolerate milk-based formula or breast milk, guardian or parent agreement to feed the assigned study formula ad libitum according to the study design No evidence of significant cardiac, respiratory, ophthalmologic, gastro-intestinal, hematologic, or metabolic disease; milk-protein allergy; or a maternal medical history known to have proven adverse effects on the fetus, tuberculosis, HIV, perinatal infections, or substance abuse 61-74% European American 60-80% mothers married Mean mother's age about 29 years Mean mother's education about 14 years	Fish oil/fungal oil and egg-derived triglyceride supplemented formulas	9-11 days after birth until 12 months of age

Amount	Results	Conclusion*
Fish oil and fungal oil supplemented preterm formula: 0.46 g AA/100 g total fatty acids ≤0.04 g EPA/100 g total fatty acids 0.13 g DHA/100 g total fatty acids	The vocabulary expression score at 14 months was significantly higher in the fish/fungal group than in the egg-TG group (p<0.05). Smiling and laughter was significantly higher in the control group than in the egg-TG group (p=0.05). No other development, cognition, vocabulary, or temperament outcomes presented were significantly difference between the formula groups.	N
Egg-derived triglyceride supplemented preterm formula: 0.45 g AA/100 g total fatty acids No detected EPA 0.14 g DHA/100 g total fatty acids	No significant differences were found between groups for weight, length, and head circumference or visual acuity.	
Control formula: No detected AA, EPA, DHA		

continued

TABLE B-1d Continued

Author	Study Type	Subjects	Exposure	Timing of Exposure
Helland et al., 2001	Randomized Controlled Trial	Pregnant women (n=590) Aged 19-35 years Oslo, Norway Single pregnancies, nulli- or primipara Intention to breastfeed No supplement of n-3 LCPUFA earlier during the pregnancy No premature births, birth asphyxia, infections, and anomalies in the infants that required special attention	Cod-liver oil supplement	17-19 weeks gestation until 3 months after delivery
McCann and Ames, 2005	Review	Summary of observational, RCTs, other experimental and animal studies	LCPUFA supplement	

Amount	Results	Conclusion*
10 mL/day cod-liver oil vs. corn oil	"There were no significant differences in gestational length or birth weight between the 2 supplement groups. Birth length, head circumference, and placental weight were also similar in the 2 supplement groups."	N
Cod-liver oil: 803 mg of EPA/ 10 mL; 1183 mg DHA/10 mL		
Corn oil: 0 mg of EPA/ 10 mL; 8.3 mg DHA/10 mL		
	"Evidence from chronic dietary restriction rodent studies . . . shows that the addition of DHA to diets of animals whose brain concentration of DHA have been severely reduced restored control performance levels."	B
	"Formula comparison and maternal supplementation studies in humans and ALA dietary restriction studies in nonhuman primates both link the availability of n-3 LCPUFAs to the development of visual attention" and higher DHA status to enhanced neuromotor development.	
	RCTs in humans have often shown no effect of "LCPUFA supplementation on cognitive or behavioral performance and some reviewers have considered that, overall, the evidence was insufficient to conclude that LCPUFA supplementation benefited development."	

continued

TABLE B-1d Continued

Author	Study Type	Subjects	Exposure	Timing of Exposure
Koletzko et al., 2001	Review	Studies published in full or in abstract form	LCPUFA supplement	Prenatal and postnatal periods
Makrides and Gibson, 2000	Review	Summary of the evidence	LCPUFA supplement	During pregnancy and lactation

Amount	Results	Conclusion*
	"Breastfeeding, which supplies preformed LCPUFA, is the preferred method of feeding for healthy infants and is strongly supported."	B
	"Infant formulas should contain at least 0.2% of total fatty acids as DHA and 0.35% as AA; formulas for preterm infants should include at least 0.35% DHA and 0.4% AA."	
	There is an absence of published studies showing direct functional benefits of supplementation of LCPUFA and studies to determine if the variability in LCPUFA status among pregnant women is related to functions in either the mother or infant.	
	"It seems prudent for pregnant and lactating women to include some food sources of DHA in their diet."	
	"There appears to be no detectable reduction in plasma n-3 LCPUFA concentrations during pregnancy, whereas there is a clear decline during the early postpartum period."	B
	"Results of randomized clinical studies suggest that n-3 LCPUFA supplementation during pregnancy does not affect the incidences of pregnancy-induced hypertension and preeclampsia without edema."	
	"n-3 LCPUFA supplementation may cause modest increases in the duration of gestation, birth weight, or both."	
	"To date there is little evidence of harm as a result of n-3 LCPUFA supplementation during either pregnancy or lactation."	

continued

TABLE B-1d Continued

Author	Study Type	Subjects	Exposure	Timing of Exposure
Leary et al., 2005	Cohort	Mother-child pairs (n=6944) Bristol, England Avon Longitudinal Study of Parents and Children (ALSPAC)	Diet	During pregnancy, unspecified

Amount	Results	Conclusion*
Carbohydrate (g) 182-218, 218-258, >258	After adjusting for sex, child's age for blood pressure, and maternal pregnancy energy intake, a significant inverse association was found between omega-3 fatty	N
Protein (g) 55-66, 66-79, >79	acids and offspring blood pressure at age 7.5 years (p=0.04).	
Total fat (g) 55-68, 68-84, >84	After adjusting for sex, child's age for blood pressure, and maternal pregnancy energy intake, there were no	
Saturated fat (g) 21-27, 27-35, >35	significant differences in offspring blood pressure at age 7.5 years based on maternal intake of carbohydrate, protein, total fat, saturated fat, polyunsaturated fat,	
Polyunsaturated fat (g)	monounsaturated fat, calcium, potassium, magnesium, protein/carbohydrate or animal protein.	
9-12, 12-16, >16	After adjusting for measurement factors, current anthropometry, maternal and social factors, birth weight, and	
Monounsaturated fat (g)	gestation, there was a significant positive association found between maternal intake of carbohydrates and	
19-24, 24-30, >30	offspring blood pressure at 7.5 years (p=0.04).	
Calcium (mg) 759-938, 939-1127, >1127	After adjusting for measurement factors, current anthropometry, maternal and social factors, birth weight, and gestation, there were no significant differences between	
Potassium (mg) 2177-2582, 2583-3021, >3021	the tertiles of maternal intake of protein, total fat, saturated fat, polyunsaturated fat, monounsaturated fat, calcium, potassium, magnesium, protein/carbohydrate, animal protein, or omega-3 fatty acid and offsprings'	
Magnesium (mg) 207-254, 255-308, >308	systolic blood pressure at age 7.5 years.	
Protein/carbohydrate 0.26-0.30, 0.31-0.35, >0.35		
Animal protein (g) 35-44, 44-53, >53		
Omega-3 fatty acids (g) 0.03-0.09, 0.10-0.27, >0.27		

continued

TABLE B-1d Continued

Author	Study Type	Subjects	Exposure	Timing of Exposure
Oken et al., 2005	Cohort	Mother-infant pairs (n=135) Aged <30 years (n=16) Aged 30-34 years (n=53) Aged ≥35 years (n=31) 82% White; 18% non-White 80% college or graduate degree Massachusetts Singleton pregnancy, were able to complete forms in English, did not plan to move out of the study area before delivery Project Viva	Seafood	Second trimester of pregnancy
Colombo et al., 2004	Cohort	Infants (n=70) Mean gestation 39.29 weeks Mean birth weight 3248.57 g Mean APGAR score (1 min) 7.94 Mean APGAR score (5 min) 8.80 Mean education (11.77 years for mother and 11.88 for father) 77% African American 21% Caucasian 1% Hispanic Kansas	DHA-enriched egg	24-28 weeks gestation until delivery

Amount	Results	Conclusion*
Number of servings/week: Canned tuna fish (3-4 oz/serving) Shrimp/lobster/ scallop/clam (1 serving) Dark meat fish (3-5 oz/serving) Other fish (3-5 oz/serving) 6 responses from never or less than 1/month to 1 or more servings/day	After controlling for maternal hair mercury level, age, race/ethnicity, education, marital status, infant sex, gestational age at birth, birth weight for gestational age, breast-feeding duration and age at cognitive testing: Each 1 serving/week increase of fish intake increases the VRM score by 4 points (%novelty preference; 95% CI 1.3-6.7). After controlling for maternal seafood intake, age, race/ethnicity, education, marital status, infant sex, gestational age at birth, birth weight for gestational age, breast-feeding duration, and age at cognitive testing: Each 1 ppm increase in maternal hair mercury levels decreases the VRM score by 7.5 points (%novelty preference; 95% CI −13.7 to −1.2).	B
This study is a follow-up to an RCT High-DHA eggs: 135 mg DHA/ egg Ordinary eggs: 35 mg DHA/egg	"Infant red blood cell DHA level was unrelated to subsequent attentional measures, but maternal red blood cell DHA was consistently predictive of later attentional outcomes." "Infants whose mothers had higher levels of DHA at birth showed accelerated developmental courses in attention across the 1st year." Percent of time spent looking in orienting increased over time in both the high- and low-DHA groups, but it was larger in the high-DHA group compared to the low-DHA group at 4, 6, and 8 months. Percent of time spent looking in sustained attention declined over time in both groups, but it was smaller in the high-DHA group compared to the low-DHA group at 4, 6, and 8 months. Percent of time spent looking in attention termination was larger at 4 months in the low-DHA group compared to the high-DHA group, and then declined and leveled off at 6 months in both groups.	B

continued

TABLE B-1d Continued

Author	Study Type	Subjects	Exposure	Timing of Exposure
Daniels et al., 2004	Cohort	Infants (n=1054) Mothers' mean age = 29 years Majority of mothers with at least an O (moderate) level education Bristol, UK Singleton, term births Avon Longitudinal Study of Parents and Children (ALSPAC)	Seafood	Maternal fish intake: 32 weeks of gestation Breastfeeding practices: 15 months after birth Infant fish intake: 6 and 12 months after birth Total mercury concentration: Cord blood at birth
Sakamoto et al., 2004	Cohort	Pregnant women (n=63) Aged 21-41 years Japan Planning to deliver at Munakata Suikokai General Hospital, Fukuoka Healthy	Maternal blood and umbili- cal cord blood lipids	Umbilical cord blood at birth and maternal blood 1 day after parturi- tion before breakfast

Amount	Results	Conclusion*
Maternal fish intake categories (during pregnancy): 1 = Rarely/never 2 = 1 meal/2 weeks 3 = 1-3 meals/week 4 = 4+ meals/week Child fish intake categories (6 months of age): 1 = Rarely/never 2 = 1+ meal/week Child fish intake categories (12 months of age): 1 = Rarely/never 2 = 1+ meal/week	Children whose mothers ate 1-3 fish meals/week and 4+ fish meals/week had significantly lower odds of low MCDI scores for social activity (OR=0.6, 95% CI 0.5-0.8 and OR=0.7, 95% CI 0.5-0.9, respectively) than the children whose mothers rarely or never ate fish during pregnancy. Children whose mothers ate 1-3 fish meals/week and 4+ fish meals/week had significantly lower odds of low DDST scores for language (OR=0.7, 95% CI 0.5-0.9 and OR=0.7, 95% CI 0.5-0.9, respectively) than the children whose mothers rarely or never ate fish during pregnancy. Children who ate 1+ fish meals/week had significantly lower odds of low MCDI scores for vocabulary comprehension (OR=0.7, 95% CI 0.5-0.8) and social activity (OR=0.7, 95% CI 0.6-0.9) and total DDST scores (OR=0.8, 95% CI 0.6-0.9). All other odds ratios presented were nonsignificant.	B
Unspecified	In all cases, fetal RBC-Hg levels (13.4 ng/g) were statistically higher than maternal RBC-Hg levels (8.41 ng/g) (p<0.01). "A strong correlation was observed in RBC-Hg between mothers and fetuses (r=0.92, p<0.001)." "Maternal RBC-Hg concentrations showed significant correlation coefficients with maternal plasma EPA (r=0.36, p<0.001) and DHA (r=0.33, p<0.005) concentrations." "Fetal RBC-Hg concentrations showed a significant positive correlation with fetal plasma EPA (r=0.32, p<0.05) and DHA (r=0.35, p<0.01)."	N/A

continued

TABLE B-1d Continued

Author	Study Type	Subjects	Exposure	Timing of Exposure
Willatts et al., 2003	Cohort	Mother and infant pairs (n=96) Term pregnancy and infant birth weight >2499 g Dundee	DHA and AA content in maternal red blood cells	34-36 weeks gestation
Cheruku et al., 2002	Cohort	Pregnant women (n=17) Men aged 29 years in the high-DHA group Men aged 24 years in the low-DHA group White (n=14) Hispanic (n=3) Windham, CT ≥4 hours of crib time in the first and second days postpartum No history of chronic hypertension, hyperlipidemia, renal or liver disease, heart disease, thyroid disorders, multiple gestations, or pregnancy-induced complications No drugs that affect the respiration of newborns, such as magnesium sulfate and butorphanol	Maternal plasma DHA	Day 1 and day 2 postpartum

Amount	Results	Conclusion*
Absolute DHA and AA levels in blood unspecified	After adjusting for maternal education, social class, birth weight, gestation, type of feeding at birth, and infant age at time of assessment: "There was a significant negative relation between maternal DHA and peak look duration ($p<0.05$), and a significant positive relation between maternal DHA and visual acuity ($p<0.01$)" at 4 months of age. The relation between AA and peak look duration and visual acuity at 4 months of age were not significant. "These results suggest that higher maternal DHA status is related to more efficient information processing and improved visual acuity development in 4-month-old infants."	B
High-DHA group (maternal plasma): >3.0% by weight of total fatty acids Low-DHA group (maternal plasma): ≤3.0% by weight of total fatty acids	On day 2 postpartum, the low-DHA group had significantly higher sleep-wake transition (% of time in crib) and less wakefulness (% time in crib) than the high-DHA group ($p<0.05$). There was a significant group effect for active sleep time ($p=0.004$) and active:quick sleep time ($p=0.001$), these times being shorter in the high-DHA group than in the low-DHA group. "Differences in the prenatal supply of LCPUFAs, especially DHA, may modify brain phospholipids and affect neural function."	B

continued

TABLE B-1d Continued

Author	Study Type	Subjects	Exposure	Timing of Exposure
Haggerty et al., 2002	Cohort	Mothers, smokers (n=11) Mothers, nonsmokers (n=13) Aberdeen, Scotland Uncomplicated, full-term pregnancies Perfusion on term placentas delivered vaginally or by elective Caesarean section from otherwise uncomplicated pregnancies	Placental tissue lipids	Within 20 minutes of delivery
Innis et al., 2001	Cohort	Infants (n=83) Term Birth weight 2500-4500 g Mean mother's age of 32 years British Colombia Intend to breast-feed for 3 months, no solid foods for at least the first 4 months after birth No mothers with substance abuse, communicable diseases, metabolic or physiologic problems, infections likely to influence fetal growth, or multiple births No infants with evidence of metabolic or physical abnormalities	Fatty acids in blood from infants and milk from mothers	2 months of age

Amount	Results	Conclusion*
Unspecified	The rates of transfer of LA and AA per perfused area were not different between the groups; "neither was the rate of placental transfer of ALA and DHA affected by smoking during pregnancy."	N/A
	"In the non-smoking control group the placenta selectively transferred polyunsaturated fatty acids to the fetus in the order DHA > AA > ALA > LA. The order of selectivity was unaltered in placentas from smokers, but the addition of ethanol to the perfusion medium altered the order of selectivity to AA > ALA > LA > DHA."	
	"The presence of ethanol in the perfusate at a concentration of 2 mg/ml significantly reduced ($p<0.01$) the absolute rate of transfer of ALA and DHA."	
Infant DHA: (g/100 g fatty acids) Plasma phospholipids = 2.2-8.0 RBC PE = 6.3-13.0 PC = 1.4-4.6 Infant AA: (g/100 g fatty acids) Plasma phospholipids = 8.1-15.8 RBC PE = 20.2-27.8 PC = 5.6-9.7 Mother's milk: (g/100 g milk fatty acids) DHA = 0.10-2.50 AA = 0.20-0.81 LA = 6.30-21.50 LNA = 0.50-4.10	"The ability to correctly discriminate a retroflex compared with dental phonetic contrast at 9 months of age was positively correlated with the plasma phospholipid DHA ($p<0.02$) and the RBC PE at 2 months of age ($p=0.02$)." "There were no significant correlations between the infants' AA status and the ability to discriminate the native or nonnative language contrasts." "There were no significant correlations between the infant DHA or AA status at 2 months of age and test scores for novelty preference, or the job search task, with adjustments for covariates included in the model."	B

continued

TABLE B-1d Continued

Author	Study Type	Subjects	Exposure	Timing of Exposure
Otto et al., 2001	Cohort	Pregnant women (n=57) Mean age around 30 years Southern Limburg, Netherlands No metabolic, cardiovascular, neurologic, or renal disorders No medications, except multivitamins and iron supplements Singleton pregnancy Term delivery No blood transfusions in the perinatal period	Plasma phospholipids	36-37 weeks gestation; 2-5 days after delivery; 1, 2, 4, 8, 16, 32, 64 weeks postpartum
Williams et al., 2001	Cohort	Boys and girls (n=435) Mean age of 3.5 years Born in last 6 months of the Avon Longitudinal Study of Parents and Children (ALSPAC) enrollment period Healthy term infants	Seafood	During pregnancy for the mothers and at 4 weeks, 4 months, and 6 months for the infants

Amount	Results	Conclusion*
Absolute amount not specified	"After delivery, total fatty acids in plasma phospholipids decreased significantly over time in the lactating and nonlactating women (p<0.0001)." "The amounts of ALA, DHA, and total n-3 fatty acids showed significant downward trends postpartum in both groups, whereas the amounts of EPA and DPA increased significantly after delivery."	N/A
Oily fish consumption categories: 1 = Never or rarely 2 = Once every 2 weeks 3 = More than once every 2 weeks White fish = cod, haddock, plaice, and fish fingers Oily fish = pilchards, sardines, mackerel, tuna, herring, kippers, trout, and salmon	After adjusting for breastfeeding, sex, maternal education, maternal age, housing tenure, financial difficulties, maternal smoking, number of older siblings in household, child care, maternal job status, mother is a vegetarian, mother's fish eating habits: "Mothers who ate oily fish at least once every 2 weeks during pregnancy were more likely to have children who achieved foveal steroacuity than were the mothers who never ate oily fish (OR=1.57, 95% CI 1.00-2.45)," but this was not significant.	B

continued

TABLE B-1d Continued

Author	Study Type	Subjects	Exposure	Timing of Exposure
Haggerty et al., 1999	Cohort	Pregnant women (n=10) Mean age of 31.3 years In last trimester of pregnancy 31-38 weeks gestational age Aberdeen, Scotland Healthy	Fatty acid composition of maternal perfusate	31-38 weeks gestation
Haggerty et al., 1997	Cohort	Term placentae (n=9) Mean weight of 566 g Delivered vaginally or by elective caesarean section Uncomplicated pregnancies Nonsmokers	Placental tissue lipids	Within 20 minutes of delivery
Al et al., 1995	Cohort	Pregnant women (n=110) Aged 19-43 years Maastricht, Netherlands Caucasian Singleton pregnancy DBP <90 mmHg No metabolic, cardiovascular, neurological or renal disorder	Maternal venous and umbilical vein fatty acid profiles	10, 14, 18, 22, 26, 30, 32, 34, 36, 38, 40 weeks gestation; after delivery; 6 months after delivery

Amount	Results	Conclusion*
Unspecified	"When perfused with fatty acids in the ratios found in maternal circulating triglyceride, the human placenta selectively transfers PUFA to the fetus in the order: DHA > ALA > LA > AA."	N/A
	"The ultimate source of fatty acids for the placenta is important for estimates of the likely supply of individual PUFA/LCPUFA to the fetus in utero."	
	"The biggest determinant of transfer of individual fatty acids from the mother to fetus is the supply of fatty acids available in the maternal circulation."	
Unspecified	"The order of selectivity for placental transfer to the fetal circulation was DHA > ALA > LA > oleic acid, whilst the proportion of AA transferred was actually lower than that for oleic acid."	N/A
	"There was no evidence of chain elongation of LA or ALA to any LCPUFA of the n-6 or n-3 series in the perfused placenta."	
Absolute amount not specified	"The average amount of total fatty acid in maternal venous plasma phospholipids increased significantly (p<0.0001) during pregnancy, but the rise in total fatty acids became less pronounced towards the end of gestation (p<0.0001)."	N/A
	Total fatty acids increased from 1238.11 mg/L at week 10 to 1867.84 mg/L at week 40 of gestation, and all of the fatty acid families showed a similar course.	
	"The mean amount of total fatty acids in umbilical plasma phospholipids was substantially lower (p<0.0001) than all maternal values" for all fatty acid families.	
	"In contrast to the absolute amounts of AA and DHA, the mean relative amounts of AA and DHA in umbilical plasma phospholipids were significantly (p<0.0001) higher than all maternal values."	

continued

TABLE B-1d Continued

Author	Study Type	Subjects	Exposure	Timing of Exposure
Clandinin et al., 1980b	Cohort	Male infants (n=14) Female infants (n=7) Died within 3 days of birth Toronto, Canada Infants died from intrapartum asphyxia, congenital heart disease, sudden infant death syndrome, diaphragmatic hernia, and accidental causes Infants were of normal body weight and weight for length, with the exception of two infant males; infants had normal head circumference, with the exception of one infant male No infections or gastrointestinal disorders, apparently normally nourished, and growing reasonably well until the time of death	Tissue fatty acid content from frontal and occipital brain lobes and cerebellum	16 hours postmortem
Bjerve et al., 1993	Case-control	Cases = adults (n=156) Controls = normal human serum stored at –80 degrees C Aged >40 years Nord-Trondelag, Norway Previously undiagnosed diabetic patients Preterm infants (n=21) Very low birth weight, with birth weight <1500 g seen consecutively at the Department of Pediatrics	Seafood and dietary DHA and AA intake	10 weeks for adults and 1 year for the preterms

Amount	Results	Conclusion*
	"Postnatal brain growth, expressed as wet weight of brain tissue, increased during the postpartum period, but was not as rapid as intrauterine brain growth."	N/A
	"In contrast to the fatty acid components, postpartum levels of LA increased 4-fold relative to prenatal levels; postpartum brain levels of AA do not differ from those observed in brain during the third trimester."	
	"Chain elongation-desaturation of AA and LA to longer-chain homologues does not occur at maximal rates for several weeks postnatally or, alternatively, that these long-chain homologues if synthesized in extracerebral tissues may not be directed into synthesis of brain tissue during this early period of infant development."	
Number of fish meals per week: <2, 2, 3, and ≥4 Mean AA intake of these groups: (g/day) 1.22, 1.19, 1.31, 1.59	"After controlling for age, gender, BMI, alcohol intake, and smoking, there was a statistically significant positive correlation based on individual observations between increasing number of fish meals and the concentration of plasma phospholipid EPA (p<0.001) and DHA (p<0.001)."	B
	After controlling for APGAR score and weight at 1 year, 82% of the variance in MDI was explained by a model including the inverse of both DHA and EPA (p=0.0001).	
	After controlling for weight at 1 year, 64% of the variance in PDI was explained by a model including the inverse of DHA (p=0.0001).	

continued

TABLE B-1d Continued

Author	Study Type	Subjects	Exposure	Timing of Exposure
Uauy et al., 1990	Case-control	Case = infants fed formula by day 10 (n=32) Control = infants fed their own mother's milk from birth (n=10) Birth weight appropriate for gestational age, able to receive enteral feedings, free of major neonatal morbidity by day 10	Human milk and milk formula	Day 10 until 36 weeks old
Makrides et al., 1994	Cross-sectional	Male infants (n=16) Female infants (n=19) Died between weeks 2 and 48 South Australia All but two born at term	Human milk and milk formula	Within 48 weeks of birth

Amount	Results	Conclusion*
Human milk: 12.7 g/100 g AA, 1.5 g/100 g n-6 > C18, 0.8 g/100 g ALA, 0.5 g/100 g n-3>C18	"Group C was comparable to the human milk-fed group, but Group A had lower DHA and n-3 LCPUFA in plasma and RBC membranes." "Cone function was not affected by dietary essential fatty acids."	N/A
Formula A: 24.2 g/100 g AA, 0.0 g/100 g n-6 > C18, 0.5 g/100 g ALA, 0.0 g/100 g n-3>C18	"Rod electroretinogram thresholds were significantly higher for Group A relative to the human milk-fed infants and Group C and significantly correlated with RBC n-3 LCPUFA ($p<0.0001$)." "Rod electroretinogram amplitude was significantly lower for Group A relative to the human milk-fed infants and Group C and related to plasma DHA and total n-3 LCPUFA ($p<0.0001$)."	
Formula B: 20.8 g/100 g AA, 0.0 g/100 g n-6 > C18, 2.7 g/100 g ALA, 0.0 g/100 g n-3>C18		
Formula C: 20.4 g/100 g AA, 0.1 g/100 g n-6 > C18, 1.4 g/100 g ALA, 1.0 g/100 g n-3>C18		
Breast-feeding index = length of breastfeeding as a % of age at death: Breast-fed: ≥85% Formula fed: <30% LA in formula ranged from 12.0% to 15.0% and ALA in formula ranged from 1.0% to 1.6%	Erythrocyte fatty acid composition of tissues were significantly lower in total saturated fatty acids ($p<0.05$), AA ($p<0.05$), and DHA ($p<0.05$) and significantly higher in DGLA ($p<0.05$), EPA ($p<0.05$), and DPA ($p<0.05$) for infants fed formula compared to those fed from the breast. Cortex fatty acid composition of tissues were significantly higher in 22:4n-6 ($p<0.05$), 22:5n-6 ($p<0.05$), and total n-6 ($p<0.005$) and lower in DHA ($p<0.005$) and total n-3 ($p<0.005$) for infants fed formula compared to those fed from the breast. There were no significant differences in retina fatty acid composition of tissues between the formula-fed and breast-fed infants.	B

continued

TABLE B-1d Continued

Author	Study Type	Subjects	Exposure	Timing of Exposure
Farquharson et al., 1992	Cross-sectional	Term infants (n=20) Preterm infants (n=2) Greater Glasgow Health Board area Died within 43 weeks of birth Previously well infants who died suddenly in the home, "cot deaths"	Human milk and milk formula	Within 43 weeks of birth
Martinez, 1992	Cross-sectional	Infants born at different gestational ages and died soon after birth of acute causes that were not related to the central nervous system Not fed but mothers well-nourished Infants nourished in utero and after birth	PUFA supplementation and PUFA-enriched formula	After infant died (they died shortly after birth)

Amount	Results	Conclusion*
Breast milk or the formula milks SMA Gold Cap and/or White Cap, Cow and Gate Premium, or Osterfeed	"Breast fed infants had greater concentrations of DHA in their cerebral cortex phospholipids than either the mixed fed group or the older SMA and CGOST groups." "No significant differences in phospholipid fatty acid content of cerebral cortex were found between the age-comparable SMA and CGOST groups."	N/A
Prenatal fatty acid amounts not specified	"Long-chain fatty acids accumulate in the human brain during the brain's growth spurt unless a serious imbalance in the supply of LA and ALA occurs." "The active formation of synaptic structures and dendritic arborizations increases significantly between 31 weeks of gestation and term." "It seems highly desirable to enrich parenteral lipids and milk formulas with DHA to provide between 0.5% and 1% of total fatty acids similar to those in human milk." "A total n-6/n-3 fatty acid ratio between 5 and 7 seems appropriate according to our analysis of human milk from others consuming complete, balanced Mediterranean diets rich in fish."	B

continued

TABLE B-1d Continued

Author	Study Type	Subjects	Exposure	Timing of Exposure
Kodas et al., 2004	Animal	2 generations of female Wistar rats	ALA-deficient diet	Control group: Control diet at birth to 60 days after birth
				Deficient group: Deficient diet at birth to 60 days after birth
				Diet reversed group 1: Control diet at day of birth until 60 days after birth
				Diet reversed group 2: Deficient diet until day 7 of life and then control diet from day 7 to day 60 of life
				Diet reversed group 3: Deficient diet until day 14 of life and then control diet from day 14 to day 60 of life
				Diet reversed group 4: Deficient diet until day 21 of life and then control diet from day 21 to day 60 of life

Amount	Results	Conclusion*
ALA-deficient diet: 6% fat African peanut oil	The fatty acid composition of phosphatidylcholine in the hippocampus of 2-month-old rats was as follows:	B
<6 mg ALA/100 g diet 1200 mg LA/100 g diet	AA was not significantly different among the different diet groups; DHA was significantly higher in the control group and all diet reversed groups compared to the deficient group (p<0.05); n-6:n-3 was significantly lower in the control group and all diet reversed groups compared to the deficient group (p<0.05); these differences were not significant between the control group and the diet reversed groups.	
Control diet: 60% peanut oil, 40% rapeseed oil		
200 mg ALA/100 g diet 1200 mg LA/100 g diet	The fatty acid composition of phosphatidylethanolamine in the hippocampus of 2-month-old rats was as follows:	

AA was significantly lower in the control group and all diet reversed groups compared to the deficient group (p<0.05); DHA was significantly higher in the control group and all diet reversed groups compared to the deficient group (p<0.05); n-6:n-3 was significantly lower in the control group and all diet reversed groups compared to the deficient group (p<0.05); these differences were not significant between the control group and the diet reversed groups.

The fatty acid composition of phosphatidylserine in the hippocampus of 2-month-old rats was as follows:

AA was not significantly different among the different diet groups; DHA was significantly higher in the control group and all diet reversed groups compared to the deficient group (p<0.05); n-6:n-3 was significantly lower in the control group and all diet reversed groups compared to the deficient group (p<0.05); these differences were not significant between the control group and the diet reversed groups; and

Basal 5-HT levels were significantly higher in the deficient group compared with the control group (p<0.05); there were no significant differences in basal 5-HT levels between the diet reversed groups 1, 2, and 3 and the control group; there were no significant differences in basal 5-HT levels between the diet reversed group 4 and the control group, deficient group, and all other diet reversed groups.

continued

TABLE B-1d Continued

Author	Study Type	Subjects	Exposure	Timing of Exposure
Korotokova et al., 2004	Animal	Pregnant Sprauge-Dawley rats	n-6:n-3 diet, n-3 diet, and n-6 diet	10 days before delivery
				10-16 days of lactation, dam fed water with ovalbumin or just water

Amount	Results	Conclusion*
n-6:n-3 diet (in mol%):	In the pups not exposed to ovalbumin:	B
7.0% soybean oil 56.0% LA, 6.2% ALA, 9.0% n-6:n-3	Delayed-type hypersensitivity responses against ovalbumin, as well as against human serum ovalbumin were not significantly different between the dietary groups;	
n-3 diet (in mol%): 7.0% linseed oil	IgG anti-avalbumin and IgG anti-human serum ovalbumin antibodies were not significant different between the three diet groups;	
14.0% LA, 33.0% ALA, 0.4% n-6:n-3	IgM anti-ovalbumin antibodies in the n-3 diet group are significantly higher than those in the n-6:n-3 diet group (p<0.05); and	
n-6 diet (in mol%): 7.0% sunflower oil 65.0% LA, 0.3% ALA, 216.0% n-6:n-3	IgM anti-human serum ovalbumin antibodies in the n-3 diet group are significantly higher that those in the n-6:n-3 diet group (p<0.05).	
	In the pups exposed to ovalbumin:	
	Delayed-hypersensitivity responses against ovalbumin were significantly higher in the n-6:n-3 diet group compared to the n-3 diet group and the n-6 diet group, while delayed-hypersensitivity responses to human serum ovalbumin were significantly higher in the n-6:n-3 diet group compared to the n-3 diet group (p<0.05);	
	IgG anti-human serum ovalbumin antibodies were significantly higher in the n-6:n-3 diet group than those in the n-3 diet group (p<0.05); and	
	IgM anti-human serum ovalbumin antibodies in the n-3 diet group are significantly lower than those in the n-6:n-3 diet group and the n-6 diet group (p<0.05).	
	Those in the n-3 diet group exposed to ovalbumin have significantly lower IgG ovalbumin, IgG anti-human serum ovalbumin, IgM anti-ovalbumin, and IgM anti-human serum ovalbumin antibodies than those not exposed to ovalbumin (p<0.05).	
	Those in the n-6 diet group exposed to ovalbumin have significantly lower IgG ovalbumin and IgM anti-ovalbumin antibodies than those not exposed to ovalbumin (p<0.05).	

continued

TABLE B-1d Continued

Author	Study Type	Subjects	Exposure	Timing of Exposure
Levant et al., 2004	Animal	Adult female Long-Evans rats	LCPUFA-deficient diet	Control diet: Day 1 of pregnancy until end of study Deficient diet: Day 1 of pregnancy until postnatal day 21. Postnatal day 21, half on deficient diet were changed to remediation diet and half stayed on deficient diet

Amount	Results	Conclusion*
Control diet: 0.35 kg/5 kg diet from soybean oil; no detected AA, EPA, DPA, or DHA	"Rats raised on the deficient diet exhibited a decrease in brain DHA content to 80% of control animals at maturity (p<0.05)" and an "increase in DPA content to 575% of control animals at maturity (p<0.001)." The remediation diet restored brain DHA and DPA content to levels similar to those on the control diet.	A
Deficient diet: 0.35 kg/5 kg diet from sunflower oil; no detected AA, EPA, DPA, or DHA	Catalepsy score was significantly lower in the deficient diet group compared to the control group (p<0.05) and the remediation diet group (p<0.05). In a test of locomotor activity in a novel environment, the deficient diet group exhibited 187% of the activity of the control diet group during the 2-hour observation (p<0.05); results were similar between the deficient diet group and the remediation diet group.	
Remediation diet: 0.3275 kg/5 kg diet from sunflower oil and 0.0225 kg/5 kg diet from fish oil 0.1 g/100 g fatty acids AA, 1.6 g/100 g fatty acids EPA, 0.4 g/100 g fatty acids DPA, 3.5 g/100 g fatty acids DHA	In the test of amphetamine-stimulated locomotor activity, the deficient diet group exhibited 144% of the activity of the control group (p<0.05).	

continued

TABLE B-1d Continued

Author	Study Type	Subjects	Exposure	Timing of Exposure
Neuringer et al., 1986	Animal	Adult female rhesus monkeys	n-3-deficient diet	2 months before conception and throughout pregnancy

*B = Evidence of a benefit; N = Evidence of no association or no clear association; N/A = A conclusion is not available; these data are presented for background information only; A = Evidence of an adverse effect.

Amount	Results	Conclusion*

Semipurified diet:
Deficient in n-3
  fatty acids
Safflower oil was
  sole fat source
High n-6:n-3 ratio
 	
Controls:
Soybean oil was
  sole fat source
High in LA
	At all ages, animals of the "deficient group had considerably lower levels of n-3 fatty acids in tissue phospholipids than their controls."
	
	Based on the occipital cortex, perinatal 22:5n-6 (p<0.01) and total n-6 (p<0.05) were significantly higher and perinatal DHA (p<0.01) and total n-3 (p<0.01) were significantly lower in the deficient group compared to the control group.
	
	Based on the occipital cortex, 22:4n-6 (p<0.01), 22:5n-6 (p<0.01), and total n 6 (p<0.01) at 22 months were significantly higher and DHA (p<0.01) and total n-3 (p<0.01) at 22 months were significantly lower in the deficient group compared to the control group.
	
	Based on the frontal cortex, perinatal 22:5n-6 (p<0.01) was significantly higher and perinatal DHA (p<0.01) and total n-3 (p<0.01) were significantly lower in the deficient group compared to the control group.
	
	Based on the frontal cortex, 22:5n-6 (p<0.01) and total n-6 (p<0.01) at 22 months were significant higher and DHA (p<0.01) and total n-3 (p<0.01) at 22 months were significantly lower in the deficient group compared to the control group.
		N/A

TABLE B-1e Studies on Allergies: Effects on Infants and Children of
Mothers Who Increase Seafood and/or Omega-3 Fatty Acid Intake

Author	Study Type	Subjects	Exposure	Timing of Exposure
Denburg et al., 2005	Randomized Controlled Trial	Pregnant women (n=83) Booked for delivery at St. John of God Hospital Subiaco, Western Australia With confirmed allergy No smoking, other medical problems, complicated pregnancies, seafood allergy; normal dietary intake did not exceed two meals of fish per week	Fish-oil supplement	20 weeks of pregnancy until delivery

Amount	Results	Conclusion*
Fish oil group: 3.7 g of n-3 PUFA 56.0% as DHA and 27.7% as EPA

Placebo group: 2.6 g olive oil 26 g/day oleic acid | Infants of those in the fish oil group had a significantly higher %CD34 expression than infants of those in the placebo group (p<0.002).

There was no significant difference between the two groups with respect to expression of all cytokine and chemokine receptors.

There was a significant association found between CD34+ in cord blood and AEDS (OR=3.93; 95% CI 1.05-14.64, p=0.042) at one year of age; however, there were no significant associations found for food allergy, moderate severe AEDS, asthma, chronic cough, or recurrent wheeze.

There were significant associations found between cord blood progenitor responsiveness to IL-5 and AEDS (OR=1.09, 95% CI 1.00-1.18, p=0.039) and recurrent wheeze (OR=1.11, 95% CI 1.02-1.21, p=0.022) at one year of age; however, there were no significant associations found for food allergy, moderate severe AEDS, asthma, or chronic cough. | B |

continued

TABLE B-1e Continued

Author	Study Type	Subjects	Exposure	Timing of Exposure
Dunstan et al., 2003a	Randomized Controlled Trial	Pregnant women (n=83) Atopic women Booked for delivery at St. John of God Hospital Subiaco, Western Australia Physician-diagnosed allergic rhinitis and/or asthma Allergic to house dust mites, grass pollens, molds, cat, dog, feathers, and cockroach and/or asthma No medical problems, no smoking, no complicated pregnancies, no seafood allergy; normal diet did not exceed two meals of fish per week	Fish-oil supplement	20 weeks of pregnancy until delivery
Dunstan et al., 2003b	Randomized Controlled Trial	Pregnant women (n=83) Atopic women Booked for delivery at St. John of God Hospital Subiaco, Western Australia Physician-diagnosed allergic rhinitis and/or asthma Allergic to house dust mites, grasses, molds, cat, dog, feathers, and cockroach and/or asthma No medical problems, no smoking, no complicated pregnancies, no seafood allergy; normal diet did not exceed two meals of fish per week; no preterm deliveries	Fish-oil supplement	20 weeks of pregnancy until delivery

Amount	Results	Conclusion*
Fish oil group: Four 1 g fish oil capsules/day 3.7 g of n-3 PUFA 56.0% as DHA and 27.7% as EPA	Neonatal in vitro IL-10 response to cat allergen was significantly lower in the fish oil group than in the placebo group (p=0.046). At birth, no significant differences were found in the neonates' cytokine response to allergens and mitogens in the two groups at birth.	B
Placebo group: Four 1 g olive oil capsules/day 66.6% n-9 oleic acid and <1.0% n-3 PUFA	IFN-γ responses to OVA were detected more frequently in the control group than in the fish oil group (p=0.009). There were no significant differences found in the frequency of detectable IL-5, IL-10, or IL-13 responses between the two groups. "The detection of a lymphoproliferative response to allergens also tended to be lower in the fish oil group compared with the control group," although this difference was not always significant (OR=4.48, 95% CI 0.87-23.07 for response to OVA allergen and OR=2.02, 95% CI 0.69-5.88 for response to cat).	
Fish oil group: Four 1 g fish oil capsules/day 3.7 g of n-3 PUFA 56.0% as DHA and 27.7% as EPA	IL-13 levels were significantly lower (p=0.025) in neonates whose mothers received fish-oil supplements in pregnancy compared to the placebo group. There were no significant differences in IFN-γ levels in cord plasmas or in IgE in plasma between the two groups.	B
Placebo group: Four 1 g olive oil capsules/day 66.6% n-9 oleic acid and <1.0% n-3 PUFA	There were no significant differences in the frequency of lymphocyte subsets for total T cells, T helper cells, T suppressor cells, NK cells, and B cells between the two groups. After adjusting for parity, gender, and delivery method, there were significant associations between cord plasma IL-13 levels and neonatal red cell membrane DHA levels (β=-0.25, 95% CI -0.49 to -0.01) and total n-3 fatty acid levels (β=-2.70, 95% CI -5.35 to -0.05).	

continued

TABLE B-1e Continued

Author	Study Type	Subjects	Exposure	Timing of Exposure
Hawkes et al., 2002	Randomized Controlled Trial	Women (n=120) Aged 20-42 years, mean about 30 years Delivered full-term single-ton infants, intended to breast-feed ≥12 weeks Adelaide, South Australia No known history of inflammatory disorders, not currently taking anti-inflammatory medication or fish-oil supplements Excluded women who had ceased lactating by 4 weeks postpartum	DHA supplement	Day 3- week 12 postpartum

Amount	Results	Conclusion*
Asked to limit fish and seafood intake to a maximum of 1 meal/week	"There was no significant difference between the dietary groups in mean rank concentrations of IL-6 or TNF-α in the aqueous phase of milk" at 4 weeks postpartum.	N
Placebo: 500 mg placebo oil	"There was no significant difference in mean rank concentrations between the dietary groups for any of the cytokines produced by cells isolated from human milk or peripheral blood after in vitro stimulation with lipopolysaccharide or in the absence of stimulation" at 4 weeks postpartum.	
Low-DHA capsule group: 70 mg EPA/day, 300 mg DHA/ day		
High DHA capsule group: 140 mg EPA/ day, 600 mg DHA/day		

continued

TABLE B-1e Continued

Author	Study Type	Subjects	Exposure	Timing of Exposure
Hodge et al., 1998	Randomized Controlled Trial	Boys and girls (n=39) Aged 8-12 years Sydney, Australia Asthmatic with a history of episodic wheeze in the last 12 months, AHR to histamine	Omega-3 diet and omega-6 diet	6 months

Amount	Results	Conclusion*
Omega-3 diet group: Canola oil and canola-based margarines and salad dressings to replace usual oils and margarines Supplement capsules = 0.18 g EPA and 0.12 g DHA/capsule 4 capsules/day = 1.20 g omega-3/ day	"There was no significant change in spirometric function, dose-response ratio to histamine or asthma severity score at either 3 or 6 months in either group."	N
Omega-6 diet group: Sunflower oil and sunflower oil-based margarines and salad dressings to replace usual oils and margarines Supplement capsules = 0.45 g safflower oil, 0.45 g palm oil, 0.10 g olive oil/capsule No EPA or DHA		

continued

TABLE B-1e Continued

Author	Study Type	Subjects	Exposure	Timing of Exposure
Newson et al., 2004	Cohort	Children (n=1238 with cord blood fatty acid data and eczema at 18 to 30 months data; n=2945 with maternal blood fatty acid data and eczema data; n=2764 with maternal blood fatty acid data and wheezing data) Bristol, England Avon Longitudinal Study of Parents and Children (ALSPAC)	Cord blood and maternal blood red cell fatty acid analysis	20 weeks of pregnancy and at delivery

*B = Evidence of a benefit; N = Evidence of no association or no clear association.

Amount	Results	Conclusion*
Cord blood (percentages of total red blood cell membrane phospholipid): Medians: 0.02 ALA, 0.11 EPA, 0.22 DPA, 2.00 DHA, 4.65 LA, and 7.80 AA	After controlling for sex, gestational age at birth, birth weight, mother's age, education level, housing tenure, parity, ethnicity, smoking in pregnancy, maternal atopic disease, child's head circumference at birth, child's crown to heel length at birth, mother's BMI, breast-feeding in first 6 months, and day care use in first 6 months:	N
	All associations between fatty acid exposure (based on cord blood levels and maternal blood levels) and eczema at 18 to 30 months were found to be nonsignificant;	
Maternal blood (percentages of total red blood cell membrane phospholipid): Medians: 0.14 ALA, 0.23 EPA, 0.60 DPA, 2.02 DHA, 11.16 LA, and 5.88 AA	All associations between fatty acid exposure (based on both cord blood levels and maternal blood levels) and wheezing at 30 to 42 months of age were found to be nonsignificant;	
	LA:ALA levels in cord blood were significantly associated with later-onset wheeze (OR–1.30, 95% CI 1.04-1.61), as was the ratio of ALA:sum of n-3 products (OR=0.86, 95% CI 0.75-0.99); and	
	No other significant associations were found between fatty acid exposure and transient infant wheeze, later-onset wheeze, or persistent wheeze.	

TABLE B-1f Studies on Visual Acuity: Effects on Infants Supplemented with Omega-3 Fatty Acids in Formula

Author	Study Type	Subjects	Exposure	Timing of Exposure
Simmer, 2005	Cochrane Review	9 Randomized Controlled Trials	LCPUFA-supplemented formula	
Gibson et al., 2001	Review	Randomized Controlled Trials (11 on preterm and 10 on term infants) Involving healthy preterm infants fed preterm formula Involving healthy term infants fed formulas from near birth Systematic literature review	DHA-supplemented formula	
Uauy et al., 2001	Review	Summary of Random-ized Controlled Trials on preterm and term infants	LCPUFA-supplemented formula	

Amount	Results	Conclusion*
	"There is little evidence from randomized trials of LCPUFA supplementation to support the hypothesis that LCPUFA supplementation confers a benefit for visual or general development of term infants."	N
	"Minor effects on VEP acuity have been suggested, but appear unlikely when all studies are reviewed."	
	"Benefits of adding DHA to formulas (with or without AA) on VEP acuity have been reported in some studies, whereas other studies have failed to detect a benefit of LC-PUFA supplementation."	B
	There is evidence supporting "the view that dietary essential fatty acid supply affects visual development of preterm and term infants."	B

continued

TABLE B-1f Continued

Author	Study Type	Subjects	Exposure	Timing of Exposure
SanGiovanni et al., 2000a	Meta-analysis	Studies done in industrialized countries Healthy, term infants Randomized studies: DHA supplemented (n=114) DHA-free (n=87) Nonrandomized studies: Milk-fed/behavioral-based (n=117 at 2 months; n=148 at 4 months) Milk-fed/electrophysiological tasks (n=146 at 4 months) DHA-free/behavioral-based (n=174 at 2 months; n=113 at 4 months) DHA-free/electrophysiological tasks (n=108 at 4 months) All study designs: DHA-supplemented/behavioral-based at 2 months (n=219) DHA-supplemented/electrophysiological tasks at 4 months (n=265) DHA-free/behavioral-based at 2 months (n=86) DHA-free/electrophysiological tasks at 4 months (n=109)	DHA-supplemented formula	

Amount	Results	Conclusion*
	Based on behavioral tests of visual acuity, the randomized studies showed a significant difference in the estimates for those fed DHA-supplemented formula vs. those fed unsupplemented formula at 2 months of age (p≤0.0005). This difference was not significant at any other age presented.	B
	Based on behavioral tests of visual acuity, the non-randomized studies showed a significant difference in the estimates for those fed human milk vs. those fed unsupplemented formula at 2 months of age (p≤0.0005) and 4 months of age (p<0.05) This difference was not significant at any other age presented.	
	Based on electrophysiological tests of visual acuity, the randomized studies showed a significant difference in the estimates for those fed (DHA-supplemented) formula vs. those fed unsupplemented formula at 7 months of age (p≤0.05). This difference was not significant at any other age presented.	
	Based on electrophysiological tests of visual acuity, the nonrandomized studies showed a significant difference in the estimates for those fed human milk vs. those fed unsupplemented formula at 4 months of age (p≤0.0005), 5 months of age (p≤0.05), and 7 months of age (p≤0.05). This difference was not significant at any other age presented.	

continued

TABLE B-1f Continued

Author	Study Type	Subjects	Exposure	Timing of Exposure
SanGiovanni et al., 2000b	Meta-analysis	5 original papers (4 prospective trials) 4 review chapters Preterm infants Randomized studies: DHA-supplemented/behavioral-based (n=48 at 2 months; n=70 at 4 months) DHA-supplemented/VEP at 4 months (n=13) DHA-free/behavioral-based (n=49 at 2 months; n=56 at 4 months) DHA-free/VEP at 4 months (n=28) All study designs: DHA-supplemented/behavioral-based at 4 months (n=80) DHA-supplemented/VEP at 4 months (n=37) DHA-free/behavioral-based at 4 months (n=87) DHA-free/VEP at 4 months (n=43)	DHA-supplemented formula	

Amount	Results	Conclusion*
	Based on behavioral tests of visual acuity, the randomized comparisons (between those fed DHA-supplemented formula and those fed unsupplemented formula) showed significant differences at 2 and 4 months of age (p≤0.001). This difference was not significant at any other age presented.	B

continued

TABLE B-1f Continued

Author	Study Type	Subjects	Exposure	Timing of Exposure
Hoffman et al., 2003	Randomized Controlled Trial	Infants (n=61) Healthy, term, singleton infants Birth weight appropriate for gestational age Breast-fed to 4-6 months North Dallas area, TX 95% White No family history of milk protein allergy; genetic or familial eye disease; vegetarian or vegan maternal dietary patterns; maternal metabolic disease, anemia, or infection; presence of a congenital malformation or infection; jaundice; perinatal asphyxia; meconium aspiration; or any perinatal event that resulted in placement in the neonatal intensive care unit	AA/DHA-supplemented formula	Enrolled at 6.5 weeks of age until 12 months of age (during time of weaning)

Amount	Results	Conclusion*
Commercial formula (Enfamil with iron) or commercial formula supplemented with 0.36% of total fatty acids as DHA and 0.72% as AA	There were no significant differences in VEP acuity before weaning in the two groups, but at 12 months the supplemented group had significantly better VEP acuity than infants in the commercial formula group ($p<0.0005$).	B
	There was a trend of better stereoacuity in the supplemented group compared to the commercial group at 9 months ($p=0.12$) and 12 months ($p=0.13$).	

continued

TABLE B-1f Continued

Author	Study Type	Subjects	Exposure	Timing of Exposure
Birch et al., 2002	Randomized Controlled Trial	Infants (n=65) Healthy, term, singleton births Birth weight appropriate for gestational age Weaned from breast-feeding at 6 weeks of age Dallas area, TX Mean maternal age about 30 years 75-78% White Majority of mothers with at least a college degree No family history of milk protein allergy; genetic or familial eye disease; vegetarian or vegan maternal dietary patterns; maternal metabolic disease, anemia, or infection; presence of a congenital malformation or infection; jaundice; perinatal asphyxia; meconium aspiration; or any perinatal event that resulted in placement in the neonatal intensive care unit	AA/DHA-supplemented formula	6 weeks of age to 52 weeks of age

Amount	Results	Conclusion*
Commercial formula (Enfamil with iron) or commercial formula supplemented with 0.36% of total fatty acids as DHA and 0.72% as AA	There were no significant differences in VEP acuity at age 6 weeks between the two groups. The control group had significantly poorer visual acuity at week 17 (p<0.003), week 26 (p<0.001), and week 52 (p<0.001) compared to the supplemented group.	B

continued

TABLE B-1f Continued

Author	Study Type	Subjects	Exposure	Timing of Exposure
Innis et al., 2002	Randomized Controlled Trial	Infants (n=194) Premature Healthy, very low birth weight infants (846-1560 g), formula-fed Multi-center study (16 neonatal centers in North America) Not small for gestational age or >24 days postnatal age when full enteral feeds ≥375 kJ/kg/day were achieved No necrotizing enterocolitis or other gastrointestinal disease, impaired visual or ocular status, or a history of underlying disease or congenital malformation that could interfere with growth Reference group = term infants whose mothers anticipated breastfeeding for at least 4 months	AA/DHA-supplemented formula	Preterm formulas: At least 28 days after enteral intake of 375 kJ/kg/day reached

Term formulas: After hospital discharge until 57 weeks of age |

Amount	Results	Conclusion*
Preterm formula 1 = Control formula (no AA or DHA)	At 57 weeks, visual acuity of the breast-fed term infants was significantly higher than in the premature infants, but not at 48 weeks; at 48 or 57 weeks, visual acuity was not significantly different among the premature infant groups.	N
Preterm formula 2 = DHA formula (0.34% fatty acids as DHA)		
Preterm formula 3 = DHA+AA formula (0.33% fatty acids as DHA, 0.60% fatty acids as AA)		
Term formula = no AA or DHA		
Breast-fed term infants = no solid foods during the study unless otherwise instructed by their physicians		

continued

TABLE B-1f Continued

Author	Study Type	Subjects	Exposure	Timing of Exposure
Van Wezel-Meijler et al., 2002	Randomized Controlled Trial	Infants (n=42) Preterm, admitted to neo-natal intensive- or high-care unit of hospital Birth weight <1750 g Leiden, Netherlands Mothers not breast-feeding Normal neurological ex-amination throughout the neonatal period Repeated ultrasound of the brain being normal or showing, at most, minor abnormalities No abnormalities of the central nervous system; abnormal neurological examination or occur-rence of seizures; any systemic disease with potential negative influ-ence on future growth or development; serious nutritional or gastro-intestinal problems preventing initiation of enteral feeding after the first week postpartum or complete enteral feeding after the third week postpartum; reti-nopathy of prematurity grade 3 or more	AA/DHA-supplemented formula	2-3 weeks after birth until weighing 3000 g

Amount	Results	Conclusion*
Supplemented preterm formula: 4.4 g fat/100 mL 0.015 g/100 mL of added DHA (microalgae) 0.031 g/100 mL of added AA (fungi) Control formula: 4.4 g fat/100 mL No addition of AA and DHA	There were no significant differences found in Flash VEP at 3 and 12 months between the two groups. There were no significant differences found in visual acuity at 3, 6, 12, or 24 months between the two groups.	N

continued

TABLE B-1f Continued

Author	Study Type	Subjects	Exposure	Timing of Exposure
Makrides et al., 2000	Randomized Controlled Trial	Infants (n=73 in formula groups; n=63 in breast-fed group) White Full-term and appropriate weight for gestational age Mean mothers' education was mid-secondary school level for formula-fed infants and completion of second-ary school for breast-fed infants No congenital disease or complications during pregnancy	AA/DHA-supplemented formula	Age at entry not specified, up to 34 weeks of age
Bougle et al., 1999	Randomized Controlled Trial	Infants (n=40) Mean age about 33 weeks Enrolled the 2nd day of enteral feeding Healthy, appropriate weight for gestational age Premature Free of respiratory, meta-bolic or neurological disease; malformations; infections; intrauterine asphyxia Fed by digestive route within the first 7 days of life	LCPUFA-supplemented formula	Within the first 2 days of enteral feed-ing, then for 30 days

Amount	Results	Conclusion*
Placebo formula (% total fatty acids): 16.8% LA, 1.5% ALA	After adjusting for gender, postconceptional age, birth weight, and maternal smoking, there were no significant differences in VEP between any of the groups at 16 or 34 weeks of age.	N
DHA formula (% total fatty acids): 16.80% LA, 1.20% ALA, 0.10% EPA, 0.35% DHA		
DHA+AA formula (% total fatty acids): 16.60% LA, 0.34% AA, 1.00% ALA, 0.34% DHA		
Breast milk (% total fatty acids, mean±SE): 13.40±2.90% LA, 0.39±0.07% AA, 0.95±0.32% ALA, 0.09±0.03% EPA, 0.20±0.07% DHA		
Breast milk (% total fatty acids, mean±SE): 14.1±2.0% LA, 0.4±0.2% GLA, 0.9±0.2% AA, 0.5±0.1% ALA, 0.5±0.1% DHA	There were no significant differences between the groups based on electrophysiological data, except that the maturation of the motor nerve conduction was significantly slower in the Formula B group than in the breast milk group and the Formula A group ($p<0.05$).	N
Formula A (% total fatty acids): 14.1% LA, 1.3% ALA		
Formula B (% total fatty acids): 17.7% LA, 0.4% GLA, 0.1% AA, 1.2% ALA, 0.1% EPA, 0.6% DHA		

continued

TABLE B-1f Continued

Author	Study Type	Subjects	Exposure	Timing of Exposure
Carlson et al., 1999	Randomized Controlled Trial	Infants (n=119)	AA/DHA-supplemented formula	<8 days of age until about 12 months of age
				Infants fed supplemented formula near birth received commercial formula from term less 3 months until 12 months of age; infants fed supplemented formula near term received commercial formula from term less 3 months to term less 1 month, and then supplemented formula until 12 months of age

Amount	Results	Conclusion*
Commercially avail-able standard formula contained no EPA or DHA	Compared to the infants not supplemented, "only those supplemented near birth had higher acuity at 2 months (p<0.02) and a trend toward higher acuity at 6 months (p<0.07)."	B
Supplemented formula 0.13% DHA and 0.40% AA from egg phospholipids	Infants supplemented at birth "also had higher acuity than those supplemented at term at 2 months (p<0.05)." "First year acuity continued to increase (p<0.05) between consecutive ages until 6 months" in those supplemented at birth and 9 months in those un-supplemented and supplemented at term. "All groups had similar acuity at 9 and 12 months."	

continued

TABLE B-1f Continued

Author	Study Type	Subjects	Exposure	Timing of Exposure
Birch et al., 1998	Randomized Controlled Trial	Infants (n=108) Healthy, term, birth weight appropriate for gestational age Singleton births Dallas, TX 75% White, 12% Black, 12% Hispanic, 1% other Mean maternal age 29 years 67.6% mothers completed at least 2 years of college No family history of milk protein allergy; genetic or familial eye disease; vegetarian or vegan maternal dietary patterns; maternal metabolic disease, anemia, or infection; presence of a congenital malformation or infection; jaundice; perinatal asphyxia; meconium aspiration; or any perinatal event that resulted in placement in the neonatal intensive care unit	AA/DHA- enriched formula	0-4 days postpartum through 17 weeks of age
Carlson et al., 1996a	Randomized Controlled Trial	Infants (n=58) Born at term (37-43 weeks) Birth weight 747-1275 g Memphis, TN Predominantly Black No growth retardation in utero and no medical problems likely to influence long-term growth and development Mothers education mean of about 12 years	DHA- supplemented formula	24 hours after birth; end point not specified

Amount	Results	Conclusion*
Enfamil + iron Enfamil + iron + 0.35% DHA Enfamil + iron + 0.36% DHA + 0.72% AA	Visual acuity was significantly poorer in the control group than in the DHA or DHA+AA groups and the breast-fed group. At 6, 17, 26, and 52 weeks the association between RBC AA and sweep VEP was not statistically significant. The association was also nonsignificant for RBC EPA. At 6, 17, 26, and 52 weeks, the association between RBC DHA was significantly associated with lower sweep VEP (p<0.001, p–0.01, p–0.05, p<0.001, respectively). At 6, 17, and 52 weeks, the association between RBC n-3:n-6 was significantly associated with lower sweep VEP (p<0.001, p=0.03, p<0.001, respectively); the association was not statistically significant at 26 weeks.	B
Formula with AA+DHA = 2 g AA/100 g total fatty acids; 0.1 g DHA/100 g total fatty acids Formula without DHA = 2.2 g ALA/100 g total fatty acids	"Term infants fed formulas with added AA and DHA had higher grating acuity at 2 months of age but not at 4, 6, 9, or 12 months of age compared with infants fed an unsupplemented formula."	B

continued

TABLE B-1f Continued

Author	Study Type	Subjects	Exposure	Timing of Exposure
Carlson et al., 1996b	Randomized Controlled Trial	Infants (n=59) Memphis, TN Maternal mean age about 22.5 year No intraventricular or periventricular hemorrhage > grade 2; a history of maternal cocaine or alcohol abuse; congenital anomalies likely to affect long-term growth and development; or intrauterine growth retardation Full enteral feeding of 418 kJ/kg/day by 6 weeks of age and tolerated enteral feeding thereafter	EPA/DHA-supplemented formula (marine oil)	Between 3-5 days post-partum until 2 months from expected term of 48±1 week post-menstrual age
Carlson et al., 1993	Randomized Controlled Trial	Infants (n=67) Birth weight 748-1398 g Mean gestational age 29 weeks Memphis, TN Did not require mechanical ventilation; have intraventricular hemorrhage > grade 2; have retinopathy of prematurity > stage 2; require surgical intervention for necrotizing enterocolitis; have severe intrauterine growth retardation; or a history of maternal substance abuse Predominantly Black and from lower socioeconomic groups Maternal age about 23 years	EPA/DHA-supplemented formula (marine oil)	Preterm formula from when infant tolerated enteral intakes >462 kJ/kg body weight/ day for 5-7 days (≈3 weeks of age) until discharge Term formula from discharge until 9 months

Amount	Results	Conclusion*
Standard preterm formula = LA at 2.5% of total fatty acid	"Visual acuity improved significantly between successive ages of 0 and 2 months, 2 and 4 months . . . Between 6 and 12 months visual acuity plateaued."	B
Marine-oil supplemented formula = 0.20% DHA and 0.06% EPA of total fatty acids		
Commercially available standard formula contained no EPA or DHA	Visual acuity development was significantly higher in the marine-oil group compared to the control group at 2 months (p<0.014) and 4 months (p<0.002).	B
Marine-oil supplemented formula contained 0.2% DHA and 0.3% EPA of total fatty acids	There were no significant differences found at the other ages reported.	

continued

TABLE B-1f Continued

Author	Study Type	Subjects	Exposure	Timing of Exposure
Birch et al., 1992	Randomized Controlled Trial	Male infants (n=32) Female infants (n=41) Born 27-33 weeks gestation Birth weight 1000-1500 g No respirator treatment for more than 7 days or congenital infections; gross congenital malformations; retinopathy of prematurity; or grade III or IV intracranial hemorrhages	EPA/DHA-supplemented formula (soy/ marine oil)	10 days of age until 6 months of age
Lauritzen et al., 2001	Review	Summary of the literature (animal, observational, RCTs)	DHA-supplemented formula	

Amount	Results	Conclusion*
Soy/marine oil-supplemented formula (preterm/follow-up formula, g/100 g lipids): LA = 20.4/18.1 ALA = 1.4/1.4 EPA+DHA = 1.0/0.9	There were significant differences in VEP acuity for the different formula groups ($p<0.025$), with the corn oil group having poorer VEP acuity than the soy/marine oil group ($p<0.05$) at 36 weeks. The corn oil group ($p<0.05$) and the soy oil group ($p<0.05$) had significantly poorer VEP acuity than the soy/marine oil group at 57 weeks.	B
Corn oil-based formula (preterm/follow-up formula, g/100 g lipids): LA = 24.2/21.1 ALA = 0.5/0.5 EPA+DHA = 0.0/0.0		
Soy oil-based formula (preterm/follow-up formula, g/100 g lipids): LA = 20.8/20.3 ALA = 2.7/2.8 EPA+DHA = 0.0/0.1		
	"Observational studies in general show better retinal function in breast-fed infants than in infants fed formula without DHA, but approximately half of the intervention studies show no effect." Animal studies do offer evidence that DHA plays a role in retinal function, but these results cannot easily be extrapolated to humans. 4 RCTs with "preterm infants have all shown a positive effect of dietary DHA on visual development;" the results from term infants are not as conclusive. More data is needed to see if the "variation in DHA content of human milk has a functional effect."	B

continued

TABLE B-1f Continued

Author	Study Type	Subjects	Exposure	Timing of Exposure
Williams et al., 2001	Cohort	Boys and girls (n=435) Mean age of 3.5 years Born in last 6 months of the Avon Longitudinal Study of Parents and Children (ALSPAC) enrollment period Healthy term infants	Seafood (mother) and breast milk (child)	Seafood = during pregnancy (mother) Breast milk = until 4 months of age (child)

Amount	Results	Conclusion*
Oily fish consumption categories: 1 = Never or rarely 2 = Once every 2 weeks 3 = More than once every 2 weeks White fish = cod, haddock, plaice, and "fish fingers" Oily fish = pilchards, sardines, mackerel, tuna, herring, kippers, trout, and salmon	After adjusting for breast-feeding, sex, maternal education, maternal age, housing tenure, financial difficulties, maternal smoking, number of older siblings in household, child care, maternal job status, mother being vegetarian, mother's fish-eating habits: "Mothers who ate oily fish at least once every 2 weeks during pregnancy were more likely to have children who achieved foveal stereoacuity than were the mothers who never ate oily fish (OR=1.57, 95% CI 1.00-2.45)," but this was not significant; and "The results of this study suggest that for full-term infants, breast-feeding is associated with enhanced stereopsis at age 3.5 years, as is a maternal DHA-rich antenatal diet, irrespective of later infant feeding practice."	B

continued

TABLE B-1f Continued

Author	Study Type	Subjects	Exposure	Timing of Exposure
Carlson et al., 1986	Cohort	Infants (n=27) Born on or before 32 weeks gestation (range 24-32 weeks) University of Mississippi Medical Center Weighed <1500 g at birth and were on full feedings of at least 60 kcal/ kg without intravenous supplementation Free of major congenital malformations and did not have any ongoing major disease process Discharged at about 1800 g	Human milk and milk formula	Delivery to an average of 7 weeks later

Amount	Results	Conclusion*
Expressed, previously frozen milk produced by their own mothers or formula	Based on phosphatidylethanolamine composition of fatty acids (in mol%): EPA was significantly lower (p<0.005) in those breast-fed after the feedings than in the pre-study samples; LA and DPA were significantly higher (p<0.001) and DHA was significantly lower (p<0.005) in those breast-fed after the feedings than in the preterm cord blood; LA was significantly higher (p<0.005) and EPA was significantly lower (p<0.005) in those formula-fed after the feedings than in the pre-study samples; LA was significantly higher (p<0.005) and DHA was significantly lower (p<0.001) in those formula-fed compared to those breast-fed; LA (p<0.005) and DPA (p<0.001) were significantly higher and AA (p<0.005) and DHA (p<0.001) were significantly lower in those formula-fed after the feedings than in the preterm cord blood; LA was significantly higher (p<0.005) and EPA was significantly lower (p<0.005) in those formula-fed after the feedings than in the pre-study samples.	N/A
Infants fed formula started with enteral feeding with Portagen and then Enfamil Premature and Similac Special Care as tolerated. Those followed after discharge were fed term formulas also produced by Enfamil and Similac		
Human milk (in mol%, mean±SE): LA = 16.00±1.30, AA = 0.59±0.04, ALA = 0.62±0.04, EPA = 0.03±0.00, DPA = 0.09±0.03, DHA = 0.19±0.03	Based on phosphatidylcholine composition of fatty acids (in mol%): LA was significantly higher (p<0.005) in those breast-fed after the feedings than in the pre-study samples; LA was significantly higher (p<0.005) and AA (p<0.001) and DHA (p<0.005) were significantly lower in those breast-fed after the feedings than in the preterm cord blood; LA was significantly higher (p<0.001) and AA was significantly lower (p<0.001) in those formula-fed after the feedings than in the pre-study samples; LA was significantly higher (p<0.005) and AA and DHA were significantly lower (p<0.001) in those formula-fed compared to those breast-fed; LA was significantly higher (p<0.005) and AA and DHA were significantly lower (p<0.001) in those formula-fed after the feedings than in the preterm cord blood.	
Portagen (in mol%, mean±SE): LA = 8.1, AA = None, ALA = Trace, EPA = None, DPA = None, DHA = None		
Enfamil Premature (in mol%, mean±SE): LA = 22.4, AA = None, ALA = 0.6, EPA = None, DPA = None, DHA = None	Based on phosphatidylserine composition of fatty acids (in mol%): LA and DHA were significantly higher (p<0.005) in those breast-fed after the feedings than in the preterm cord blood; AA was significantly lower (p<0.005) in those breast-fed after the feedings than in the pre-study samples; LA and DHA were significantly higher (p<0.005) in those formula-fed after the feedings than in the pre-study samples; AA was significantly lower (p<0.005) and DHA was significantly higher (p<0.025) in those formula-fed after the feedings than in the pre-study samples.	
Similac Special Care (in mol%, mean±SE): LA = 17.4, AA = None, ALA = 0.9, EPA = None, DPA = None, DHA = None		

continued

TABLE B-1f Continued

Author	Study Type	Subjects	Exposure	Timing of Exposure
Putnam et al., 1982	Cohort	Infants (n=40) Enrolled at birth Well-baby clinic at the University of South Florida Medical Clinics At least 90% of energy from human milk or formula before sample collection	Human milk and milk formula	3 weeks of age to 6 months of age Breast milk collected at 8 weeks and infants' blood drawn between 4.5 and 6 months of age

Amount	Results	Conclusion*
Mothers were encouraged to follow the recommendations of the American Academy of Pediatrics Committee on Nutrition (food other than human milk or humanized formula be omitted from infant's diet until he/she was 4-6 months of age)	"Human milk-fed infants had lower concentrations of membrane LA than SMA-fed infants despite the equivalent relative intakes of dietary LA."	N/A

"These diets did not influence the relative contributions of PE, PC, Sp, and PS to erythrocyte membrane phospholipid nor did they influence the lipid phosphorous/cholesterol ratio."

Significant differences in fatty acid composition of infant erythrocyte ethanolamine are as follows (weight % of total fatty acid methyl esters):

Human milk (% of total, mean): 15.80±0.61 LA, 0.60±0.03 AA, 0.80±0.09 ALA, 0.10±0.03 EPA, 0.10±0.01 DPA, 0.10±0.01 DHA

Infants fed human milk had significantly higher AA (p<0.05), DPA (p<0.05), and DHA (p<0.001) than those fed SMA formula; and

Enfamil + iron (% of total, mean): 45.1 LA, No AA, 5.0 ALA, No EPA, No DPA, No DHA

Infants fed human milk had significantly higher AA (p<0.01) and significantly lower LA (p<0.001), ALA (p<0.001), EPA (p<0.05), and DHA (p<0.001) than those fed Enfamil formula with iron.

SMA formula (% of total, mean): 14.0 LA, No AA, 1.2 ALA, No EPA, No DPA, No DHA

continued

TABLE B-1f Continued

Author	Study Type	Subjects	Exposure	Timing of Exposure
Sanders and Naismith, 1979	Cross-sectional	Infants (n=18) Aged 14 weeks Fed from birth a modified cow's milk formula or had been breast-fed Participated in an earlier study	Human milk and milk formula	14 weeks of age
Neuringer et al., 1984	Animal	Adult female rhesus monkeys	Diet deficient in n-3 fatty acids	2 months before conception and throughout pregnancy

*N = Evidence of no association or no clear association; B = Evidence of a benefit; N/A = A conclusion is not available; these data are presented for background information only.

Amount	Results	Conclusion*
Breast milk (% total fatty acids, mean±SE): LA = 6.90±0.81, ALA = 0.80±0.05, EPA = 0.20±0.08, DPA = 0.52±0.27, DHA = 0.59±0.23 Milk formula (% total fatty acids, mean): LA = 1.60, ALA = 0.70, EPA = 0.08, DPA = 0.11, DHA = 0.02	LA, AA, DHA are significantly lower in the formula-fed infants than in the breast-fed infants (p<0.01, p<0.05, p<0.01, respectively). EPA and DPA are significantly higher in the formula-fed infants than in the breast-fed infants (p<0.05). "The minimum requirement of the young infant for LA is substantially less than 1% of the dietary energy, the value most widely quoted."	N/A
Experimental group: Semipurified diet deficient in n-3 fatty acids Safflower oil sole fat source 76.0% LA, 0.3% GLA, 0.2% DGLA, 0.3% ALA, 225.0% n-6:n-3 of total fatty acids Control group: Soy bean oil sole fat source 53.1% LA, 0.0% GLA, 0.3% DGLA, 7.7% ALA, 7.0% n-6:n-3 of total fatty acids	AA and total n-6 fatty acids were significantly higher in the experimental group infants compared to the control group infants (p<0.005). ALA, EPA, DPA, DHA and total n-3 fatty acids are all significantly lower in the experimental group infants compared to the control group infants (p<0.001). At 4, 8, and 12 weeks, the visual acuity threshold in the experimental group was significantly lower than in the control group (p<0.05, p<0.0005, p<0.005, respectively).	B

TABLE B-1g Studies on Cognitive and Motor Development: Effects on Infants Supplemented with Omega-3 Fatty Acids in Formula

Author	Study Type	Subjects	Exposure	Timing of Exposure
Cohen et al., 2005	Review	Aggregated 8 randomized controlled trials (1 study of maternal dietary supplementation and 7 studies of formula supplementation)	n-3 supplement	
Simmer and Patole, 2005	Cochrane Review	11 randomized controlled trials	LCPUFA-supplemented formula	
Simmer, 2005	Cochrane Review	9 randomized controlled trials	LCPUFA-supplemented formula	

Amount	Results	Conclusion*
	An increase in maternal intake of DHA during pregnancy of 1 g/day will increase child IQ by 0.8-1.8 points.	B
	"Prenatal maternal DHA intake increasing the child plasma (RBC) DHA phospholipid fraction by 1% has the same impact on cognitive development as formula DHA supplementation that increases the child's plasma (RBC) DHA phospholipid fraction by 1%."	
	"Because typical DHA intake associated with fish consumption is well under 1 g/day, changes in fish consumption will result in IQ effects amounting to a fraction of a point," but they are not clinically detectable.	
	"No long-term benefits were demonstrated for infants receiving formula supplemented with LCPUFA. There was no evidence that supplementation of formula with n-3 and n-6 LCPUFA impaired the growth of preterm infants."	N
	"There is little evidence from randomized trials of LCPUFA supplementation to support the hypothesis that LCPUFA supplementation confers a benefit for visual or general development of term infants."	N
	"Minor effects on VEP acuity have been suggested, but appear unlikely when all studies are reviewed."	

continued

TABLE B-1g Continued

Author	Study Type	Subjects	Exposure	Timing of Exposure
Gibson et al., 2001	Review	Randomized controlled trials (11 on preterm and 10 on term infants) Involving healthy preterm infants fed preterm formula Involving healthy term infants fed formulas from near birth Systematic literature review	LCPUFA-supplemented formula	
Uauy et al., 2001	Review	Summary of random-ized controlled trials on preterm and term infants	AA/DHA-supplemented formula	
Carlson and Neuringer, 1999	Review	Summary of animal studies and random-ized controlled trials Based on a session from the AOCS 1996 meet-ing: *PUFA in Infant Nutrition: Consensus and Controversies*	Neural DHA accumulation	

Amount	Results	Conclusion*
	"Although there are still some concerns on safety issues regarding the addition of LCPUFA to preterm infant formula, the evidence in support of a beneficial effect of such supplementation on visual function is relatively compelling."	B
	"It seems that the possible negative effects of n-3 LCPUFA on growth of preterm infants have been overcome through improved study design and/or the addition of a balance of n-6 and n-3 LCPUFA."	
	"There is also mixed evidence for the support of an effect of dietary LCPUFA on more global measures of development (Bayley's Scales of Infant Development or Brunet-Lezine test)."	
	"Evidence for a beneficial effect of AA+DHA supplementation on CNS development is strong."	B
	"The preliminary information on cognitive development is insufficient to fully establish a relationship between LCPUFA and mental development."	
	Studies in deficient monkeys suggest that "lower brain accumulation of DHA may influence neural domains such as sensation, motivation or temperament, but not cognition."	B
	"The most consistent effect identified to date in human and animal studies has been that of look duration and tests of visual attention."	
	"A limited number of behavioral studies in animals and humans address the question of neural DHA accumulation and developmental measures other than vision."	

continued

TABLE B-1g Continued

Author	Study Type	Subjects	Exposure	Timing of Exposure
Bouwstra et al., 2005	Randomized Controlled Trial	Infants (n=256 to 446, depending on assessment) Term, healthy Groningen, Netherlands University and Martini Hospitals in Groningen and at midwife clinics No congenital disorders that interfered with adequate functioning in daily life; infants from multiple births; infants whose mothers did not have mastery of the Dutch language or suffered from significant illness or disability; adopted or foster infants; or formula-fed infants who had received human milk >5 days	LCPUFA-supplemented formula	Birth to 2 months of age

Amount	Results	Conclusion*
Control formula (in mol%): 11.56 LA, 1.27 ALA Supplemented formula (in mol%): 11.00 LA, 0.18 GLA, 0.03 DGLA, 0.39 AA, 1.30 ALA, 0.06 EPA, 0.23 DHA Breastfed (in mol%, mean±SE): 13.62±4.24 LA, 0.11±0.03 GLA, 0.34±0.06 DGLA, 0.34±0.06 AA, 1.11±0.35 ALA, 0.06±0.04 EPA, 0.19±0.11 DHA	"The groups did not show statistically significant differences in clinical neurological condition, neurological optimality score, fluency score, and the psychomotor and mental development indices at 18 months."	N

continued

TABLE B-1g Continued

Author	Study Type	Subjects	Exposure	Timing of Exposure
Clandinin et al., 2005	Randomized Controlled Trial	Infants (n=361) Preterm Multi-site study First phase: Gestational age ≤35 weeks postmenstrual age <10 total days of enteral feeding of >30 mL/kg/day No congenital abnormalities of the gastrointestinal tract, hepatitis, hepatic or biliary pathology, necrotizing enterocolitis confirmed before enrollment, or history of underlying disease or congenital malformations likely to interfere with evaluation Second phase: Successful completion of the first phase, ≥80% of enteral intake from study formula during hospitalization, and 100% caloric intake from study formula at completion of the first phase	Algal-DHA- and fish-DHA-supplemented formulas, human milk	Premature formula: ≥14 days of age until at/near hospital discharge (40 weeks of age) Discharge formula: 40 weeks until 53 weeks postmenstrual age Term formula: 53 weeks until 92 weeks postmenstrual age

Amount	Results	Conclusion*
Control formula: No DHA or AA	At 118 weeks, breast-fed term infants had significantly higher MDI and PDI scores compared to the control formula group, the algal-DHA formula group, and the fish-DHA formula group (p<0.05).	B
Algal-DHA formula: 17 mg DHA/100 kcal from algal oil, 34 mg AA/100 kcal from fungal oil 0.3% fatty acids from DHA, 0.6% fatty acids from AA	At 118 weeks, the algal-DHA formula group had a higher MDI score (p=0.056), although it was not significant, and a significantly higher PDI score (p<0.05) compared to the control formula group.	
Fish-DHA formula: 17 mg DHA/100 kcal from tuna fish oil, 34 mg AA/100 kcal from fungal oil 0.3% fatty acids from DHA, 0.6% fatty acids from AA	At 118 weeks, the fish-DHA formula group had significantly higher MDI and PDI scores (p<0.05) compared to the control formula group.	
Worldwide human milk: 0.3% DHA and 0.6% AA (weight of fatty acids)		

continued

TABLE B-1g Continued

Author	Study Type	Subjects	Exposure	Timing of Exposure
Jensen et al., 2005	Randomized Controlled Trial	Pregnant women (n=227) Aged 18-40 years Houston, TX White (75% DHA group; 79% control group) African American (19% DHA group; 13% control group) Women plan to breast-feed exclusively for ≥4 months Infant gestational age >37 weeks Infant birth weight 2500-4200 g No chronic maternal disorders; major congenital anomalies and obvious gastroin-testinal or metabolic disorders of the infant	DHA supplement	Within 5 days after delivery until 4 months postpartum
Fewtrell et al., 2004	Randomized Controlled Trial	Infants (n=238) Preterm Glasgow, UK Birth weight ≤2000 g Mean maternal age about 29 years Social class 1 or 2 (18% in controls; 27% in LCPUFA group) Mothers with degree or higher (2% in con-trols; 7% in LCPUFA group)	LCPUFA-supplemented formula	Preterm formu-las: when pedia-trician decided that preterm formula should be started, to discharge Discharge formulas: from discharge until 9 months after term

Amount	Results	Conclusion*
High-DHA capsule (algal triacylglycerol): 0.8% LA and 41.7% DHA by weight 200 mg DHA/day Control capsule (soy and corn oil): 56.3% LA, 3.9% ALA by weight	There were no significant differences in visual acuity from the Teller Acuity Card at 4 or 8 months of age or from the Sweep VEP at 4 months of age between the two groups. There were no significant differences in mean transient VEP latency at 4 and 8 months of age between the two groups; but the transient VEP amplitude was significantly lower in the infants of the high-DHA capsule group compared to the infants of the control capsule group (p<0.03). There were no significant differences in Gesell Gross Motor, CAT, or CLAMS DQ scores at 12 and 30 months of age or in Bayley MDI at 30 months of age between the two groups; but Bayley PDI at 30 months of age was 8.4 points higher in infants of the high-DHA capsule group compared to infants of the control capsule group.	N
LCPUFA-supplemented formulas (g/100 g fat): 12.30 LA, 0.04 AA, 1.50 ALA, 0.10 EPA, 0.50 DHA Control formulas (g/100 g fat): 11.5 LA, 1.6 ALA, no AA, EPA, or DHA	At 18 months of age, the Bayley MDI and PDI scores did not differ significantly between the groups. At 9 months of age, overall development scores and individual subscale scores did not differ significantly between the groups.	N

continued

TABLE B-1g Continued

Author	Study Type	Subjects	Exposure	Timing of Exposure
Bouwstra et al., 2003	Randomized Controlled Trial	Infants (n=397) Term, healthy Groningen, Netherlands University and Martini Hospitals in Groningen and at midwife clinics No congenital disorders that interfered with adequate functioning in daily life; infants from multiple births; infants whose mothers did not have mastery of the Dutch language or suffered from significant illness or disability; adopted or foster infants; or formula-fed infants who had received human milk >5 days	LCPUFA-supplemented formula	Birth to 2 months of age

Amount	Results	Conclusion*
Control formula (in mol%): 11.56 LA, 1.27 ALA Supplemented formula (in mol%): 11.00 LA, 0.18 GLA, 0.03 DGLA, 0.39 AA, 1.30 ALA, 0.06 EPA, 0.23 DHA Breast-fed (in mol%, mean±SE): 13.62±4.24 LA, 0.11±0.03 GLA, 0.34±0.06 DGLA, 0.34±0.06 AA, 1.11±0.35 ALA, 0.06±0.04 EPA, 0.19±0.11 DHA	After controlling for profession of mother's partner requiring a university or vocational-college education, Obstetrical Optimality Score, and age at assessment: The control formula group had a significantly lower OR of occurrence of normal-optimal general movements at age 3 months when compared to the breast-fed infants (OR=0.55; p=0.038); and Those in the supplemented formula group had a significantly lower OR of occurrence of normal-optimal general movements at age 3 months when compared to the breast-fed infants (OR=0.42; p=0.006), but the OR was not significant when compared to the control formula group (OR=0.77; p=0.41). After controlling for marital status, family history of diabetes, gestational age at birth, condition of perineum, and age at assessment: The control formula group had a significantly higher OR of mildly abnormal general movements at age 3 months when compared to the breast-fed infants (OR=2.03; p=0.039); and The supplemented formula group had a significantly lower OR of mildly abnormal general movements at age 3 months when compared to the control formula group (OR=0.49; p=0.032), but the OR was not significant when compared to the breast-fed infants (OR=0.94; p=0.87).	B

continued

TABLE B-1g Continued

Author	Study Type	Subjects	Exposure	Timing of Exposure
Helland et al., 2003	Randomized Controlled Trial	Pregnant women (n=48 in cod-liver oil group; n=36 in corn oil group) Aged 19-35 years Oslo, Norway Healthy women with, singleton pregnancy, nulli- or primiparous, intention to breast-feed No supplement of n-3 LCPUFA earlier during pregnancy, premature births, birth asphyxia, general infections, or anomalies in the infants that required special attention	Cod-liver oil supplement	From 18 weeks of pregnancy until 3 months after delivery
Fewtrell et al., 2002	Randomized Controlled Trial	Infants (n=195 formula-fed; n=88 breast-fed) Preterm Birth weight <1750 g Nottingham and Leicester, UK No congenital malformation known to affect neurodevelopment Mothers decided not to breast-feed by 10 days of age; tolerated enteral feeds at that time (for randomized groups) Social class 1 or 2 (19% in controls; 26% in LCPUFA group; 33% in breast-fed group)	LCPUFA-supplemented formula	10 days of age until discharge

Amount	Results	Conclusion*

Cod-liver oil:
10 mL/day
1183 mg DHA,
  803 mg EPA
 	
Corn oil:
10 mL/day
4747 mg LA, 92 mg
  ALA
	K-ABC scores were significantly higher for the subset MPCOMP among children from the cod-liver oil group compared to the corn oil group (p=0.049). The scores for the other subtests (SEQPROC, SIMPROC, NONVERB) were also higher in the cod-liver oil group compared to the corn oil group, but they were not significant.	B

LCPUFA-
  supplemented
  formula (g/100 g
  fat):
12.00 LA, 0.31 AA,
  0.60 ALA, 0.04
  EPA, 0.17 DHA
 	
Control formula
  (g/100 g fat):
10.6 LA, 0.7 ALA, no
  detected AA, EPA,
  DHA
	There were no significant differences in KPS quotients at 9 months of age and neurological status at 9 or 18 months of age between the two formula groups.
	
	There were no significant differences found in Bayley MDI or PDI at 18 months of age between the two formula groups.
	
	Breast-fed infants had significantly higher KPS quotients (overall, adaptive, gross motor, fine motor, and personal-social) at 9 months of age (p<0.005) and significantly higher Bayley MDI and PDI at 18 months of age (p<0.005) compared to the control formula-fed infants.
	
	Breast-fed infants had significantly higher KPS quotients (overall, adaptive, gross motor, fine motor, and personal-social) at 9 months of age (p<0.005; p<0.05 for gross motor quotient) and significantly higher Bayley MDI and PDI at 18 months of age (p<0.005) compared to the LCPUFA-supplemented formula infants.
		N

continued

TABLE B-1g Continued

Author	Study Type	Subjects	Exposure	Timing of Exposure
Van Wezel-Meijler et al., 2002	Randomized Controlled Trial	Infants (n=42) Preterm, admitted to neonatal intensive- or high-care unit of hospital Birth weight <1750 g Leiden, Netherlands Mothers not breast-feeding Normal neurological ex- amination throughout the neonatal period Repeated ultrasound of the brain being normal or show- ing, at most, minor abnormalities No abnormalities of the central nervous system; abnormal neurological examina- tion or occurrence of seizures; any systemic disease with potential negative influence on future growth or development; serious nutritional or gastro- intestinal problems preventing initiation of enteral feeding after the first week post- partum or complete enteral feeding after the third week post- partum; retinopathy of prematurity grade 3 or more	AA/DHA-supplemented formula	2-3 weeks after birth until weighing 3000 g

Amount	Results	Conclusion*
Supplemented pre-term formula: 4.4 g fat/100 mL 0.015 g/100 mL of added DHA (microalgae) 0.031 g/100 mL of added AA (fungi) Control formula: 4.4 g fat/100 mL No addition of DHA and AA	There were no significant differences found in Bayley MDI and PDI at 3, 6, 12, or 24 months between the two groups. There were no significant differences found in myelination at 3 and 12 months between the two groups.	N

continued

TABLE B-1g Continued

Author	Study Type	Subjects	Exposure	Timing of Exposure
Auestad et al., 2001	Randomized Controlled Trial	Infants (n=294 formula-fed; n=165 breast-fed) Kansas City, MO; Little Rock, AR; Pittsburgh, PA; Tucson, AZ Good health, term status, either ≤9 days of age (formula group) or ≤11 days of age and currently breast-feeding (breast-feeding group), birth weight ≥2500 g, 5-minute APGAR score ≥7, ability to tolerate milk-based formula or breast milk, guardian or parent agreement to feed the assigned study formula ad libitum according to the study design No evidence of significant cardiac, respiratory, ophthalmologic, gastrointestinal, hematologic, or metabolic disease; milk-protein allergy; or a maternal medical history known to have proven adverse effects on the fetus, tuberculosis, HIV, perinatal infections, or substance abuse 61-74% European American 60-80% mothers married Mean mothers' age about 29 years Mean mothers' education about 14 years	Fish oil/fungal oil and egg-derived triglyceride-supplemented formulas	9-11 days after birth until 12 months of age

Amount	Results	Conclusion*
Fish oil and fungal oil-supplemented preterm formula: 0.46 g AA/100 g total fatty acids ≤0.04 g EPA/100 g total fatty acids 0.13 g DHA/100 g total fatty acids Egg-derived triglyceride-supplemented preterm formula: 0.45 g AA/100 g total fatty acids No detected EPA 0.14 g DHA/100 g total fatty acids Control formula: No detected AA, EPA, DHA	The vocabulary expression score at 14 months was significantly higher in the fish/fungal group than in the egg-TG group (p<0.05). Smiling and laughter was significantly higher in the control group than in the egg-TG group (p=0.05). No other development, cognition, vocabulary, or temperament outcomes presented were significantly different between the formula groups.	B

continued

TABLE B-1g Continued

Author	Study Type	Subjects	Exposure	Timing of Exposure
O'Connor et al., 2001	Randomized Controlled Trial	Infants (n=470) Preterm Birth weight 750-1800 g Cleveland, OH; Kansas City, MO; Little Rock, AR; Nottingham and Leeds, UK; Louisville, KY; Portland, OR; New York, NY; Santiago, Chile White (n=81 controls; n=80 fish/fungal; n=85 egg-TG) No serious congenital abnormalities that could affect growth and development; major surgery before randomization; periventricular/intra-ventricular hemor-rhage greater than grade II; maternal incapacity; liquid ventilation; asphyxia resulting in severe and permanent neurologic damage; or uncontrolled systemic infection at the time of enrollment	Fish oil/fungal oil and egg-derived triglyc-eride/fish oil-supplemented formulas	In hospital formula from within 72 hours of first enteral feeding until term-corrected age

Post-discharge formula from term-corrected age until 12 months of age |

Amount	Results	Conclusion*
All in g/100 g total fatty acids (mean±SE) In-hospital control: 16.0±0.9 LA, 2.4±0.1 ALA, no AA, EPA, DHA In-hospital AA+DHA (fish/fungal oil): 16.80±1.00 LA, 2.60±0.30 ALA, 0.43±0.02 AA, 0.08±0.01 EPA, 0.27±0.04 DHA In-hospital AA+DHA (egg-TG/fish oil): 17.50±0.90 LA, 2.50±0.30 ALA, 0.41±0.00 AA, no EPA, 0.24±0.01 DHA Post-discharge control: 19.1±1.1 LA, 2.4±0.2 ALA, no AA, EPA, DHA Post-discharge AA+DHA (fish/fungal oil): 19.50±0.70 LA, 2.40±0.20 ALA, 0.43±0.01 AA, no EPA, 0.16±0.01 DHA Post-discharge AA+DHA (egg-TG/fish oil): 20.30±0.40 LA, 2.40±0.20 ALA, 0.41±0.02 AA, no EPA, 0.15±0.02 DHA	The mean novelty preference of the egg-TG/fish oil formula group was significantly greater than the control group (p=0.02) and the fish/fungal formula group (p=0.003) at 6 months corrected age. Using a Bonferroni adjusted alpha level of 0.0083, the difference between the fish/fungal formula group and the egg-TG/fish formula group was statistically significant. "Vocabulary comprehension did not differ among the 3 study formula groups at either 9 or 14 months corrected age in either the intent-to-treat or sub-group analysis."	B

continued

TABLE B-1g Continued

Author	Study Type	Subjects	Exposure	Timing of Exposure
Birch et al., 2000	Randomized Controlled Trial	Infants (n=56) Healthy, term, birth weight appropriate for gestational age Singleton births Dallas, TX Predominantly White About 65% mothers had a college or postgraduate education No family history of milk protein allergy; genetic or familial eye disease; vegetarian or vegan maternal dietary patterns; maternal metabolic disease, anemia; or infection; presence of a congenital malformation or infection; jaundice; perinatal asphyxia; meconium aspiration; or any perinatal event that resulted in placement in the neonatal intensive care unit	AA-enriched formula	0-4 days of age to 17 weeks of age
Lucas et al., 1999	Randomized Controlled Trial	Infants (n=309 formula-fed; n=138 breast-fed) Healthy, term, singleton pregnancies, appropriate size for gestational age Nottingham and Leicester, UK Mean maternal age about 27 years 93.5% married About 70% with no higher school qualifications	LCPUFA-supplemented formula	Birth until 6 months of age

Amount	Results	Conclusion*
Enfamil + iron Enfamil + iron + 0.35% DHA Enfamil + iron + 0.36% DHA + 0.72% AA	The mean Bayley MDI score at 18 months was significantly higher in the DHA/AA-supplemented formula group than in the control formula group ($p<0.05$). The mean Bayley PDI score at 18 months was not statistically different among the three groups ($p=0.13$). The mean Behavioral Rating Scale score at 18 months was not statistically different among the three groups ($p=0.30$).	B
LCPUFA-supplemented formula: 15.90% LA, 0.30% AA, 1.40% ALA, 0.01% EPA, 0.32% DHA Control formula: 12.4% LA, 1.1% ALA	There were no significant differences in Bayley MDI and PDI at 18 months or in Knobloch, Passamanick, and Sherrard's test at 9 months between the two formula groups. There were no significant differences in stools to 6 months, crying time (minutes/day) to 6 months, or formula intake to 6 months between the two formula groups. There were no significant differences in the OR of infection-related outcomes or the prescription of antibiotics at 9 months between the two formula groups.	N

continued

TABLE B-1g Continued

Author	Study Type	Subjects	Exposure	Timing of Exposure
Scott et al., 1998	Randomized Controlled Trial	Infants (n=274) Healthy, full-term Kansas, MO; Portland, OR; Seattle, WA No prematurity, intra-uterine growth re-tardation, congenital anomalies, 5-minute APGAR score <7, or other significant perinatal medical complications	AA/DHA-supplemented formula	Those random-ized, formula from first week after delivery Those exclu-sively breast-feeding, breast milk for first 3 months and then supple-mentation with Similac + iron Solid food supplementation at 4 months
Willatts et al., 1998a	Randomized Controlled Trial	Infants (n=44) Term UK Mothers from a single maternity hospital	LCPUFA-supplemented formula	Birth to 4 months of age

Amount	Results	Conclusion*
Control formula: No added LCPUFA	There were no significant differences in Bayley scores among the groups for either the Mental Index or the Motor Index.	A
DHA formula group (fish oil): 0.2wt% DHA	After controlling for maternal education and site, when comparing all four groups, the vocabulary comprehension score at 14 months was significantly lower in the DHA formula group compared to the breast-feeding group (p=0.017).	
DHA+AA formula group (egg yolk phospholipid): 0.12wt% DHA, 0.43wt% AA	After controlling for maternal education and site, when comparing only the three formula groups, the vocabulary production score at 14 months was significantly lower in the DHA formula group compared to the control formula group (p=0.027). No other reported associations between MacArthur Communicative Development Inventories at 14 months and the formula groups and those breast-feeding were found to be significant.	
Unsupplemented for- mula (g/100 g fat): 11.40 LA, 0.70 ALA, <0.10 AA, no DHA	The median quartiles for entire problem intention score (p=0.035) and the cover step intention score (p=0.032) were significantly higher in the LCPUFA-supplemented group compared to the unsupplemented group.	B
LCPUFA-supplement- ed formula (g/100 g fat): 11.50-12.80 LA, 0.60-0.65 ALA, 0.30-0.40 AA, 0.15-0.25 DHA	The median quartiles for entire problem intentional solutions score (p=0.021) and cover step intentional solutions (p=0.005) were significantly higher in the LCPUFA-supplemented group compared to the unsupplemented group. There were no significant differences in the median quartiles for the barrier step or cloth step for either the intention score or the intentional solutions score.	

continued

TABLE B-1g Continued

Author	Study Type	Subjects	Exposure	Timing of Exposure
Willatts et al., 1998b	Randomized Controlled Trial	Infants (n=40) Term Birth weight 2500-4000 g Dundee, UK Mean maternal age about 27 years Mean maternal education about 17 years Demonstrated either an early or late peak fixation on the habituation assessment undertaken at 3 months of age	LCPUFA-supplemented formula	Birth to 4 months of age
Carlson and Werkman, 1996	Randomized Controlled Trial	Infants (n=59) Mean gestational age about 28 weeks Birth weight 747-1275 g Predominantly Black Memphis, TN Mean mothers' education about 12 years No need for mechanical ventilation at that time; intraventricular hemorrhage > grade 2; retinopathy of prematurity > stage 2; surgery for necrotizing enterocolitis; weight < the fifth percentile for gestational age; history of maternal substance abuse	DHA-supplemented formula	Preterm formula from 3 days to 2 months of age Term formula from 2 months to 12 months of age

Amount	Results	Conclusion*
Unsupplemented formula (g/100 g fat): 11.40 LA, 0.70 ALA, <0.10 AA, no DHA LCPUFA-supplemented formula (g/100 g fat): 11.50-12.80 LA, 0.60-0.65 ALA, 0.30-0.40 AA, 0.15-0.25 DHA	There were no significant differences in 9-month problem-solving scores (intention score and number of solutions) between the two groups. For those who had an early peak fixation at 3 months, there were no significant differences in 9-month problem-solving score (intention score or intentional solutions) between the two groups (p=0.18). For those who had a late peak fixation at 3 months, the number of intentional solutions was significantly higher in the LCPUFA-supplemented group compared to the unsupplemented group (p<0.02).	B
All in g/100 g total fatty acids Preterm control formula: 21.20 LA, 2.40 ALA, no EPA or DHA Preterm DHA-supplemented formula: 21.20 LA, 2.40 ALA, 0.06 EPA, 0.20 DHA Term formula: 34.30 LA, 4.80 ALA, no EPA or DHA	At 12 months of age, the DHA-supplemented group had statistically more number of looks to familiar (p<0.05) and less seconds of time/novel looks (p<0.05) compared to the controls. No other statistically significant results were reported on visual attention.	B

continued

TABLE B-1g Continued

Author	Study Type	Subjects	Exposure	Timing of Exposure
Werkman and Carlson, 1996	Randomized Controlled Trial	Infants (n=67) Mean gestational age 29 weeks Birth weight 748-1398 g Can tolerate enteral; intakes >462 kJ/kg body weight/day for 5-7 days Predominantly Black Memphis, TN Mean maternal age 23 years Mean mothers' education about 11.5 years No need for mechanical ventilation at that time; intraventricular hemorrhage > grade 2; retinopathy of prematurity > stage 2; surgery for necrotizing enterocolitis; weight < the fifth percentile for gestational age; history of maternal substance abuse	DHA-supplemented formula	Preterm formula until discharge Term formula from discharge until 9 months past term Other foods gradually added to diet at about 4 months past term Mixed diet, including whole cow's milk from 9 to 12 months
Agostoni et al., 1995	Randomized Controlled Trial	Infants (n=86) Mothers' mean age = about 30 years Gestational age between 37-42 weeks, weight at birth appropriate for gestational age Milan, Italy APGAR score better than 7 at 5 minutes, absence of disease	LCPUFA-supplemented formula	Within 3 days until 4 months of age

Amount	Results	Conclusion*
All in g/100 g total fatty acids	"Diet did not significantly influence look duration during familiarization, but there was a trend toward shorter look duration in DHA-supplemented infants compared to the controls."	B
Preterm control formula:		
19.1 LA, 3.0 ALA, no EPA or DHA	At 6.5 months of age, the DHA-supplemented group had a statistically higher number of total looks ($p<0.01$), number of looks to novel ($p<0.01$), and number of looks to familiar ($p<0.05$) compared to the controls.	
Preterm DHA-supplemented formula:		
18.7 LA, 3.1 ALA, 0.3 EPA, 0.2 DHA	At 9 months of age, the DHA-supplemented group had a statistically higher number of total looks ($p<0.01$), number of looks to novel ($p<0.01$), number of looks to familiar ($p<0.05$), and less seconds for average time/look ($p<0.05$) compared to the controls.	
Term control formula:		
33.2 LA, 4.8 ALA, no EPA or DHA		
Term DHA-supplemented formula:	At 12 months, the DHA-supplemented group had a statistically shorter novel time as a percentage of total time ($p<0.05$), more seconds of time to familiar ($p<0.05$), and a higher number of total looks ($p<0.01$), number of looks to novel ($p<0.05$), and number of looks to familiar ($p<0.05$) compared to the controls.	
32.6 LA, 4.9 ALA, 0.3 EPA, 0.2 DHA		
	No other significant results were reported for visual attention.	
Supplemented formula (g/100 g fat):	The mean developmental quotient (DQ) at 4 months for those in the standard formula group was statistically lower from the DQ in the supplemented formula group ($p<0.05$) and the breast-feeding group ($p<0.05$).	B
10.80 LA, 0.30 GLA, 0.73 ALA, 0.44 AA, 0.05 EPA, 0.30 DHA		
Standard formula (g/100 g fat):	There was no statistical difference between the mean DQ at 4 months of the supplemented formula group and the breast-feeding group.	
11.10 LA, 0.70 ALA		
Human milk (g/100 g fat):		
6.9-16.4 LA, 0.1-0.9 GLA, 0.7-1.3 ALA, 0.2-1.2 AA, 0.0-0.6 EPA, 0.1-0.6 DHA		

continued

TABLE B-1g Continued

Author	Study Type	Subjects	Exposure	Timing of Exposure
McCann and Ames, 2005	Review	Summary of observational, RCTs, other experimental and animal studies	DHA status and LCPUFA-supplemented formula	
Bryan et al., 2004	Review	Summary of the literature (all designs)	PUFA from breast milk or formula	
Jacobson, 1999	Review	Mostly 2 prospective longitudinal studies Detroit study on effects of prenatal exposure to alcohol Michigan study of effects of pre- and postnatal exposure to PCBs	LCPUFA-supplemented formula	

Amount	Results	Conclusion*
	"Evidence from chronic dietary restriction rodent studies . . . shows that the addition of DHA to diets of animals whose brain concentration of DHA have been severely reduced restored control performance levels."	B
	"Formula comparison and maternal supplementation studies in humans and ALA dietary restriction studies in nonhuman primates both link the availability of n-3 LCPUFAs to the development of visual attention" and higher DHA status to enhanced neuromotor development.	
	RCTs in humans have often shown no effect of "LCPUFA supplementation on cognitive or behavioral performance and some reviewers have considered that, overall, the evidence was insufficient to conclude that LCPUFA supplementation benefited development."	
	"There is moderate evidence that PUFAs, and long-chain omega-3 PUFAs in particular, from either breast milk or supplemented infant formula, are beneficial in the development of visual acuity and cognitive performance in infants."	B
	"There is very limited empirical evidence, due to the small number of extant studies, for the beneficial effects of PUFAs, and omega-3 PUFAs in particular, on cognitive performance in older children."	
	"Evidence suggest that omega-3 PUFAs may have a role in the control of the symptoms of neurological disorders such as ADHD and dyslexia."	
	"Any comparisons between breastfed and supplemented groups should include measures of maternal IQ and quality of parenting on which these groups tend to differ."	B
	"Animal and human studies indicating a relation between LCPUFA supplementation and enhanced visual acuity and shorter visual fixations may, in fact, represent relatively independent effects of supplementation on both acuity and cognitive processing speed."	

continued

TABLE B-1g Continued

Author	Study Type	Subjects	Exposure	Timing of Exposure
Daniels et al., 2004	Cohort	Infants (n=1054) Mothers' mean age = 29 years Majority of mothers with at least an O level (moderate) education Bristol, UK Singleton, term births Avon Longitudinal Study of Parents and Children (ALSPAC)	Seafood	Maternal fish intake: 32 weeks of gestation Breast-feeding practices: 15 months after birth Infant fish intake: 6 and 12 months after birth Total mercury concentration: Cord blood at birth
Innis et al., 2001	Cohort	Infants (n=83) Term Birth weight 2500-4500 g Mean mothers' age 32 years British Columbia Intend to breast-feed for 3 months, no solid foods for at least the first 4 months after birth No mothers with substance abuse, communicable diseases, metabolic or physiologic problems, infections likely to influence fetal growth, or multiple births No infants with evidence of metabolic or physical abnormalities	Fatty acids in blood from infants and milk from mothers	2 months of age

Amount	Results	Conclusion*
Maternal fish intake categories (during pregnancy): 1 = Rarely/never 2 = 1 meal/2 weeks 3 = 1-3 meals/week 4 = 4+ meals/week	Children whose mothers ate 1-3 fish meals/week and 4+ fish meals/week had significantly lower odds of low MCDI scores for social activity (OR=0.6, 95% CI 0.5-0.8 and OR=0.7, 95% CI 0.5-0.9, respectively) than the children whose mothers rarely or never ate fish during pregnancy.	B
Child fish intake categories (6 months of age): 1 = Rarely/never 2 = 1+ meal/week	Children whose mothers ate 1-3 fish meals/week and 4+ fish meals/week had significantly lower odds of low DDST scores for language (OR=0.7, 95% CI 0.5-0.9 and OR=0.7, 95% CI 0.5-0.9, respectively) than the children whose mothers rarely or never ate fish during pregnancy.	
Child fish intake categories (12 months of age): 1 = Rarely/never 2 = 1+ meal/week	Children who ate 1+ fish meals/week had significantly lower odds of low MCDI scores for vocabulary comprehension (OR=0.7, 95% CI 0.5-0.8) and social activity (OR=0.7, 95% CI 0.6-0.9) and total DDST score (OR=0.8, 95% CI 0.6-0.9). All other odds ratios presented were nonsignificant.	
Infant DHA: (g/100 g fatty acids) Plasma phospholipids = 2.2-8.0 RBC PE = 6.3-13.0 PC = 1.4-4.6	"The ability to correctly discriminate a retroflex compared with dental phonetic contrast at 9 months of age was positively correlated with the plasma phospholipid DHA (p<0.02) and the RBC PE at 2 months of age (p=0.02)."	B
Infant AA: (g/100 g fatty acids) Plasma phospholipids = 8.1-15.8 RBC PE = 20.2-27.8 PC = 5.6-9.7	"There were no significant correlations between the infants' AA status and the ability to discriminate the native or nonnative language contrasts." "There were no significant correlations between the infant DHA or AA status at 2 months of age and test scores for novelty preference, or the job search task, with adjustments for covariates included in the model."	
Mother's milk: (g/100 g milk fatty acids) DHA = 0.10-2.50 AA = 0.20-0.81 LA = 6.30-21.50 LNA = 0.50-4.10		

continued

TABLE B-1g Continued

Author	Study Type	Subjects	Exposure	Timing of Exposure
Kodas et al., 2004	Animal	2 generations of female Wistar rats	ALA-deficient diet	Control group: Control diet at birth to 60 days after birth
				Deficient group: Deficient diet at birth to 60 days after birth
				Diet reversed group 1: Control diet at day of birth until 60 days after birth
				Diet reversed group 2: Deficient diet until day 7 postpartum and then control diet from day 7 to day 60 postpartum
				Diet reversed group 3: Deficient diet until day 14 postpartum and then control diet from day 14 to day 60 postpartum
				Diet reversed group 4: Deficient diet until day 21 postpartum and then control diet from day 21 to day 60 postpartum

Amount	Results	Conclusion*
ALA-deficient diet: 6% fat African pea- nut oil <6 mg ALA/100 g of diet 1200 mg LA/100 g of diet Control diet: 60% peanut oil, 40% rapeseed oil 200 mg ALA/100 g of diet 1200 mg LA/100 g of diet	The fatty acid composition of phosphatidylcholine in the hippocampus of 2-month-old rats was as follows: AA was not significantly different among the different diet groups; DHA was significantly higher in the control group and all diet reversed groups compared to the deficient group (p<0.05); n-6:n-3 was significantly lower in the control group and all diet reversed groups compared to the deficient group (p<0.05). These differences were not significant between the control group and the diet reversed groups. The fatty acid composition of phosphatidylethanolamine in the hippocampus of 2-month-old rats was as follows: AA was significantly lower in the control group and all diet reversed groups compared to the deficient group (p<0.05); DHA was significantly higher in the control group and all diet reversed groups compared to the deficient group (p<0.05); n-6:n-3 was significantly lower in the control group and all diet reversed groups compared to the deficient group (p<0.05). These differences were not significant between the control group and the diet reversed groups. The fatty acid composition of phosphatidylserine in the hippocampus of 2-month-old rats was as follows: AA was not significantly different among the different diet groups; DHA was significantly higher in the control group and all diet reversed groups compared to the deficient group (p<0.05); n-6:n-3 was significantly lower in the control group and all diet reversed groups compared to the deficient group (p<0.05). These differences were not significant between the control group and the diet reversed groups. Basal 5-HT levels were significantly higher in the deficient group compared with the control group (p<0.05); there were no significant differences in basal 5-HT levels between the diet reversed groups 1, 2, and 3 and the control group; there were no significant differences in basal 5-HT levels between the diet reversed group 4 and the control group, deficient group, and all other diet reversed groups.	B

continued

TABLE B-1g Continued

Author	Study Type	Subjects	Exposure	Timing of Exposure
Levant et al., 2004	Animal	Adult female Long-Evans rats	AA/EPA/DPA/DHA-deficient diet	Control diet: Day 1 of pregnancy until end of study Deficient diet: Day 1 of pregnancy until postnatal day 21. Postnatal day 21, half on deficient diet were changed to remediation diet and half stayed on deficient diet
Chalon et al., 2001	Animal	Male rats 2-3 months old	ALA-deficient diet	2-3 months of age

Amount	Results	Conclusion*
Control diet: 0.35 kg/5 kg diet from soybean oil; no detected AA, EPA, DPA, or DHA	"Rats raised on the deficient diet exhibited a decrease in brain DHA content to 80% of control animals at maturity (p<0.05)" and an "increase in DPA content to 575% of control animals at maturity (p<0.001)."	A
Deficient diet: 0.35 kg/5 kg diet from sunflower oil; no detected AA, EPA, DPA, or DHA	The remediation diet restored brain DHA and DPA content to levels similar to those on the control diet. Catalepsy score was significantly lower in the deficient diet group compared to the control group (p<0.05) and the remediation diet group (p<0.05).	
Remediation diet: 0.3275 kg/5 kg diet from sunflower oil and 0.0225 kg/5 kg diet from fish oil AA = 0.1 g/100 g fatty acids EPA = 1.6 g/100 g fatty acids DPA = 0.4 g/100 g fatty acids DHA = 3.5 g/100 g fatty acids	In a test of locomotor activity in a novel environment, the deficient diet group exhibited 187% of the activity of the control diet group during the 2-hour observation (p<0.05); results were similar between the deficient diet group and the remediation diet group. In the test of amphetamine-stimulated locomotor activity, the deficient diet group exhibited 144% of the activity of the control group (p<0.05).	
ALA-deficient diet: 1200 mg LA/100 g diet, <6 mg ALA/100 g diet African peanut oil	"Intake of PUFA constitutes an environmental factor able to act on the central nervous system function." "Chronic dietary deficiency in ALA in rats induces abnormalities in several parameters of the mesocortical and mesolimbic dopaminergic systems."	B
Diet balanced in n-6 and n-3 PUFA: 1200 mg LA/100 g diet, 200 mg ALA/100 g African peanut oil and rapeseed oil	"It is proposed that strong links exist among PUFA status, neurotransmission processes, and behavioral disorders in humans."	

continued

TABLE B-1g Continued

Author	Study Type	Subjects	Exposure	Timing of Exposure
de la Presa, Owens, and Innis, 1999	Animal	Newborn male piglets Birth weight >1 kg <12 hours old	GLA/AA/DHA-supplemented formula	<12 hours old to 18 days of age
Delion et al., 1996	Animal	2 generations of female Wistar rats	ALA-deficient diet	2 weeks before mating (second generation)

*B = Evidence of a benefit; N = Evidence of no association or no clear association; A = Evidence of an adverse effect.

Amount	Results	Conclusion*
4 formula diets (all in g/100 g):	There were no significant differences in brain weight, brain protein, DNA, cholesterol or phospholipid concentrations, or CNPase activity among the different diet groups.	B
Diet 1 (Diet D-): 1.6 LA, 0.1 ALA, no GLA, AA, or DHA	Piglets fed formulas with AA and DHA had significantly higher frontal cortex dopamine, HVA, norepinephrine, tryptophan and serotonin concentrations than piglets fed formulas without AA and DHA.	
Diet 2 (Diet D+): 1.9 LA, 0.1 GLA, 0.4 AA, 0.1 ALA, 0.3 DHA	The concentrations of all frontal cortex monoamines and metabolites in piglets fed Diet 2 formula were not different from those of piglets fed Diets 3 and 4.	
Diet 3 (Diet C-): 15.6 LA, 1.5 ALA, no GLA, AA, or DHA	The inclusion of AA and DHA in Diet 4 had no significant effect on any of the frontal cortex monoamines or metabolites measured, compared to Diet 3.	
Diet 4 (Diet C+): 16.4 LA, 0.1 GLA, 0.4 AA, 1.6 ALA, 0.3 DHA		
ALA-deficient diet: 6% fat as peanut oil 6 mg ALA/100 g diet 1200 mg LA/100 g diet	In the control diet group, n-3 (mostly DHA) levels reached a maximum in the stratium and a minimum in the frontal cortex at 12 months of age and remained unchanged during aging in the cerebellum.	N
Control diet: 60% peanut oil, 40% rapeseed oil 200 mg ALA/100 g diet 1200 mg LA/100 g diet	"In the deficient diet group, DHA content considerably reduced as compared with controls." No specific effects of the deficient diet were found on the proportion of any phospholipid classes. In the control diet group, dopamine levels reached a maximum at 6 months of age, were decreased up to 12 months of age, and then stabilized in the stratium and frontal cortex. However, "the levels were not diet related in the stratium but were dramatically reduced in the frontal cortex of deficient rats and remained unchanged throughout all ages." In the control diet group, 5-HT levels increased between 2 and 6 months of age in the stratium and then stabilized; they did not change in the frontal cortex or cerebellum during aging.	

TABLE B-1h Studies on Allergies: Effects on Infants Supplemented with Omega-3 Fatty Acids in Formula

Author	Study Type	Subjects	Exposure	Timing of Exposure
Calder, 2001	Review	Summary of animal studies and human trials	Fish-oil supplement	
Field et al., 2001	Review	Summary of animal studies and human trials	AA/DHA-supplemented formula	

Amount	Results	Conclusion*
	"Animal studies have shown that dietary fish oil results in altered lymphocyte function and in suppressed production of proinflammatory cytokines by macrophages."	B
	"Clinical studies have reported that fish-oil supplementation has beneficial effects in rheumatoid arthritis, inflammatory bowel disease, and among some asthmatics."	
	"The effect of fatty acids during pregnancy upon the maternal immune system and upon that of the infant are not known."	
	"Recent research has been directed at the neurological, retinal, and membrane benefits of adding AA and DHA to infant formula. In adults and animals, feeding DHA affects T-cell function. However, the effect of these lipids on the development and function of the infant's immune system is not known."	N
	"The addition of small amounts of DHA and AA (at levels similar to that in human milk) to preterm infant formula can influence the concentration, proportion, maturation, and cytokine production of peripheral blood lymphocytes."	

continued

TABLE B-1h Continued

Author	Study Type	Subjects	Exposure	Timing of Exposure
Field et al., 2000	Randomized Controlled Trial	Infants (n=44) Preterm, medically stable Edmonton, AB, Canada Appropriate weight for gestational age and receive 100% daily fluid and energy requirements enterally by day 14 postpartum No major congenital infection, significant neonatal morbidity, or acute illness that precluded feeding by mouth; no mixed feedings or corticosteroids, red cell, and plasma transfusions, or intravenous lipid emulsion beyond day 8 postpartum	AA/DHA-supplemented formula	Before day 8 postpartum until day 42 postpartum

*B = Evidence of a benefit; N = Evidence of no association or no clear association.

Amount	Results	Conclusion*
Standard commercial preterm formula group (% weight of total fatty acids): 12.8 LA, 1.4 ALA, no AA or DHA Supplemented preterm formula group (% weight of total fatty acids): 12.10 LA, 1.50 ALA, 0.49 AA, 0.35 DHA	At 14 days postpartum, infants in the supplemented formula group had significantly higher hematocrit (L/L) concentrations compared to those in the human milk group (p<0.05). At 14 days postpartum, infants in the human milk group had significantly higher monocytes compared to both the standard formula group and the supplemented formula group (p<0.05). At 42 days postpartum, infants in the standard formula group had significantly higher T helper phenotypes and CD4/CD8 phenotypes compared to both the supplemented formula group and the human milk group (p<0.05). At 42 days postpartum, infants in the standard formula group had significantly lower monocytes compared to the human milk group (p<0.05). At 42 days postpartum, infants in the human milk group had significantly higher B cells compared to those in both formula groups (p<0.05). At 42 days postpartum, infants in the standard formula group had significantly higher sIL 2R production compared to the supplemented formula group (p<0.05) and significantly lower IL 10 production compared to the human milk group (p<0.05). No other reported results were found to be significant.	B

TABLE B-1i Studies on ADHD: Effects on Children Supplemented with Omega-3 Fatty Acids in Foods Other Than Exclusively Breast Milk or Infant Formula Experimental Studies in Humans

Author	Study Type	Subjects	Exposure	Timing of Exposure
Richardson, 2004	Review	Summary of RCTs	HUFA supplement	
Hirayama et al., 2004*	Randomized Controlled Trial	Children (n=40) Aged 6-12 years Recruited from a summer camp for children with psychiatric disorders Diagnosed or suspected as ADHD	DHA supplement	2 months

Amount	Results	Conclusion**
	Omega-3 fatty acids, particularly EPA, may be beneficial in the management of dyslexia, dyspraxia, and ADHD.	B
	There is no evidence that omega-6 fatty acids are beneficial in the management of dyslexia, dyspraxia, and ADHD, but positive results have been found using an omega-3:omega-6 combination for both ADHD and dyslexia.	
DHA group: Fermented soybean milk 3 times/ week (600 mg DHA/125 mL) Bread rolls 2 times/week (300 mg DHA/45 g) Steamed bread 2 times/week (600 mg DHA/60 g) Total = 3600 mg DHA, 700 mg EPA/week	Short-term visual memory was significantly improved in the control group from baseline until the end of the study (p=0.02), but not in the DHA group. The short-term visual memory was significantly better in the control group than in the DHA group (p=0.02).	A
	The number of errors of omission and commission were significantly improved in the continuous performance test in the control group from baseline until the end of the study (p=0.02 and p=0.01, respectively).	
Control group: Placebo food containing olive oil instead of DHA-rich fish oil	The number of errors of commission were significantly higher in the DHA group than in the control group (p=0.001).	

continued

TABLE B-1i Continued

Author	Study Type	Subjects	Exposure	Timing of Exposure
Harding et al., 2003*	Trial	Boys and girls (n=20) Aged 7-12 years Diagnosed with ADHD No other medication or treatment, street drugs, other nutritional or botanical supplements, co-morbid disorders	Multivitamin, multiple mineral, phytonutrients, essential fatty acid supplements	4 weeks
Stevens et al., 2003*	Randomized Controlled Trial	Boys and girls (n=47) Aged 6-13 Central Indiana = 100-mile radius of West Lafayette Those with diagnosed ADHD and those without ADHD No chronic health problems Presence of 1+ severe symptoms or several mild symptoms	PUFA supplement	4 months

Amount	Results	Conclusion**
Groups determined by parental choice Ritalin group: 5-15 mg Ritalin 2-3 times daily Supplement group: A multivitamin, multi-mineral, phytonu-trients, essential fatty acids (180 mg EPA and 120 mg DHA from salmon oil and 45 mg GLA from borage oil) and phospholipids (soy lecithin), pro-biotics, and amino acids	Both the Ritalin group and the supplement group showed significant gains in the Full Scale Response Control Quotient and the Full Scale Attention Control Quotient scores ($p \leq 0.01$ and $p \leq 0.001$, respectively). There were no significant differences in improvement between the two groups.	B
PUFA group: 8 capsules of PUFA/day 60 mg DHA, 10 mg EPA, 5 mg AA, 12 mg GLA, 3 mg vitamin E/capsule Placebo group: 8 capsules of placebo/day 0.8 g olive oil/capsule	Based on those who completed the intervention, the change in teacher hit reaction time (measured both in ms and T-score) was significantly greater in the PUFA group than in the placebo group ($p=0.05$ and $p=0.02$, respectively) at 4 months. At baseline, there were no significant differences in parents' DBD and teachers' DBD scores between the two groups; after 4 months of treatment the number of children who improved on the parents' DBD attention and oppositional/defiant disorder scales was significantly higher in the PUFA group than in the placebo group ($p=0.09$ and $p=0.02$, respectively). No other significant differences were found between the two groups.	B

continued

TABLE B-1i Continued

Author	Study Type	Subjects	Exposure	Timing of Exposure
Richardson and Puri, 2002*	Randomized Controlled Trial	Boys and girls (n=41) Aged 8-12 years Northern Ireland Referred to a school for children with specific literacy problems No official diagnosis of ADHD or any other psychiatric disorder; use of fatty acid supplements in last 6 months; consumption of oily fish >2 times/week; history of any other neurological or major psychiatric disorder or other significant medical problems; not in treatment for ADHD	HUFA supplement	12 weeks

Amount	Results	Conclusion**
Supplement group: 186 mg EPA/day, 480 mg DHA/day, 96 mg GLA/day, 60 IU vitamin E/day, 864 mg LA/day, 42 mg AA/day, 8 mg thyme oil/day Placebo: Olive oil	At 3 months, the mean psychosomatic ADHD sub- scale, mean Conners' ADHD index score, and mean DSM inattention score were significantly lower in the supplemented group than in the placebo group ($p=0.05$, $p=0.03$, $p=0.05$, respectively). At 12 weeks, the improvements were significantly greater for the supplemented group compared to the placebo group for the cognitive problems ($p=0.01$), the anxious/shy subscales ($p=0.04$), and the Conners' index global scale ($p=0.02$).	B

continued

TABLE B-1i Continued

Author	Study Type	Subjects	Exposure	Timing of Exposure
Brue et al., 2001	Randomized Controlled Trial	Boys and girls (n=51) Aged 4-12 years Referred by parents, pediatricians, psychologists, psychiatrists, and educators ADHD diagnosed by a physician or psychologist No serious and preexisting medical or psychological condition or taking a stimulant medication other than Ritalin	Essential fatty acid supplement	Two 12-week trials

Amount	Results	Conclusion**
Trial 1: Treatment Group and Ritalin + Treatment Group: 10 mg Ginkgo biloba, 200 mg Melissa officinalis, 30 mg Grapine, 35 mg dimethylamino-ethanol, 100 mg 1-glutamine	Based on parent and teacher reports from Trial 1, there were no significant differences in inattentiveness or hyperactive-impulsive subscales between any of the treatment groups and their respective controls.	N
Placebo Group and Ritalin + Placebo Group: 200 mg Slippery elm supplement	Based on parent reports from Trial 2, those in the double treatment + EFA group had a significantly lower hyperactive-impulsive subscale score than the double treatment group (p=0.03).	
Trial 2: Double Treatment Group and Ritalin + Double Treatment Group: 20 mg Ginkgo biloba, 400 mg Melissa officinalis, 60 mg Grapine, 70 mg dimethylamino-ethanol, 200 mg 1-glutamine	Based on teacher reports from Trial 2, those in the Ritalin + double treatment + EFA group had a significantly higher inattentive subscale score than the Ritalin + double treatment group (p=0.04). Based on teacher reports from Trial 2, those in the double treatment + EFA group had a significantly higher hyperactive-impulsive subscale score than the double treatment group (p=0.04).	
Double Treatment + EFA Group and Ritalin + Double Treatment + EFA Group: 20 mg Ginkgo biloba, 400 mg Melissa officinalis, 60 mg Grapine, 70 mg dimethylamino-ethanol, 200 mg 1-glutamine, 1000 mg flaxseed		

continued

TABLE B-1i Continued

Author	Study Type	Subjects	Exposure	Timing of Exposure
Voigt et al., 2001*	Randomized Controlled Trial	Boys and girls (n=63) Aged 6-12 years 100% White in DHA group; 85% White in placebo group Texas No ineffective treatment with stimulant medication; treatment with other psychotropic medications; previous diagnosis of other childhood psychiatric disorders; use of dietary supplements; occurrence of a significant life event within 6 months; history of head injury or seizures; receipt of special education services for mental retardation or a pervasive developmental disorder; premature birth; exposure to tobacco, alcohol, or other drugs in utero; diagnosis of a disorder of lipid metabolism or other chronic medical condition Previous diagnosis of ADHD Being treated successfully with stimulant medication	Algae-derived triglyceride supplement	4 months

Amount	Results	Conclusion**
Algae-derived TG capsule: 345 mg DHA/day	Between baseline and 4 months, TOVA errors of omission significantly increased (p=0.03-0.01) and color trails 1 (p=0.03-0.01) and color trails 2 (p=0.001) significantly decreased for the supplemented group. Between baseline and 4 months, TOVA errors of commission (p<0.0003) and color trails 2 (p<0.0003) significantly decreased and TOVA total response time (p=0.03-0.01) significantly increased for the placebo group. "There were no differences between groups at any time on any behavior measure by the parental Conners' Rating Scales."	N

continued

TABLE B-1i Continued

Author	Study Type	Subjects	Exposure	Timing of Exposure
Stevens et al., 1995*	Case-control	Cases = boys with ADHD (n=53) Control = healthy boys (n=43) Aged 6-12 years North central Indiana Primarily White	Plasma fatty acid analysis	At time of visit
Mitchell et al., 1987*	Case-control	Cases = hyperactive children (n=48) Controls = from two local primary schools (n=49) Boys and girls Mean age about 9 years 92% European About 95% mothers in top three socioeconomic groups Auckland, New Zealand	Serum fatty acid levels	At time of visit
Mitchell et al., 1983*	Case-control	Cases = from a residential school for "maladjusted" children (n=23) Controls = from a normal intermediate school (n=20) Boys and girls Aged 10-13 years for controls Aged 7.5-13 years for cases Auckland, New Zealand	Level of red blood cell essential fatty acids	At time of visit

*Included in Schachter HM, Kourad K, Merali Z, Lumb A, Tran K, Miguelez M. 2005. *Effects of Omega-3 Fatty Acids on Mental Health. Summary, Evidence Report/Technology Assessment No. 116 (Prepared by the University of Ottawa Evidence-based Practice Center under Contract No. 290-02-0021).* Rockville, MD: Agency for Healthcare Research and Quality.

**B = Evidence of a benefit; A = Evidence of an adverse effect; N = Evidence of no association or no clear association.

Amount	Results	Conclusion**
Omega-3 fatty acids as continuous variables	Boys with ADHD had significantly lower mean levels of plasma AA, EPA, and DHA than the controls (p<0.02, p<0.02, p<0.03, respectively). Boys with ADHD had significantly lower mean levels of red blood cell AA (p<0.02), 22:4n-6 (p<0.03), and DHA (p<0.06), and significantly higher mean levels of red blood cell 22:5n-6 (p<0.05) compared to the controls.	B
Omega-3 fatty acids as continuous variables	The mean level of DHA from nonfasting blood samples was significantly lower in the hyperactive children than in the controls (p=0.045). The mean levels of DGLA and AA from nonfasting blood samples were significantly lower in the hyperactive children than in the controls (p=0.007 and p=0.027, respectively). No significant differences in blood serum n-3 or n-6 fatty acids were found.	B
Omega-3 fatty acids as continuous variables	The mean levels of LA, DGLA, and AA from fasting blood samples were lower in the "maladjusted" children than in the normal children (0.05<p<0.01), although the differences were not significant. The mean level of 22:5n-6 from fasting blood samples was higher in the "maladjusted" children than in the normal children (0.05<p<0.1), although this difference was not significant. No other significant differences were found between the two groups in terms of fatty acid levels in fasting blood samples.	N

TABLE B-1j Studies on Allergies and Asthma: Effects on Children
Supplemented with Omega-3 Fatty Acids in Foods Other Than
Exclusively Breast Milk or Infant Formula

Author	Study Type	Subjects	Exposure	Timing of Exposure
Peat et al., 2004	Randomized Controlled Trial	Pregnant women (n=616) Mean age about 29 years About 47% tertiary educated Sydney, Australia At least one parent or sibling with current asthma or frequent wheeze; fluency in English; a telephone at home; residence within 30 km of the recruitment center No pet at home; vegetarian diet; multiple births; or less than 36 weeks gestation The Childhood Asthma Prevention Study (CAPS)	Tuna-fish oil supplement	Child's age of 6 months to 3 years
Hodge et al., 1998*	Randomized Controlled Trial	Boys and girls (n=39) Aged 8-12 years Sydney, Australia Asthmatic with a history of episodic wheeze in the last 12 months and airway hyper-responsiveness to histamine No other significant diseases; taking regular oral corticosteroids or with known aspirin or dietary salicylate sensitivity	EPA/DHA supplement	6 months

Amount	Results	Conclusion**
Intervention group: 500 mg/day tuna fish oil 184 mg omega-3 fatty acids Placebo group: Sunola oil 83% monounsaturated oil	At 3 years of age, there were no significant differences in prevalence of asthma, wheezing, eczema, and atopy between the intervention group and the placebo group. However, those in the intervention group had significantly lower prevalence of mild or moderate coughing (p=0.03) and atopic coughing (p=0.003) than the placebo group.	N
Omega-3 group: 0.18 g EPA and 0.12 g DHA/capsule 4 capsules/day = 1.2 g omega-3/day Omega-6 group: 0.45 g safflower oil, 0.45 g palm oil, 0.10 g olive oil/capsule No EPA or DHA	"There was no significant change in spirometric function, dose response ratio to histamine or asthma severity score at either 3 or 6 months in either group." "There were no significant differences between groups in TNFα production over time (p=0.22)." "Dietary enrichment of omega-3 fatty acids over 6 months increased plasma levels of these fatty acids, reduced stimulated tumour necrosis factor α production, but had no effect on the clinical severity of asthma in these children."	N

continued

TABLE B-1j Continued

Author	Study Type	Subjects	Exposure	Timing of Exposure
Denny et al., 2003	Review	18 cross-sectional studies 4 case-control studies 3 cohort studies	Dietary PUFA	
Smit et al., 1999	Review	All epidemiological evidence	Seafood	

Amount	Results	Conclusion**
	"Very few studies investigated the effects of polyunsaturated fatty acids (PUFAs) on chronic obstructive pulmonary disease (COPD) and asthma, and the results of those that were found showed conflicting results."	N
	"It is very difficult to draw any conclusions on the true impact of dietary PUFA intake on respiratory health."	
	"The evidence in this review suggests that diet does play a role in asthma and COPD, but the causality of association cannot be confirmed because of the observational nature of most of the studies."	
	"The findings of several large studies in adults suggest that high fish intake has beneficial effects on lung function."	B
	"The relationship between fish intake and respiratory symptoms and clinical disease is less evident."	

continued

TABLE B-1j Continued

Author	Study Type	Subjects	Exposure	Timing of Exposure
Peat et al., 1998*	Review	Longitudinal cohort studies and cross-sectional studies	Diet	

Amount	Results	Conclusion**
	In cross-sectional studies, the risk factors for presence in: 1. Airway narrowing are atopy, family history of asthma, gender (male), and parental smoking; 2. Airway size are low birth weight, parental smoking, and diet (low magnesium or antioxidant intake); 3. Airway hyperresponsiveness are atopy, family history of asthma, high allergen exposure, and diet (high sodium/magnesium or low omega-3 fatty acid intake). In longitudinal studies, the risk factors for ongoing conditions from: 1. Airway narrowing are atopy early in childhood, gender (female), parental smoking, symptoms that begin before age 5, persistent wheeze in childhood in the absence of respiratory infection, and reduced expiratory flow rate; 2. Airway size are atopy, gender (female), and airway hyperresponsiveness; 3. Airway hyperresponsiveness are atopy in early childhood, airway hyperresponsiveness in childhood, reduced expiratory flow rate, and gender (female). Important future longitudinal studies will be those that divide the broad spectrum of asthma into phenotypic groups.	B

continued

TABLE B-1j Continued

Author	Study Type	Subjects	Exposure	Timing of Exposure
Takemura et al., 2002*	Case-control	Cases = currently asthmatic students (n=1673) Controls = students who were never asthmatic (n=22,109) Boys and girls Elementary and junior high school students Aged 6-15 years, Tokorozawa City, Japan Tokorozawa Childhood Asthma and Pollinosis Study	Seafood	

Amount	Results	Conclusion**
Fish intake categories: 1 = Almost none 2 = 1-2 times/month 3 = 1-2 times/week 4 = ≥3-4 times/week Serving size unspecified; cited that "most of the variation is explained by frequency of use rather than differences in serving sizes"	After adjusting for age, gender, parental history of asthma: The OR for current asthma was slightly significantly higher for those who ate fish 1-2 times/week compared to those who ate fish 1-2 times/month (OR=1.133, 95% CI 1.021-1.258); and Although the ORs for current asthma were not significant for those who ate fish almost never (OR=0.957, 95% CI 0.725-1.263) and ≥3-4 times/week (OR=1.334, 95% CI 0.907-1.963) compared to those who ate fish 1-2 times/month, there was a significant positive trend with an increase of fish consumption (p for trend = 0.0078). After adjusting for age, gender, parental history of asthma, and vegetable and fruit intake: The OR for current asthma was slightly significantly higher for those who ate fish 1-2 times/week compared to those who ate fish 1-2 times/month (OR=1.117, 95% CI 1.005-1.241); and Although the ORs for current asthma were not significant for those who ate fish almost never (OR=1.039, 95% CI 0.785-1.376) and ≥3-4 times/week (OR=1.319, 95% CI 0.896-1.943) compared to those who ate fish 1-2 times/month, there was a significant positive trend with an increase of fish consumption (p for trend = 0.0349).	A

continued

TABLE B-1j Continued

Author	Study Type	Subjects	Exposure	Timing of Exposure
Hodge et al., 1996*	Case-control	Boys and girls (n=468) Aged 8-11 Sydney, Australia With airway hyperre-sponsiveness, wheeze in the last 12 months, and 3-in-5 sample of children with no airway hyperrespon-siveness or wheeze in the last 12 months	Seafood	In the past year
Ellwood et al., 2001	Ecological	Children Aged 6-7 and 13-14 years 53 countries The International Study of Asthma and Allergies in Childhood (ISAAC) Data from FAO Food Balance Sheet	PUFA and seafood intake	

Amount	Results	Conclusion**
Total fish intake/week Ever eat fresh fish, fresh oily fish, or fresh non-oily fish	There were no significant differences in total fish intake between children with normal airways (1.2 servings, 95% CI 1.0-1.3), airway hyperresponsiveness (1.2 servings, 95% CI 0.9-1.5), wheeze (1.2 servings, 95% CI 0.8-1.5) and current asthma (1.0 servings, 95% CI 0.8-1.2). Significantly fewer children with asthma ever ate oil fish compared to children with normal airways (p<0.05); however, there was no significant difference between those with current asthma and normal children who ate exclusively oily fish. After adjusting for atopy, parental asthma, parental smoking, ethnicity, country of birth, early respiratory illness, and sex: Children who ate oily fish had a significantly lower OR of current asthma when compared to children who did not eat oily fish (OR-0.26, 95% CI 0.09 0.72); and There were no other significant associations found between type of fish (fresh fish, oily fish, non-oily fish) and airway hyperresponsiveness, wheeze, or current asthma.	B
Percentage of total energy consumed as PUFA: 3%-12% Range of fish intake not reported	There were no significant associations found between total PUFA intake (% of total fat) for current wheezing, severe wheezing, allergic rhinoconjunctivitis, and atopic eczema. There was a significant inverse association found between all fish (fresh and frozen) consumption and asthma, allergic rhinoconjunctivitis, and atopic eczema, for the 13- to 14-year old age group; the same inverse association remained for the 6- to 7-year-old age group, but the association was weaker.	B

continued

TABLE B-1j Continued

Author	Study Type	Subjects	Exposure	Timing of Exposure
Satomi et al., 1994*	Ecological	Boys and girls (n=7742) Aged 6-11 years Japan 1st-, 3rd-, 5th-grade students Coastal schools = fish harvest and consumption are high Inland schools = located far from sea but close to the coast school district	Seafood	

*Included in Schachter HM, Reisman J, Tran K, Dales B, Kourad K, Barnes D, Sampson M, Morrison A, Gaboury I, Blackman J. 2004. *Health Effects of Omega-3 Fatty Acids on Asthma. Summary, Evidence Report/Technology Assessment No. 91 (Prepared by the University of Ottawa Evidence-based Practice Center under Contract No. 290-02-0021). AHRQ Publication No. 04-E013-2.* Rockville, MD: Agency for Healthcare Research and Quality.

**N = Evidence of no association or no clear association; B = Evidence of a benefit; A = Evidence of an adverse effect.

Amount	Results	Conclusion**
Fish consumption categories: Very often = ≥4-5 times/week Relatively often = 2-3 times/week Often = 1 time/week Infrequently = 1-2 times/month Seldom = <1 time/month	Coastal school children who ate reddish fish (sardine, mackerel, pike) very often had a significantly lower prevalence of history of asthma than those who seldom ate reddish fish (p<0.01). There were no other significant differences for these children based on consumption of pale fish, shellfish, fish-paste, seaweed, and dried fish. Inland school children who ate pale fish (flatfish, sea bream, turbot) and seaweed very often had significantly higher prevalence of history of asthma than those who seldom ate pale fish and seaweed (p<0.01; 0.01<p<0.05, respectively). There were no other significant differences for these children based on reddish fish, shellfish, fish-paste, and dried fish.	B

REFERENCES

Agostoni C, Trojan S, Bellu R, Riva E, Giovannini M. 1995. Neurodevelopmental quotient of healthy term infants at 4 months and feeding practice: The role of long-chain polyunsaturated fatty acids. *Pediatric Research* 38(2):262–266.

Al MDM, van Houwelingen AC, Kester ADM, Hasaart THM, de Jong AEP, Hornstra G. 1995. Maternal essential fatty acid patterns during normal pregnancy and their relationship to the neonatal essential fatty acid status. *British Journal of Nutrition* 74(1):55–68.

Auestad N, Halter R, Hall RT, Blatter M, Bogle ML, Burks W, Erickson JR, Fitzgerald KM, Dobson V, Innis SM, Singer LT, Montalto MB, Jacobs JR, Qiu W, Bornstein MH. 2001. Growth and development in term infants fed long-chain polyunsaturated fatty acids: A double-masked, randomized, parallel, prospective, multivariate study. *Pediatrics* 108(2): 372–381.

Birch EE, Birch DG, Hoffman DR, Uauy R. 1992. Dietary essential fatty acid supply and visual acuity development. *Investigations in Ophthalmology and Visual Science* 33(11):3242–3253.

Birch EE, Hoffman DR, Uauy R, Birch DG, Prestidge C. 1998. Visual acuity and the essentiality of docosahexaenoic acid and arachidonic acid in the diet of term infants. *Pediatric Research* 44(2):201–209.

Birch EE, Garfield S, Hoffman DR, Uauy R, Birch DG. 2000. A randomized controlled trial of early dietary supply of long-chain polyunsaturated fatty acids and mental development in term infants. *Developmental Medicine and Child Neurology* 42(3):174–181.

Birch EE, Hoffman DR, Castaneda YS, Fawcett SL, Birch DG, Uauy RD. 2002. A randomized controlled trial of long-chain polyunsaturated fatty acid supplementation of formula in term infants after weaning at 6 wk of age. *American Journal of Clinical Nutrition* 75(3):570–580.

Bjerve KS, Brubakk AM, Fougner KJ, Johnsen H, Midthjell K, Vik T. 1993. Omega-3 fatty acids: Essential fatty acids with important biological effects, and serum phospholipid fatty acids as markers of dietary omega 3-fatty acid intake. *American Journal of Clinical Nutrition* 57(Suppl 5):801S–805S.

Bougle D, Denise P, Vimard F, Nouvelot A, Penneillo MJ, Guillois B. 1999. Early neurological and neuropsychological development of the preterm infant and polyunsaturated fatty acids supply. *Clinical Neurophysiology* 110(8):1363–1370.

Bouwstra H, Dijck-Brouwer DA, Wildeman JA, Tjoonk HM, van der Heide JC, Boersma ER, Muskiet FA, Hadders-Algra M. 2003. Long-chain polyunsaturated fatty acids have a positive effect on the quality of general movements of healthy term infants. *American Journal of Clinical Nutrition* 78(2):313–318.

Bouwstra H, Dijck-Brouwer DA, Boehm G, Boersma ER, Muskiet FA, Hadders-Algra M. 2005. Long-chain polyunsaturated fatty acids and neurological developmental outcome at 18 months in healthy term infants. *Acta Paediatric* 94(1):26–32.

Bouzan C, Cohen JT, Connor WE, Kris-Etherton PM, Gray GM, Konig A, Lawrence RS, Savitz DA, Teutsch SM. 2005. A quantitative analysis of fish consumption and stroke risk. *American Journal of Preventive Medicine* 29(4):347–352.

Brue AW, Oakland TD, Evans RA. 2001. The use of a dietary supplement combination and an essential fatty acid as an alternative and complementary treatment for children with attention-deficit/hyperactivity disorder. *The Scientific Review of Alternative Medicine* 5(4):187–194.

Bryan J, Osendarp S, Hughes D, Calvaresi E, Baghurst K, van Klinken J-W. 2004. Nutrients for cognitive development in school-aged children. *Nutrition Reviews* 62(8):295–306.

Bulstra-Ramakers MT, Huisjes HJ, Visser GH. 1995. The effects of 3g eicosapentaenoic acid daily on recurrence of intrauterine growth retardation and pregnancy induced hypertension. *British Journal of Obstetrics and Gynaecology* 102(2):123–126.

Calder PC. 2001. Polyunsaturated fatty acids, inflammation, and immunity. *Lipids* 36(9):1007–1024.

Carlson SE, Neuringer M. 1999. Polyunsaturated fatty acid status and neurodevelopment: A summary and critical analysis of the literature. *Lipids* 34(2):171–178.

Carlson SE, Werkman SH. 1996. A randomized trial of visual attention of preterm infants fed docosahexaenoic acid until two months. *Lipids* 31(1):85–90.

Carlson SE, Rhodes PG, Ferguson MG. 1986. Docosahexaenoic acid status of preterm infants at birth and following feeding with human milk or formula. *American Journal of Clinical Nutrition* 44(6):798–804.

Carlson SE, Werkman SH, Rhodes PG, Tolley EA. 1993. Visual-acuity development in healthy preterm infants: Effect of marine-oil supplementation. *American Journal of Clinical Nutrition* 58(1):35–42.

Carlson SE, Ford AJ, Werkman SH, Peeples JM, Koo WW. 1996a. Visual acuity and fatty acid status of term infants fed human milk and formulas with and without docosahexaenoate and arachidonate from egg yolk lecithin. *Pediatric Research* 39(5):882–888.

Carlson SE, Werkman SH, Tolley EA. 1996b. Effect of long-chain n-3 fatty acid supplementation on visual acuity and growth of preterm infants with and without bronchopulmonary dysplasia. *American Journal of Clinical Nutrition* 63(5):687–697.

Carlson SE, Werkman SH, Montalto MB, Tolley EA. 1999. Visual acuity development of preterm (PT) infants fed docosahexaenoic acid (DHA) and arachidonic acid (ARA): Effect of age at supplementation. *Pediatric Research* 45:279A.

Chalon S, Vancassel S, Zimmer L, Guilloteau D, Durand G. 2001. Polyunsaturated fatty acids and cerebral function: Focus on monoaminergic neurotransmission. *Lipids* 36(9):937–944.

Cheruku SR, Montgomery-Downs HE, Farkas SL, Thoman EB, Lammi-Keefe CJ. 2002. Higher maternal plasma docosahexaenoic acid during pregnancy is associated with more mature neonatal sleep-state patterning. *American Journal of Clinical Nutrition* 76(3):608–613.

Clandinin MT, Chappell JE, Leong S, Heim T, Swyer PR, Change GW. 1980b. Extrauterine fatty acid accretion in infant brain: Implications for fatty acid requirements. *Early Human Development* 4(2):131–138.

Clandinin MT, Van Aerde JE, Merkel KL, Harris CL, Springer MA, Hansen JW, Diersen-Schade DA. 2005. Growth and development of preterm infants fed infant formulas containing docosahexaenoic acid and arachidonic acid. *Journal of Pediatrics* 146(4):461–468.

Clausen T, Slott M, Solvoll K, Drevon CA, Vollset SE, Henriksen T. 2001. High intake of energy, sucrose, and polyunsaturated fatty acids is associated with increased risk of preeclampsia. *American Journal of Obstetrics and Gynecology* 185(2):451–458.

Cohen JT, Bellinger DC, Connor WE, Shaywitz BA. 2005. A quantitative analysis of prenatal intake of n-3 polyunsaturated fatty acids and cognitive development. *American Journal of Preventive Medicine* 29(4):366–374.

Colombo J, Kannass KN, Shaddy DJ, Kundurthi S, Maikranz JM, Anderson CJ, Blaga OM, Carlson SE. 2004. Maternal DHA and the development of attention in infancy and toddlerhood. *Child Development* 75(4):1254–1267.

Daniels JL, Longnecker MP, Rowland AS, Golding J, the ALSPAC Study Team. 2004. Fish intake during pregnancy and early cognitive development of offspring. *Epidemiology* 15(4):394–402.

de Groot RH, Hornstra G, van Houwelingen AC, Roumen F. 2004. Effect of alpha-linolenic acid supplementation during pregnancy on maternal and neonatal polyunsaturated fatty acid status and pregnancy outcome. *American Journal of Clinical Nutrition* 79(2):251–260.

de la Presa Owens S, Innis SM. 1999. Docosahexaenoic and arachidonic acid prevent a decrease in dopaminergic and serotoninergic neurotransmitters in frontal cortex caused by a linoleic and α-linolenic acid deficient diet in formula-fed piglets. *Journal of Nutrition* 129(11):2088–2093.

Delion S, Chalon S, Guilloteau D, Besnard J-C, Durand G. 1996. α-linolenic acid dietary deficiency alters age-related changes of dopaminergic and serotoninergic neurotransmission in the rat frontal cortex. *Journal of Neurochemistry* 66(4):1582–1591.

Denburg JA, Hatfield HM, Cyr MM, Hayes L, Holt PG, Sehmi R, Dunstan JA, Prescott SL. 2005. Fish oil supplementation in pregnancy modifies neonatal progenitors at birth in infants at risk of atopy. *Pediatric Research* 57(2):276–281.

Denny SI, Thompson RL, Margetts BM. 2003. Dietary factors in the pathogenesis of asthma and chronic obstructive pulmonary disease. *Current Allergy and Asthma Reports* 3(2):130–136.

Dunstan JA, Mori TA, Barden A. 2003a. Fish oil supplementation in pregnancy modifies neonatal allergen-specific immune responses and clinical outcomes in infants at high risk of atopy: A randomized, controlled trial. *Journal of Allergy and Clinical Immunology* 112(6):1178–1184.

Dunstan JA, Mori TA, Barden A. 2003b. Maternal fish oil supplementation in pregnancy reduces interleukin-13 levels in cord blood of infants at high risk of atopy. *Clinical and Experimental Allergy* 33(4):442–448.

Ellwood P, Asher MI, Bjorksten B, Burr M, Pearce N, Robertson CF. 2001. Diet and asthma, allergic rhinoconjunctivitis and atopic eczema symptom prevalence: An ecological analysis of the International Study of Asthma and Allergies in Childhood (ISAAC) data. ISAAC Phase One Study Group. *European Respiratory Journal* 17(3):436–443.

Farquharson J, Jamieson EC, Logan RW, Cockburn MD, Patrick WA. 1992. Infant cerebral cortex phospholipid fatty-acid composition and diet. *Lancet* 340(8823):810–813.

Fewtrell MS, Morley R, Abbott A, Singhal A, Isaacs EB, Stephenson T, MacFadyen U, Lucas A. 2002. Double-blind, randomized trial of long-chain polyunsaturated fatty acid supplementation in formula fed to preterm infants. *Pediatrics* 110(1):73–82.

Fewtrell MS, Abbott RA, Kennedy K, Singhal A, Morley R, Caine E, Jamieson C, Cockburn F, Lucas A. 2004. Randomized, double-blind trial of long-chain polyunsaturated fatty acid supplementation with fish oil and borage oil in preterm infants. *Journal of Pediatrics* 144(4):471–479.

Field CJ, Thomson CA, Van Aerde JE, Parrott A, Euler A, Lien E, Clandinin MT. 2000. Lower proportion of CD45R0+ cells and deficient interleukin-10 production by formula-fed infants, compared with human-fed, is corrected with supplementation of long-chain polyunsaturated fatty acids. *Journal of Pediatric Gastroenterology and Nutrition* 31(3):291–299.

Field CJ, Clandinin MT, Van Aerde JE. 2001. Polyunsaturated fatty acids and T-cell function: Implications for the neonate. *Lipids* 36(9):1025–1032.

Gibson RA, Chen W, Makrides M. 2001. Randomized trials with polyunsaturated fatty acid interventions in preterm and term infants: Functional and clinical outcomes. *Lipids* 36(9):873–883.

Grandjean P, Bjerve KS, Weihe P, Steuerwald U. 2001. Birthweight in a fishing community: Significance of essential fatty acids and marine food contaminants. *International Journal of Epidemiology* 30(6):1272–1278.

Haggarty P, Page K, Abramovich DR, Ashton J, Brown D. 1997. Long-chain polyunsaturated fatty acid transport across the perfused human placenta. *Placenta* 18(8):635–642.

Haggarty P, Ashton J, Joynson M, Abramovich DR, Page K. 1999. Effect of maternal polyunsaturated fatty acid concentration on transport by the human placenta. *Biology of the Neonate* 75(6):350–359.

Haggarty P, Abramovich DR, Page K. 2002. The effect of maternal smoking and ethanol on fatty acid transport by the human placenta. *British Journal of Nutrition* 87(3):247–252.

Harding KL, Judah RD, Gant C. 2003. Outcome-based comparison of Ritalin versus food-supplement treated children with AD/HD. *Alternative Medicine Review* 8(3):319–330.

Harper V, MacInnes R, Campbell D, Hall M. 1991. Increased birth weight in northerly islands: Is fish consumption a red herring? *British Medical Journal* 303(6795):166.

Haugen G, Helland I. 2001. Influence of preeclampsia or maternal intake of omega-3 fatty acids on the vasoactive effect of prostaglandin F-two-alpha in human umbilical arteries. *Gynecologic and Obstetrical Investigations* 52(2):75–81.

Hawkes JS, Bryan D-L, Makrides M, Neumann MA, Gibson RA. 2002. A randomized trial of supplementation with docosahexaenoic acid–rich tuna oil and its effects on the human milk cytokines interleukin 1β, interleukin 6, and tumor necrosis factor. *American Journal of Clinical Nutrition* 75(4):754–760.

Helland IB, Saugstad OD, Smith L, Saarem K, Solvoll K, Ganes T, Drevon CA. 2001. Similar effects on infants of n-3 and n-6 fatty acids supplementation to pregnant and lactating women. *Pediatrics* 108(5):e82. [Online]. Available: http://www.pediatrics.org/cgi/content/full/108/5/e82 [accessed August 22, 2005].

Helland IB, Smith L, Saarem K, Saugstad OD, Drevon CA. 2003. Maternal supplementation with very-long-chain n-3 fatty acids during pregnancy and lactation augments children's IQ at 4 years of age. *Pediatrics* 111(1):39–44.

Hibbeln JR. 2002. Seafood consumption, the DHA content of mothers' milk and prevalence rates of postpartum depression: A cross-national, ecological analysis. *Journal of Affective Disorders* 69(1–3):15–29.

Hibbeln JR, Salem N Jr. 1995. Dietary polyunsaturated fatty acids and depression: When cholesterol does not satisfy. *American Journal of Clinical Nutrition* 62(1):1–9.

Hirayama S, Hamazaki T, Terasawa K. 2004. Effect of docosahexaenoic acid-containing food administration on symptoms of attention deficit/hyperactivity disorder—a placebo-controlled double-blind study. *European Journal of Clinical Nutrition* 58(3):467–473.

Hodge L, Salome CM, Peat JK, Haby MM, Xuan W, Woolcock AJ. 1996. Consumption of oily fish and childhood asthma risk. *Medical Journal of Australia* 164(3):137–140.

Hodge L, Salome CM, Hughes JM, Liu-Brennan D, Rimmer J, Allman M, Pang D, Armour C, Woolcock AJ. 1998. Effect of dietary intake of omega-3 and omega-6 fatty acids on severity of asthma in children. *European Respiratory Journal* 11(2):361–365.

Hoffman DR, Birch EE, Castaneda YS, Fawcett SL, Wheaton DH, Birch DG, Uauy R. 2003. Visual function in breast-fed term infants weaned to formula with or without long-chain polyunsaturated at 4 to 6 months: A randomized clinical trial. *Journal of Pediatrics* 142(6):669–677.

Holman RT, Johnson SB, Ogburn PL. 1991. Deficiency of essential fatty acids and membrane fluidity during pregnancy and lactation. *Proceedings of the National Academy of Sciences of the United States of America* 88(11):4835–4839.

Innis SM, Gilley J, Werker J. 2001. Are human milk long-chain polyunsaturated fatty acids related to visual and neural development in breast-fed term infants? *Journal of Pediatrics* 139(4):532–538.

Innis SM, Adamkin DH, Hall RT, Kalhan SC, Lair C, Lim M, Stevens DC, Twist PF, Diersen-Schade DA, Harris CL, Merkel KL, Hansen JW. 2002. Docosahexaenoic acid and arachidonic acid enhance growth with no adverse effects in preterm infants fed formula. *Journal of Pediatrics* 140(5):547–554.

Jacobson SW. 1999. Assessment of long-chain polyunsaturated fatty acid nutritional supplementation on infant neurobehavioral development and visual acuity. *Lipids* 34(2):151–160.

Jensen CL, Voigt RG, Llorente AM, Peters SU, Prager TC, Zou Y, Fraley JK, Heird WC. 2004. Effect of maternal docosahexaenoic acid (DHA) supplementation on neuropsychological and visual status of former breast-fed infants at five years of age. *Pediatric Research* (abstract) 55:181A.

Jensen CL, Voigt RG, Prager TC, Zou YL, Fraley JK, Rozelle JC, Turcich MR, Llorente AM, Anderson RE, Heird WC. 2005. Effects of maternal docosahexaenoic acid intake on visual function and neurodevelopment in breastfed term infants. *American Journal of Clinical Nutrition* 82(1):125–132.

Kesmodel U, Olsen SF, Salvig JD. 1997. Marine n-3 fatty acid and calcium intake in relation to pregnancy induced hypertension, intrauterine growth retardation, and preterm delivery. A case-control study. *Acta Obstetricia et Gynecologica Scandinavica* 76(1):38–44.

Kodas E, Galineau L, Bodard S, Vancassel S, Guilloteau D, Besnard J-C, Chalon S. 2004. Serotoninergic neurotransmission is affected by n-3 polyunsaturated fatty acids in the rat. *Journal of Neurochemistry* 89(3):695–702.

Koletzko B, Agostoni C, Carlson SE, Clandinin T, Hornstra G, Neuringer M, Uauy R, Yamashiro Y, Willatts P. 2001. *Acta Paediatrica* 90(4):460–464.

Lauritzen L, Hansen HS, Jorgensen MH, Michaelsen KF. 2001. The essentiality of long chain n-3 fatty acids in relation to development and function of the brain and retina. *Progress in Lipid Research* 40(1–2):1–94.

Leary SD, Ness AR, Emmett PM, Davey Smith G, Headley JE, ALSPAC Study Team. 2005. Maternal diet in pregnancy and offspring blood pressure. *Archives of Disease in Childhood* 90(5):492–493.

Levant B, Radel JD, Carlson SE. 2004. Decreased brain docosahexaenoic acid during development alters dopamine-related behaviors in adult rats that are differentially affected by dietary remediation. *Behavioural Brain Research* 152(1):49–57.

Llorente AM, Jensen CL, Voigt RG, Fraley JK, Berretta MC, Heird WC. 2003. Effect of maternal docosahexaenoic acid supplementation on postpartum depression and information processing. *American Journal of Obstetrics and Gynecology* 188(5):1348–1353.

Lucas A, Stafford M, Morley R, Abbott R, Stephenson T, MacFadyen U, Elias A, Clements H. 1999. Efficacy and safety of long-chain polyunsaturated fatty acid supplementation of infant-formula milk: A randomised trial. *Lancet* 354(9194):1948–1954.

Lucas M, Dewailly E, Muckle G, Ayotte P, Bruneau S, Gingras S, Rhainds M, Holub BJ. 2004. Gestational age and birth weight in relation to n-3 fatty acids among Inuit (Canada). *Lipids* 39(7):617–626.

Makrides M, Gibson RA. 2000. Long-chain polyunsaturated fatty acid requirements during pregnancy and lactation. *American Journal of Clinical Nutrition* 71(1 Suppl):307S–311S.

Makrides M, Neumann MA, Byard RW, Simmer K, Gibson RA. 1994. Fatty acid composition of brain, retina, and erythrocytes in breast- and formula-fed infants. *American Journal of Clinical Nutrition* 60(2):189–194.

Makrides M, Neumann MA, Simmer K, Gibson RA. 2000. A critical appraisal of the role of dietary long-chain polyunsaturated fatty acids on neural indices of term infants: A randomized, controlled trial. *Pediatrics* 105(1 Part 1):32–38.

Martinez M. 1992. Tissue levels of polyunsaturated fatty acids during early human development. *Journal of Pediatrics* 120(3 Part 2):S129–S138.

McCann JC, Ames BN. 2005. Is docosahexaenoic acid, an n-3 long-chain polyunsaturated fatty acid, required for development of normal brain function? An overview of evidence from cognitive and behavioral tests in humans and animals. *American Journal of Clinical Nutrition* 82(2):281–295.

Mitchell EA. 1987. Clinical characteristics and serum essential fatty acid levels in hyperactive children. *Clinical Pediatrics* 26(8):406–411.

Mitchell EA, Lewis S, Cutler DR. 1983. Essential fatty acids and maladjusted behaviour in children. *Prostaglandins, Leukotrienes and Medicine* 12(3):281–287.

Neuringer M, Connor WE, Van Petten C, Barstad L. 1984. Dietary omega-3 fatty acid deficiency and visual loss in infant rhesus monkeys. *Journal of Clinical Investigations* 73(1):272–276.

Neuringer M, Connor WE, Lin DS, Barstad L, Luck S. 1986. Biochemical and functional effects of prenatal and postnatal ω3 fatty acid deficiency on retina and brain in rhesus monkeys. *Proceedings of the National Academy of Science* 83(11):4021–4025.

Newson RB, Shaheen SO, Henderson AJ, Emmett PM, Sherriff A, Calder PC. 2004. Umbilical cord and maternal blood red cell fatty acids and early childhood wheezing and eczema. *Journal of Allergy and Clinical Immunology* 114(3):531–537.

O'Connor DL, Hall R, Adamkin D, Auestad N, Castillo M, Connor WE, Connor SL, Fitzgerald K, Groh-Wargo S, Hartman EE, Jacobs J, Janowsky J, Lucas A, Margeson D, Mena P, Neuringer M, Nesin M, Singer L, Stephenson T, Szabo J, Zemon V. 2001. Growth and development in preterm infants fed long-chain polyunsaturated fatty acids: A prospective, randomized controlled trial. *Pediatrics* 108(2):259–371.

Oken E, Kleinman KP, Olsen SF, Rich-Edwards JW, Gillman MW. 2004. Associations of seafood and elongated n 3 fatty acid intake with fetal growth and length of gestation: Results from a US pregnancy cohort. *American Journal of Epidemiology* 160(8):774–783.

Oken E, Wright RO, Kleinman KP, Bellinger D, Hu H, Rich-Edwards JW, Gillman MW. 2005. Maternal fish consumption, hair mercury, and infant cognition in a US cohort. *Environmental Health Perspectives* 113(10):1376–1380.

Olsen SF, Secher NJ. 1990. A possible preventive effect of low-dose fish oil on early delivery and pre-eclampsia: Indications from a 50-year old controlled trial. *British Journal of Nutrition* 64(3):599–609.

Olsen SF, Secher NJ. 2002. Low consumption of seafood in early pregnancy as a risk factor for preterm delivery: Prospective cohort study. *British Medical Journal* 324(7335):447–450.

Olsen SF, Hansen HS, Sommer S, Jensen B, Sorensen TI, Secher NJ, Zachariassen P. 1991. Gestational age in relation to marine n-3 fatty acids in maternal erythrocytes: A study of women in the Faroe Islands and Denmark. *American Journal of Obstetrics and Gynecology* 164(5 Part 1):1203–1209.

Olsen SF, Sorensen JD, Secher NJ, Hedegaard M, Henriksen TB, Hansen HS, Grant A. 1992. Randomised controlled trial of effect of fish-oil supplementation on pregnancy duration. *Lancet* 339(8800):1003–1007.

Olsen SF, Secher NJ, Tabor A, Weber T, Walker JJ, Gluud C, Fish Oil Trials In Pregnancy (FOTIP) Team. 2000. Randomised clinical trials of fish oil supplementation in high risk pregnancies. *British Journal of Obstetrics and Gynecology* 107(3):382–395.

Onwude JL, Lilford RJ, Hjartardottir H, Staines A, Tuffnell D. 1995. A randomized double blinded placebo controlled trial of fish oil in high risk pregnancy. *British Journal of Obstetrics and Gynaecology* 102(2):95–100.

Otto SJ, van Houwelingen AC, Badart-Smook A, and Hornstra G. 2001. Comparison of the peripartum and postpartum phospholipid polyunsaturated fatty acid profiles of lactating and nonlactating women. *American Journal of Clinical Nutrition* 73(6):1074–1079.

Otto SJ, de Groot RH, Hornstra G. 2003. Increased risk of postpartum depressive symptoms is associated with slower normalization after pregnancy of the functional docosahexaenoic acid status. *Prostaglandins, Leukotrienes and Essential Fatty Acids* 69(4):237–243.

Peat JK. 1998. Asthma: A longitudinal perspective. *Journal of Asthma* 35(3):235–241.

Peat JK, Mihrshahi S, Kemp AS, Marks GB, Tovey ER, Webb K, Mellis CM, Leeder SR. 2004. Three-year outcomes of dietary fatty acid modification and house dust mite reduction in the Childhood Asthma Prevention Study. *Journal of Allergy & Clinical Immunology* 114(4):807–813.

People's League of Health. 1942. Nutrition of expectant and nursing mothers. *Lancet* 2:10–12.

Putnam JC, Carlson SE, DeVoe PW, Barness LA. 1982. The effect of variations in dietary fatty acids on the fatty acid composition of erythrocyte phosphatidylcholine and phosphatidylethanolamine in human infants. *American Journal of Clinical Nutrition* 36(1):106–114.

Richardson AJ. 2004. Clinical trials of fatty acid treatment in ADHD, dyslexia, dyspraxia and the autistic spectrum. *Prostaglandins, Leukotrienes and Essential Fatty Acids* 70(4):383–390.

Richardson AJ, Puri BK. 2002. A randomized double-blind, placebo-controlled study of the effects of supplementation with highly unsaturated fatty acids on ADHD-related symptoms in children with specific learning difficulties. *Progress in Neuropsychopharmacology and Biological Psychiatry* 26(2):233–239.

Sakamoto M, Kubota M, Liu XJ, Murata K, Nakai K, Satoh H. 2004. Maternal and fetal mercury and n-3 polyunsaturated fatty acids as a risk and benefit of fish consumption to fetus. *Environmental Science and Technology* 38(14):3860–3863.

Salvig JD, Olsen SF, Secher NJ. 1996. Effects of fish oil supplementation in late pregnancy on blood pressure: A randomised controlled trial. *British Journal of Obstetrics and Gynaecology* 103(6):529–533.

Sanders TA, Naismith DJ. 1979. A comparison of the influence of breast-feeding and bottle-feeding on the fatty acid composition of the erythrocytes. *British Journal of Nutrition* 41(3):619–623.

SanGiovanni JP, Berkey CS, Dwyer JT, Colditz GA. 2000a. Dietary essential fatty acids, long-chain polyunsaturated fatty acids, and visual resolution acuity in healthy fullterm infants: A systematic review. *Early Human Development* 57(3):165–188.

SanGiovanni JP, Parra-Cabrera S, Colditz GA, Berkey CS, Dwyer JT. 2000b. Meta-analysis of dietary essential fatty acids and long-chain polyunsaturated fatty acids as they relate to visual resolution acuity in healthy preterm infants. *Pediatrics* 105(6):1292–1298.

Satomi H, Minowa M, Hatano S, Nagakura T, Iikura Y. 1994. An epidemiological study of the preventive effect of dietary fish on bronchial asthma. *Koshu Eisei In Kenkyu Hokoku/Bulletin of the Institute of Public Health* 43(3):305–314.

Schiff E, Ben-Baruch G, Barkai G, Peleg E, Rosenthal T, Mashiach S. 1993. Reduction of thromboxane A2 synthesis in pregnancy by polyunsaturated fatty acid supplements. *American Journal of Obstetrics and Gynecology* 168(1 Part 1):122–124.

Scott DT, Janowsky JS, Carroll RE, Taylor JA, Auestad N, Montalto MB. 1998. Formula supplementation with long-chain polyunsaturated fatty acids: Are there developmental benefits? *Pediatrics* 102(5):E59.

Sibai BM. 1998. Prevention of preeclampsia: A big disappointment. *American Journal of Obstetrics and Gynecology* 179(5):1275–1278.

Simmer K. 2005. Longchain polyunsaturated fatty acid supplementation in infants born at term. *Cochrane Library* Issue 2. [Online]. Available: http://www.cochrane.org/cochrane/revabstr/AB000376.htm [accessed October 18, 2005].

Simmer K, Patole S. 2005. Longchain polyunsaturated fatty acid supplementation in preterm infants. *Cochrane Library* Issue 2. [Online]. Available: http://www.cochrane.org/cochrane/revabstr/AB000375.htm [accessed October 18, 2005].

Sindelar CA, Scheerger SB, Plugge SL, Eskridge KM, Wander RC, Lewis NM. 2004. Serum lipids of physically active adults consuming omega-3 fatty acid-enriched eggs or conventional eggs. *Nutrition Research* 24(9):731–739.

Smit HA, Grievink L, Tabak C. 1999. Dietary influences on chronic obstructive lung disease and asthma: A review of the epidemiological evidence. *Proceedings of the Nutrition Society* 58(2):309–319.

Smuts CM, Borod E, Peeples JM, Carlson SE. 2003a. High-DHA eggs: Feasibility as a means to enhance circulating DHA in mother and infant. *Lipids* 38(4):407–414.

Smuts CM, Huang M, Mundy D, Plasse T, Major S, Carlson SE. 2003b. A randomized trial of docosahexaenoic acid supplementation during the third trimester of pregnancy. *Obstetrics and Gynecology* 101(3):469–479.

Stevens L, Zhang W, Peck L, Kuczek T, Grevstad N, Nahori A, Zentall SS, Arnold LE, Burgess JR. 2003. EFA Supplementation in children with inattention, hyperactivity, and other disruptive behaviors. *Lipids* 38(10):1007–1021.

Stevens LJ, Zentall SS, Deck JL, Abate ML, Watkins BA, Lipp SR, Burgess JR. 1995. Essential fatty acid metabolism in boys with attention-deficit hyperactivity disorder. *American Journal of Clinical Nutrition* 62(4):761–768.

Takemura Y, Sakurai Y, Honjo S, Tokimatsu, Gibo M, Hara T, Kusakari A, Kugai N. 2002. The relationship between fish intake and the prevalence of asthma: The Tokorozawa childhood asthma and pollinosis study. *Preventive Medicine* 34(2):221–225.

Timonen M, Horrobin D, Jokelainen J, Laitinen J, Herva A, Rasanen P. 2004. Fish consumption and depression: The Northern Finland 1966 birth cohort study. *Journal of Affective Disorders* 82(3):447–452.

Troisi RJ, Willett WC, Weiss ST. 1995. A prospective study of diet and adult-onset asthma. *American Journal of Respiratory Critical Care* 151(5):1401–1408.

Uauy R, Birch DG, Birch EE, Tyson JE, Hoffman. 1990. Effect of dietary omega-3 fatty acids on retinal function of very-low-birth-weight neonates. *Pediatric Research* 28(5):485–492.

Uauy R, Hoffman DR, Peirano P, Birch DG, Birch EE. 2001. Essential fatty acids in visual and brain development. *Lipids* 36(9):885–895.

van Wezel-Meijler G, Van Der Knaap MS, Huisman J, Jonkman EJ, Valk J, Lafeber HN. 2002. Dietary supplementation of long-chain polyunsaturated fatty acids in preterm infants: Effects on cerebral maturation. *Acta Paediatrica* 91(9):942–950.

Velzing-Aarts FV, van der Klis FRM, Muskiet FAJ. 1999. Umbilical vessels of preeclamptic women have low contents of both n-3 and n-6 long-chain polyunsaturated fatty acids. *American Journal of Clinical Nutrition* 69(2):293–298.

Voigt RG, Llorente M, Jensen CL, Fraley K, Berretta MC, Heird WC. 2001. A randomized, double-blind, placebo-controlled trial of docosahexaenoic acid supplementation in children with attention-deficit/hyperactivity disorder. *Journal of Pediatrics* 139(2):189–196.

Wang YP, Kay HH, Killam AP. 1991. Decreased levels of polyunsaturated fatty acids in preeclampsia. *American Journal of Obstetrics and Gynecology* 164(3):812–818.

Werkman SH, Carlson SE. 1996. A randomized trial of visual attention of preterm infants fed docosahexaenoic acid until nine months. *Lipids* 31(1):91–97.

Willatts P, Forsyth JS, DiModugno MK, Varma S, Colvin M. 1998a. Effect of long-chain polyunsaturated fatty acids in infant formula on problem solving at 10 months of age. *Lancet* 352(9129):688–691.

Willatts P, Forsyth JS, DiModugno MK, Varma S, Colvin M. 1998b. Influence of long-chain polyunsaturated fatty acids on infant cognitive function. *Lipids* 33(10):973–980.

Willatts P, Forsyth S, Mires G, Ross P. 2003. *Maternal DHA status in late pregnancy is related to infant look duration and acuity at age 4 months.* Poster presented at the meeting of the Society for Research in Child Development, Tampa, FL.

Williams MA, Zingheim RW, King IB, Zebelman AM. 1995. Omega-3 fatty acids in maternal erythrocytes and risk of preeclampsia. *Epidemiology* 6(3):232–237.

Williams C, Birch EE, Emmett PM, Northstone K. 2001. Stereoacuity at age 3.5 y in children born full-term is associated with prenatal and postnatal dietary factors: A report from a population-based cohort study. *American Journal of Clinical Nutrition* 73(2):316–322.

Studies on Adult Chronic Diseases

TABLE B-2a Secondary Prevention Studies with Cardiovascular Outcomes

Author	Study Type	Subjects	Exposure
Hooper et al., 2006	Meta-analysis	48 randomized controlled trials 41 cohorts Omega-3 intake for ≥6 months in adults Primary and secondary prevention	n-3 supplement

Amount	Results	Conclusion**
High omega-3 fat vs. low omega-3 fat/control Intake differed by 0.1-0.6 g omega-3/day among the two groups (absolute levels not specified)	Based on RCTs, no significant differences were found between the high omega-3 fat group and the low omega-3 fat/control group with regards to risk of mortality (n=15 RCTs; RR=0.87, 95% CI 0.73-1.03), cardiovascular events (n=18 RCTs; RR=0.95, 95% CI 0.82 1.12), cancer or death from cancer (n=10 RCTs; RR=1.07, 95% CI 0.88-1.30), or stroke (n=9 RCTs; RR=1.17, 95% CI 0.91-1.51). Based on cohorts, no significant differences were found between the high omega-3 fat group and the low omega-3 fat/control group with regards to risk of cardiovascular events (n=7 cohorts; RR=0.91, 95% CI 0.73-1.13), cancer or death from cancer (n=7 cohorts; RR=1.02, 95% CI 0.87-1.19), or stroke (n=4 cohorts; RR=0.87, 95% CI 0.72-1.04). Based on three cohorts, those in the low omega-3 fat/control group had a significantly higher risk of mortality compared to those in the high omega-3 fat group (RR=0.65, 95% CI 0.48-0.88).	N

continued

TABLE B-2a Continued

Author	Study Type	Subjects	Exposure
Hooper et al., 2005	Cochrane Review	48 randomized controlled trials 41 cohorts Primary and secondary prevention	n-3 supplement or advice

Amount	Results	Conclusion**
	Based on RCTs, no significant differences were found between those randomized to n-3 supplementation or advice and those not randomized to n-3 supplementation or advice with regards to total mortality (n=44 RCTs; RR=0.87, 95% CI 0.73-1.03), combined cardiovascular events (n=31 RCTs; RR=0.95, 95% CI 0.82-1.12), cancers (n=10 RCTs; RR=1.07, 95% CI 0.88-1.30), cardiovascular deaths (n=44 RCTs; RR=0.85, 95% CI 0.68-1.06), fatal myocardial infarction (n=38 RCTs; RR=0.86, 95% CI 0.60-1.25), non-fatal myocardial infarction (n=26 RCTs; RR=1.03, 95% CI 0.70 1.50), sudden death (n=37 RCTs; RR=0.85, 95% CI 0.49-1.48), angina (n=25 RCTs; RR=0.78, 95% CI 0.59-1.02), stroke (n=26 RCTs; RR=1.17, 95% CI 0.91-1.51), heart failure (n=20 RCTs; RR=0.51, 95% CI 0.31-0.85), peripheral vascular events (n=17 RCTs; RR=0.26, 95% CI 0.07-1.06), and re-vascularization (n=23 RCTs; RR=1.05, 95% CI 0.97-1.12).	N
	Based on cohort studies, no significant differences were found between those randomized to n-3 supplementation or advice and those not randomized to n-3 supplementation or advice with regards to combined cardiovascular events (n=7 cohorts; RR=0.91, 95% CI 0.73-1.13), cancers (n=10 cohorts; RR=1.02, 95% CI 0.87-1.19), nonfatal myocardial infarction (n=4 cohorts; RR=0.93, 95% CI 0.69-1.26), stroke (n=4 cohorts; RR=0.87, 95% CI 0.72-1.04), peripheral vascular events (n=1 cohort; RR=0.94, 95% CI 0.84-1.04), and revascularization (n=2 cohorts; RR=1.07, 95% CI 0.76-1.50).	
	Based on cohort studies, significant differences were found between those randomized to n-3 supplementation or advice and those not randomized to n-3 supplementation or advice with regards to total mortality (n=3 cohorts; RR=0.65, 95% CI 0.48-0.88), cardiovascular deaths (n=11 cohorts; RR=0.79, 95% CI 0.63-0.99), fatal myocardial infarction (n=2 cohorts; RR=0.42, 95% CI 0.21-0.82), and sudden death (n=1 cohort; RR=0.44, 95% CI 0.21-0.91).	

continued

TABLE B-2a Continued

Author	Study Type	Subjects	Exposure
Konig et al., 2005	Meta-analysis	7 observational studies (primary prevention) 4 RCTs (secondary prevention)	Seafood
Burr et al., 2005	Review	Review of two randomized controlled trials (Burr et al., 1989, 2003 below) Secondary prevention	Dietary advice
Harper and Jacobson, 2005	Review	Systematic literature review of 14 randomized controlled trials Northern Europe, Southern Europe, India Excluded if trial involved >1 intervention unless in a prospective 2×2 design Patients followed for ≥1 year Secondary prevention	6 on fish oil 2 on fish 5 on ALA suppl. 2 on ALA-enriched diets

Amount	Results	Conclusion**
Servings/week, a continuous number 1 serving = 100 g	Among those with no preexisting CHD (from observational studies), the linear regression model showed that each one serving increase in fish consumption per week reduces one's risk of CHD death by 0.039 (95% CI –0.066 to –0.011) but does not significantly change one's risk of nonfatal MI by (ΔRR=0.0083, 95% CI –0.012 to 0.028). "The information available is insufficient for the purposes of quantitatively analyzing the impact of fish consumption on CHD risk for individuals with preexisting CHD" (from RCTs).	B
See Burr et al., 1989, 2003 below	"It appeared that fish oil, which protected post-MI male patients in DART, increased the risk of cardiac death in men with angina, being particularly associated with sudden death." "The apparently conflicting findings may be attributable to the different clinical conditions of the subjects . . . together with different effects of dietary fish and fish oil." "The evidence supports a role for fish oil (EPA or DHA) or fish in secondary prevention, because the clinical trials have demonstrated a reduction in total mortality, CHD death, and sudden death." "Evidence from these trials had indicated that EPA plus DHA supplementation in the range of 0.5-1.8 g/day provides significant benefit." "The data on the plant-based n-3 PUFA, ALA, is very promising. However, the existing studies were small, and a large randomized controlled trial is needed before recommendations can be definitely made for CHD prevention." "The data for ALA show possible reductions in sudden death and nonfatal myocardial infarction, suggesting other potential cardioprotective mechanisms other than a predominately antiarrhythmic role."	N B

continued

TABLE B-2a Continued

Author	Study Type	Subjects	Exposure
Leaf et al., 2005	Randomized Controlled Trial	Men and women (n=402) Mean age about 65 years 18 US centers Had a cardioverter defibrillator implanted because of a history of cardiac arrest, sustained ventricular tachycardia, or syncope with inductive, sustained ventricular tachycardia or ventricular fibrillation during electrophysiologic studies Follow-up of 12 months Secondary prevention	n-3 supplement

Amount	Results	Conclusion**
Treatment: Four 1 g gelatin capsules of an ethyl ester concentrate of n-3 fatty acids (2.6 g EPA+DHA) Placebo: Four 1 g capsules of olive oil	After controlling for sex, left ventricular ejection fraction (continuous), New York Heart Association class III congestive heart failure, history of myocardial infarction, history of prior defibrillator therapies for ventricular tachycardia or ventricular fibrillation, time from implanted cardioverter/defibrillator implant (continuous), and sustained ventricular tachycardia as the indication for the implanted cardioverter defibrillator: The intent-to-treat analysis provided a significant relative risk of time to first event of 0.67 (95% CI 0.47-0.95, p=0.024) for all confirmed events among those in the treatment group compared to the placebo group; The on-treatment analysis (for all who had taken any of their prescribed supplements) provided a significant relative risk of time to first event of 0.67 (95% CI 0.46-0.98, p=0.037) for all confirmed events among those in the treatment group compared to the placebo group; and The on-treatment analysis (for all on-treatment at least 11 months) provided a significant relative risk of time to first event of 0.52 (95% CI 0.32-0.83, p=0.0060) for all confirmed events among those in the treatment group compared to the placebo group. Similar results were found when probable events were also included.	B

continued

TABLE B-2a Continued

Author	Study Type	Subjects	Exposure
Raitt et al., 2005	Randomized Controlled Trial	Men and women (n=200) Mean age about 62 Patients at six medical centers in the United States Receiving an implantable cardioverter defibrillator for an electrocardiogram-documented episode of sustained ventricular tachycardia or ventricular fibrillation that was not the result of acute myocardial infarction or a revisible cause or who had a preexisting implantable cardioverter defibrillator and had received implantable cardioverter/defibrillator therapy for an electrocardiogram-documented episode of sustained ventricular tachycardia or ventricular fibrillation within the last 3 months No class I or class II antiarrhythmic medications; ≥1 fatty fish meal/week; flaxseed oil, cod-liver oil, or fish-oil supplements in the last month Follow-up of 2 years Secondary prevention	n-3 supplement

Amount	Results	Conclusion**
Treatment: 1.8 g/day fish oil (42% EPA and 30% DHA) Placebo: Olive oil (73% oleic acid, 12% palmitic acid, 0% EPA+DHA)	There was a significant difference in the number of patients hospitalized for neurological conditions among those assigned to the placebo compared to those assigned to the treatment (p=0.04). However, there were no other significant differences found in mortality, hospitalizations, coronary revascularization, myocardial infarction, cancer, and diarrhea between the two groups. There were no significant differences in the time to first episode of implantable cardioverter/defibrillator therapy for ventricular tachycardia or ventricular fibrillation after randomization between the two groups (p=0.19). However, among those with qualified arrhythmia at the time of study entry, those assigned to fish oil had significantly greater incidence of ventricular tachycardia or ventricular fibrillation treated by the implantable cardioverter defibrillator compared to those assigned to placebo (p=0.007).	A

continued

TABLE B-2a Continued

Author	Study Type	Subjects	Exposure
Baer et al., 2004	Randomized Crossover Trial	Men (n=50) Aged 25-60 years All races Beltsville, MD In good health, with no hypertension, hyperlipidemia, diabetes, peripheral vascular disease, gout, liver or kidney disease, or endocrine disorders Fasting plasma HDL-c >0.65 mmol/L, triacylglycerol <3.39 mmol/L, and 85-120% of their sex-specific ideal BMI No lipid-lowering drugs, blood pressure medication, or dietary supplements, or eating habits inconsistent with the study protocol 30-week intervention (six diets for 5 weeks each) Primary prevention	Diet

Amount	Results	Conclusion**
Diets 1-5: 38.9% energy from fat, 15% energy from protein, 46.1% energy from digestible carbohydrates	After 5 weeks on the stearic acid diet, the least squares mean plasma fibrinogen levels were significantly higher than after 5 weeks on all other diets (p<0.05).	N
Diet 6: 30.4% energy from fat, 54.6% energy from carbohydrate	After 5 weeks on the trans fatty acid diet, the least squares mean plasma C-reactive protein levels were significantly higher than after 5 weeks on all other diets (p<0.05).	
Diet 1 (carbohydrate diet): 8.5% of energy from fat replaced by digestible carbohydrate	After 5 weeks on the oleic acid diet, the least squares mean plasma interleukin 6 levels were significantly lower than after 5 weeks on all other diets, except for the trans fatty acid + stearic acid diet (p<0.05).	
Diet 2 (oleic acid diet): 8% of energy enriched with oleic acid	After 5 weeks on the trans fatty acids diet, the least squares mean plasma C-reactive protein levels were significantly higher than after 5 weeks on the carbohydrate diet, the oleic diet, and the trans fatty acid + stearic acid diet (p<0.05).	
Diet 3 (LMP diet): 8% of energy enriched with lauric (L), myristic (M), and palmitic (P) acids		
Diet 4 (stearic acid diet): 8% of energy enriched with stearic acid	After 5 weeks on the oleic acid diet, the least squares mean plasma interleukin 6 levels were significantly lower than after 5 weeks on the trans fatty acid diet, stearic acid diet, or the LMP diet (p<0.05).	
Diet 5 (trans fatty acid diet): 8% of energy enriched with trans fatty acids	After 5 weeks on the oleic acid diet, the least squares mean plasma E-selectin levels were significantly lower than after 5 weeks on all other diets, except for the carbohydrate diet (p<0.05).	
Diet 6 (trans fatty acid + stearic acid diet): 4% energy enriched with trans fatty acids and 4% of energy enriched with stearic acid	After 5 weeks on the trans fatty acids diet, the least squares mean plasma E-selectin levels were significantly higher than after 5 weeks on all other diets (p<0.05).	
	There were no other significant differences reported between the diets with regards to fibrinogen, C-reactive protein, interleukin 6, or E-selectin levels.	

continued

TABLE B-2a Continued

Author	Study Type	Subjects	Exposure
Burr et al., 2003	Randomized Controlled Trial	Men (n=3114) Aged <70 years South Wales, UK Being treated with angina Mortality ascertained at 3-9 years after enrollment No exertional chest pain or discomfort; men awaiting coronary artery by-pass surgery, men who already ate oily fish twice a week, men who could not tolerate oily fish or fish oil, men who appeared to be unsuitable on other grounds (e.g., other serious illness, likelihood of moving out of area) The Diet and Angina Randomized Trial (DART 2) Follow-up of 3 years (after last subject was recruited) Secondary prevention	Dietary advice

Amount	Results	Conclusion**
Fish advice = eat at least 2 portions of oily fish each week or take up to 3 g of fish oil as a partial or total substitute	Those given fish advice had significantly higher percentage of cardiac deaths (p=0.02) and sudden deaths (p=0.02) compared to those who did not receive fish advice. There was not a significant difference in the number of total deaths between these two groups.	A
Fruit/vegetable advice = eat 4-5 portions of fruit and vegetables and drink at least 1 glass of natural orange juice daily, and also increase the intake of oats	No significant differences were found between the fruit/vegetable advice group and the no fruit/vegetable advice group for total number of deaths, number of cardiac deaths, or number of sudden deaths.	
Both = a combination of both of these forms of advice	After adjusting for age, smoking, previous MI, history of high blood pressure, diabetes, BMI, serum cholesterol, medication, and fruit advice or fish advice:	
Sensible eating = non-specific advice that did not include either form of advice	Those who received fish advice had a slightly significant higher hazard ratio for cardiac deaths (HR=1.26, p=0.047) and a significant higher hazard ratio for sudden death (HR=1.54, p=0.025), compared to those who did not receive fish advice.	
	There were no significant associations found between those who received fruit/vegetable advice vs. those who did not and all deaths, cardiac deaths, or sudden deaths.	

continued

TABLE B-2a Continued

Author	Study Type	Subjects	Exposure
Marchioli et al., 2002	Randomized Controlled Trial	Men and women (n=11,323) No age limits Gruppo Italiano per lo Studio della Sopravivivenza nell'Infarto miocardico-Prevenzione (GISSI trial) Recent MI Follow-up of 3.5 years (about 38,418 person-years) Secondary prevention	n-3 supplement

Amount	Results	Conclusion**
n-3 fatty acids group = 1 g/day Vitamin E group = 300 mg/day Combination group Control group	After adjusting for age, sex, complications after myocardial infarction, smoking habits, history of diabetes mellitus and arterial hypertension, total blood cholesterol, HDL cholesterol, fibrinogen, leukocyte count, and claudication intermittens: Those who received n-3 fatty acids had a significantly lower relative risk of death, nonfatal MI, and nonfatal stroke at 9 months, 12 months, and 42 months of follow-up than the controls (RR=0.76, 95% CI 0.60-0.97 at 9 months, RR=0.79, 95% CI 0.63 0.98 at 12 months, and RR=0.85, 95% CI 0.74-0.98 at 42 months). The relative risks at 3 and 6 months of follow-up were also lower in the n-3 fatty acid group compared to the controls, but they were not significant. Those who received n-3 fatty acids had a significantly lower relative risk of CVD death, nonfatal MI, and nonfatal stroke at 9 months (RR=0.75, 95% CI 0.58-0.97), 12 months (RR=0.78, 95% CI 0.62-0.99), and 42 months (RR=0.80, 95% CI 0.68-0.94) of follow-up than the controls. The relative risks at 3 and 6 months of follow-up were also lower in the n-3 fatty acid group compared to the controls, but they were not significant.	B

continued

TABLE B-2a Continued

Author	Study Type	Subjects	Exposure
Ness et al., 2002	Randomized Controlled Trial	Men (n=2033) Aged <70 years 21 hospitals in south Wales and south-west England Survived an MI Diet and Reinfarction Trial (DART) 21,147 person-years of follow-up Secondary prevention	Dietary advice

Amount	Results	Conclusion**
Fish advice = eat at least 2 portions of fatty fish each week and as much other fish as they could manage (using fish oil capsule as a partial or total replacement if necessary) Fat advice = aimed at reducing total fat and increasing the polyunsaturated to saturated fat ratio Fiber advice = eat at least 6 slices of wholemeal bread per day or an equivalent amount of cereal fiber	After adjusting for myocardial infarction, angina, hypertension at baseline; x-ray evidence of cardiomegaly, pulmonary congestion or pulmonary edema at baseline; and treatment with β-blockers, other anti-hypertensives, digoxin/antiarrhythmics, or anticoagulants: Those who received fish advice had a significantly lower hazard ratio for all-cause mortality at 0-2 years of follow-up (HR=0.73, 95% CI 0.56-0.95) and a significantly higher hazard ratio at 2-5 years of follow-up (HR=1.31, 95% CI 1.01-1.71) compared to those who did not receive fish advice. However, there were no significant differences between the two groups and all-cause mortality after 5 years of follow-up; Those who received fish advice had a significantly lower hazard ratio for coronary heart disease at 0-2 years of follow-up (HR=0.68, 95% CI 0.51-0.91) compared to those who did not receive fish advice. After 2 years of follow-up, there were no significant differences between the two groups and their risk of coronary heart disease; and There were no significant differences between those who received fish advice vs. those who did not and risk of stroke throughout 10 years of follow-up.	N

continued

TABLE B-2a Continued

Author	Study Type	Subjects	Exposure
Nilsen et al., 2001	Randomized Controlled Trial	Men and women (n=300) Aged >18 years Central Hospital in Rogaland, Stavanger, Norway Suffered from acute MI Discontinued regular supplementation of other fish oil products No assumed noncompliance; expected survival <2 years because of severe heart failure; ongoing gastrointestinal bleeding or verified stomach ulcer; thrombocytopenia or blood platelets <100×109/L; liver insufficiency; participation in any other study; residence outside the recruitment area Mean follow-up time of 1.5 years Secondary prevention	n-3 supplement
GISSI Investigators, 1999*	Randomized Controlled Trial	Men and women (n=11,324) No age limits Recent MI (≤3 months) No contraindications to the dietary supplements; were able to provide informed written consent, had no unfavorable short-term outlook (e.g., overt congestive heart failure, cancer, etc.) 42 months of follow-up Gruppo Italiano per lo Studio della Sopravivivenza nell'Infarto miocardico-Prevenzione (GISSI trial) Secondary prevention	n-3 supplement

Amount	Results	Conclusion**
Fish oil = 850-880 mg EPA+DHA/capsule Control = same amount in corn oil 2 capsules twice a day	When compared to the corn oil group, there were no significant associations found between fish oil and fatal cardiac events and resuscitations, nonfatal cardiac events, revascularization, total mortality, time to first event, or cardiac event or revascularization.	N
n-3 PUFA alone vs. vitamin E alone vs. combination of the two vs. no supplement (control) Absolute amounts not specified	In the four-way analysis, those who received n-3 PUFA had a significantly lower relative risk of death, nonfatal MI, and nonfatal stroke (RR=0.85, 95% CI 0.74-0.98) and cardiovascular death, nonfatal MI, and nonfatal stroke (RR=0.80, 95% CI 0.68-0.95) compared to the controls. In the four-way analysis, those who received n-3 PUFA had a significantly lower relative risk of all fatal events (RR=0.80, 95% CI 0.67-0.94), all cardiovascular deaths (RR=0.70, 95% CI 0.56-0.87), cardiac death (RR=0.65, 95% CI 0.51-0.82), coronary death (RR=0.65, 95% CI 0.51-0.84), and sudden death (RR=0.55, 95% CI 0.40-0.76). Similar results were also found in the two-way analysis.	B

continued

TABLE B-2a Continued

Author	Study Type	Subjects	Exposure
Singh et al., 1997	Randomized Controlled Trial	Men and women (n=360) Mean age of 48.5 years Admitted to the Medical Hospital and Research Center, Moradabad Clinical diagnosis of acute MI in the preceding 24 hours Indian Experiment of Infarct Survival (IEIS-4) Secondary prevention	n-3 supplement
Burr et al., 1989	Randomized Controlled Trial	Men (n=2033) Aged <70 years South Wales, UK From those admitted to 21 hospitals for acute MI No diabetes, those awaiting cardiac surgery, or those who already intended to eat one of the intervention diets 2 years of follow-up The Diet and Reinfarction Trial (DART) Follow-up of 2 years Secondary prevention	Dietary advice

Amount	Results	Conclusion**
Fish oil = 1.08 g/day EPA + 0.72 g/day DHA Mustard oil = 2.9 g/day ALA Placebo = 100 mg/day aluminum hydroxide	Compared to the placebo group, those in the fish oil group had significantly lower relative risks of angina pectoris (RR=0.42, 95% CI 0.22-0.77), total arrhythmias (RR=0.46, 95% CI 0.21-0.98), total cases with poor left ventricular function (RR=0.48, 95% CI 0.28-0.82), NYHA class III and IV heart failure (RR=0.44, 95% CI 0.18-0.88), and total cardiac events (RR=0.70, 95% CI 0.29-0.90). Compared to the placebo group, the fish oil group also had lower relative risks of ventricular ectopic beats (>8/minute and >3 consecutively), left ventricular enlargement, hypotension, sudden cardiac death, total cardiac death, and nonfatal reinfarction, but these were not significant. Serious concerns have been raised about the performance and conclusions of this trial and other related publications by this investigator.	B
Fat advice = reduce fat to 30% of total energy and increase polyunsaturated to saturated ratio to 1.0 Fish advice = consume at least 2 weekly portions of 200-400 g fatty fish (or 0.15 g of MaxEPA capsules daily if one could not tolerate fish) Fiber advice = increase intake of cereal fiber to 18 g daily	Total mortality and IHD mortality was significantly lower in the fish advice group than in the non-fish advice group (p<0.05 and p<0.01, respectively). There were no significant differences in nonfatal MI or IHD events in the fish advice group and the non-fish advice group. There were no significant differences in total mortality, IHD deaths, nonfatal MI, or IHD events between the fat advice group and the non-fat advice group or between the fiber advice group and the non-fiber advice group. After controlling for history of MI, angina, or hypertension; X-ray evidence of cardiomegaly, pulmonary congestion, or pulmonary edema; and treatment (at entry) with β-blockers, other antihypertensives, digoxin/antiarrhythmics, or anticoagulants; those in the fish advice group had a significantly lower relative risk of all deaths than those not in the fish advice group (p<0.05); similar results were also found in the unadjusted comparison.	B

continued

TABLE B-2a Continued

Author	Study Type	Subjects	Exposure
He et al., 2004b	Meta-analysis	13 cohort studies from 11 independent studies English language 222,364 participants 3032 coronary heart disease deaths Average of 11.8 years of follow-up Primary prevention	Seafood

Amount	Results	Conclusion**
Categories of fish intake: 1 = Never-<1 time/month 2 = 1-3 times/month 3 = 1 time/week 4 = 2-4 times/week 5 = ≥5 times/week	Based on pooled relative risks of CHD mortality, those who ate fish 1 time/week, 2-4 times/week, and ≥5 times/week had significantly lower risk of CHD mortality than those who never ate fish (RR=0.85, 95% CI 0.76-0.96; RR=0.77, 95% CI 0.66-0.89; RR=0.62, 95% CI 0.46-0.82, respectively). Those who ate fish 1-3 times/month also had a lower relative risk compared to those who never ate fish, but it was not significant (RR=0.89, 95% CI 0.79-1.01). "Each 20-g/day increase in fish intake was related to a 7% lower risk of CHD mortality (p for trend = 0.03)."	B

continued

TABLE B-2a Continued

Author	Study Type	Subjects	Exposure
Whelton et al., 2004	Meta-analysis	14 cohort studies 5 case-control studies Conducted in adult humans English language Published before May 2003 Primary and secondary prevention	Seafood

Amount	Results	Conclusion**
Consumed fish on a regular basis vs. consumed little or no fish Level of fish consumption: <2, 2-<4, ≥4 portions per week	In 6 cohort studies, those consuming any amount of fish had a significantly lower risk of coronary heart disease mortality compared to those who ate no fish; in seven cohort studies no significant associations were found between fish consumption and coronary heart disease mortality. Based on pooled estimates from a random-effects model, those who ate any fish (pooled RR=0.83, 95% CI 0.76-0.90), those who ate <2 portions of fish/week (pooled RR=0.83, 95% CI 0.75-0.92), and those who ate 2 <4 portions of fish/week (pooled RR=0.75, 95% CI 0.62-0.92) had a significantly lower risk of coronary heart disease mortality compared to those who ate no fish; a significant difference was not found between those who ate ≥4 portions of fish/week and those who never ate fish. In one cohort study and five case-control studies those consuming any amount of fish had a significantly lower risk of total coronary heart disease compared to those who ate no fish; in one cohort study, those who ate fish had a significantly higher risk of total coronary heart disease compared to those who ate no fish (RR≈1.8, 95% CI 1.2-3.2); in five cohort studies no significant associations were found between fish consumption and total coronary heart disease. Based on pooled estimates from a random-effects model, those who ate any fish (pooled RR=0.86, 95% CI 0.81-0.92), those who ate <2 portions of fish/week (pooled RR=0.85, 95% CI 0.80-0.91), and those who ate 2-<4 portions of fish/week (pooled RR=0.83, 95% CI 0.69-0.99) had a significantly lower risk of total coronary heart disease compared to those who ate no fish; a significant difference was not found between those who ate ≥4 portions of fish/week and those who never ate fish.	B

continued

TABLE B-2a Continued

Author	Study Type	Subjects	Exposure
Calder, 2004	Review	Primary and secondary prevention studies in humans (n=25)	Seafood or n-3 supplement
Marckmann and Gronbaek, 1999	Review	Prospective cohort studies (n=9) Letter (n=1) Short report (n=1) Sample size and length of follow-up varied between studies Primary prevention	Seafood

Amount	Results	Conclusion**
	"Substantial evidence from epidemiological and case-control studies indicates that consumption of fish, fatty fish, and long-chain n-3 PUFAs reduces the risk of cardiovascular mortality."	B
	"Secondary prevention studies using long-chain n-3 PUFAs in patients post-myocardial infarction have shown a reduction in total and cardiovascular mortality."	
	"Long-chain n-3 PUFAs have been shown to decrease blood triacylglycerol (triglyceride) concentrations, to decrease production of chemoattractants, growth factors, adhesion molecules, inflammatory eicosanoids and inflammatory cytokines, to lower blood pressure, to increase nitric oxide production, endothelial relaxation and vascular compliance, to decrease thrombosis and cardiac arrhythmias and to increase heart rate variability."	
	Both Krohout (1985) and Daviglus (1997) showed a significant inverse relationship between fish intake (g/day) and risk of coronary heart disease (p for trend <0.05 and p for trend − 0.04, respectively).	N
	"Our overall conclusion is that individuals at low risk of CHD and with healthy lifestyles do not gain any additional protection against CHD from eating fish. On the other hand, high-risk individuals appear to benefit in a dose-dependent manner from increasing their fish consumption up to an optimum of 40-60 g."	

continued

TABLE B-2a Continued

Author	Study Type	Subjects	Exposure
Iso et al., 2006	Cohort	Men (n=19,985) Women (n=21,593) Aged 40-59 years Japan (Iwate Prefecture, Akita, Nagano, Okinawa) The Japan Public Health Center-based Study Cohort I No myocardial infarction, angina pectoris, stroke, or cancer at baseline 477,325 person-years of follow-up Primary prevention	Seafood

Amount	Results	Conclusion**
One serving = 100 g for fresh fish, 20 g for dried or salted fish, 20 g for salted fish roe, 20 g for salted fish preserves n-3 amounts per serving = 1.22 g for fresh fish and shellfish, 0.40 g for dried fish, 0.52 g for salted eggs, and 0.11 g for salted fish gut Quintiles of fish and n-3 intakes: 1 (low) = mean of 23 g/day 2 = mean of 51 g/day 3 = mean of 78 g/day 4 = mean of 114 g/day 5 (high) = mean of 180 g/day	After adjusting for age; sex; cigarette smoking; alcohol intake; BMI; histories of hypertension and diabetes; medication use for hypercholesterolemia; education level; sports at leisure time; quintiles of dietary intake of fruits, vegetables, saturated fat, monounsaturated fat, n-6 polyunsaturated fat, cholesterol; total energy; and public health center: Those in the 5th quintile of fish intake had a significantly lower HR of definite MI (HR=0.44, 95% CI 0.24-0.81) and nonfatal coronary events (HR=0.43, 95% CI 0.23-0.81) than those in the 1st quintile. Those in the 2nd, 3rd, and 4th quintiles also had lower hazard ratios of definite MI and nonfatal coronary events, but they were not significant; No significant associations were found between quintiles of fish intake and coronary heart disease, total MI, sudden cardiac death, or fatal coronary events; Those in the 5th quintile of n-3 intake had significantly lower HRs of coronary heart disease (HR=0.58, 95% CI 0.35-0.97), total MI (HR=0.43, 95% CI 0.24-0.78), definite MI (HR=0.35, 95% CI 0.18-0.66), and nonfatal coronary heart disease (HR=0.33, 95% CI 0.17-0.63) than those in the 1st quintile; Those in the 4th quintile of n-3 intake had a significantly lower HR of nonfatal coronary events (HR=0.57, 95% CI 0.34-0.98) than those in the 1st quintile. However, there were no significant associations found between n-3 intake and coronary heart disease, total MI, or definite MI, sudden cardiac death, or fatal coronary events when comparing the 4th quintile to the 1st quintile; and Those in the 3rd quintile of n-3 intake had significantly lower HRs of definite MI (HR=0.59, 95% CI 0.37-0.94) and nonfatal coronary events (HR=0.61, 95% CI 0.38-0.97) than those in the 1st quintile. However, there were no significant associations found between n-3 intake and coronary heart disease, total MI, sudden cardiac death, or fatal coronary events when comparing the 3rd quintile to the 1st quintile.	B

continued

TABLE B-2a Continued

Author	Study Type	Subjects	Exposure
Mozaffarian et al., 2004	Cohort	Men and women (n=4815) Aged ≥65 years From Medicare eligibility lists in 4 US communities Cardiovascular Health Study (CHS) Free of atrial fibrillation at baseline Follow-up of 12 years Primary prevention	Seafood

Amount	Results	Conclusion**
Categories of fish intake (tuna/other or fried fish/fish sandwich): 1 = <1 time/month 2 = 1-3 times/month 3 = 1-4 times/week 4 = ≥5 times/week	After adjusting for age, gender, race, education, diabetes, BMI, prevalent coronary heart disease, prevalent valvular heart disease, smoking status, pack-years of smoking, leisure-time activity, total caloric intake, alcohol, saturated fat, beef/pork, fruits, vegetables, cereal fiber, systolic blood pressure, diastolic blood pressure, left ventricular systolic function at baseline, treated hypertension, C-reactive protein: Those who ate tuna/other fish 1-4 times/week or ≥5 times/week had significantly lower HR of atrial fibrillation than those who ate tuna/other fish <1 time/month (HR=0.72, 95% CI 0.57-0.90 and HR=0.70, 95% CI 0.53-0.93, respectively). Those who ate tuna/other fish 1-3 times/month also had a lower HR of atrial fibrillation than those who ate tuna/other fish <1 time/month, but it was not significant. There was no significant association found between fried fish/fish sandwich intake and the risk of atrial fibrillation.	B

continued

TABLE B-2a Continued

Author	Study Type	Subjects	Exposure
Mozaffarian et al., 2003	Cohort	Men and women (n=3910) Aged ≥65 years From Medicare eligibility lists in 4 US communities Cardiovascular Health Study (CHS) Free from CVD at baseline Follow-up of 9.3 years Primary prevention	Seafood

Amount	Results	Conclusion**
Categories of fish intake (tuna/other or fried fish/fish sandwich): 1 = <1 time/month 2 = 1-3 times/month 3 = 1 time/week 4 = 2 times/week 5 = ≥3 times/week	After adjusting for age, gender, education, diabetes, current smoking, pack-years of smoking, BMI, systolic blood pressure, LDL-C, HDL-C, triglycerides, C-reactive protein, and intake of saturated fat, alcohol, beef/pork, fruits, and vegetables: Those who ate tuna/other fish 2 times/week and ≥3 times/week had a significantly lower RR of total IHD death than those who ate tuna/other fish <1 time/month (RR=0.53, 95% CI 0.30-0.96 and RR=0.47, 95% CI 0.27-0.82, respectively). Those who ate tuna/other fish 1-3 times/month and 1 time/week also had lower RR of total IHD death compared to those who ate tuna/other fish <1 time/month, but they were not significant; Those who ate tuna/other fish ≥3 times/week had a significantly lower RR of arrhythmic IHD death than those who ate tuna/other fish <1 time/month (RR=0.32, 95% CI 0.15-0.70). The other categories of intake also showed lower RR of arrhythmic IHD death compared to the 1st category of intake but they were not significant; and There were no significant associations found between tuna/other fish intake and nonfatal MI and between fried fish/fish sandwiches and total IHD death, arrhythmic IHD death, or nonfatal MI. After adjusting for age, gender, education, diabetes, current smoking, and pack-years of smoking: Those who ate tuna/other fish ≥3 times/week had a significantly lower RR of total IHD death and arrhythmic IHD death than those who ate tuna/other fish <1 time/month (RR=0.51, 95% CI 0.31-0.83 and RR=0.42, 95% CI 0.21-0.84, respectively). There were no other significant associations found between the other categories of tuna/other fish intake and the risk of death from total IHD, arrhythmic IHD, or nonfatal MI; and Those who ate fried fish/fish sandwiches ≥3 times/week had a significantly higher RR of nonfatal MI death than those who ate fried fish/fish sandwiches <1 time/month (RR=2.30, 95% CI 1.18-4.46). There were no other significant associations found between the other categories of fried fish/fish sandwich intake and the risk of death from total IHD, arrhythmic IHD, or nonfatal MI.	B

continued

TABLE B-2a Continued

Author	Study Type	Subjects	Exposure
Osler et al., 2003	Cohort	Men (n=4513) Women (n=3984) Aged 30-70 years Copenhagen County, Denmark general population MONICA 1 = born in 1922, 1932, 1942, or 1952; examined in 1982 MONICA 2 = born in 1927, 1937, 1947, or 1957; examined in 1987 MONICA 3 = born in 1922, 1932, 1942, 1952, or 1962; examined in 1992 No CHD in the preceding 5 years before enrollment (fatal or nonfatal CHD as an end point) 52,607 person-years of follow-up for men 48,596 person-years of follow-up for women Primary prevention	Seafood

Amount	Results	Conclusion**
Categories of fish intake: 1 = Never 2 = ≤1 time/month 3 = 2 times/month 4 = 1 time/week 5 = ≥2 times/week	After adjusting for smoking status, physical activity, alcohol, educational status, healthy diet score, total cholesterol, total cholesterol, BMI: Those who consumed fish 2 times/month had a significant lower HR of all-cause mortality compared to those who ate fish 1 time/week (HR=0.84, 95% CI 0.73-0.96). No other significant differences were found between categories of fish consumption and all-cause mortality, CHD mortality and morbidity, and CHD mortality.	B

continued

TABLE B-2a Continued

Author	Study Type	Subjects	Exposure
Hu et al., 2002	Cohort	Women (n=84,688) Aged 30-55 years Nurses living in the United States Nurses' Health Study Exclude those who left 10 or more items blank on the dietary questionnaire, those with reported total food intakes judged to be implausible, and those who had a history of cancer, angina, myocardial infarction, coronary revascularization, stroke, or other cardiovascular disease at baseline Follow-up of 16 years Primary prevention	Seafood

Amount	Results	Conclusion**
Serving sizes: Dark-meat fish = 3-5 oz (1.51 g EPA/DHA) Canned tuna = 3-4 oz (0.42 g EPA/DHA) Other fish = 3-5 oz (0.48 g EPA/DHA) Shrimp/lobster/scallops = 3.5 oz (0.32 g EPA/DHA) Categories of fish intake: 1 = <1 time/month 2 = 1-3 times/month 3 = 1 time/week 4 = 2-4 times/week 5 = ≥5 times/week	After adjusting for age, time periods, smoking status, BMI, alcohol intake, menopausal status and postmenopausal hormone use, vigorous to moderate activity, number of times aspirin was used per week, multivitamin use, vitamin E supplement use, history of hypertension, hypercholesterolemia, diabetes, and intake of transfat, the ratio of polyunsaturated fat to saturated fat, and dietary fiber: Those in categories 2-5 of fish intake all had significantly lower RR of coronary heart disease compared to those in category 1 (RR=0.79, 95%CI 0.64-0.97; RR=0.72, 95% CI 0.59-0.88; RR=0.72, 95% CI 0.57-0.91; RR=0.69, 95% CI 0.52-0.93, respectively) (p for trend = 0.007); Those in categories 3 and 5 of fish intake had significantly lower RR of fatal CHD compared to those in category 1 (RR=0.65, 95% CI 0.46-0.91 and RR=0.55, 95% CI 0.33-0.91, respectively). Those in categories 2 and 4 also had lower RRs but they were not significant (p for trend = 0.01); and Those in categories 3 and 4 had significantly lower RR of nonfatal MI compared to those in category 1 (RR=0.75, 95% CI 0.59-0.96 and RR=0.71, 95% CI 0.53-0.96, respectively). Those in categories 2 and 5 also had lower RRs but they were not significant (p for trend = 0.10); and Similar results were found when the model did not also adjust for intake of transfat, the ratio of polyunsaturated fat to saturated fat, and dietary fiber.	B

continued

TABLE B-2a Continued

Author	Study Type	Subjects	Exposure
Nagata et al., 2002	Cohort	Men (n=13,355) Women (n=15,724) Aged 35 years or older Takayama, Gifu, Japan No history of cancer, stroke, or ischemic heart disease Follow-up of 7 years (201,160 person-years) Primary prevention	Seafood or n-3 supplement

Amount	Results	Conclusion**
Quintiles of fish intake (median g/day): Quintile 1 = 46.2 for men, 36.6 for women Quintile 2 = 68.1 for men, 53.9 for women Quintile 3 = 86.8 for men, 68.8 for women Quintile 4 = 111.9 for men, 88.1 for women Quintile 5 = 157.8 for men, 122.4 for women Quintiles of fish oil intake (medium mg/day): Quintile 1 = 410 for men, 332 for women Quintile 2 = 602 for men, 486 for women Quintile 3 = 788 for men, 635 for women Quintile 4 = 1051 for men, 832 for women Quintile 5 = 1582 for men, 1253 for women	After adjusting for age, total energy intake, marital status, BMI, smoking status, alcohol intake, coffee intake, exercise, and history of hypertension and diabetes mellitus: There were no significant associations between quintiles of fish intake and risk of all-cause mortality among men or women; Men in the 2nd quintile of fish oil intake had a significantly lower HR of all-cause mortality than men in the 1st quintile of fish oil intake (HR=0.82, 95% CI 0.67-0.99). Men in the higher quintiles of fish oil intake also had lower HR of all-cause mortality compared to men in the 1st quintile of fish oil intake, but they were not significant; and Women in the 5th quintile of fish oil intake had a significantly lower HR of all-cause mortality than women in the 1st quintile of fish oil intake (HR=0.77, 95% CI 0.62-0.94). Women in the other quintiles of fish oil intake also had lower HR of all-cause mortality compared to women in the 1st quintile of fish oil intake, but they were not significant. There were no significant associations found between quintiles of fish oil intake and cardiovascular disease mortality among men or women.	N

continued

TABLE B-2a Continued

Author	Study Type	Subjects	Exposure
Yuan et al., 2001	Cohort	Men (n=18,244) Aged 45-64 years Shanghai, China No history of cancer Follow-up of 12 years (179,466 person-years) Primary prevention	Seafood

Amount	Results	Conclusion**
Fresh fish = 0.57 g n-3 fatty acids/100 g Salted fish = 0.44 g n-3 fatty acids/100 g Shellfish = 0.36 g n-3 fatty acids/100 g	After controlling for age, total energy intake, level of education, BMI, current smoker at recruitment, average number of cigarettes smoked/day, number of alcoholic drinks consumed/week, history of diabetes, and history of hypertension:	B
Fish and shellfish categories (g/week): 1 = <50 (<1 serving/week) 2 = 50-<100 (1 serving/week) 3 = 100-<150 (2 servings/week) 4 = 150-<200 (3 servings/week) 5 = ≥200 (≥4 servings/week)	Those in the 2nd and 5th categories of fish/shellfish intake had significantly lower RR of acute myocardial infarction mortality than those in the 1st category (RR=0.55, 95% CI 0.33-0.91 and RR=0.41, 95% CI 0.22-0.78, respectively) (p for trend = 0.03). Similar results were found for the categories of fish only, but there were no associations found between shellfish only and risk of acute myocardial infarction mortality; and	
Quintiles of n-3 fatty acid intake (g/week): 1 = <0.27 2 = 0.27-0.43 3 = 0.44-0.72 4 = 0.73-1.09 5 = ≥1.10	Those in the 2nd, 4th, and 5th quintiles of n-3 fatty acid intake had significantly lower RR of acute myocardial infarction mortality than those in the 1st quintile (RR=0.39, 95% CI 0.20-0.75; RR=0.53, 95% CI 0.29-0.97; RR=0.43, 95% CI 0.23-0.81, respectively). Those in the 3rd quintile also had a lower RR compared to the 1st quintile, but it was not significant (RR=0.67, 95% CI 0.42-1.08). There were no significant associations between fish intake and other ischemic heart disease mortality or stroke mortality or between n-3 fatty acid intake and other ischemic heart disease mortality.	

continued

TABLE B-2a Continued

Author	Study Type	Subjects	Exposure
Gillum et al., 2000	Cohort	Men and women (n=8825) White (n=7421) Black (n=1404) Aged 25-74 years US general population (civilian, non-institutionalized) excluding Alaska, Hawaii, and reservation lands of American Indians National Health and Nutrition Examination Survey (NHANES) I Epidemiologic Follow-up Study No history of heart disease at baseline No unknown baseline fish consumption, systolic blood pressure, serum cholesterol concentration, history of diabetes, cigarette smoking status, alcohol intake, body mass index, history of heart disease, nonrecreational physical activity, or educational attainment Average follow-up of 18.8 years Primary prevention	Seafood
Oomen et al., 2000	Cohort	Men Aged 50-69 years Finland (n=1088), Italy (n=1097), Netherlands (n=553) cohorts of the Seven Countries Study Free of CHD at baseline Follow-up of 20 years Primary prevention	Seafood

Amount	Results	Conclusion**
Categories of fish consumption: 1 = Never 2 = <1 occasion/week 3 = 1 occasion/week 4 = >1 occasion/week	After adjusting for baseline age, smoking, history of diabetes, education < high school graduate, systolic blood pressure, serum cholesterol concentration, BMI, alcohol intake, and physical activity: Among White men, those who ate fish 1 occasion/week had a significantly lower RR of all-cause mortality (RR=0.76, 95% CI 0.63-0.91) and noncardiovascular disease mortality (RR=0.68, 95% CI 0.53-0.88) compared to those who never ate fish. No other comparisons between categories of fish consumption, and all-cause, cardiovascular disease, or noncardiovascular disease, mortality were significant; There were no significant associations found between fish intake and all-cause, cardiovascular disease, and noncardiovascular disease mortality among Black men, White women, or Black women; and There were no significant associations found between fish intake and incidence of coronary heart disease among White or Black men or women.	B
Finland fish consumption: 1 = 0-19 g/day 2 = 20-39 g/day 3 = ≥40 g/day Italy fish consumption: 1 = 0 g/day 2 = 1-19 g/day 3 = 20-39 g/day 4 = ≥40 g/day Netherlands fish consumption: 1 = 0 g/day 2 = 1-19 g/day 3 = ≥20 g/day	After adjusting for age, BMI, cigarette smoking, and intake of energy, vegetables, fruit, alcohol, meat, butter, and margarine, there were no significant associations found between total fish consumption and the risk of 20-year CHD mortality in any of the three countries. Similar results were found when the model did not adjust for intake of vegetables, fruit, alcohol, meat, butter, and margarine. After stratifying by country cohort and pooling the data, the overall RR for CHD mortality for intake of 1-19 g/day of fatty fish was 0.57 (95% CI 0.40-0.80) and for intake of ≥20 g/day of fatty fish was 0.87 (95% CI 0.59-1.27) compared to no fatty fish consumption.	N

continued

TABLE B-2a Continued

Author	Study Type	Subjects	Exposure
Albert et al., 1998	Cohort	Men (n=20,551) Aged 40-84 years US physicians Physicians' Health Study Free of MI, stroke, transient ischemic attack, or cancer at baseline 2-by-2 factorial design to receive aspirin, beta carotene, both active drugs, or both placebo 11 years of follow-up (253,777 person-years) Primary prevention	Seafood

Amount	Results	Conclusion**
Categories of fish intake: <1 meal per month 1-3 meals per month 1-<2 meals per week 2-5 meals per week ≥5 meals per week	After adjusting for age, those who ate fish 1-<2 meals per week, 2-<5 meals per week, and ≥5 meals per week had a significantly lower RR of sudden death than those who ate fish only <1 per month (RR=0.42, 95% CI 0.21-0.88; RR=0.46, 95% CI 0.23-0.93; RR=0.34, 95% CI 0.14-0.83, respectively) (p for trend = 0.03). After combining the higher quartiles of fish consumption, those who ate fish ≥1 per week had a significantly lower relative risk of sudden death than those who ate fish only <1 per month (RR=0.44, 95% CI 0.22-0.86) (p for trend = 0.006). After adjusting for age, aspirin, and beta carotene treatment assignment, evidence of cardiovascular disease prior to 12-month questionnaire, BMI, smoking status, history of diabetes, history of hypertension, history of hypercholesterolemia, alcohol consumption, vigorous exercise, and vitamin E, vitamin C, and multivitamin use: Those who ate fish 1-<2 meals per week and ≥5 meals per week had a significantly lower RR of sudden death than those who ate fish only <1 per month (RR=0.47, 95% CI 0.23-0.98 and RR=0.39, 95% CI 0.15-0.96, respectively) (p for trend = 0.11); and After combining the higher quartiles of fish consumption, those who ate ≥1 fish meal per week had a significantly lower RR of sudden death than those who ate only <1 fish meal per month (RR=0.48, 95% CI 0.24-0.96) (p for trend = 0.03).	B

continued

TABLE B-2a Continued

Author	Study Type	Subjects	Exposure

Daviglus et al., 1997	Cohort	Men (n=1822)
		Aged 40-55 years
		Chicago, IL
		Employed for at least 2 years at the
		    Western Electric Company Hawthorne
		    Works in Chicago; occupations related
		    to manufacturing telephones
		Chicago Western Electric Study
		Free of CVD at baseline
		Follow-up of 30 years
		Primary prevention
			Seafood

Mann et al., 1997	Cohort	Men (n=4102)
		Women (n=6700)
		Vegetarians and their nonvegetarian
		    friends and family
		Aged 16-79 years
		UK
		No cancer at entry
		Excluded those who failed to provide
		    full information concerning smoking
		    habits, height, weight, and employ-
		    ment category
		Follow-up of 13.3 years (over 143,000
		    person-years)
		Primary prevention
			Seafood

Rodriquez et al., 1996	Cohort	Men (n=3310) Aged 45-68 years Oahu, Hawaii Japanese ancestry Current smokers Honolulu Heart Program Free of CHD, stroke, cancer at baseline Follow-up of 23 years Primary prevention	Seafood

Amount	Results	Conclusion**
Categories of fish intake: 1 = 0 g/day 2 = 1-17 g/day 3 = 18-34 g/day 4 = ≥35 g/day	After controlling for baseline age and education, religion, systolic blood pressure, serum cholesterol, number of cigarettes smoked per day, BMI, presence or absence of diabetes, presence or absence of electrocardiographic abnormalities, and daily intake of energy, cholesterol, saturated, monounsaturated, and polyunsaturated fatty acids, total protein, carbohydrate, alcohol, iron, thiamine, riboflavin, niacin, vitamin C, beta carotene, and retinol: Those who consumed fish had a lower relative risk of death from MI, CVD, CHD, and all causes. However, the only significant differences were between the 4th category of fish consumption compared to the 1st category for death from overall MI (RR=0.56, 95% CI 0.33-0.93), all CHD (RR=0.62, 95% CI 0.40-0.94), and nonsudden death from MI (RR=0.33, 95% CI 0.12-0.91).	B
Categories of fish intake: 1 = None 2 = <1 time/week 3 = ≥1 time/week	After adjusting for age, sex, smoking, and social class, there were no significant associations found between fish intake and the risk of death from ischemic heart disease or all causes (for those with no evidence of preexisting disease at the time of recruitment).	N
Categories of fish intake: 1 = Almost never 2 = <2 times/week 3 = 2-4 times/week 4 = Almost daily 5 = >1 time/day Low = <2 times/week High = ≥2 times/week	After adjusting for age, years lived in Japan, total calories/day, alcohol intake, physical activity, years smoked, hypertension, and serum cholesterol, glucose, and uric acid levels: In the high-smoking group, those with high fish intake had a significantly lower risk of CHD mortality compared to those with low fish intake (RR=0.5, 95% CI 0.28-0.91). There was no significant association found between fish intake and CHD mortality among past smokers (p=0.6).	N

continued

TABLE B-2a Continued

Author	Study Type	Subjects	Exposure
Ascherio et al., 1995	Cohort	Men (n=44,895) Aged 40-75 years US health professionals Health Professional Follow-up Study Free of known CVD at baseline; no previous diagnosis of MI, angina, stroke, transient ischemic attack, peripheral arterial disease, or had undergone coronary artery surgery 6 years of follow-up (242,029 person-years) Primary prevention	Seafood

Amount	Results	Conclusion**
Quintiles of n-3 fatty acids (g/day): 0.01-0.11, 0.12-0.19, 0.20-0.28, 0.29-0.41, 0.42-6.52 Category of fish intake: 1 = <1 time/month 2 = 1-3 times/month 3 = 1 time/week 4 = 2-3 times/week 5 = 4-5 times/week 6 = ≥6 times/week	There were no significant associations found between dietary intake of n-3 fatty acids and the risk of coronary artery bypass grafting, nonfatal MI, fatal CHD, any MI, or any CHD. After controlling for age, those in the 4th category of fish intake had a significantly lower RR of nonfatal MI compared to those in the 1st category (RR=0.65, 95% CI 0.45-0.94). Those in the 2nd, 4th, and 5th categories of fish intake had significantly lower RR of any MI compared to those in the 1st category (RR=0.67, 95% CI 0.46-0.99; RR=0.69, 95% CI 0.51-0.94; RR=0.65, 95% CI 0.47-0.92, respectively). After controlling for age, BMI, smoking habits, alcohol consumption, history of hypertension, history of diabetes, history of hypercholesterolemia, family history of MI before 60 years of age, and profession: Those in the 5th and 6th categories of fish intake had a significantly higher RR of coronary artery bypass grafting than those in the 1st category (RR=1.71, 95% CI 1.09-2.68 and RR=1.65, 95% CI 1.03-2.64, respectively); Those in the 2nd and 4th categories of fish intake had a significantly lower RR of nonfatal MI than those in the 1st category (RR=0.62, 95% CI 0.39-1.00 and RR=0.67, 95% CI 0.46-0.97, respectively); Those in the 5th category of fish intake had a significantly lower relative risk of fatal CHD than those in the 1st category (RR=0.54, 95% CI 0.29-1.00); Those in the 2nd, 4th, and 5th categories of fish intake had a significantly lower RR of any MI than those in the 1st category (RR=0.66, 95% CI 0.44-0.97; RR=0.69, 95% CI 0.51-0.94; RR=0.65, 95% CI 0.46-0.92, respectively); and No other significant associations were found between fish intake and CHD.	B

continued

TABLE B-2a Continued

Author	Study Type	Subjects	Exposure
Kromhout et al., 1995	Cohort	Men (n=137) Women (n=135) Aged 64-87 years for men Aged 64-85 years for women Rotterdam, Netherlands All patients of the same general practice Follow-up of 17 years Primary prevention	Seafood
Salonen et al., 1995	Cohort	Men (n=1833) Aged 42, 48, 54, or 60 years Eastern Finland Kuopio Ischaemic Heart Disease Risk Factor Study (KIHD) No CHD, history of cerebrovascular stroke, claudication, or cancer at baseline Mean follow-up time for AMI for individuals of 5 years Mean follow-up time for death of 6 years Primary prevention	Seafood

Amount	Results	Conclusion**
Fish intake = yes or no	After adjusting for age, gender, prevalence of MI and angina pectoris, systolic blood pressure, total cholesterol, smoking, alcohol and energy intake/body weight, those who ate fish had a significant lower RR of CHD mortality than those who did not eat fish (RR=0.51, 95% CI 0.29-0.89). The difference in CHD mortality between the fish eaters and the non-fish eaters became apparent after 5 years of follow-up.	B
Continuous variable = g/day Binary variable = <30 or ≥30 g/day	After adjusting for age, examination year, ischemic exercise ECG, and maximal oxygen uptake, family history of CHD, cigarette-years, mean systolic blood pressure, diabetes, socioeconomic status, place of residence, dietary iron intake, and serum apolipoprotein B, HDL-cholesterol, and ferritin concentrations: Each one unit (g/day) increase in fish intake significantly increased the risk of fatal or non-fatal AMI (RR=1.004, 95% CI 1.001-1.007). There were no significant associations between fish intake (as a continuous variable) and death from CHD, CVD, or all causes; and Those who consumed ≥30 g/day of fish had a significantly higher risk of fatal or nonfatal AMI compared to those who consumed >30 g/day (RR=1.87, 95% CI 1.13-3.09). There was no significant association found between fish intake ≥30 g/day and CHD, CVD, or all-cause mortality. Similar results were found when the model only adjusted for age, examination year, ischemic exercise ECG, and maximal oxygen uptake.	A

continued

TABLE B-2a Continued

Author	Study Type	Subjects	Exposure
Dolecek, 1992	Cohort (nested in an RCT)	Men (n=6250) Aged 35-57 years 22 US clinical centers Multiple Risk Factor Intervention Trial (MRFIT) Only included those in the usual care group for this analysis At high risk of developing CHD because of smoking status, diastolic blood pressure, and serum cholesterol levels Follow-up of 10.5 years Primary prevention	Seafood
Fraser et al., 1992	Cohort	Men and women (n=26,473) Mean age 51 years (men) Mean age 53 years (women) California Non-Hispanic White Adventists The Adventist Health Study No history of heart disease or diabetes at baseline; almost no current smokers (although some past smokers) Follow-up of 6 years Primary prevention	Seafood

Amount	Results	Conclusion**
Quintiles of fish n-3s: Quintile 1 = mean of 0.000 g Quintile 2 = mean of 0.009 g Quintile 3 = mean of 0.046 g Quintile 4 = mean of 0.153 g Quintile 5 = mean of 0.664 g	After adjusting for age, race, smoking, baseline diastolic blood pressure, high density lipoprotein, low density lipoprotein, and alcohol: A one-unit increase in fish n-3 consumption, expressed in grams, significantly decreased one's risk of CVD mortality ($\beta=-0.9598$, $p<0.01$) and CHD mortality ($\beta=-0.93388$, $p<0.05$); however there were no significant associations found between fish n-3 consumption and risk of mortality from cancer or all causes; and A one-unit increase in fish n-3 consumption, expressed as % kcal, significantly decreased one's risk of CVD mortality ($\beta=-0.4499$, $p<0.01$), CHD mortality ($\beta=-0.4715$, $p<0.05$), and all-cause mortality ($\beta=-0.2590$, $p<0.05$); however there was no significant association found between fish n-3 consumption and risk of mortality from cancer.	B
Categories of fish intake: 1 = None 2 = 0<x<1 time/week 3 = ≥1 time/week	After stratifying for age, sex, smoking, exercise, relative weight, and high blood pressure, no significant RRs were found for definite nonfatal MI, definite fatal CHD, or fatal CHD as determined by death certificate, based on fish intake. However, there seemed to be a trend of lower RRs for higher intakes of fish.	N

continued

TABLE B-2a Continued

Author	Study Type	Subjects	Exposure
Kromhout et al., 1985	Cohort	Men (n=852) Aged 40-59 years Zutphen, Netherlands The Zutphen Study (Dutch contribution to the Seven Countries Study) Free of CHD at baseline Follow-up of 20 years Primary prevention	Seafood

Amount	Results	Conclusion**
Categories of fish intake: 1 = 0 g/day 2 = 1-14 g/day 3 = 15-29 g/day 4 = 30-44 g/day 5 = ≥45 g/day	After adjusting for age, systolic blood pressure, serum total cholesterol, cigarette smoking, subscapular skinfold thickness, physical activity, energy intake, dietary cholesterol, prescribed diet, and occupation: Those in category 4 of fish intake had a significantly lower RR of death from coronary heart disease than those in the 1st category (RR=0.36, 95% CI 0.14-0.93); and Those in the 2nd, 3rd, and 5th fish consumption categories also had lower RRs of death from coronary heart disease than those in the 1st category, but they were not significant (p for trend = <0.05).	B

continued

TABLE B-2a Continued

Author	Study Type	Subjects	Exposure
Albert et al., 2002	Case-control (nested)	Cases (n=94) = sudden death occurred (first manifestation of CVD) Controls (n=184) = free of confirmed CVD Men Aged 40-84 years US physicians Physicians' Health Study Free of MI, stroke, transient ischemic attacks, or cancer at baseline 2-by-2 factorial design to receive aspirin, beta carotene, both active drugs, or both placebo 17 years of follow-up (time from study enrollment to sudden death = 0.7-16.9 years) Primary prevention	Baseline blood fatty acid levels

Amount	Results	Conclusion**
Quartiles of n-3 fatty acids (% total fatty acids): 2.12-4.32, 4.33-5.19, 5.20-6.07, 6.08-10.2	After adjusting for age and smoking status: The RR of sudden death was significantly lower for those in the 3rd and 4th quartiles of n-3 fatty acid intake (RR=0.37, 95% CI 0.17-0.83 and RR=0.31, 95% CI 0.13-0.75, respectively) compared to those in the 1st quartile (p for trend = 0.004). After adjusting for assignment to aspirin and beta carotene treatment or placebo, BMI, history of diabetes, history of hypertension, history of hypercholesterolemia, alcohol consumption, frequency of vigorous exercise and parental history of MI before the age of 60: The RR of sudden death was significantly lower for those in the 3rd and 4th quartiles of n-3 fatty acid intake (RR=0.28, 95% CI 0.09-0.87 and RR=0.19, 95% CI 0.05-0.71, respectively) compared to those in the 1st quartile (p for trend = 0.007). After adjusting for assignment to aspirin and beta carotene treatment or placebo, BMI, history of diabetes, history of hypertension, history of hypercholesterolemia, alcohol consumption, frequency of vigorous exercise, parental history of myocardial infarction before the age of 60, trans unsaturated fatty acid and monounsaturated fatty acid levels: The RR of sudden death was significantly lower for those in the 3rd and 4th quartiles of n-3 fatty acids (RR=0.19, 95% CI 0.05-0.69 and RR=0.10, 95% CI 0.02-0.48, respectively) compared to those in the 1st quartile (p for trend = 0.001).	B

continued

TABLE B-2a Continued

Author	Study Type	Subjects	Exposure
Martinez-Gonzalez et al., 2002	Case-control	Cases = suffered first definite AMI; admitted to hospital (n=171) Controls = admitted to same hospital during same month for unrelated conditions (n=171) Men and women Aged <80 years Three tertiary hospitals of Pamplona, Spain No history of angina pectoris, a previous diagnosis of CHD, or other prior diagnosis of major cardiovascular disease Secondary prevention	Seafood
Sasazuki et al., 2001	Case-control	Cases = first episode of AMI (n=632) Controls = residents from same municipalities as the cases (n=1214) Men and women Aged 40-79 years 22 collaborating hospitals in Fukuoka City, Japan, and in 21 adjacent municipalities Fukuoka Heart Study Secondary prevention	Seafood

Amount	Results	Conclusion**
Categories of fish intake: 1 = <60 g/day 2 = 60-77 g/day 3 = 77-106 g/day 4 = 106-142 g/day 5 = >142 g/day	After adjusting for age, hospital, gender, smoking, BMI, high blood pressure, high blood cholesterol, diabetes, leisure-time physical activity, socioeconomic status, and total energy: Those in the 3rd and 5th categories of fish intake had significantly lower ORs of first MI compared to those in the 1st category (OR=0.28, 95% CI 0.10-0.77 and OR=0.31, 95% CI 0.11-0.85, respectively). Those in the 2nd and 4th categories of fish intake also had lower ORs compared to those in the 1st category, but they were not significant. Those in the three upper quintiles of fish intake had a significantly lower OR of a first MI compared to those in the lower quintile (OR=0.36, 95% CI 0.15-0.87). After further adjusting for olive oil, fiber, fruits, vegetables, alcohol, meat/meat products, and white bread/rice/pasta intake, this association was not significant (OR=0.37, 95% CI 0.13-1.03).	B
Categories of fish consumption (men and women): Low = <2/week Intermediate = 2-3/week High = 4+/week	After adjusting for smoking, alcohol use, sedentary job, leisure-time physical activity, hyperlipidemia, hypertension, diabetes mellitus, angina pectoris, and obesity: Men who consumed intermediate and high levels of fish had a significantly lower RR of acute MI compared to those who consumed low levels of fish (RR=0.5, 95% CI 0.3-0.8 and RR=0.6, 95% CI 0.4-0.9, respectively); and The relative risks for acute MI based on fish consumption were not significant among women. Similar results were found when also adjusting for fruit and tofu intake.	B

continued

TABLE B-2a Continued

Author	Study Type	Subjects	Exposure
Tavani et al., 2001	Case-control	Cases = first episode of nonfatal AMI; admitted to hospital (n=507) Controls = admitted to same hospital for unrelated conditions (n=478) Men and women Aged 25-79 years Greater Milan, Italy area Secondary prevention	Seafood
Siscovick et al., 1995	Case-control	Case = primary cardiac arrest patients (n=334) Controls = from community (n=493) Men and women Aged 25-74 years Married Seattle and suburban King County, WA Free of prior clinical heart disease, major comorbidities, and use of fish-oil supplements On average, 4 months between the date of cardiac arrest and in-person interview Primary prevention	Seafood

Amount	Results	Conclusion**
Mixed Mediterranean fish = 0.94 g of n-3 per portion Other fish = 0.49 g of n-3/portion Canned tuna, mackerel, and sardines = 0.34 g of n-3/portion Categories of n-3 PUFA: Lowest = <0.81 g/week Intermediate = 0.81-1.28 g/week Highest = >1.28 g/week Categories of total fish and fresh fish: 1 = <1 portion/week 2 = 1-<2 portions/week 3 = ≥2 portions/week Categories of canned fish: 1 = 0 portions/week 2 = >0-<1 portion/week 3 = ≥1 portion/week	After adjusting for age; sex; education; BMI; cholesterol; smoking; coffee, alcohol, meat, vegetables, fruit, and calorie intake; physical activity; hyperlipidemia; diabetes; hypertension; and family history of AMI in first-degree relative: Those who consume an intermediate or high level of n-3 PUFAs had a significantly lower OR of AMI compared to those who consumed a low level of n-3 PUFAs (OR=0.67, 95% CI 0.47-0.96 and OR=0.67, 95% CI 0.47-0.95, respectively). Those who consume two or more portions of total fish/week had a significantly lower OR of AMI compared to those who consume less than one portion/week (OR=0.68, 95% CI 0.47-0.98). Those who consume 1-<2 portions/week of total fish also had a lower OR of AMI than those who consume <1 portion/week, but it was not significant. There were no significant associations found between fresh fish intake and canned fish intake and the risk of AMI. Similar results were found when the model only adjusted for age and sex.	B
Average serving size = 3 oz of fish Quartiles of n-3 fatty acids (g/month): Quartile 1 = 0.12-1.95 Quartile 2 = 1.96-4.05 Quartile 3 = 4.06-7.40 Quartile 4 = 7.41-12.72	After adjusting for age, current smoking, former smoking, family history of MI or sudden death, fat intake scale, hypertension, diabetes mellitus, physical activity, weight, height, and education: Those in quartiles 2, 3, and 4 of dietary n-3 fatty acid intakes all had significantly lower ORs of primary cardiac arrest compared to those who never consumed fish (OR=0.7, 95% CI 0.6-0.9; OR=0.5, 95% CI 0.4-0.8; OR=0.4, 95% CI 0.2-0.7, respectively). Those in the 1st quartile also had a lower OR of primary cardiac arrest compared to those who never consumed fish, but it was not significant.	B

continued

TABLE B-2a Continued

Author	Study Type	Subjects	Exposure
Gramenzi et al., 1990	Case-control	Cases = an acute MI (n=287) Controls = acute disorders unrelated to ischemic heart disease (n=649) Women Aged 22-69 years for cases Aged 21-69 years for controls 30 hospitals in northern Italy No chronic or digestive conditions; cardiovascular, malignant, hormonal, or gynecological disease; or any disorder that was potentially related to consumption of alcohol or smoking Primary prevention	Seafood

Amount	Results	Conclusion**
Tertiles of fish intake (# portions/week): Tertile 1 = <1 Tertile 2 = 1 Tertile 3 = >1	After adjusting for age, area of residence, education, smoking, hyperlipidemia, diabetes, hypertension, and BMI, the OR for MI was 0.8 for the 2nd tertile of fish intake and 0.7 for the 3rd tertile of fish intake, compared to the 1st tertile (p<0.05). After adjusting for age, area of residence, education, smoking, hyperlipidemia, diabetes, hypertension, BMI, carrots, green vegetables, fresh fruit, meat, ham and salami, butter, total fat score, coffee, and alcohol, the OR for MI was 1.0 for the 2nd tertile of fish intake and 0.8 for the 3rd tertile of fish intake, compared to the 1st tertile, and they were not significant.	B

continued

TABLE B-2a Continued

Author	Study Type	Subjects	Exposure
Bang et al., 1971	Ecological	Men (n=61) Women (n=69) Aged >30 years Eskimos in the northwest coast of Greenland, compared to Danish controls Most are hunters and/or fishermen Primary prevention	Plasma total lipids, lipoproteins, cholesterol, and triglycerides

*Included in Balk E, Chung M, Lichtenstein A, Chew P, Kupelnick B, Lawrence A, DeVine D, Lau J. 2004. *Effects of Omega-3 Fatty Acids on Cardiovascular Risk Factors and Intermediate Markers of Cardiovascular Disease. Summary, Evidence Report/Technology Assessment No. 93 (Prepared by the Tufts-New England Medical Center Evidence-based*

Amount	Results	Conclusion**

Total lipids (g/L±SD):
  Eskimo men = 6.17±0.89
  Eskimo women =
    6.13±0.88
  Danish men = 7.12±1.24
  Danish women =
    7.29±1.16
Cholesterol (g/L±SD):
  Eskimo men = 2.33±0.35
  Eskimo women =
    2.22±0.43
  Danish men = 2.73±0.49
  Danish women =
    2.86±0.49
Triglycerides (g/L±SD):
  Eskimo men = 0.57±0.28
  Eskimo women =
    0.44±0.13
  Danish men = 1.29±0.62
  Danish women =
    1.08±0.51
Pre-β-lipoproteins
    (g/L±SD):
  Eskimo men = 0.48±0.31
  Eskimo women =
    0.43±0.33
  Danish men = 1.70±0.86
  Danish women =
    1.08±0.51
β-lipoproteins (g/L±SD):
  Eskimo men = 4.38±0.93
  Eskimo women =
    4.15±0.89
  Danish men = 5.11±1.16
  Danish women =
    5.31±1.32
α-lipoproteins (g/L±SD):
  Eskimo men = 4.02±1.39
  Eskimo women =
    3.91±1.41
  Danish men = 2.78±0.82
  Danish women =
    3.64±0.94
	Among males, the Eskimos had significantly lower plasma total lipids ($p<0.001$), cholesterol ($p<0.001$), triglycerides ($p<0.001$), pre-β-lipoproteins ($p<0.001$), β-lipoproteins ($p<0.001$), and α-lipoproteins ($p<0.001$) compared to the Danes. However, the differences in total lipids and cholesterol among men 31-40 years and β-lipoproteins among men 31-50 years between the Eskimos and the Danes were not significant.
	
	Among women, the Eskimos had significantly lower plasma total lipids ($p<0.001$), cholesterol ($p<0.001$), triglycerides ($p<0.001$), pre-β-lipoproteins ($p<0.001$), and β-lipoproteins ($p<0.001$). However, the difference in β-lipoproteins among women 31-50 years between the Eskimos and the Danes was not significant.
	
	There were no significant differences in α-lipoproteins among the female Eskimos and Danes.
		B

Practice Center, Boston, MA). AHRQ Publication No. 04-E010-1. Rockville, MD: Agency for Healthcare Research and Quality.
  **N = Evidence of no association or no clear association; B = Evidence of a benefit; A = Evidence of an adverse effect.

TABLE B-2b Studies on Stroke

Author	Study Type	Subjects	Exposure
Hooper et al., 2005	Cochrane Review	48 RCTs At least 6 months of omega-3 fatty acids vs. placebo or control 26 cohorts (47 analyses) Follow-up of 4-25 years	n-3 supplement
Bouzan et al., 2005	Meta-analysis	5 cohort studies 1 case-control study	Seafood
He et al., 2004a	Meta-analysis	9 cohorts (from 8 studies) English language	Seafood

Amount	Results	Conclusion**
	Based on RCTs, no significant association was found between omega-3 intake and risk of total stroke based on a meta-analysis (RR=1.17, 95% CI 0.91-1.51) or sensitivity analysis (RR=0.87, 95% CI 0.72-1.04).	N
Servings/week, a continuous variable	In the linear regression model, for each one-unit increase in servings/week of fish, the change in the risk ratio of total stroke is -0.20 (95% CI -0.066 to 0.027), but this is not significant. In the quadratic regression model, for each one-unit increase in servings/week of fish, the change in the risk ratio of total stroke is 0.0037 (95% CI -0.0096 to 0.017), but this is not significant.	N
Categories of fish consumption: 1 = <1 time/month 2 = 1-3 times/month 3 = 1 time/week 4 = 2-4 times/week 5 = ≥5 times/week	Based on pooled RRs, those who consumed fish 1 time/week, 2-4 times/week, and ≥5 times/week had significantly lower RR of stroke compared to those who consumed fish <1 time/month (RR=0.87, 95% CI 0.77-0.98; RR=0.82, 95% CI 0.72-0.94; and RR=0.69, 95% CI 0.54-0.88, respectively); the RR was not significant for those who consumed fish 1-3 times/month compared to those who consumed fish <1 time/month. Based on pooled RRs, those who consumed fish 1-3 times/month, 1 time/week, 2-4 times/week, and ≥5 times/week had significantly lower RR of ischemic stroke compared to those who consumed fish <1 time/month (RR=0.69, 95% CI 0.48-0.99; RR=0.68, 95% CI 0.52-0.88; RR=0.66, 95% CI 0.51-0.87; and RR=0.65, 95% CI 0.46-0.93, respectively). There were no significant associations found between fish consumption and hemorrhagic stroke.	B

continued

TABLE B-2b Continued

Author	Study Type	Subjects	Exposure
Mozaffarian et al., 2005	Cohort	Men and women (n=4778) Aged ≥65 years 4 US communities From Medicare eligibility lists Free of known cerebrovascular disease at baseline Cardiovascular Health Study (CHS) 12 years of follow-up	Seafood

Amount	Results	Conclusion**
Categories of tuna/ other fish intake: 1 = <1 time/month 2 = 1-3 times/month 3 = 1-4 times/week 4 = ≥5 times/week	After adjusting for age, sex, education, diabetes, coronary heart disease, smoking status, pack-years of smoking, aspirin use, BMI, leisure-time physical activity, alcohol use, total caloric intake, systolic blood pressure, LDL-c, HDL-c, triglyceride, and C-reactive protein levels:	B
Categories for fried fish/fish sandwich intakes: 1 = <1 time/month 2 = 1-3 times/month 3 = ≥1 time/week	Those who consumed tuna/other fish 1-4 times/ week had a significantly lower risk of total stroke and ischemic stroke compared to those who consumed tuna/other fish <1 time/month (HR=0.74, 95% CI 0.56-0.98 and HR=0.73, 95% CI 0.54-0.98, respectively). Those who consumed tuna/ other fish 1-3 times/month and ≥5 times/week also had lower risks of total stroke and ischemic stroke compared to those who consumed tuna/other fish <1 time/month, but they were not significant; Those who consumed fried fish/fish sandwiches ≥1 time/week had significantly higher risk of total stroke and ischemic stroke compared to those who consumed fried fish/fish sandwiches <1 time/month (HR=1.33, 95% CI 1.05-1.68 and HR=1.39, 95% CI 1.08-1.79, respectively); and There were no significant associations found between tuna/other fish intake or fried fish/fish sandwich intake and the risk of hemorrhagic stroke.	

continued

TABLE B-2b Continued

Author	Study Type	Subjects	Exposure
Sauvaget et al., 2003	Cohort	Men (n=14,209) Women (n=22,921) Aged 34-103 years Nagasaki and Hiroshima, Japan The Life Span Study Atomic bomb survivors and their non-exposed controls No prevalent cases of cancer, self-reported cases of stroke, ischemic heart disease, and both stroke and ischemic heart disease Follow-up of 16 years	Seafood

Amount	Results	Conclusion**
Categories of fish intake: 1 = Never 2 = ≤1 time/week 3 = 2-4 times/week 4 = Almost daily Tertiles of fish intake: Low – 11-18 g/day Moderate = 30 g/day High = 46-65 g/day	After adjusting for sex, birth cohort, city, radiation dose, self-reported BMI, smoking status, alcohol habits, education level, history of diabetes, and hypertension: There was no significant association found between fish (except broiled) intake and the risk of total stroke mortality, when fish intake was defined as never, ≤1 time/week, 2-4 times/week, and almost daily; however, there was a significant trend (p=0.046); Those who ate broiled fish almost daily had a significantly lower RR of total stroke mortality compared to those who never ate broiled fish (HR=0.60, 95% CI 0.37-0.98); Those who ate moderate and high levels of fish products had significantly lower RRs of total stroke (RR=0.85, 95% CI 0.75-0.97 and RR=0.85, 95% CI 0.75-0.98, respectively) and intracerebral hemorrhage (RR=0.70, 95% CI 0.54-0.91 and RR=0.70, 95% CI 0.54-0.92, respectively) compared to those who ate low levels of fish products; and There were no significant associations between intake (defined as low, moderate, and high) of fish products and cerebral infarction.	B

continued

TABLE B-2b Continued

Author	Study Type	Subjects	Exposure
He et al., 2002*	Cohort	Men (n=43,671) Aged 40-75 years US health professionals Health Professional Follow-up Study No previously diagnosed stroke, MI, coronary artery surgery, angina pectoris, peripheral arterial disease, diabetes mellitus, transient ischemic attack, or other cardiovascular disease Follow-up of 12 years	Seafood and dietary n-3 fatty acid intake

Amount	Results	Conclusion**

Serving sizes:
Dark-meat fish =
  3-5 oz (1.60 g n-3)
Canned tuna = 3-4 oz
  (0.41 g n-3)
Other fish = 3-5 oz
  (0.56 g n-3)
Shrimp/lobster/scallops
  = 3.5 oz (0.26 g n-3)
 	
Categories of fish
  intake:
1 = <1 time/month
2 = 1-3 times/month
3 = 1 time/week
4 = 2-4 times/week
5 = ≥5 times/week
 	
Quintiles of n-3 fatty
  acids:
1 = <0.05 g/day
2 = 0.05-<0.2 g/day
3 = 0.2-<0.4 g/day
4 = 0.4-<0.6 g/day
5 = ≥0.6 g/day
	After adjusting for BMI, physical activity, history of hypertension, smoking status, use of aspirin, fish oil, multivitamins, intake of total calories, total fat, saturated fat, trans-unsaturated fat, alcohol, potassium, magnesium, total servings of fruits and vegetables, and hypercholesterolemia at baseline:
	
	Those in the higher quintiles of cumulative fish consumption all had significantly lower RR of ischemic stroke compared to those who consumed fish <1 time/month (RR=0.57, 95% CI 0.35-0.95; RR=0.56, 95% CI 0.37-0.84; RR=0.55, 95% CI 0.36-0.85; and RR=0.54, 95% CI 0.31-0.94, respectively);
	
	Those in the 4th quintile of cumulative fish intake had a significantly lower RR of total stroke than those in the 1st quintile (RR=0.67, 95% CI 0.46-0.96). The other quintiles also had lower relative risks compared to the 1st quintile, but they were not significant;
	
	There were no significant associations found between cumulative fish intake and the risk of hemorrhagic stroke; similar results were found for most recent fish intake;
	
	Those in the 2nd, 3rd, and 4th quintiles of n-3 PUFA intake had significantly lower RRs of ischemic stroke compared to those in the first quintile (RR=0.56, 95% CI 0.35-0.88; RR=0.63, 95% CI 0.40-0.98; RR=0.54, 95% CI 0.32-0.91, respectively). Those in the 5th quintile also had a lower RR of ischemic stroke compared to those in the 1st quintile, but it was not significant; and
	
	There were no significant associations found between n-3 PUFA intake and total stroke or hemorrhagic stroke.
		B

continued

TABLE B-2b Continued

Author	Study Type	Subjects	Exposure
Iso et al., 2001*	Cohort	Women (n=79,839) Aged 34-59 years US nurses Nurses' Health Study No history of cancer, angina, myocardial infarction, coronary revascularization, stroke, other cardiovascular diseases before baseline; or a history of physician-diagnosed diabetes or high serum cholesterol levels Follow-up of 14 years (1,086,261 person-years)	Seafood and dietary n-3 fatty acid intake

Amount	Results	Conclusion**

Serving sizes:
Dark-meat fish =
  3-5 oz (1.51 g
  EPA/DHA)
Canned tuna = 3-4 oz
  (0.42 g EPA/DHA)
Other fish = 3-5 oz
  (0.48 g EPA/DHA)
Shrimp/lobster/scal-
  lops = 3.5 oz (0.32 g
  EPA/DHA)
 	
Categories of fish
  intake:
1 = <1 time/month
2 = 1-3 times/month
3 = 1 time/week
4 = 2-4 times/week
5 = ≥5 times/week
 	
Quintiles of n-3 PUFAs
  (median in grams):
1 = 0.077 g/day
2 = 0.118 g/day
3 = 0.171 g/day
4 = 0.221 g/day
5 = 0.481 g/day
	After adjusting for Joules, BMI, alcohol intake, menopausal status and postmenopausal hormone use, vigorous exercise, usual aspirin use, multivitamin use, history of hypertension, and frequency of total fruit and vegetable intake and for intake of saturated fat, trans-unsaturated fat, linoleic acid, animal protein, and calcium:
	
	Those who consume 2-4 servings of fish/week had a signficantly lower RR of thrombotic infarction than those who ate fish <1 time/month (RR=0.52, 95% CI 0.27-0.99). Although all other categories of higher fish consumption had lower RRs of thrombotic infarction than the 1st category, they were not significant;
	
	Those who ate fish 2 or more times per week had sigificantly lower RR of lacunar infarction than those who ate fish <1 time/month (RR=0.28, 95% CI 0.12-0.67). Although all other categories of higher fish consumption had lower RRs of lacunar infarction than the 1st category, they were not significant;
	
	There were no significant associations found between fish consumption and total stroke, ischemic stroke, large-artery occlusive infarction, hemorrhagic stroke, subarachnoid hemorrhage, or intraparenchymal hemorrhage;
	
	Those in quintile 3 of omega-3 PUFA intake had a significantly lower RR of total stroke (RR=0.69, 95% CI 0.53-0.89), ischemic stroke (RR=0.67, 95% CI 0.47-0.98), and thrombotic infarction (RR=0.64, 95% CI 0.43-0.95) compared to those in quintile 1;
	
	Those in quintile 5 of omega-3 PUFA intake had a significantly lower RR of total stroke (RR=0.72, 95% CI 0.53-0.99) and lacunar infarction (RR=0.37, 95% CI 0.19-0.73) compared to those in quintile 1; and
	
	There were no significant associations found between omega-3 PUFA intake and large-artery occlusive infarction, hemorrhagic stroke, subarachnoid hemorrhage, or intraparenchymal hemorrhage.
		B

continued

TABLE B-2b Continued

Author	Study Type	Subjects	Exposure
Yuan et al., 2001	Cohort	Men (n=18,244) Aged 45-64 years Shanghai, China No history of cancer Follow-up of 12 years (179,466 person-years) Primary prevention	Seafood and dietary n-3 fatty acid intake

Amount	Results	Conclusion**
Fresh fish = 0.57 g n-3 fatty acids/100 g Salted fish = 0.44 g n-3 fatty acids/100 g Shellfish = 0.36 g n-3 fatty acids/100 g Fish and shellfish categories (g/week): 1 = <50 (<1 serving/week) 2 = 50-<100 (1 serving/week) 3 = 100-<150 (2 servings/week) 4 = 150-<200 (3 servings/week) 5 = ≥200 (≥4 servings/week) Quintiles of n-3 fatty acids: (g/week) 1 = <0.27 2 = 0.27-0.43 3 = 0.44-0.72 4 = 0.73-1.09 5 = ≥1.10	After controlling for age, total energy intake, level of education, BMI, current smoker at recruitment, average number of cigarettes smoked per day, number of alcoholic drinks consumed per week, history of diabetes, and history of hypertension: There were no significant associations found between fish consumption and risk of stroke mortality; and Those in the 3rd quintile of n-3 fatty acid intake had significantly lower RR of stroke mortality compared to those in the 1st quintile (RR=0.76, 95% CI 0.58-0.98). Those in the 2nd, 4th, and 5th quintiles also had lower RRs of stroke mortality compared to those in the 1st quintile, but they were not significant.	B

continued

TABLE B-2b Continued

Author	Study Type	Subjects	Exposure
Gillum et al., 1996*	Cohort	Men and women (n=5192) Aged 45-74 years White (n=4410) Black (n=782) National Health and Nutrition Examination Survey (NHANES) I No history of stroke at baseline Excluded those with unknown baseline fish consumption, systolic blood pressure, serum cholesterol level, diabetes history, number of cigarettes smoked, BMI, history of heart disease, or educational attainment Average follow-up of 12 years	Seafood
Orencia et al., 1996*	Cohort	Men (n=1847) Aged 40-55 years Employed at least 2 years at the Hawthorne Works of the Western Electric Co. in Chicago, IL 65% first- or second-generation Americans, predominantly of German, Polish, or Bohemian ancestry Chicago Western Electric Study Free of CHD and stroke at baseline Follow-up of 30 years (46,426 person-years)	Seafood

Amount	Results	Conclusion**
Categories of fish consumption: 1 = Never 2 = <1 time/week 3 = 1 time/week 4 = >1 time/week	After adjusting for baseline age, smoking, history of diabetes, history of heart disease, education less than high school graduate, systolic blood pressure, serum albumin concentration, serum cholesterol concentration, BMI, alcohol intake, and physical activity: White women aged 45-74 years who ate fish >1 time/week had a significantly lower RR of acute stroke incidence compared to those who never ate fish (RR=0.55, 95% CI 0.32-0.93); Significant RRs were not found when the women were separated and analyzed based on different age groups (45-64 years and 65-74 years) or for White men; and Black men and women who ate any fish had a significantly lower RR of acute stroke incidence (RR=0.51, 95% CI 0.30-0.88) and stroke death (RR=0.26, 95% CI 0.11-0.64) compared to those who never ate fish.	B
Categories of fish consumption: 1 = None 2 = 1-17 g/day 3 = 18-34 g/day 4 = ≥35 g/day	After adjusting for age, systolic blood pressure, cigarette smoking, serum cholesterol, diabetes, ECG abnormalities, table salt use, alcohol intake, iron, thiamine, riboflavin, niacin, vitamin C, beta-carotene, retinol, total energy, polyunsaturated fatty acids, carbohydrates, and total protein, there were no significant associations found between fish consumption and risk of fatal and nonfatal stroke.	N

continued

TABLE B-2b Continued

Author	Study Type	Subjects	Exposure
Morris et al., 1995*	Cohort	Men (n=21,185) Aged 40-84 years US physicians Physicians' Health Study No history of MI, stroke, transient ischemic attacks, cancer, liver or renal disease, peptic ulcer, gout, current use of aspirin, other platelet-active drugs, or nonsteroidal anti-inflammatory agents Follow-up of 4 years	Seafood and dietary n-3 fatty acid intake

Amount	Results	Conclusion**
Categories of fish: 1 = Canned tuna 2 = Dark-meat fish (4-6 oz) 3 = Other fish (4-6 oz) 4 = Shrimp, lobster, or scallops	After adjusting for each level of fish consumption, age, aspirin and beta-carotene assignment, smoking, alcohol consumption, obesity, diabetes mellitus, vigorous exercise, parental history of MI before age 60 years, history of hypertension, history of hypercholesterolemia, vitamin supplement use, and saturated fat intake:	B
Categories of fish intake: 1 = <1 meal/week 2 = 1 meal/week 3 = 2 4 meals/week 4 = ≥5 meals/week	Those who consumed 1 fish meal/week had a significantly higher RR of total MI (RR=1.5, 95% CI 1.1-2.1) and cardiovascular deaths (RR=2.6, 95% CI 1.4-4.8) compared to those who consume fish <1 meal/week;	
Quintiles of n-3 fatty acids intake (g/week): 1 = <0.5 2 = 0.5-<1.0 3 = 1.0-<1.7 4 = 1.7-<2.3 5 = ≥2.3	No other significant RRs of total myocardial infarction, nonfatal myocardial infarction, stroke, cardiovascular deaths, or total cardiovascular events were found based on weekly fish consumption; Those in the 2nd quintile of omega-3 fatty acid intake had a higher RR of total MI than those in the 1st quintile (RR=1.6, 95% CI 1.1-2.4); and No other significant RR of total MI, nonfatal MI, stroke, cardiovascular deaths, or total cardiovascular events were found based on weekly omega-3 fatty acid intake.	

continued

TABLE B-2b Continued

Author	Study Type	Subjects	Exposure
Keli et al., 1994*	Cohort	Men (n=552) Aged 50-69 years Zutphen, Netherlands The Zutphen Study (Dutch contribution to the Seven Countries Study) Free of stroke at baseline Follow-up of 15 years	Seafood

Kromann and Green, 1980	Cohort	Men and women (n=1800)
		All ages
		Born in Greenland and/or with Green-
		  landic mothers in the Upernavik
		  district, northwest Greenland
		5-10% persons of other origin
		Follow-up of 25 years (40,472
		  person-years)
			Diet

Amount	Results	Conclusion**
Categories of fish consumption: Low = ≤20 g/day High = >20 g/day	Fish consumption (g/day) was significantly different in those who did not suffer from a stroke (18.3±19.8) than those who did (12.8±12.3) after 15 years of follow-up (p<0.05). After adjusting for age, average systolic blood pressure 1960-1970, average serum cholesterol 1960-1970, cigarette smoking until 1970, and intake of energy and vegetable protein, alcohol consumption, and prescribed diet in 1970: Those who consumed >20 g/day of fish had a lower, but not statistically significant, HR of stroke incidence than those who ate ≤20 g/day of fish (HR=0.49, 95% CI 0.24-1.01); Those who always consumed fish did not have a significantly lower HR of stroke incidence than those who ate fish "not always" (HR=0.71, 95% CI 0.38-1.33).	B
This population is mainly occupied with whaling and sealing, fowling, and to a lesser degree fishing	Summarizes the disease patterns of cancer, "apoplexy," epilepsy, peptic ulcer, acute myocardial infarction, rheumatic fever, chronic polyarthritis, chronic pyelonephritis, chronic glomerulonephritis, diabetes mellitus, psoriasis, psychosis, multiple sclerosis, and thyrotoxicosis.	N
The traditional diet is supplemented with Danish food	The pattern of disease in this study "differs from that of Western Europe, as we have found frequent occurrence of apoplexy and grand mal epilepsy, but rare or nonoccurrence of acute myocardial infarction, diabetes mellitus, thyrotoxicosis, bronchial asthma, multiple sclerosis and psoriasis."	

continued

TABLE B-2b Continued

Author	Study Type	Subjects	Exposure
Caicoya, 2002*	Case-control	Cases (n=440) = incident cases of stroke Controls (n=473) = no acute stroke, living in study area at time of study Aged 40-85 years Asturias, Spain (a northern region)	Seafood and dietary n-3 fatty acid intake
Jamrozik et al., 1994	Case-control	Cases (n=501) = stroke, drawn from the register of acute cerebrovascular events compiled as part of the Perth Community Stroke Study (PCSS) Controls (n=931) = drawn from electoral rolls for the study area of the PCSS Men and women Perth, Western Australia	Seafood

Amount	Results	Conclusion**
Categories of fish consumption (based on the 20th, 50th, and 80th percentiles): 1 = Noneaters, eaters of ≤11.2 g/day 2 = 11.3 g/day < x < 28.7 g/day 3 = 28.8 g/day ≤ x < 46.5 g/day 4 = ≥46.5 g/day Categories of n-3 fatty acid intake: 20th percentile = 115 mg/day 50th percentile = 328 mg/day 80th percentile = 660 mg/day	After adjusting for hypertension, alcohol intake, atrial fibrillation, and peripheral artery disease: Those who ate 1-22.5 g of fish/day had a significantly lower OR of stroke compared to those who never ate fish (OR=0.30, 95% CI 0.12-0.78). No significant ORs for stroke were found for those who consumed 23-45, 46-90, or 91-250 g of fish/day; and Those who ate >46.5 g of fish/day had a significantly higher OR of cerebral infarction compared to those who never ate fish (OR=1.98, 95% CI 1.08-3.45). No significant ORs for cerebral infarction were found for those who consumed 11.3-28.7 or 28.8-46.5 g of fish/day; and There was no significant association found between intake of n-3 fatty acids (mg/day) and risk of stroke.	B
Consumption of fish >2 times/month	After adjusting for alcohol and tobacco use, history of hypertension, claudication (for first ever stroke), diabetes mellitus (for primary intracerebral hemorrhage), previous stroke or transient ischemic attack, use of reduced-fat or skim milk: Eating fish >2 times/month significantly lowered the odds of a first-ever stroke (OR=0.60, 95% CI 0.36-0.99) and primary intracerebral hemorrhage (OR=0.42, 95% CI 0.19-0.90), compared to not eating fish >2 times/month. No significant ORs were found for all strokes and ischemic stroke based on consuming fish >2 times/month.	B

continued

TABLE B-2b Continued

Author	Study Type	Subjects	Exposure
Skerrett and Hennekens, 2003	Review	Review of observational studies, randomized trials, and biological studies	Seafood or n-3 supplements
Zhang et al., 1999	Ecological	36 countries Data from the World Health Statistics Annual (WHO) and Food Balance Sheets (FAO) Mortality data age-standardized to 45-74 years, and averaged over latest available 3 years	Seafood

*Included in Wang C, Chung M, Balk E, Kupelnick B, DeVine D. 2004. *Effects of Omega-3 Fatty Acids on Cardiovascular Disease. Evidence Report/Technology Assessment No. 94 (Prepared by the Tufts-New England Medical Center Evidence-based Practice Center, Boston, MA under contract no. 290-02-0022). AHRQ Publication No. 04-E009-2.* Rockville, MD: Agency for Healthcare Research and Quality.

**N = Evidence of no association or no clear association; B = Evidence of a benefit.

Amount	Results	Conclusion**
	"Ecologic/cross-sectional and case-control studies have generally shown an inverse association between consumption of fish and fish oils and stroke risk. Results from five prospective studies have been less consistent, with one showing no association, one showing a possible inverse association, and three demonstrating a significantly inverse association."	B
	"Consumption of fish several times per week reduces the risk of thrombotic stroke but does not increase the risk of hemorrhagic stroke."	
	"Fish consumption was independently, significantly, and inversely associated with mortality from all causes, ischemic heart disease, and stroke in both sexes." The statistics for these associations are $p<0.001$, $0.01<p<0.001$, and $0.05<p<0.001$, respectively.	B

TABLE B-2c Studies on Lipid Profile

Author	Study Type	Subjects	Exposure
Dunstan et al., 2003	Randomized Controlled Trial	Women (n=83) Booked for delivery at St. John of God Hospital, Subiaco, Western Australia Atopic pregnancy Allergic women No smoking, other medical problems, complicated pregnancies, preterm delivery, seafood allergy; normal diet intake did not exceed two meals of fish per week From 20 weeks of pregnancy to delivery	n-3 supplement
Christensen et al., 1999	Randomized Controlled Trial	Men (n=35) Women (n=25) Medical staff, bank employees, and students at institutions in Aalborg, Denmark No medications, no known diseases Follow-up of 12 weeks	n-3 supplement

Amount	Results	Conclusion**

Fish oil group:
1.0 g fish oil/capsule,
  4 capsules/day
3.7 g n-3
  PUFA/capsule
(56% DHA,
  27.7% EPA)
 	
Placebo group:
1 g olive oil/capsule,
  4 capsules/day
(66.6% n-9 oleic
  acid, <1% n-3
  PUFA)
	"Levels of n-6 PUFA AA were significantly lower in the fish oil group ($15.02\pm1.44\%$, $p<0.001$), compared with the placebo group ($17.45\pm1.17\%$). There was no difference in the levels of oleic acid between the groups."
	
	"Interleukin-13 levels were significantly lower (geometric mean 9.61, 95% CI 5.46-16.93, $p=0.025$) in neonates whose mothers received fish-oil supplements in pregnancy compared to the placebo group (geometric mean 26.32, 95% CI 13.44-51.55)."
	
	"There were no significant differences in the frequency of lymphocyte subsets between the two groups with respect to total T cells, T helper cells, T suppressor cells, NK cells, and B cells."
		B

High n-3 group: 10 capsules 6.6 g/day n-3 PUFA (3 g EPA/2.9 g DHA) Low n-3 group: 3 capsules n-3, 7 capsules of olive oil 2 g/day n-3 PUFA 0.9 g EPA/0.8 g DHA Placebo group: 10 capsules Olive oil	n-3 PUFA in granulocytes (both for EPA and DHA) and in platelets (both for EPA and DHA) were significantly higher after supplementation, compared to before supplementation, for those in the high n-3 group and the low n-3 group ($p<0.01$). Plasma triacylglycerols were significantly lower after supplementation, compared to before supplementation, for those in the high n-3 group ($p<0.01$) and the low n-3 group ($p<0.05$). The changes in DHA in granulocytes and plasma triacylglyercols after supplementation were significantly higher in the high n-3 group compared to the placebo group ($p<0.05$). The changes in EPA in granulocytes and EPA and DHA in platelets were significantly higher in the high n-3 group than in the low n-3 group and the placebo group ($p<0.05$).	B

continued

TABLE B-2c Continued

Author	Study Type	Subjects	Exposure
Vericel et al., 1999	Randomized Controlled Trial	Men and women (n=20) Aged 70-83 years France Diastolic blood pressure <95 mmHg and systolic blood pressure <180 mmHg No metabolic, malignant, or degenerative diseases Follow-up of 42 days	n-3 supplement
Leng et al., 1998*	Randomized Controlled Trial	Men and women (n=120) Mean age about 66 years Edinburgh, UK Intermittent claudication on the Edinburgh Claudication Questionnaire An ankle brachial pressure index ≤0.9 in at least one limb No clinical evidence of critical ischemia; unstable angina or a MI within the previous 3 months; severe intercurrent illnesses including severe liver disorders, malignancy, or epilepsy; concurrent treatment with anticoagulants, other oils, lithium, or phemothiazines; pregnant or actively trying to conceive; already participating in a clinical trial Follow-up of 2 years	n-3 supplement

Amount	Results	Conclusion**
RO-PUFA treatment capsule: 600 mg oil = 150 mg DHA, 30 mg EPA, 1900 ppm alpha-tocopherol	"The composition of platelet total phospholipids was not affected by the low supplementation of RO-PUFA or sunflower oil." "Neither the GSH-Px activities nor the enzyme levels were affected by any supplement of oil."	N
Control capsule: 600 mg sunflower oil and 600 ppm alpha-tocopherol	Compared to baseline, RO-PUFA significantly increased platelet phosphatidylethanolamine DHA (2.7 ± 0.2 mol% to 3.4 ± 0.1 mol%, $p<0.001$).	
Polyunsaturated fatty acids group: 280 mg GLA, 45 mg EPA/capsule 2 capsules twice/day for first 2 weeks, 3 capsules twice daily thereafter	Among completers, VLDL was significantly higher in the polyunsaturated fatty acids group at 6 months ($p\leq0.05$) and HDL was significantly higher at 24 months ($p\leq0.01$) compared to the placebo group. At baseline, hematocrit (%) and fibrin D-dimer (ng/ml) were significantly lower in the polyunsaturated fatty acids group compared to the placebo group ($p\leq0.05$).	B
Placebo group: 500 mg sunflower oil 2 capsules twice/day for first 2 weeks, 3 capsules twice daily thereafter	At 6 months, hematocrit (%) was significantly higher in the polyunsaturated fatty acids group compared to the placebo group ($p\leq0.01$). There were no significant differences in hemostatis factors at 24 months between the two groups.	

continued

TABLE B-2c Continued

Author	Study Type	Subjects	Exposure
Luo et al., 1998*	Randomized Controlled Trial (crossover)	Men (n=10) Mean age of 54 years Patients of the Department of Diabetes outpatient clinic (diabetics) Type II diabetes, a fasting plasma glucose of 7.84-14.0 mmol/L, HbA1c <10.5%, plasma triacylglycerol of 1.72-4.6 mmol/L No abnormal renal, hepatic, and thyroid functions; gastrointestinal disorders Follow-up of 2 months while on each supplement	n-3 supplement

Amount	Results	Conclusion**

Fish oil group:
6 g fish oil
30% n-3 fatty acids;
  18% EPA, 12%
  DHA
2 capsules 3 times/
  day
 	
Sunflower oil group:
6 g sunflower oil
65% n-6 fatty acids;
  0.2% n-3 fatty
  acids
2 capsules 3 times/
  day
 	
Recommended to
  consume 55% of
  calories as carbo-
  hydrates, 15% as
  protein, 30% as fat
	There were no significant differences in fasting plasma glucose, insulin, or HbA1c between the two groups.
	
	After 2 months of sunflower oil and fish oil treatments, the fish oil treatment significantly lowered triacylglycerols and lipoprotein(a) compared to the the sunflower oil treatment ($p<0.05$ and $p<0.02$, respectively). There were no other significant differences between the two treatments in the other fasting circulating lipid and lipoprotein concentrations measured.
		B

continued

TABLE B-2c Continued

Author	Study Type	Subjects	Exposure
Dunstan et al., 1997*	Randomized Controlled Trial	Men (n=40) Women (n=15) Aged 30-65 years Perth, Australia With treated noninsulin-dependent diabetes mellitus Nonsmokers, not taking fish-oil supplements or eating >1 fish meal/week, sedentary for the previous 6 months Excluded if taking insulin or medication for lipid disorders; drinking >30 ml alcohol/day; had a previous history or evidence of heart, liver, or renal disease; neuropathy; retinopathy; or had asthma or any orthopedic disorder that precluded exercise participation Follow-up of 8 weeks	Diet (includes seafood) and exercise

Amount	Results	Conclusion**
Group 1: Low-fat diet ($\leq$30% energy from fat) + moderate exercise (55-65% of Vo_2max)	After adjusting for baseline age, sex, and change in body weight: Relative to no fish and light exercise, fish and moderate exercise (Group 3) significantly lowered serum triglycerides (-1.21 ± 0.28; p=0.0001) and significantly raised HDL_2 (0.08$\pm$0.03, p=0.02);	B
Group 2: Low-fat diet ($\leq$30% energy from fat) + light exercise (heart rate <100 bpm)	Relative to no fish and light exercise, fish and light exercise (Group 4) significantly lowered serum triglycerides (-1.22 ± 0.28; p=0.0001) and significantly raised HDL_2 (0.08$\pm$0.03, p=0.02); and	
Group 3: Low-fat diet with the inclusion of 1 fish meal daily (3.6 g n-3/day) + moderate exercise (55-65% of Vo_2max)	Relative to no fish and light exercise, no fish and moderate exercise (Group 1) significantly lowered serum triglycerides (-0.68 ± 0.29; p=0.03).	
Group 4: Low-fat diet with the inclusion of 1 fish meal daily (3.6 g n-3/day) + light exercise (heart rate <100 bpm)		

continued

TABLE B-2c Continued

Author	Study Type	Subjects	Exposure
Schaefer et al., 1996*	Randomized Controlled Trial	Men and women (n=22) Mean age of 63 (all >40 years, all women postmenopausal) Plasma LDL-cholesterol within the 10th and 90th percentile for their age and sex No medication known to affect plasma lipoprotein cencentrations; no endocrine, liver, or kidney disease Nonsmokers, did not consume alcohol regularly Follow-up of 24 weeks National Cholesterol Education Program (NCEP) Step 2 diet	Seafood

Amount	Results	Conclusion**
Baseline diet: 14.1±2.2 % energy from saturated fat 14.5±1.0 % energy from monounsaturated fat 4.1±0.2 % energy from LA 0.7±0.2 % energy from ALA <0.01 % energy from AA, EPA, DHA each	Those on the high-fish diet significantly lowered their total cholesterol, LDL-C, HDL-C, apolipoprotein B, apolipoprotein A-I (p<0.0001), and postprandial tricylglycerols (p<0.05). There were no significant changes found for VLDL-C, TC:HDL-C, (triacylglycerols, lipoprotein(a), or LDL particle score.	B
High-fish diet: 4.5±0.7 % energy from saturated fat 11.6±1.4 % energy from monounsaturated fat 7.0±0.4 % energy from LA 1.9±0.6 % energy from ALA 0.1±0.1 % energy from AA 0.2±0.1 % energy from EPA 0.5±0.2 % energy from DHA	Those on the low-fish diet significantly lowered their total cholesterol, LDL-C, HDL-C, apolipoprotein B, apolipoprotein A-I (p<0.0001), and significantly increased their LDL particle score (p<0.05). There were no significant changes found for VLDL-C, TC:HDL-C, triacylglycerols, postprandial triacylglycerols, and lipoprotein(a).	
Low-fish diet: 4.0±0.4 % energy from saturated fat 10.8±0.9 % energy from monounsaturated fat 7.1±0.8 % energy from LA 2.0±0.2 % energy from ALA <0.02 % energy from AA <0.02 % energy from EPA 0.1±0.1 % energy from DHA		

continued

TABLE B-2c Continued

Author	Study Type	Subjects	Exposure
Eritsland et al., 1995*	Randomized Controlled Trial	Men (n=523) Women (n=78) Aged 36-81 years Oslo, Norway With stenosing coronary artery disease Referred for coronary artery bypass grafting Follow-up of 6 months Reference group (for serum Lp(a)): Men (n=79) Women (n=20) Aged 25-81 years Apparently healthy Current or retired employees attending a regular health check-up	n-3 supplement
Sacks et al., 1995	Randomized Controlled Trial	Men and women (n=59) Aged 30-75 years Boston, MA Had narrowing of ≥30% lumen diameter of a major coronary artery, a total cholesterol concentration <250 mg/dL, and triglyceride level <350 mg/dL No congestive heart failure, liver, renal, or serious gastrointestinal disease, insulin-dependent diabetes mellitus, current cigarette smoking, or alcohol intake >14 drinks/week Follow-up of 2.4 years	n-3 supplement

Amount	Results	Conclusion**
n-3 PUFA group: 4 capsules/day Each capsule = 1 g n-3 PUFA (51% EPA, 32% DHA) + 3.7 IU alpha-tocopherol	Serum EPA, DHA, and total n-3 concentrations significantly increased in the n-3 PUFA group between baseline and the 6-month assessment (p<0.001). The changes in serum EPA, DHA, and total n-3 concentrations from baseline to the 6-month assessment were also significantly higher in the n-3 PUFA group compared to the control group (p<0.001).	B
	Among those who had a baseline Lp(a) of ≥20 mg/dL, the change in serum Lp(a) levels from baseline to the 6-month assessment was significantly different in the n-3 PUFA group (29.7 mg/dL to 28.7 mg/dL) than in the control group (30.3 mg/dL to 30.8 mg/dL) (p=0.023). There were no significant differences in the change of serum Lp(a) found between the two groups among those who had a baseline Lp(a) of <20 mg/dL.	
Fish oil group: 12 capsules/day 500 mg n-3 fatty acids/capsule (240 mg EPA, 160 mg DHA, 100 mg mostly DPA) 6 g of n-3 fatty acids/day	From baseline to follow-up, there was a significant increase in body weight, LDL-C, apolipoprotein B, and Lp(a), and a significant decrease in triglycerides among those in the fish oil group (p<0.01; p<0.05 for lipoprotein Lp(a)).	B
	From baseline to follow-up there was a significant increase in body weight (p<0.01), cholesterol (p<0.05), and apolipoprotein B (p<0.01) among those in the control group.	
Control group: 12 capsules of olive oil/day	The change in triglycerides from baseline to follow-up was significantly different among the fish oil group (−28±53 mg/dL) and the control group (6±35 mg/dL) (p<0.01).	
	After 2.4 years of supplementation, the fish oil group had significantly higher EPA, DPA, DHA, and EPA+DPA+DHA (p<0.0001) and significantly lower palmitic acid (p=0.048), oleic acid (p=0.0009), and arachidonic acid (p=0.001) in the adipose tissue compared to the control group.	

continued

TABLE B-2c Continued

Author	Study Type	Subjects	Exposure
Mori et al., 1994*	Randomized Controlled Trial	Men (n=120) Aged 30-60 years Perth, Australia Eating not more than one fish meal/week or drinking more than an average of 30 mL alcohol/day (3 standard drinks) With high-normal blood pressure and elevated serum cholesterol No history of unstable heart, renal, or liver disease, hypercholesterolemia, asthma, or any major allergies Follow-up of 12 weeks	Seafood and n-3 supplements

Amount	Results	Conclusion**
Seven dietary groups:	Among those in Groups 1-5, there were significant differences between the groups in the change in percentage of daily fat intake from polyunsaturated fatty acids (change (%) = -4.5, 0.9, -7.1, 0.9, and -1.9, respectively; p<0.001).	B
40% total energy from fat and: 1 = placebo 2 = fish (1 fish meal/day)		
3 = fish-oil capsules (0.8 g/day DHA, 2.6 g n-3/day)	Among those in Groups 6-7, there were significant differences between the groups in the change in percentage of daily fat intake from polyunsaturated fatty acids (change (%) = 13.0 and 18.9, respectively; p<0.01).	
4 = fish (1 fish meal/day) and fish-oil capsules (0.8 g/day DHA, 2.6 g n-3/day)		
5 = twice the dosage of fish-oil capsules (1.6 g/day DHA, 5.2 g n-3/day)	Among those in Groups 1-5, there were significant differences between the groups in regards to the change in cholesterol (change (mg/d) = 124.3, -33.8, 188.3, 103.4, and 58.7, respectively; p<0.01).	
30% total energy from fat and: 6 = control group 7 = fish (1 fish meal/day)	There were no significant changes in % of energy from total fat, % of daily fat from monounsaturated fatty acids or saturated fatty acids, total carbohydrate, total protein, or fiber intake.	
Fish meals included: Greenland turbot fillets (160 g/day) = 1.5 g/day DHA, 3.5 g/day total n-3 fatty acids		
Canned sardines (95 g/day) = 1.7 g/day DHA, 4.1 g/day total n-3 fatty acids		
Tuna (90 g/day) = 1.3 g/day DHA, 3.2 g/day total n-3 fatty acids		
Salmon (90 g/day) = 2.4 g/day DHA, 3.8 g/day total n-3 fatty acids		

continued

TABLE B-2c Continued

Author	Study Type	Subjects	Exposure
Vandongen et al., 1993	Randomized Controlled Trial	Men (n=120) Aged 30-60 years Perth, Australia BMI <33 kg/m^2, SBP 130-159 mmHg, DBP 80-99 mmHG, serum cholesterol 5.2-6.9 mmol/L, nonsmoking, not taking any medication, no significant illness or allergic disorder Eating ≤1 fish meal and drinking <210 mL alcohol/week Follow-up of 12 weeks	Seafood and n-3 supplements

Amount	Results	Conclusion**
Seven dietary groups:	A significant group effect was found for the change in heart rate (p<0.01 for supine; p = 0.06 for erect) from baseline to end of intervention.	B
40% total energy from fat and:		
1 = placebo	No significant differences were found between groups in SBP, DBP, weight, 24-hour urine potassium levels, sodium, blood glucose, or blood insulin from baseline to end of intervention.	
2 = fish (1 fish meal/day)		
3 = fish-oil capsules (1.3 g n-3/day)		
4 = fish (1 fish meal/day) and fish-oil capsules (1.3 g n-3/day)		
5 = twice the dosage of fish-oil capsules (2.6 g n-3/day)		
30% total energy from fat and:		
6 = control group		
7 = fish (1 fish meal/ day)		
Fish meals included:		
Greenland turbot fillets (≈160 g/day) 3.5 g/day total n-3 fatty acids		
Canned sardines (95 g/day) 4.1 g/ day total n-3 fatty acids		
Tuna (90 g/day) ≈3.2 g/day total n-3 fatty acids		
Salmon (90 g/day) 3.8 g/day total n-3 fatty acids		

continued

TABLE B-2c Continued

Author	Study Type	Subjects	Exposure
Cobiac et al., 1991*	Randomized Controlled Trial	Men (n=31) Aged 30-60 years Adelaide, South Australia Mildly hyperlipidemic and normotensive No history of heart disease, hypertension, bleeding disorders, liver or renal disorders, gout, diabetes, recent cerebrovascular accident, or obesity No steroids, nonsteroidal anti-inflammatory drugs, aspirin, beta-blockers, allopurinol, or cardiac glycosides No excessive alcohol intake (>40 g/day) or smoked >20 cigarettes/day Follow-up of 8 weeks	Seafood and n-3 supplementation
Hanninen et al., 1989*	Randomized Controlled Trial	Men (n=100) Mean age of 23.5 years Kuopio, Finland Healthy students Follow-up of 12 weeks	Seafood

Amount	Results	Conclusion**
Fish treatment: 1 kg (raw) Atlantic salmon + 150 g sardines in sild oil per week 4.5 g EPA+DHA/day	After the fish treatment (compared to baseline values), cholesterol, triglycerides, VLDL-C, LDL-C, VLDL triglycerides, Apo A-I, and Apo A-II were significantly lower and HDL, Apo A-I:Apo A-II, and HDL-C:Apo A-I were significantly higher ($p<0.05$).	B
Fish-oil treatment: 105 g MaxEPA/week 4.6 g EPA+DHA/day Continued with meats as during baseline	After the fish-oil treatment (compared to baseline values), triglycerides, VLDL-C, VLDL triglycerides, Apo A-I, Apo-AII, and Apo A-I:Apo B were significantly lower, and HDL-C, Apo A-I:Apo A-II, and HDL-C:Apo A-I were significantly higher ($p<0.05$).	
Control diet: Continuation of baseline diet	After the control treatment (compared to baseline values), lipids, LDL-C, and Apo A-I were significantly lower and HDL-C:Apo A-I was significantly higher ($p<0.05$).	
	The changes in triglycerides, VLDL-C, VLDL triglycerides, and HDL-C:Apo A-I in the fish and fish-oil groups were significantly greater than the changes in the control group ($p<0.05$, $p=0.002$ for HDL-C:Apo A-I); the change in HDL-C was significantly greater in the fish-oil group than in the control group ($p<0.05$).	
	The changes in fibrinogen, thromboxane, and bleeding time after treatment were significantly different in the fish group compared to the control group ($p<0.05$).	
Fish meal groups: 0.9, 1.5, 2.3, or 3.8 fish meals/week	Those who ate 3.8 fish meals/week lowered their serum triglycerides and apolipoprotein B significantly ($p<0.02$ and $p<0.05$, respectively) after eating the fish diet for 12 weeks; there were no significant changes after 12 weeks for those who ate 0.9, 1.5, and 2.3 fish meals/week.	B
Controls: 1 fish meal/2 weeks		
Meals = Finnish freshwater fish (rainbow trout, vendace, and perch) and brack- ish water fish (Baltic herring) Portion size = 150 g	There were no significant changes in serum cholesterol, serum apolipoprotein A-I, hemoglobin, thrombocytes, vitamin E, or vitamin A after eating the fish diets for 12 weeks.	

continued

TABLE B-2c Continued

Author	Study Type	Subjects	Exposure
Dewailly et al., 2001	Cohort	Men and women (n=426) Aged 18-74 years Permanent residents of Nunavik, Canada Inuit Excluded households of only non-Inuit persons, persons not related to an Inuit, and institutionalized persons	Plasma phospho-lipid com-position; seafood; diet

*Included in Balk E, Chung M, Lichtenstein A, Chew P, Kupelnick B, Lawrence A, DeVine D, Lau J. 2004. *Effects of Omega-3 Fatty Acids on Cardiovascular Risk Factors and Intermediate Markers of Cardiovascular Disease. Summary, Evidence Report/Technology Assessment No. 93. (Prepared by the Tufts-New England Medical Center Evidence-based Practice Center, Boston, MA). AHRQ Publication No. 04-E010-1.* Rockville, MD: Agency for Healthcare Research and Quality.

**B = Evidence of a benefit; N = Evidence of no association or no clear association.

Amount	Results	Conclusion**
Plasma phospholipids = relative percentages of total fatty acids by weight Fish and marine mammal intake from 24-hour recalls Consumption of traditional and market food stuffs from a food frequency questionnaire	After adjusting for age, sex, waist girth, smoking status, and alcohol intake: EPA, DHA, EPA+DHA, EPA:AA, and n-3:n-6 are positively associated with total cholesterol (p=0.0001); EPA (p=0.005), DHA (p=0.0003), EPA+DHA (p=0.0007), EPA:AA (p=0.002), and n-3:n-6 (p=0.003) are positively associated with LDL; EPA (p=p=0.0001), DHA (p=0.004), EPA+DHA (p=0.0001), EPA:AA (p=0.0001), and n-3:n-6 (p=0.0001) are positively associated with HDL; EPA (p=0.04) and EPA:AA (p=0.05) are negatively associated with total cholesterol:HDL; EPA (p=0.0001), EPA+DHA (p=0.0003), EPA:AA (p=0.0002), and n-3:n-6 (p=0.001) are negatively associated with triacylglycerols; and EPA (p=0.02), DHA (p=0.01), EPA+DHA (p=0.008), EPA:AA (p=0.02), and n-3:n-6 (p=0.008) are positively associated with glucose.	N

TABLE B-2d Studies on Blood Pressure

Author	Study Type	Subjects	Exposure
Hooper et al., 2005	Cochrane Review	7 studies (2743 participants) After 6 months of supplementation	n-3 supplement
Geleijnse et al., 2002*	Meta-analysis	36 RCTs (22 with double-blinded design) Adult study populations (mean age ≥18 years) Published after 1966 No sick/hospitalized populations, including renal and diabetic patients Mean trial duration of 11.7 weeks (range = 3-52 weeks)	n-3 supplement

Amount	Results	Conclusion*
	"Neither [systolic or diastolic blood pressure] were significantly affected by omega-3 supplementation" (SBP mean difference = 1.03 mmHg, 95% CI –3.30 to 1.25, p=0.18; DBP mean difference = –0.23 mmHg, 95% CI 1.10-0.64, p=0.92).	N
Doses of fish oil: <1.0 g/day in 1 trial 1.0 1.9 g/day in 5 trials 2.0-2.9 g/day in 4 trials 3.0-15.0 g/day in 26 trials mean dose = 3.7 g/day	In the univariate analysis: Based on all trials, fish oil decreased SBP and DBP significantly more among those >45 years of age compared to those ≤45 years of age (p=0.023 for SBP and p=0.020 for DBP) and in those with hypertension compared to those without hypertension (p=0.008 for SBP and p=0.041 for DBP). Fish oil also decreased SBP and DBP more in populations with males and females compared to those with only males and among those with a BMI >26.8kg/m² compared to those with BMI ≤26.8 kg/m², but the differences were not significant; and Based on double-blinded trials, fish oil decreased SBP and DBP significantly more among those with hypertension compared to those without hypertension (p=0.005 for SBP and p=0.010 for DBP). Fish oil also decreased SBP and DBP more among those >45 years of age compared to those ≤45 years of age; in populations with males and females compared to those with only males, and among those with a BMI >26.8kg/m² compared to those with BMI ≤26.8 kg/m², but the differences were not significant. After adjusting for age, percent males, baseline BP, study design, and fish oil dose: Fish oil decreased SBP and DBP more among those >45 years of age compared to those ≤45 years of age, in populations with males and females compared to those with only males, in those with hypertension compared to those without hypertension, and among those with a BMI >26.8kg/m² compared to those with BMI ≤26.8 kg/m², but the differences were not significant.	N

continued

TABLE B-2d Continued

Author	Study Type	Subjects	Exposure
Ness et al., 1999	Randomized Controlled Trial	Men (n=2033) Aged <70 years From 21 hospitals in South Wales and the south west of England Diet and Reinfarction Trial (DART) Suffered from recent MI Excluded if they already intended to eat one of the study diets, if they had serious illnesses (e.g., diabetes, cancer, or renal function), if they were being considered for cardiac surgery, if they were participating in a local cohort study, if they planned to live outside the study area, if they were averse to one of the proposed diets Follow-up of 2 years	Dietary advice
Vericel et al., 1999	Randomized Controlled Trial	Men and women (n=20) Aged 70-83 years France Diastolic blood pressure <95 mmHg and systolic blood pressure <180 mmHg No metabolic, malignant, or degenerative diseases Follow-up of 42 days	n-3 supplement
Leng et al., 1998*	Randomized Controlled Trial	Men and women (n=120) Mean age about 66 years Edinburgh Intermittent claudication on the Edinburgh Claudication Questionnaire An ankle brachial pressure index ≤0.9 in at least one limb No clinical evidence of critical ischemia; unstable angina or a myocardial infarction within the previous 3 months; severe intercurrent illnesses including severe liver disorders, malignancy, or epilepsy; concurrent treatment with anticoagulants, other oils, lithium, or phemothiazines; pregnant or actively trying to conceive; already participating in a clinical trial Follow-up of 2 years	n-3 supplement

Amount	Results	Conclusion*
Eight dietary regimes: 1 = Fat advice 2 = Fish advice 3 = Fiber advice 4 = Fat and fish advice 5 = Fat and fiber advice 6 = Fish and fiber advice 7 = Fat, fish, and fiber advice 8 = No advice	After adjusting for 5-year age group and BP at baseline: At 6 months, those who received fish advice had lower SBP and DBP than those who did not receive fish advice (difference in SBP = -0.61, 95% CI -2.15 to 0.92 and difference in DBP = -0.50, 95% CI -1.47 to 0.46), but the differences were not significant; and At 2 years, those who received fish advice had higher SBP and DBP than those who did not receive fish advice (difference in SBP = 0.40, 95% CI -1.33 to 2.13 and difference in DBP = 0.19, 95% CI -0.88 to 1.26), but the differences were not significant.	B
RO-PUFA treatment capsule: 600 mg oil = 150 mg DHA, 30 mg EPA, 1900 ppm alpha-tocopherol Control capsule: 600 mg sunflower oil and 600 ppm alpha-tocopherol	Compared to baseline, RO-PUFA significantly lowered systolic blood pressure (145.5±5.1 mmHg to 131.5±4.5 mmHg, p<0.001). There was no significant change in diastolic blood pressure.	B
Polyunsaturated fatty acids group: 280 mg GLA, 45 mg EPA/capsule 2 capsules twice/day for first 2 weeks, 3 capsules twice/day thereafter Placebo group: 500 mg sunflower oil 2 capsules twice/day for first 2 weeks, 3 capsules twice/day thereafter	There were no significant differences in systolic blood pressure or diastolic blood pressure between the two groups at baseline or at 6 months. At 24 months systolic blood pressure was significantly lower in the polyunsaturated fatty acids group compared to the placebo group (150.1±3.5 mmHg vs. 161.8±3.1 mmHg, p≤0.05).	B

continued

TABLE B-2d Continued

Author	Study Type	Subjects	Exposure
Vandongen et al., 1993	Randomized Controlled Trial	Men (n=120) Aged 30-60 years Perth, Australia BMI <33 kg/m², SBP 130-159 mmHg, DBP 80-99 mmHG, serum cholesterol 5.2-6.9 mmol/L, nonsmoking, not taking any medication, no significant illness or allergic disorder Eating ≤1 fish meal and drinking <210 mL alcohol/week Follow-up of 12 weeks	Seafood and n-3 supplements

Amount	Results	Conclusion*
Seven dietary groups: 40% total energy from fat and: 1 = placebo 2 = fish (1 fish meal/day) 3 = fish-oil capsules (1.3 g n-3/day) 4 = fish (1 fish meal/day) and fish-oil capsules (1.3 g n-3/day) 5 = twice the dosage of fish-oil capsules (2.6 g n-3/day) 30% total energy from fat and: 6 = control group 7 = fish (1 fish meal/day) Fish meals included: Greenland turbot fillets (≈160 g/day) ≈3.5 g/day total n-3 fatty acids Canned sardines (≈95 g/day) ≈4.1 g/day total n-3 fatty acids Tuna (≈90 g/day) ≈3.2 g/day total n-3 fatty acids Salmon (≈90 g/day) ≈3.8 g/day total n-3 fatty acids	There was a significant difference in change in heart rate (bpm) from baseline until the end of the intervention between the groups (p<0.01). Heart rate went down in Groups 2, 3, 4, 5, and 7 and heart rate went up in Groups 1 and 6.	B

continued

TABLE B-2d Continued

Author	Study Type	Subjects	Exposure
Cobiac et al., 1991*	Randomized Controlled Trial	Men (n=31) Aged 30-60 years Adelaide, South Australia Mildly hyperlipidemic and normotensive No history of heart disease, hypertension, bleeding disorders, liver or renal disorders, gout, diabetes, recent cerebrovascular accident, or obesity No steroids, nonsteroidal anti-inflammatory drugs, aspirin, beta-blockers, allopurinol, or cardiac glycosides No excessive alcohol intake (>40 g/day) or smoked >20 cigarettes/day Follow-up of 8 weeks	Seafood and n-3 supplementation
Dewailly et al., 2001	Cohort	Men and women (n=426) Aged 18-74 years Permanent residents of Nunavik, Canada Inuit Excluded households of only non-Inuit persons, persons not related to an Inuit, and institutionalized persons	Plasma phospholipid composition; seafood; diet

Amount	Results	Conclusion*
Fish treatment: 1 kg (raw) Atlantic salmon + 150 g sardines in sild oil per week 4.5 g EPA+DHA/day Fish-oil treatment: 105 g MaxEPA/week 4.6 g EPA+DHA/day Continued with meats as during baseline Control diet: Continuation of baseline diet	After fish treatment, compared to baseline values, systolic and diastolic blood pressure were significantly lower (p<0.05). After the fish-oil treatment, compared to baseline values, systolic blood pressure was significantly lower (p<0.05). After the control treatment, compared to baseline values, diastolic blood pressure was significantly lower (p<0.05). There were no significant differences between the changes in the three treatment groups.	B
Plasma phospholipids = relative percentages of total fatty acids by weight Fish and marine mammal intake from 24-hour recalls Consumption of traditional and market food stuffs from a food frequency questionnaire	After adjusting for age, sex, waist girth, smoking status, and alcohol intake, no significant associations were found between EPA, DHA, EPA+DHA, EPA:AA or n-3:n-6 and systolic blood pressure or diastolic blood pressure.	N

continued

TABLE B-2d Continued

Author	Study Type	Subjects	Exposure
Appleby et al., 2002	Cross-sectional	Men (n=2351) Women (n=8653) Aged 20-78 years UK European Prospective Investigation into Cancer and Nutrition (EPIC)—Oxford Cohort Free of cancer at baseline	Diet

*Included in Balk E, Chung M, Lichtenstein A, Chew P, Kupelnick B, Lawrence A, DeVine D, Lau J. 2004. *Effects of Omega-3 Fatty Acids on Cardiovascular Risk Factors and Intermediate Markers of Cardiovascular Disease. Summary, Evidence Report/Technology Assessment No. 93. (Prepared by the Tufts-New England Medical Center Evidence-based Practice Center, Boston, MA). AHRQ Publication No. 04-E010-1.* Rockville, MD: Agency for Healthcare Research and Quality.

Amount	Results	Conclusion*
Four diet groups: Meat eaters Fish eaters = ate fish but no meat Vegetarians = ate neither meat nor fish but did eat dairy products and/or eggs Vegans = did not eat any meat, fish, eggs, or dairy products	After adjusting for age, there were significant differences between the diet groups in regards to SBP among men (p<0.005), SBP among women (p<0.005), DBP among men (p<0.005) and DBP among women (p<0.0001). After adjusting for age and BMI, the only significant difference in blood pressure was for DBP among women (p<0.01). After adjusting for age, BMI, alcohol intake and vigorous exercise (for men), and hormone exposure (for women), the only significant difference in blood pressure was for DBP among women (p<0.01). After adjusting for age, BMI, alcohol intake and vigorous exercise (for men), hormone exposure (for women), protein, carbohydrate, total fat, saturated fat and polyunsaturated fat, energy, P/S ratio, and NSP intake, the only significant difference in blood pressure was for DBP among women (p=0.02). After adjusting for age, BMI, alcohol intake and vigorous exercise (for men), hormone exposure (for women), protein, carbohydrate, total fat, saturated fat and polyunsaturated fat, energy, P/S ratio, and NSP intake, sodium (from food only), potassium, calcium, and magnesium intakes, the only significant difference in blood pressure was for DBP among women (p=0.02). After adjusting for age, the prevalence of self-reported hypertension for meat eaters, fish eaters, vegetarians, and vegans was 15.0%, 9.8%, 9.8%, and 5.8% for men, respectively, and 12.1%, 9.6%, 8.9%, and 7.7% for women, respectively. After adjusting for age and BMI, the prevalence of self-reported hypertension for meat eaters, fish eaters, vegetarians, and vegans was 12.9%, 9.3%, 9.5%, and 6.1% for men, respectively, and 10.6%, 9.7%, 8.7%, and 8.3% for women, respectively.	B

**N = Evidence of no association or no clear association; B = Evidence of a benefit.

TABLE B-2e Studies on Arrhythmia

Author	Study Type	Subjects	Exposure
Leaf et al., 2003	Review	Clinical trials (n=6 analyses) Animal and laboratory studies (for potential mechanisms)	n-3 supplement
Christensen et al., 1999	Randomized Controlled Trial	Men (n=35) Women (n=25) Medical staff, bank employees, and students at institutions in Aalborg, Denmark No medications, no known diseases 12 weeks of follow-up	n-3 supplement
Christensen et al., 1996	Randomized Controlled Trial	Men and women (n=49) Aged ≤75 years Aalborg Hospital, Denmark Discharged after MI and ventricular ejection fraction <0.40 No pacemakers or permanent tachyarrhythmias, or serious non-cardiac disease Follow-up of 12 weeks	n-3 supplement

Amount	Results	Conclusion*
	From the randomized controlled trials, "the evidence has been strengthened that fish oil fatty acids can prevent sudden cardiac death in humans, and this may prove to be their major cardiac benefit."	B
	From the randomized controlled trials, there were no significant associations found between fish oil fatty acids and the reduction of nonfatal MIs.	
	"If there is a family history of sudden cardiac death, then the supplement should be increased to 1 to 2 g of EPA plus DHA."	
	"These n-3 fatty acids are antiarrhythmis and can prevent sudden cardiac death in humans."	
High n-3 group: 10 capsules 6.6 g/day n-3 PUFA 3 g EPA/2.9 g DHA	There were no significant differences between the three diet groups in regards to the changes in six heart rate variability indexes from before to after supplementation.	B
Low n-3 group: 3 capsules n-3, 7 capsules of olive oil 2 g/day n-3 PUFA 0.9 g EPA/0.8 g DHA		
Placebo group: 10 capsules Olive oil		
n-3 fatty acid group: 5.2 g n-3 PUFA 4.3 g EPA and DHA	After n-3 polyunsaturated fatty acid treatment, the mean heart rate variability, defined as standard deviation of all normal RR intervals in 24-hour Holter recording, was significantly higher compared to baseline (124 ms vs. 115 ms, p=0.04).	A
Placebo group: Olive oil	The mean difference in heart rate variability, defined as standard deviation of all normal RR intervals in 24-hour Holter recording, was significantly different after n-3 polyunsaturated fatty acid treatment (mean difference = –8.3, 95% CI –16 to –1) compared to after the control treatment (mean difference = 9.4, 95% CI –2 to 20, p=0.01).	

continued

TABLE B-2e Continued

Author	Study Type	Subjects	Exposure
Frost and Vestergaard, 2005	Cohort	Men (n=22,528) Women (n=25,421) Aged 50-64 years Born in Denmark, living in the Copenhagen and Aarhus areas No previous cancer diagnosis in the Danish Cancer Registry No hospitalization before baseline with endocrine diseases or cardiovascular diseases other than hypertension Follow-up of 5.7 years (128,131 person-years for men and 147,251 person-years for women)	Seafood
Christensen et al., 1997	Cross-sectional	Men and women (n=52) Aged 48-75 years Discharged after MI from Aalborg Hospital, Denmark Echocardiography performed within the first week after MI Left ventricular ejection fraction ≤40% No implanted pacemaker, no permanent tachyarrhythmias, no serious noncardiac disease Using baseline data from Christensen et al., 1996	Platelet fatty acids; seafood

*B = Evidence of a benefit; A = Evidence of an adverse effect; N = Evidence of no association or no clear association.

Amount	Results	Conclusion*
Frequency of fish consumption: Never, <1 time/month, 1 time/month, 2-3 times/month, 1 time/week, 2-4 times/week, 5-6 times/week, 1 time/day, 2-3 times/day, 4-5 times/day, 6-7 times/day, ≥8 times/day	After adjusting for age, sex, height, BMI, smoking, consumption of alcohol, total energy intake, systolic blood pressure, treatment for hypertension, total serum cholesterol, and level of education: Those in Quintile 5 of n-3 PUFA from fish had a significantly higher hazard rate ratio of atrial fibrillation or flutter, when compared to those in Quintile 1 (HRR=1.34, 95% CI 1.02-1.76); and	N
Quintiles of n-3 PUFA from fish (g/day): Quintile 1 = 0.16±0.08 Quintile 2 = 0.36±0.06 Quintile 3 = 0.52±0.07 Quintile 4 = 0.74±0.10 Quintile 5 = 1.29±0.47	The association between n-3 PUFA from fish and risk of atrial fibrillation or flutter was not significant for any other quintiles when compared to Quintile 1, however there was a positive trend (p=0.006).	
3 groups of DHA content in platelets: 1 = <2.26% 2 = 2.26-3.14% 3 = >3.14% Fish intake: 1 = 0 times/week 2 = 1 time/week 3 = ≥2 times/week	The standard deviation of all normal RR intervals in the entire 24-hour recording was higher in those who ate fish at least 1 time/week (122 ms for those who ate fish 1 time/week and 119 ms for those who ate fish ≥2 times/week), compared to those who ate fish 0 times per week (103 ms), but these differences were not significant. The standard deviations of all normal RR intervals in the entire 24-hour recording for those in the first, second, and third tertile of DHA contents in platelets were approximately 98 ms, 116 ms, and 140 ms, respectively.	A

TABLE B-2f Studies on Other Cardiac Indicators

Author	Study Type	Subjects	Exposure
Agren et al., 1997*	Randomized Controlled Trial	Men (n=55) Healthy students Kuopio, Finland Follow-up of 15 weeks	Seafood and n-3 supple- mentation
Cobiac et al., 1991*	Randomized Controlled Trial	Men (n=31) Aged 30-60 years Adelaide, South Australia Mildly hyperlipidemic and normotensive No history of heart disease, hypertension, bleeding disorders, liver or renal disor- ders, gout, diabetes, recent cerebrovas- cular accident, or obesity No steroids, nonsteroidal anti- inflammatory drugs, aspirin, beta-block- ers, allopurinol, or cardiac glycosides No excessive alcohol intake (>40 g/day) or who smoked >20 cigarettes/day Follow-up of 8 weeks	Seafood and n-3 supple- mentation

*Included in Balk E, Chung M, Lichtenstein A, Chew P, Kupelnick B, Lawrence A, DeVine D, Lau J. 2004. *Effects of Omega-3 Fatty Acids on Cardiovascular Risk Factors and Intermediate Markers of Cardiovascular Disease. Summary, Evidence Report/Technology Assessment No. 93. (Prepared by the Tufts-New England Medical Center Evidence-based Practice Center, Boston, MA).* AHRQ Publication No. 04-E010-1. Rockville, MD: Agency for Healthcare Research and Quality.
    ** N = Evidence of no association or no clear association; B = Evidence of a benefit.

Amount	Results	Conclusion **
Fish-diet group: 4.30±0.50 fish con- taining meals/week 0.38±0.04 g EPA and 0.67±0.098 g DHA/day Fish-oil group: 4 g/day 1.33 g EPA and 0.95 g DHA/day DHA-oil group: 4 g/day 1.68 g DHA/day	The change in Factor X (% of normal) from baseline to 15 weeks was significantly greater in the fish-diet group compared to the control group ($p<0.05$). The change in collagen (50 µg/ml) from baseline to 15 weeks was significantly greater in the fish-diet group and the fish-oil group when compared to the controls ($p<0.05$). No other significant associations were found between the diet groups with regards to the change in PT (ratio), APTT (ratio), Factor VII (% of normal), Factor X (% of normal), fibrinogen (g/l), prothrombin fragment 1+2 (nmol/L), tissue factor pathway inhibitor (ng/mL), platelet aggregation (%T), ADP (2.0 µmol/L), ADP (5.0 µmol/L), and collagen (50 µg/L).	N
Fish treatment: 1 kg (raw) Atlantic salmon + 150 g sardines in sild oil per week 4.5 g EPA+DHA/day Fish-oil treatment: 105 g MaxEPA/week 4.6 g EPA+DHA/day Continued with meats as during baseline Control diet: Continuation of baseline diet	The changes in fibrinogen and thromboxane were significantly lower and the change in bleeding time was significantly longer in the fish-diet group compared to the control diet group ($p<0.05$).	B

TABLE B-2g Studies on Diabetes

Author	Study Type	Subjects	Exposure
Dunstan et al., 1999*	Randomized Controlled Trial	Men and women (n=55) Mean age about 53 years Western Australia Nonsmoking, treated type II diabetes Fasting serum triglyceride >1.8 mmol/L and/or HDL-C <1.0 mmol/L and BMI <36.0 kg/m^2 Follow-up of 8 weeks	Diet (includes seafood) and exercise

Amount	Results	Conclusion**
Group 1: Low-fat diet (≤30% energy from fat) + moderate exercise (55-65% of Vo₂max)	The change in erythrocyte omega-3 fatty acids from baseline to end of intervention were significantly different for both the fish and moderate exercise (Group 3) and the fish and light exercise (Group 4) compared to the controls (p<0.05).	B
Group 2: Low-fat diet (≤30% energy from fat) + light exercise (heart rate <100 bpm)	The change in plasma tPa antigen from baseline to end of intervention were significantly different for the fish and moderate exercise (Group 3), fish and light exercise (Group 4), and no fish and moderate exercise (Group 1) groups compared to the controls (p<0.05).	
Group 3: Low-fat diet with the inclusion of 1 fish meal daily (3.6 g n-3/day) + moderate exercise (55-65% of Vo₂max)	The change in erythrocyte omega-6 fatty acids from baseline to end of intervention were significantly different for both the fish and moderate exercise (Group 3) and the fish and light exercise (Group 4) compared to the controls (p<0.05). The change in plasma factor VII from baseline to end of intervention was significantly different for the fish and light exercise group compared to the control group (p<0.05).	
Group 4: Low-fat diet with the inclusion of 1 fish meal daily (3.6 g n-3/day) + light exercise (heart rate <100 bpm)	There were no significant differences in change in plasma PAI-1 antigen or change in plasma fibrinogen from baseline to end of intervention for the three other treatment groups compared to the controls.	

continued

TABLE B-2g Continued

Author	Study Type	Subjects	Exposure
Mori et al., 1999*	Randomized Controlled Trial	Men and women (n=63) Aged 40-70 years Royal Perth Hospital, Australia Nonsmoking men and postmenopausal women Overweight, BMI >25, systolic blood pressure 125-180 mmHg, diastolic blood pressure <110 mmHg Receiving antihypertensive treatment for ≥3 months No lipid-lowering or antiinflammatory drugs, no more than 1 fish meal/week, drank <175 g alcohol/week Follow-up of 16 weeks	Seafood; diet
Sirtori et al., 1998*	Randomized Controlled Trial	Men and women (n=935) Aged 45-75 for men Aged 55-80 for women Italy (63 clinical groups) Presenting with hyperlipoproteinemias type IIb or IV, associated with at least one further risk factor No severe intercurrent ailments, kidney or renal disease, intestinal malabsorptions, duodenal ulcer nonresponsive to therapy, BMI ≥30, history of vascular or nonvascular brain disease, severe hyperlipidemia needing drug treatment, severe hypertension, myocardial infarction in the preceding 3 months, or unstable angina Follow-up of 1 year	n-3 supplement

Amount	Results	Conclusion**
Control group = weight-maintaining diet Fish group = weight-maintaining diet + fish daily (about 3.65 n-3/day) Weight loss group = energy restricted diet (to achieve 5-8 kg weight loss) Fish + weight loss group = energy restricted diet + fish daily	From baseline to end of intervention, the fish + weight loss diet significantly increased plasma phospholipid n-3 fatty acids (p<0.0001) and significantly decreased plasma phospholipid n-6 fatty acids (p<0.0001), fasting insulin (p<0.05), and insulin AUC (p<0.05) compared to the control diet. From baseline to end of intervention, the fish diet (with weight maintenance) significantly increased plasma phospholipid n-3 fatty acids (p<0.0001) and plasma phospholipid n-6 fatty acids (p<0.0001) compared to the control group. From baseline to end of intervention, the change in fasting insulin levels and insulin AUC levels was significantly different in the fish group compared to the weight loss group and the fish + weight loss group (p<0.05). There was no association found between diet group and change in fasting glucose or glucose AUC.	N
For first 2 months: Group 1 = 1530 mg EPA/1050 mg DHA Group 2 = olive oil placebo After 2 months until 6 months: Group 1 = 1020 mg EPA/700 mg DHA Group 2 = olive oil placebo Open phase from 6-12 months: 2 g/day of n-3 ethyl esters	No statistical differences could be detected between the two groups in terms of fasting glucose levels, HbA1c and insulinemia after 1 year of treatment.	N

continued

TABLE B-2g Continued

Author	Study Type	Subjects	Exposure
Grundt et al., 1995*	Randomized Controlled Trial	Men (n=51) Women (n=6) Aged 18-70 years Stavanger, Norway Outpatient center Has combined hyperlipidemia No dietary supplementation or medication containing omega-3 fatty acids during the run-in period, no antihyperlipemic medication No MI or other serious disease occurring within 3 months of enrollment, known diabetes mellitus, serious psychological disease, known drug or alcohol abuse, pregnancy or lactation Follow-up of 12 weeks	n-3 supplement
Kesavulu et al., 2002	Trial	Men and women (n=34) Nonobese, type II diabetic On oral antidiabetic drugs, but not on lipid lowering drugs or antioxidant therapy Normotensive; no other clinical complications other than diabetes, no diabetic complications Follow-up of 3 months	n-3 supplement

Amount	Results	Conclusion**
Treatment: 2 g concentrated ethylester compound 85% EPA/DHA Control: 2 g concentrated ethylester compound 85% corn oil	There were no statistical differences between the two groups or within the groups (between 2 weeks before treatment and after 12 weeks of treatment) with regards to serum glucose, plasma insulin, plasma proinsulin, insulin:glucose ratio, and proinsulin:glucose ratio.	N
Group 1 diabetics: 1 month of antidiabetic drugs alone 2 months of omega-3 supplement (1080 mg EPA and 720 mg DHA/day) along with the antidiabetic drugs Group 2 diabetics: 3 months of antidiabetic drugs alone Group 3: Non-diabetic controls	After combined therapy, fasting blood glucose and glycated hemoglobin were significantly higher in the Group 1 diabetics than in the controls (p<0.001). After 3 months of antidiabetic treatment, there were no significant differences in fasting blood glucose and glycated hemoglobin between Group 2 diabetics and the controls.	B

continued

TABLE B-2g Continued

Author	Study Type	Subjects	Exposure
Madsen et al., 2001*	Cross-sectional	Men (n=171) Women (n=98) Aged 39-77 years Aalborg, Denmark Referred for coronary angiography because of clinical suspicion of CAD; clinically stable No acute myocardial infarction in past 6 months, nonischemic cardiomyopathy, pacemaker, or permanent tachyarrhythmias	PUFA in granulocyte membranes; seafood

*Included in Balk E, Chung M, Lichtenstein A, Chew P, Kupelnick B, Lawrence A, DeVine D, Lau J. 2004. *Effects of Omega-3 Fatty Acids on Cardiovascular Risk Factors and Intermediate Markers of Cardiovascular Disease. Summary, Evidence Report/Technology Assessment No. 93. (Prepared by the Tufts-New England Medical Center Evidence-based Practice Center, Boston, MA). AHRQ Publication No. 04-E010-1.* Rockville, MD: Agency for Healthcare Research and Quality.

**B = Evidence of a benefit; N = Evidence of no association or no clear association.

Amount	Results	Conclusion**
Fish Score: (sum for lunch and dinner, can range from 2-12) 1 = never eating fish 2 = eating fish 1 time/month 3 = eating fish 2-3 times/month 4 = eating fish 1 time/week 5 = eating fish 2-3 times/week 6 = eating fish at least 1 time/day	"Subjects with CRP levels in the lower quartiles had significantly higher contents of DHA in granulocytes than subjects with CRP levels in the upper quartile" (p=0.02). There were no significant associations found between CRP and LA, ALA, AA, EPA, or DPA content in granulocyte membranes or between CRP and fish score.	N

TABLE B-2h Studies on Adult Asthma and Allergies

Author	Study Type	Subjects	Exposure
Troisi et al., 1995	Cohort	Women (n=77,866) Aged 30-55 years US nurses Nurses' Health Study No diagnosed cancer, CVD, diabetes, emphysema, chronic bronchitis, or asthma before or at time of questionnaire Follow-up of 10 years	Dietary total fat and n-3 intake
Huang et al., 2001	Cross-sectional	Men (n=582) Women (n=584) Aged 13-17 years Taiwan Uninstitutionalized The National Nutritional Survey (1993-1996)	Seafood; diet

* N = Evidence of no association or no clear association; B = Evidence of a benefit.

Amount	Results	Conclusion*
Quintiles of total fat intake (median): 1 = 51.9 g 2 = 62.7 g 3 = 69.9 g 4 = 77.0 g 5 = 87.4 g	After adjusting for age, smoking, BMI, area of residence, number of physician's visits, and quintiles of energy intake: There were no significant associations found between total fat intake, saturated fat intake, or omega-3 fat intake and the risk of asthma;	N
Quintiles of omega-3 (median): 1 = 0.05 g 2 = 0.09 g 3 = 0.13 g 4 = 0.21 g 5 = 0.36 g	Those in Quintile 3 of monounsaturated fat intake (median = 28.6 g) had a significantly lower RR of asthma than those in Quintile 1 (median = 20.1 g) (RR=0.74, 95% CI 0.59-0.93); and Those in Quintiles 2 and 4 of LA intake (median = 6 g and 11.1 g, respectively) had significantly lower RR of asthma than those in Quintile 1 (median = 4.49 g) (RR=0.71, 95% CI 0.57-0.89; RR=0.74, 95% CI 0.59-0.93; respectively).	
Quartiles of fish intake, absolute amounts unspecified	There were no significant differences found between the quartiles of all fish, shellfish, other seafood intake and prevalence of physician-diagnosed asthma (p=0.82, p=0.12, p=0.99, respectively). There was a significant difference among the quartiles of oily fish and the prevalence of physician-diagnosed asthma (quartile 1 = 1.5%, quartile 2 = 2.5%, quartile 3 = 4.6%, and quartile 4 = 4.9%; p=0.01). There were no significant differences found between the quartiles of all fish, oily fish, shellfish, other seafood intake and prevalence of physician-diagnosed allergic rhinitis (p=0.39, p=0.65, p=0.45, p=0.15, respectively).	B

TABLE B-2i Studies on Cancer

Author	Study Type	Subjects	Exposure
Stolzenberg-Solomon et al., 2002	Randomized Controlled Trial	Men (n=27,111) Aged 50-69 years Southwestern Finland Smoked ≥5 cigarettes/day Alpha-tocopherol, Beta-Carotene Cancer Prevention (ATBC) Study No history of malignancy other than nonmelanoma cancer of the skin or carcinoma in situ, severe angina upon exertion, chronic renal insufficiency, liver cirrhosis, chronic alcoholism, receipt of anticoagulant therapy, other medical problems which might limit long-term participation, and current use of supplements containing vitamin E (>20 mg/day), vitamin A (>20,000 IU/day), or beta-carotene (>6 mg/day) Follow-up of up to 13 years (260,006 person-years)	Seafood; dietary fatty acids
MacLean et al., 2006	Review	Part of a larger systematic literature review Cohorts (n=20 cohorts; 38 articles) 11 different types of cancer	Seafood; dietary fatty acids

Amount	Results	Conclusion*
Randomized to 50 mg/day of alpha-tocopherol, 20 mg/day of beta-carotene, both, or placebo Quantiles of fish intake and n-3 fish oil intake, absolute amount unspecified	After adjusting for energy intake, age, and years of smoking, there were no significant associations found between quantities of fish intake or quantiles of n-3 fish oil intake and the risk of pancreatic cancer.	N
	"For each breast, lung, and prostate cancer, there were significant associations for both increased and decreased risk and far more estimates that did not demonstrate any association." "No trend was found across many different cohorts and many different categories of omega-3 fatty acid consumption to suggest that omega-3 fatty acids reduce overall cancer risk."	N

continued

TABLE B-2i Continued

Author	Study Type	Subjects	Exposure
Terry et al., 2003	Review	7 cohort studies on breast cancer 8 cohort studies on prostate cancer 1 cohort study on endometrial cancer 19 case-control studies on breast cancer 9 case-control studies on prostate cancer 7 case-control studies on endometrial cancer 5 case-control studies on ovarian cancer	Seafood, n-3 supplement, serum phospholipids, adipose tissue, and erythrocyte membrane fatty acids

Amount	Results	Conclusion*
	"The development and progression of breast and prostate cancers appear to be affected by processes in which EPA and DHA play important roles." However, "whether the consumption of fish containing marine fatty acids can alter the risk of these cancers or of other hormone-dependent cancers is unclear."	N
	"Although there is ample evidence from in vitro and animal studies that these essential fats can inhibit the progression of tumors in various organs, particularly the breast and prostate, the evidence from epidemiologic studies is less clear."	
	"Although most of the studies did not show an association between fish consumption or marine fatty acid intake and the risk of hormone-related cancers, the results of the few studies from populations with a generally high intake of marine fatty acids are encouraging."	

continued

TABLE B-2i Continued

Author	Study Type	Subjects	Exposure
Norat et al., 2005	Cohort	Men and women (n=478,040) Aged 35-70 years 23 centers in 10 European countries European Prospective Investigation into Cancer and Nutrition (EPIC) Recruited from general population Free of cancer at baseline, other than nonmelanoma skin cancer Average follow-up of 4.8 years (2,279,075 person-years)	Seafood

Amount	Results	Conclusion*
Categories of fish intake: 1 = <10 g/day 2 = 10-20 g/day 3 = 20-40 g/day 4 = 40-80 g/day 5 = ≥80 g/day	After adjusting for age, sex, energy from nonfat sources, energy from fat sources, height, weight, occupational physical activity, smoking status, dietary fiber, alcohol intake, and stratified for center: Those in the 4th and 5th categories of fish intake had a significantly lower HR of colorectal cancer than those in the 1st category (HR=0.67, 95% CI 0.56-0.82; and HR=0.69, 95% CI 0.54-0.88, respectively). The HR for the 2nd and 3rd categories of fish intake were also lower compared to the 1st category, but they were not significant; Those in the 4th and 5th categories of fish intake had a significantly lower HR of rectal cancer than those in the 1st category (HR=0.64, 95% CI 0.47 0.88; and HR=0.49, 95% CI 0.32-0.76, respectively). The HR for the 2nd and 3rd categories of fish intake were also lower compared to the 1st category, but they were not significant; Those in the 4th category of fish intake had a significantly lower HR of colon cancer than those in the 1st category (HR=0.69, 95% CI 0.54-0.88). The HR for the 2nd, 3rd, and 5th categories of fish intake were also lower compared to the 1st category, but they were not significant; and Every 100 g increase in daily fish intake significantly lowered the HR for colorectal cancer (HR=0.70, 95% CI 0.57-0.87), colon cancer (HR=0.76, 95% CI 0.59-0.99), and rectal cancer (HR=0.61, 95% CI 0.43-0.87).	B

continued

TABLE B-2i Continued

Author	Study Type	Subjects	Exposure
Allen et al., 2004	Cohort	Men (n=18,115) Mean age at entry was 51 years Mean age at diagnosis was 75 years Hiroshima and Nagasaki, Japan Life Span Study/The Adult Health Study In Hiroshima or Nagasaki during the time of the bombs and who were residents of one of the cities in the 1950 census, or not present in either city at the time of the bombs No prostate cancer at baseline Average follow-up of 16.9 years (252,602 person-years)	Seafood
English et al., 2004	Cohort	Men and women (n=37,112) Aged 27-75 years Melbourne, Australia The Melbourne Collaborative Cohort Study Deliberately recruited Italian and Greek migrants Free of colorectal cancer, diabetes, a heart attack, or angina at baseline Average follow-up of 9 years	Seafood

Amount	Results	Conclusion*
Scores of intake for each food: 1 = Missing or <2 times/week 2 = 2-4 times/week 3 = Almost daily Total fish/broiled fish intake: Low = Score of 2 Intermediate = Score of 3-4 High = Score of ≥5	After adjusting for age, calendar period, city of residence, radiation dose, and education level: Those who ate fish almost daily had a significantly higher RR of prostate cancer compared to those who ate fish <2 times/week (RR=1.54, 95% CI 1.03-2.31). Those who ate fish 2-4 times/week also had a higher RR of prostate cancer compared to those who ate fish <2 times/week, but this association was not significant (RR=1.18, 95% CI 0.83-1.67); There were no significant associations found between broiled fish intake and risk of prostate cancer; and Those in the highest category of total fish intake had a significantly higher RR of prostate cancer compared to those in the lowest category (RR=1.77, 95% CI 1.01-3.11). Those in the intermediate category also had a higher RR of prostate cancer compared to those in the lowest category, but this association was not significant (RR=1.19, 95% CI 0.82-1.73).	A
Categories of fish intake: 1 = < 1.0 time/week 2 = 1.0-1.4 times/week 3 = 1.5-2.4 times/week 4 = 2.5+ times/week	After adjusting for sex, country of birth, and intake of energy, fat, and cereal products: There were no significant associations found between fish intake (defined by four categories) and the risk of colorectal cancer, colon cancer, or rectal cancers; and There were no significant associations found between fish intake (defined as a continuous variable) and the risk of colorectal cancer (HR=0.99, 95% CI 0.91-1.08), colon cancer (HR=1.01, 95% CI 0.90-1.12), and rectal cancer (HR=0.97, 95% CI 0.84-1.12).	N

continued

TABLE B-2i Continued

Author	Study Type	Subjects	Exposure
Folsom and Demissie, 2004	Cohort	Women (n=41,836) Aged 55-69 years Iowa Iowa Women's Health Study Group 1 = no heart disease or cancer at baseline Group 2 = no cancer at baseline, but a history of myocardial infarction, angina, or other heart disease Follow-up of 442,965 person-years	Seafood; dietary fatty acids
Augustsson et al., 2003	Cohort	Men (n=47,882) Aged 40-75 years US health professionals Health Professionals Follow-up Study No diagnosis of cancer at baseline Follow-up of 12 years	Seafood

Amount	Results	Conclusion*
Categories of fish intake: 1 = <0.5 times/week 2 = 0.5-1.0 times/week 3 = 1.0-1.5 times/week 4 = >1.5-<2.5 times/week 5 = ≥2.5 times/week Quintiles of omega-3 fatty acid intake: 1 = ≤0.05 g/day 2 = 0.06-0.10 g/day 3 = 0.11-0.16 g/day 4 = 0.17-0.26 g/day 5 = ≥0.27 g/day	After adjusting for age, energy intake, education level, physical activity, alcohol consumption, smoking status, pack-years of cigarette smoking, age at first live birth, estrogen use, vitamin use, BMI, waist/hip ratio, diabetes, hypertension, intake of whole grains, fruit and vegetables, red meat, cholesterol, and saturated fat: Among women with no cancer or heart disease at baseline, no significant associations were found between frequency of fish intake and risk of cancer mortality or breast cancer; and Among women with no cancer or heart disease at baseline, no significant associations were found between quintiles of omega-3 fatty acid intake and risk of total mortality or breast cancer incidence.	N
Categories of fish consumption: 1 = <2 times/month 2 = 2 times/month to 1 time/week 3 = 2-3 times/week 4 = >3 times/week	After adjusting for age, calories, fatty acids, lycopene, retinol, vitamin D, and physical activity: Those who ate fish >3 times/week had a significantly lower RR of metastatic prostate cancer than those who ate fish <2 times/month (RR=0.56, 95% CI 0.37-0.86). No other comparisons for metastatic prostate cancer were significant; There were no significant associations found between total fish consumption and all prostate cancer or advanced prostate cancer; and Each additional 0.5 g/day of marine fatty acids was associated with a RR of 0.76 (95% CI 0.58-0.98) for metastatic prostate cancer. "When fish intake was analyzed as a continuous variable, an increase in three servings of fish per week was associated with a RR of 0.75 (95% CI 0.60-0.94) for metastatic prostate cancer."	B

continued

TABLE B-2i Continued

Author	Study Type	Subjects	Exposure

Holmes et al., 2003	Cohort	Women (n=88,647)
		Aged 30-55 years
		US nurses
		Nurses' Health Study (NHS)
		No diagnosed cancer other than
		    nonmelanoma skin cancer prior to
		    1980
		Follow-up of 18 years
			Seafood

Amount	Results	Conclusion*
Categories of fish intake: 1 = ≤0.13 servings/day 2 = 0.14-0.20 servings/day 3 = 0.21-0.27servings/day 4 = 0.28-0.39 servings/day 5 = ≥0.40 servings/day	After adjusting for age, 2-year time period, total energy intake, alcohol intake, parity and age at first birth, BMI at age 18, weight change since age 18, height in inches, family history of breast cancer, history of benign breast disease, age at menarche, menopausal status, age at menopause and hormone replacement therapy use, and duration of menopause: There was no significant association found between fish intake and the risk of breast cancer for the whole cohort or when premenopausal women and postmcnopausal women were analyzed separately; and Similarly nonsignificant results were found when fish intake was defined as no intake, <1 serving/day and ≥1 serving/day.	N

continued

TABLE B-2i Continued

Author	Study Type	Subjects	Exposure
Stripp et al., 2003	Cohort	Women (n=23,693) Aged 50-64 years Copenhagen and Aarhus, Denmark Diet, Cancer and Health study No diagnosis of cancer at baseline Median follow-up of 4.8 years	Seafood

Amount	Results	Conclusion*
Lean fish = ≤8 g/100 g Fatty fish = >8 g/100 g	After adjusting for parity, benign breast tumor, years of school, use of hormone replacement therapy, duration of HRT use, BMI, and alcohol:	A

Percentiles of lean fish
  intake:
  5th percentile = 7 g/day
  25th percentile =
    16 g/day
  75th percentile =
    32 g/day
  95th percentile =
    56 g/day
Percentiles of fatty fish
  intake:
  5th percentile = 2 g/day
  25th percentile =
    6 g/day
  75th percentile =
    19 g/day
  95th percentile =
    39 g/day
Percentiles of fried fish
  intake:
  5th percentile = 5 g/day
  25th percentile =
    13 g/day
  75th percentile =
    30 g/day
  95th percentile =
    55 g/day
Percentiles of boiled fish
  intake:
  5th percentile = 0 g/day
  25th percentile =
    4 g/day
  75th percentile =
    11 g/day
  95th percentile =
    23 g/day
Percentiles of processed
  fish intake:
  5th percentile = 2 g/day
  25th percentile =
    6 g/day
  75th percentile =
    19 g/day
  95th percentile =
    40 g/day
	Every 25 g/day increase in total fish consumption significantly increased the risk of breast cancer (IRR=1.13, 95% CI 1.03-1.23); and
	
	The risk of breast cancer is also increased for every 25 g/day increase in fatty fish (IRR=1.11, 95% CI 0.91-1.34), lean fish (IRR=1.13, 95% CI 0.99-1.29), fried fish (IRR=1.09, 95% CI 0.95-1.25), boiled fish (IRR=1.09, 95% CI 0.85-1.42), and processed fish (IRR=1.12, 95% CI 0.93-1.34), but the IRR were not.	

continued

TABLE B-2i Continued

Author	Study Type	Subjects	Exposure
Takezaki et al., 2003	Cohort	Men (n=2798) Women (n=3087) Aged 40-79 years Aichi Prefecture, Japan Rural area Follow-up of 14 years	Seafood

Amount	Results	Conclusion*
Categories of fish and shellfish intake: Low = <1 time/week Middle = 1-2 times/week High = ≥3 times/week	After adjusting for age, sex, smoking, and occupation, those in the high-fish and -shellfish intake category had a significantly lower RR for incident lung cancer than those in the low category (RR=0.32, 95% CI 0.13-0.76) (p for trend = 0.003). The middle intake group also had a smaller RR but it was not significant (RR=0.99, 95% CI 0.48-2.03). After adjusting for age, sex, smoking, and occupation: Those in the middle and high categories of total fish intake (regardless of preparation method) had a significantly lower RR for incident lung cancer than those in the low category (RR=0.43, 95% CI 0.20-0.95; and RR=0.23, 95% CI 0.10-0.54; respectively); Those in the high categories of broiled and boiled fish intake had significantly lower RR for incident lung cancer than those in the low categories (RR=0.40, 95% CI 0.17-0.93; and RR=0.27, 95% CI 0.09-0.81; respectively). Those in the middle categories of broiled and boiled fish intake also had lower RR for incident lung cancer than those in the low category but they were not significant; and There were no significant associations found between raw or deep-fried fish intake and the risk of incident lung cancer. Similar results were found when the model further adjusted for drinking, exercise habit, consumption of meat, green-yellow vegetables, and salty/dried fish.	B

continued

TABLE B-2i Continued

Author	Study Type	Subjects	Exposure
Ngoan et al., 2002	Cohort	Men (n=5917) Women (n=7333) Aged >15 years Fukuoka Prefecture, Japan Follow-up of 139,390 person-years	Seafood
Ozasa et al., 2001	Cohort	Men (n=42,940) Women (n=55,308) Aged 40-79 years 19 prefectures throughout Japan Japanese Collaborative Cohort (JACC) Study No history of lung cancer Average follow-up of 92 months	Seafood
Terry et al., 2001	Cohort	Men (n=6272) Mean age of 55.6 years (baseline) Twin pairs from the Sweden Twin registry Sweden Follow-up of 30 years	Seafood

Amount	Results	Conclusion*
Categories of cuttle fish intake: Low = seldom or never Medium = 2-4 times/month High = 2-4 times or more/week Categories of fish intake: Low = 2-4 times or less/month Medium = 2-4 times/week High = 1 time or more/day	After adjusting for age, there was no significant association found between intake of fresh fish, processed fish, or cuttle fish and the risk of stomach cancer among men and women. After adjusting for age, sex, smoking, processed meat, liver, cooking or salad oil, suimono, and pickled food, there was no significant association found between intake of fresh fish, processed fish, or cuttle fish either including the first 3 years of follow-up or excluding the first 3 years of follow-up.	N
Categories of fish intake: 1 = ≤1-2 times/week 2 = 3-4 times/week 3 = Almost every day	After adjusting for age, parents' history of lung cancer, smoking status, smoking index and time since quitting smoking, there was no significant association found between fish intake and risk of lung cancer death in men or women.	N
Categories of fish intake: 1 = Never/seldom part of diet 2 = Small part of diet 3 = Moderate part of diet 4 = Large part of diet	After adjusting for age, BMI, physical activity, smoking, and consumption of alcohol, red meat, processed meat, fruit and vegetables, and milk: Those who never or seldomly ate fish had a significantly higher RR of all prostate cancers than those who made fish a moderate part of their diet (RR=2.3, 95% CI 1.2-4.5, $p<0.05$); Those who never or seldomly ate fish had a significantly higher RR of prostate cancer deaths than those who made fish a moderate part of their diet (RR=3.3, 95% CI 1.8-6.0, $p<0.01$); and No other comparisons between fish consumption and all prostate cancers or prostate cancer deaths were significant.	B

continued

TABLE B-2i Continued

Author	Study Type	Subjects	Exposure
Key et al., 1999	Cohort	Women (n=34,759) Hiroshima and Nagasaki, Japan Life Span Study In Hiroshima or Nagasaki during the time of the bombs and city residents during the 1950 census, or not in either city at the time of the bombs Follow-up of 488,989 person-years	Seafood
Kato et al., 1997	Cohort	Women (n=14,727) Aged 34-65 years New York and Florida New York University Women's Health Study No use of hormonal medication or pregnancy in preceding 6 months Follow-up of 105,044 person-years	Seafood

Amount	Results	Conclusion*
Categories of fish intake: 1 = ≤ 1 time/week 2 = 2-4 times/week 3 = ≥5 times/week 4 = Unknown	After adjusting for attained age, calendar period, city, age at time of bombing, and radiation dose: There were no significant associations found between categories of fish (not dried) intake and risk of breast cancer; and Those in the "unknown" category of dried fish intake had a significantly lower RR of breast cancer than those in the 1st category (RR=0.77, 95% CI 0.60-0.98). No other comparisons for dried fish intake were significant.	N
Quartile of fish intake, absolute amounts not specified	After adjusting for calories intake, age, place at enrollment, and highest level of education: Those in the 4th quartile of fish intake had a significantly lower RR of colorectal cancer compared to those in the 1st quartile (RR=0.49, 95% CI 0.27-0.89). The RR for those in the 2nd and 3rd quartiles were not significant (p for trend = 0.007); Those in the 4th quartile of fish protein intake had a significantly lower RR of colorectal cancer compared to those in the 1st quartile (RR=0.42, 95% CI 0.23-0.77). The RR for those in the 2nd and 3rd quartiles were also lower but not significant (p for trend = 0.016); Those in the 4th quartile of fish calcium intake had a significantly lower RR of colorectal cancer compared to those in the 1st quartile (RR=0.41, 95% CI 0.22-0.74). The RR for those in the 2nd and 3rd quartiles were also lower but not significant (p for trend = 0.001); and No significant association was found between fish fat intake and risk of colorectal cancer (p for trend = 0.056).	B

continued

TABLE B-2i Continued

Author	Study Type	Subjects	Exposure

Veierod et al., 1997	Cohort	Men (n=25,956)
		Women (n=25,496)
		Aged 16-56 years
		Norway
		Attended Norwegian health screening
		    between 1977 and 1983
		Average follow-up of 11.2 years
		    (578,047 person-years)
			Seafood; n-3
			supplements

Chiu et al., 1996	Cohort	Women (n=35,156)
		Aged 55-69 years
		Iowa
		Iowa Women's Health Study
		No self-reported history of cancer at
		    baseline or prior use of chemotherapy
		Follow-up of 7 years (233,261
		    person-years)
			Seafood

Amount	Results	Conclusion*
Cod-liver oil intake: yes or no	After adjusting for smoking status, gender, age at inclusion, and attained age:	B
Sardines, pickled herring (sandwich spread): yes or no	Those taking cod liver oil had a lower incidence rate ratio of lung cancer compared to those not taking cod liver oil (IRR=0.5, 95% CI 0.3-1.0), but it was not significant;	
Categories of fish liver intake: 1 = <1 time/week in season 2 = 1-2 times/week in season 3 = ≥3 times/week in season	Those who consumed sardines and pickled herring had a significantly higher incidence rate ratio compared to those not consuming sardines and pickled herring (IRR=1.5, 95% CI 1.1-2.2); Those who consumed fish liver ≥3 times/week in season had a significantly higher incidence rate ratio of lung cancer compared to those who consumed fish liver <1 time/week in	
Categories of main meals with fish: 1 = <1 time/week 2 = 1-2 times/week 3 = 3-4 times/week 4 = ≥5 times/week	season (IRR=2.6, 95% CI 1.2-6.0). Those who consumed fish liver 1-2 times/week in season also had a higher incidence rate ratio compared to those who consumed fish liver <1 time/week in season (IRR=1.1, 95% CI 0.7-1.7), but it was not significant; and	
	Those who consumed main meals with fish ≥5 times/week had a significantly higher incidence rate ratio of lung cancer compared to those who ate main meals with fish <1 time/week (IRR=3.0, 95% CI 1.2-7.3). Those who consumed main meals with fish 1-2 times/week and 3-4 times/week also had higher incidence rate ratios of lung cancer compared to those who consumed main meals with fish <1 time/week (IRR=1.1, 95% CI 0.6-2.2; and IRR=1.0, 95% CI 0.5-2.1), but they were not significant.	
Categories of fish intake: 1 = <4 servings/month 2 = 4-6 servings/month 3 = >6 servings/month	After adjusting for age and total energy intake, there were no significant associations found between intake of all fish or polyunsaturated fat and risk of non-Hodgkins lymphoma.	N

continued

TABLE B-2i Continued

Author	Study Type	Subjects	Exposure
Chyou et al., 1995	Cohort	Men (n=7995) Born in 1900-1919 Examined from 1965-1968 Oahu, Hawaii American men of Japanese ancestry Participated in the Honolulu Heart Program Follow-up of 24 years	Seafood
Giovannucci et al., 1994	Cohort	Men (n=47,949) Aged 40-75 years US health professionals Health Professionals Follow-up Study No diagnosed cancer at baseline	Seafood
Le Marchand et al., 1994	Cohort	Men (n=20,316) Aged <45 years Permanent resident of Hawaii Nonmilitary Japanese, Caucasian, Filipino, Hawaiian/ part Hawaiian, and Chinese No invasive cancer within 5 years before entry, no diagnosis of prostate cancer earlier than 5 years before interview Median follow-up of 6 years (between entry and diagnosis for cases)	Seafood
Chyou et al., 1993	Cohort	Men (n=7995) Born in 1900-1919 Examined from 1965-1968 Oahu, Hawaii American men of Japanese ancestry Participated in the Honolulu Heart Program Follow-up of 22 years	Seafood

Amount	Results	Conclusion*
Categories of fish intake: 1 = ≤1 serving/week 2 = 2-4 servings/week 3 = ≥5 servings/week	After adjusting for age, alcohol, number of cigarettes/day and number of years smoked: There was no significant association found between fish intake and the risk of upper aerodigestive tract cancer (RR=1.02, 95% CI 0.65-1.61 for 2-4 times/week compared to ≤1 time/week; and RR=1.37, 95% CI 0.70-2.69 for ≥5 times/week compared to ≤1 time/week).	N
Categories of fish intake (median): 1 = 8.4 g/day 2 = 20.9 g/day 3 = 31.0 g/day 4 = 47.8 g/day 5 = 83.4 g/day	After adjusting for age, there was no significant association found between fish intake and the risk of colon cancer.	N
Quantile of fish intake, absolute amounts not specified	After adjusting for age, ethnicity, and income, no significant association was found between risk of prostate cancer and quantile of fish intake at baseline.	N
Categories of fish intake: 1 = ≤1 serving/week 2 = 2-4 servings/week 3 = ≥5 servings/week	After adjusting for age and smoking, there was no significant association found between fish intake and bladder cancer (RR=0.90, 95% CI 0.59-1.39 for 2-4 times/week compared to ≤1 time/week; and RR=0.67, 95% CI 0.26-1.67 for ≥5 times/week compared to ≤1 time/week).	N

continued

TABLE B-2i Continued

Author	Study Type	Subjects	Exposure
Vatten et al., 1990	Cohort	Women (n=14,500) Aged 35-51 years Norway Participated in the National Health Screening Service Follow-up of 11-14 years (mean = 12 years)	Seafood
Willett et al., 1990	Cohort	Women (n=88,751) Aged 30-55 years US nurses Nurses' Health Study (NHS) No history of cancer, inflammatory bowel disease, or familial polyposis at baseline Follow-up of 6 years (512,488 person-years)	Seafood

Amount	Results	Conclusion*
Categories of overall fish intake: 1 = ≤2 times/week 2 = >2 times/week Categories of poached fish intake: 1 = <2 times/month 2 = 2-4 times/month 3 = ≥5 times/month	After adjusting for age: Those who ate fish >2 times/week had a higher IRR of breast cancer when compared to those who ate fish ≤2 times/week, but it was not significant (IRR=1.2, 95% CI 0.8-1.7); and Those who ate poached fish 2-4 times/month and ≥5 times/month had lower IRR of breast cancer when compared to those who ate poached fish <2 times/week, but they were not significant (IRR=0.8, 95% CI 0.5-1.1; and IRR=0.7, 95% CI 0.4-1.0; respectively).	N
Categories of fish intake: 1 = <1 time/month 2 = 1-3 times/month 3 = 1 time/week 4 = 2-4 times/week 5 = ≥5 times/week Quintiles of chicken and fish intake: 1 = <22 g/day 2 = 22-28 g/day 3 = 29-40 g/day 4 = 41-64 g/day 5 = ≥65 g/day	After adjusting for age, there was no significant association found between fish intake and incidence of colon cancer. After adjusting for age and total energy intake: Those in the 4th and 5th quintiles of chicken and fish intake had significantly lower RR of colon cancer compared to those in the 1st quintile (RR=0.47, 95% CI 0.27-0.81; and RR=0.56, 95% CI 0.34-0.92; respectively); and Those in the 2nd and 3rd quintiles of chicken and fish intake also had lower RR of colon cancer compared to those in the 1st quintile (RR=0.75, 95% CI 0.46-1.22; and RR=0.99, 95% CI 0.63-1.54; respectively), but they were not significant.	N

continued

TABLE B-2i Continued

Author	Study Type	Subjects	Exposure
Mills et al., 1989	Cohort	Men (n=about 15,000) Aged ≥25 years California Seventh-day Adventists Follow-up of 6 years (78,000 person-years)	Seafood
Kvale et al., 1983	Cohort	Men (n=13,785) Women (n=2928) Men in a probability sample of the general population of Norway A roster of male siblings, living in Norway, of migrants to the US Male and female family members of patients interviewed in a Norwegian case-control study of gastrointestinal cancer Follow-up of 11.5 years	Seafood
Pan et al., 2004	Case-control	Cases = with incident ovarian cancer (n=442) Controls = without cancer from eight provinces, except Manitoba (n=2135) Women Mean age of 55 years Canada National Enhanced Cancer Surveillance Study (NECSS)	Seafood; dietary fatty acids

Amount	Results	Conclusion*
Categories of fish intake: 1 = Never 2 = <1 time/week 3 = ≥1 time/week	After adjusting for age: Those who ate fish <1 time/week had a significantly higher RR of prostate cancer compared to those who never ate fish (RR=1.68, 95% CI 1.16-2.43); and Those who ate fish ≥1 time/week also had a higher relative risk of prostate cancer compared to those who never ate fish, but it was not significant (RR=1.47, 95% CI 0.84-2.60). After adjusting for age; education; current use of meat, poultry or fish, beans, legumes or peas, citrus fruit, dry fruit; and index of fruit, nuts, and tomatoes: No significant association was found between current use of fish and prostate cancer risk (RR=1.37, 95% CI 0.95-1.96 for <1 time/week compared to never and RR=1.57, 95% CI 0.88-2.78 for ≥1 time/week compared to never).	A
Index of frequency of fish intake (scores): 1 = <10 2 = 10-14 3 = 15-19 4 = ≥20	After adjusting for age, cigarette smoking, region, and urban/rural place of residence, no significant association was found between the fish intake (the highest score of fish intake compared to the lowest score of fish intake) and the risk of lung cancer, with either histologically verified primary tumor (β=−0.07±0.13, p=0.63) or squamous and small-cell carcinomas (β=−0.01±0.17, p=0.99).	N
Serving size=4 oz/week Quartiles of fish and fatty acid intakes, absolute amount unspecified	After adjusting for 10-year age group, province of residence, education, alcohol consumption, cigarette pack-years, BMI, total caloric intake, recreational physical activity, number of live births, menstruation years, and menopause status: There were no significant associations found between fish intake or fatty acid intake (saturated, monounsaturated, or polyunsaturated) and risk of ovarian cancer.	N

continued

TABLE B-2i Continued

Author	Study Type	Subjects	Exposure
Goldbohm et al., 1994	Case-cohort	Men (n=1688) Women (n=1812) Aged 55-69 years Netherlands Based on incident cases of colon cancer Subcohort of Netherlands Cohort Study Follow-up of over 3.3 years	Seafood; dietary fatty acids
Larsson et al., 2004	Review	Case-control, cohort, and animal studies	Seafood; n-3 supplements

*N = Evidence of no association or no clear association; B = Evidence of a benefit; A = Evidence of an adverse effect.

Amount	Results	Conclusion*
Categories of fish intake: 1 = 0 g/day 2 = 0-10 g/day 3 = 10-20 g/day 4 = >20 g/day Quintiles of fatty acids	After adjusting for age and energy: Men in the 3rd category of fish intake had a significantly lower RR of colon cancer compared to men in the 1st category of fish intake (RR=0.41, 95% CI 0.21-0.83). No other significant relative risks of colon cancer were found based on fish intake for men, women, or both sexes; and No significant associations were found between risk of colon cancer and intake of energy, fat, saturated fat, monounsaturated fat, polyunsaturated fat, or protein for among men, women, or both sexes.	B
	"Increasing evidence from animal and in vitro studies indicates that n-3 fatty acids, especially the long-chain polyunsaturated fatty acids EPA and DHA, present in fatty fish and fish oils, inhibit carcinogenesis." "The epidemiologic data on the association between fish consumption, as a surrogate marker for n-3 fatty acid intake, and cancer risk are, however, somewhat less consistent." n-3 fatty acids may modify the carcinogenic process by suppressing AA-derived eicosanoid biosynthesis; influencing transcription factor activity, gene expression, and signal transduction pathways; modulating estrogen metabolism; increasing or decreasing the production of free radicals and reactive oxygen species; and influencing insulin sensitivity and membrane fluidity.	N

TABLE B-2j Studies on Aging and Other Neurological Outcomes

Author	Study Type	Subjects	Exposure
Chen et al., 2003	Cohort	Men with incident Parkinson's disease (n=191) Women with incident Parkinson's disease (n=168) Data from Health Professionals Follow-up Study and Nurses' Health Study No Parkinson's disease, stroke, or cancer at baseline Follow-up of 2 years	Dietary fatty acids

Amount	Results	Conclusion*
Quintiles of polyunsaturated fatty acids, fish n-3 fatty acids, EPA, and DHA; absolute amounts not specified	After adjusting for baseline age, length of follow-up, smoking, energy intake, alcohol consumption, and caffeine intake:	N
	There were no significant associations found between quintiles of polyunsaturated fatty acids, fish n-3 fatty acids, EPA, or DHA and risk of Parkinson's disease.	

continued

TABLE B-2j Continued

Author	Study Type	Subjects	Exposure
Morris et al., 2003	Cohort (nested in a randomized controlled trial)	Men and women (n=815) Aged ≥65 years Chicago, IL (south-side) 62% Black, 38% White, 61% female, mean education level 11.8 years Chicago Health and Aging Project Free of Alzheimer's disease at baseline follow-up of 3 years	Seafood and dietary n-3 fatty acids

Amount	Results	Conclusion*
Quintiles of n-3 fatty acids (g/day): 0.37-1.05, 1.06-1.22, 1.23-1.39, 1.40-1.60, 1.61-4.10 Categories of fish intake: Never, 1-3 times/ month, 1 time/week, ≥2 times/week	After adjusting for age, period of observation, and fish consumption (1-3 times/months, 1 time/ week, and ≥2 times/week): There were no significant associations found between fish consumption and risk of incident Alzheimer's disease; Those in the 5th quintile of total n-3 fatty acid intake had a significantly lower RR of incident Alzheimer's disease than those in the 1st quintile (RR=0.3, 95% CI 0.1-0.7); and Those in the 4th quintile of DHA intake had a significantly lower RR of incident Alzheimer's disease than those in the 1st quintile (RR=0.3, 95% CI 0.1-0.9). After adjusting for age, period of observation, fish consumption (1-3 times/month, 1 time/week, and ≥2 times/week), sex, race, education, total energy intake, APOE-ε4, and race × APOE-ε4 interaction: The higher categories of fish intake had lower RR of incident Alzheimer's disease compared to those who never ate fish (RR=0.6, 95% CI 0.3-1.3 for 1-3 times/month; RR=0.4, 95% CI 0.2-0.9 for 1 time/week; and RR=0.4, 95% CI 0.2-0.9 for ≥2 times/week); Those in the 5th quintile of total n-3 fatty acid intake had a significantly lower RR of incident Alzheimer's disease than those in the 1st quintile (RR=0.4, 95% CI 0.1-0.9); and Those in the 4th and 5th quintiles of DHA intake had a significantly lower RR of incident Alzheimer's disease than those in the 1st quintile (RR=0.2, 95% CI 0.1-0.8; and RR=0.3, 95% CI 0.1-0.9; respectively). There were no other significant associations found between intake of n-3 fatty acids, DHA, EPA, and LA and the risk of incident Alzheimer's disease.	B

continued

TABLE B-2j Continued

Author	Study Type	Subjects	Exposure
Barberger-Gateau et al., 2002	Cohort	Men and women (n=1674) Aged ≥68 years Southwestern France Personnes Agees QUID (PAQUID study)—third wave of study Free of dementia at baseline and living at home Follow-up of 7 years	Seafood

Amount	Results	Conclusion*
Categories of fish or seafood consumption: 1 = Once a day 2 = At least once a week (but not everyday) 3 = From time to time (but not weekly) 4 = Never	After adjusting for age and sex, those who ate fish or seafood at least once a week had a significantly lower risk of being diagnosed with dementia in the 7 years of follow-up (HR=0.66, 95% CI 0.47-0.93). After adjusting for age and sex, those who ate fish or seafood at least once a week had a lower risk of developing Alzheimer's disease in the 7 years of follow-up (HR=0.69, 95% CI 0.47-1.01), with borderline significance. After adjusting for age, sex, and education, those who ate fish or seafood at least once a week had a lower risk of being diagnosed with dementia in the 7 years of follow-up (HR=0.73, 95% CI 0.52-10.3), but it was not significant. There was a "significant trend between increasing consumption of fish or seafood and decreasing incidence of dementia (p for trend = 0.0091)."	B

continued

TABLE B-2j Continued

Author	Study Type	Subjects	Exposure
Kalmijn et al., 1997a	Cohort	Men and women (n=5386) Aged >55 years Rotterdam, Netherlands Rotterdam Study About 43% former smokers, about 23% current smokers About 2% history of stroke, about 7% history of myocardial infarction Average follow-up of 2.1 years	Dietary fatty acids
Zhang et al., 2000	Cohort	Women (n=92,422 in NHS, n=95,389 in NHS II) Aged 30-55 years in NHS Aged 25-42 years in NHS II US nurses living in 11 states Nurses' Health Study (NHS) and Nurses' Health Study II (NHS II)—pooled Follow-up of 14 years in NHS and 4 years in NHS II	Seafood and dietary fatty acids

Amount	Results	Conclusion*
Tertiles of total fat intake: ≤75.5 g/day, 75.5-85.5 g/day, >85.5 g/day	After adjusting for age, sex, education, and total energy:	B
Tertiles of saturated fat intake: ≤29.0 g/day, 29.0-34.0 g/day, >34.0 g/day	Those in the 3rd tertile of total fat intake had a significantly higher RR of total dementia than those in the 1st tertile (RR=2.4, 95% CI 1.1-5.2). Those in the 2nd tertile also had a higher RR of total dementia compared to those in the 1st tertile, but it was not significant;	
Tertiles of cholesterol intake: ≤208.5 mg/day, 208.5-254.5 mg/day, >254.5 mg/day	Those in the 3rd tertile of fish intake had a significantly lower RR of total dementia (RR=0.4, 95% CI 0.2-0.9) and Alzheimer's disease without cerebrovascular disease (RR=0.3, 95% CI 0.1-0.9) than those in the 1st	
Tertiles of LA intake: ≤9.5 g/day, 9.5-15.0 g/day, >15.0 g/day	tertile. Those in the 2nd tertile also had a lower RR of total dementia and Alzheimer's disease without cerebrovascular disease compared to those in the 1st tertile, but they were not	
Tertiles of fish intake: ≤3.0 g/day, 3.0-18.5 g/day, >18.5 g/day	significant; and	
	No other significant RR were found for total dementia, Alzheimer's disease without cerebrovascular disease, or dementia with a vascular component based on daily intake of total fat, saturated fat, cholesterol, LA and fish.	
Categories of fish intake: 1 = <1 time/week 2 = 1-2.9 times/week 3 = 3-4.9 times/week	After adjusting for age, total energy, tier at birth, and pack-years of smoking:	N
Quintiles of total energy, total fat, animal fat, vegetable fat, saturated fat, monounsaturated fat, n-6 polyunsaturated fat, trans-unsaturated fat, cholesterol; absolute amounts not specified	There were no significant RR of multiple sclerosis based on one unit daily increments of oleic acid (RR=0.7, 95% CI 0.4-1.4), LA (RR=0.3, 95% CI 0.1-1.1), AA (RR=0.9, 95% CI 0.7-1.2), fish omega-3 fatty acids (RR=1.1, 95% CI 0.9-1.3), EPA (RR=1.3, 95% CI 0.9-1.9), or DHA (RR=1.1, 95% CI 0.9-1.5) ;	
	There were no significant RR of multiple sclerosis based on categories of fish and other seafood (RR=1.0, 95% CI 0.8-1.4 for category 2 compared to category 1; RR=0.9, 95% CI 0.6-1.3 for category 3 compared to category 1).	

continued

TABLE B-2j Continued

Author	Study Type	Subjects	Exposure
Kalmijn et al., 1997b	Cohort	Men (n=939) Aged 69-89 years Zutphen, Netherlands The Zutphen Elderly Study (continuation of the Zutphen Study) Follow-up of 3 years	Dietary fatty acids
Ghadirian et al., 1998	Case-control	Cases = incident MS patients (n=197) Controls = from general population (n=202) Men and women Mean age of 42 years for male cases Mean age of 37.5 years for female cases Montreal, Canada	Seafood

Amount	Results	Conclusion*
Total energy, n-6 PUFA, n-3 PUFA, fish as continuous variables	No significant differences in the change in daily intake of total energy, n-6 PUFA, n-3 PUFA, or fish from 1985-1990 were found between those with normal and impaired cognitive function.	N
Tertiles of n-3 fatty acids intake: Low = 0.0-37.5 mg/day Medium = 37.5-155.5 mg/day High = 155.5-2110.5 mg/day	Those with normal cognitive function had significantly higher mean daily intakes of energy (p=0.03), DHA (p=0.05), and fish (p=0.02); and significantly lower mean daily intakes of total fat (p=0.02), total PUFA (p=0.002), and LA (p=0.006) than those with impaired cognitive function.	
	The adjusted OR for prevalent cognitive impairment are OR=1.09 (95% CI 0.65-1.80) for medium n-3 fatty acid intake and OR=0.96 (95% CI 0.57-1.62) for high n-3 fatty acid intake compared to the low n-3 fatty acid intake (p for trend = 0.9). They are not significant.	
	The adjusted OR for cognitive decline are OR=0.85 (95% CI 0.40-1.82) for medium n-3 fatty acid intake and OR=0.78 (95% CI 0.35-1.73) for high n-3 fatty acid intake compared to the low n-3 fatty acid intake (p for trend = 0.5). They are not significant.	
100 g increments of intake/day	After adjusting for total energy and BMI, every 100 g increase in daily fish intake decreases the risk of multiple sclerosis (OR=0.91, 95% CI 0.78-1.05). For males this statistic is 1.08 (95% CI 0.84-1.40), and for females this statistic is 0.83 (95% CI 0.69-1.00).	B (females only)

continued

TABLE B-2j Continued

Author	Study Type	Subjects	Exposure
Petridou et al., 1998	Case-control	Cases = with cerebral palsy (n=91) Controls = no cerebral palsy, from same study base as the cases (series1 = closest neighbor of similar sex and age as the case; series2 = first neurological patient seen by attending physicians after a visit by the case, with a healthy sibling of similar sex and age as the case) (n=246) Children Aged about 4-9 years Athens, Greece	Seafood

* N = Evidence of no association or no clear association; B = Evidence of a benefit.

Amount	Results	Conclusion*
Categories of fish/fish product intake: 1 = <1 time/week 2 = 1 time/week 3 = >1 time/week	After adjusting for age of child, sex, maternal age at delivery, maternal age at menarche, maternal chronic disease, previous spontaneous abortions, persistent vomiting during index pregnancy, multiple pregnancy, number of obstetric visits, timing of membrane rupture in relation to index delivery, use of general anaesthesia in the index delivery, mode of delivery, abnormal placenta, head circumference, evident congenital malformation, place of index delivery, use of supplementary Fe during index pregnancy, intentional physical exercise during index pregnancy, painless delivery classes, energy intake, cereals and starchy roots, sugars and syrups, pulses and nuts/seeds, vegetables, fruits, meat and meat products, milk and milk products, and oils and fats: Each one weekly serving increase in fish and fish products during pregnancy lowered the odds of having a child with cerebral palsy (OR=0.63, 95% CI 0.37-1.08, p=0.09), but this statistic was not significant.	N

REFERENCES

Agren JJ, Vaisanen S, Hanninen O. 1997. Hemostatic factors and platelet aggregation after a fish-enriched diet or fish oil or docosahexaenoic acid supplementation. *Prostaglandins Leukotrienes & Essential Fatty Acids* 57(4–5):419–421.

Albert CM, Hennekens CH, O'Donnell CJ, Ajani UA, Carey VJ, Willett WC, Ruskin JN, Manson JE. 1998. Fish consumption and risk of sudden cardiac death. *Journal of the American Medical Association* 279(1):23–28.

Albert CM, Campos H, Stampfer MJ, Ridker PM, Manson JE, Willett WC, Ma J. 2002. Blood levels of long-chain n-3 fatty acids and the risk of sudden death. *New England Journal of Medicine* 346(15):1113–1118.

Allen NE, Sauvaget C, Roddam AW, Appleby P, Nagano J, Suzuki G, Key TJ, Koyama K. 2004. A prospective study of diet and prostate cancer in Japanese men. *Cancer Causes Control* 15(9):911–920.

Appleby PN, Davey GK, Key TJ. 2002. Hypertension and blood pressure among meat eaters, fish eaters, vegetarians and vegans in EPIC-Oxford. *Public Health Nutrition* 5(5):645–654.

Ascherio A, Rimm EB, Stampfer MJ, Giovannucci EL, Willett WC. 1995. Dietary intake of marine n-3 fatty acids, fish intake, and the risk of coronary disease among men. *New England Journal of Medicine* 332(15):977–982.

Augustsson K, Michaud DS, Rimm EB, Leitzmann MF, Stampfer MJ, Willett WC, Giovannucci E. 2003. A prospective study of intake of fish and marine fatty acids and prostate cancer. *Cancer Epidemiology, Biomarkers, and Prevention* 12(1):64–67.

Baer DJ, Judd JT, Clevidence BA, Tracy RP. 2004. Dietary fatty acids affect plasma markers of inflammation in healthy men fed controlled diets: A randomized crossover study. *American Journal of Clinical Nutrition* 79(6):969–973.

Bang HO, Dyerberg J, Nielsen AB. 1971. Plasma lipid and lipoprotein pattern in Greenlandic West-coast Eskimos. *Lancet* 1(7710):1143–1145.

Barberger-Gateau P, Letenneur L, Deschamps V, Peres K, Dartigues J-F, Renaud S. 2002. Fish, meat, and risk of dementia: A cohort study. *British Medical Journal* 325(7370):932–933.

Bouzan C, Cohen JT, Connor WE, Kris-Etherton PM, Gray GM, Konig A, Lawrence RS, Savitz DA, Teutsch SM. 2005. A quantitative analysis of fish consumption and stroke risk. *American Journal of Preventive Medicine* 29(4):347–352.

Burr ML, Fehily AM, Gilbert JF, Rogers S, Holliday RM, Sweetnam PM, Elwood PC, Deadman NM. 1989. Effects of changes in fat, fish, and fibre intakes on death and myocardial reinfarction: Diet and reinfarction trial (DART). *Lancet* 2(8666):757–761.

Burr ML, Ashfield-Watt PAL, Dunstan FDJ, Fehily AM, Breay P, Ashton T, Zotos PC, Haboubi NAA, Elwood PC. 2003. Lack of benefit of dietary advice to men with angina: Results of a controlled trial. *European Journal of Clinical Nutrition* 57(2):193–200.

Burr ML, Dunstan FD, George CH. 2005. Is fish oil good or bad for heart disease? Two trials with apparently conflicting results. *Journal of Membrane Biology* 206(2):155–163.

Caicoya M. 2002. Fish consumption and stroke: A community case-control study in Asturias, Spain. *Neuroepidemiology* 21(3):107–114.

Calder PC. 2004. n-3 fatty acids and cardiovascular disease: Evidence explained and mechanisms explored. *Clinical Science* (London, England) 107(1):1–11.

Chen H, Zhang SM, Hernan MA, Willett WC, Ascherio A. 2003. Dietary intakes of fat and risk of Parkinson's disease. *American Journal of Epidemiology* 157(11):1007–1014.

Chiu BC, Cerhan JR, Folsom AR, Sellers TA, Kushi LH, Wallace RB, Zheng W, Potter JD. 1996. Diet and risk of non-Hodgkin lymphoma in older women. *Journal of the American Medical Association* 275(17):1315–1321.

Christensen JH, Gustenhoff P, Korup E, Aaroe, J, Toft E, Moller J, Rasmussen K, Dyerberg J, Schmidt EB. 1996. Effect of fish oil on heart rate variability in survivors of myocardial infarction: A double blind randomised controlled trial. *British Medical Journal* 312(7032):677–678.

Christensen JH, Korup E, Aaroe J, Toft E, Moller J, Rasmussen K, Dyerberg J, Schmidt EB. 1997. Fish consumption, n-3 fatty acids in cell membranes, and heart rate variability in survivors of myocardial infarction with left ventricular dysfunction. *American Journal of Cardiology* 79(12):1670–1673.

Christensen JH, Christensen MS, Dyerberg J, Schmidt EB. 1999. Heart rate variability and fatty acid content of blood cell membranes: A dose-response study with n-3 fatty acids. *American Journal of Clinical Nutrition* 70(3):331–337.

Chyou PH, Nomura AM, Stemmermann GN. 1993. A prospective study of diet, smoking, and lower urinary tract cancer. *Annals of Epidemiology* 3(3):211–216.

Chyou PH, Nomura AM, Stemmermann GN. 1995. Diet, alcohol, smoking and cancer of the upper aerodigestive tract: A prospective study among Hawaii Japanese men. *International Journal of Cancer* 60(5):616–621.

Cobiac L, Clifton PM, Abbey M, Belling GB, Nestel PJ. 1991. Lipid, lipoprotein, and hemostatic effects of fish vs. fish-oil n-3 fatty acids in mildly hyperlipidemic males. *American Journal of Clinical Nutrition* 53(5):1210–1216.

Daviglus ML, Stamler J, Orencia AJ, Dyer AR, Liu K, Greenland P, Walsh MK, Morris D, Shekelle RB. 1997. Fish consumption and the 30-year risk of fatal myocardial infarction. *New England Journal of Medicine* 336(15):1046–1053.

Dewailley E, Blanchet C, Lemieux S, Sauve L, Gingras S, Ayotte P, Holub BJ. 2001. n-3 fatty acids and cardiovascular disease risk factors among the Inuit of Nunavik. *American Journal of Clinical Nutrition* 74(4):464–473.

Dolecek TA. 1992. Epidemiological evidence of relationships between dietary polyunsaturated fatty acids and mortality in the multiple risk factor intervention trial. *Proceedings of the Society for Experimental Biology and Medicine* 200(2):177–182.

Dunstan DW, Mori TA, Puddey IB, Beilin LJ, Burke V, Morton AR, Stanton KG. 1997. The independent and combined effects of aerobic exercise and dietary fish intake on serum lipids and glycemic control in NIDDM. A randomized controlled study. *Diabetes Care* 20(6):913–921.

Dunstan DW, Mori TA, Puddey IB, Beilin LJ, Burke V, Morton AR, Stanton KG. 1999. A randomised, controlled study of the effects of aerobic exercise and dietary fish on coagulation and fibrinolytic factors in type 2 diabetics. *Thrombosis and Haemostasis* 81(3):367–372.

Dunstan JA, Mori TA, Barden A. 2003. Maternal fish oil supplementation in pregnancy reduces interleukin-13 levels in cord blood of infants at high risk of atopy. *Clinical and Experimental Allergy* 33(4):442–448.

English DR, MacInnis RJ, Hodge AM, Hopper JL, Haydon AM, Giles GG. 2004. Red meat, chicken, and fish consumption and risk of colorectal cancer. *Cancer Epidemiology, Biomarkers, and Prevention* 13(9):1509–1514.

Eritsland J, Arnesen H, Berg K. 1995. Serum Lp(a) lipoprotein levels in patients with coronary artery disease and the influence of long-term n-3 fatty acid supplementation. *Scandinavian Journal of Clinical & Laboratory Investigation* 55(4):295–300.

Folsom AR, Demissie Z. 2004. Fish intake, marine omega-3 fatty acids, and mortality in a cohort of postmenopausal women. *American Journal of Epidemiology* 160(10):1005–1010.

Fraser GE, Sabate J, Beeson WL, Strahan TM. 1992. A possible protective effect of nut consumption on risk of coronary heart disease. The Adventist Health Study. *Archives of Internal Medicine* 152(7):1416–1424.

Frost L, Vestergaard P. 2005. n-3 fatty acids consumed from fish and risk of atrial fibrillation or flutter: The Danish Diet, Cancer, and Health Study. *American Journal of Clinical Nutrition* 81(1):50–54.

Geleijnse JM, Giltay EJ, Grobbe DE, Donders AR, Kok FJ. 2002. Blood pressure response to fish oil supplementation: Metaregression analysis of randomized trials. *Journal of Hypertension* 20(8):1493–1499.

Ghadirian P, Jain M, Ducic S, Shatenstein B, Morisset R. 1998. Nutritional factors in the aetiology of multiple sclerosis: A case-control study in Montreal, Canada. *International Journal of Epidemiology* 27(5):845–852.

Gillum RF, Mussolino ME, Madans JH. 1996. The relationship between fish consumption and stroke incidence. The NHANES I Epidemiologic Follow-up Study (National Health and Nutrition Examination Survey). *Archives of Internal Medicine* 156(5):537–542.

Gillum RF, Mussolino M, Madans JH. 2000. The relation between fish consumption, death from all causes, and incidence of coronary heart disease. The NHANES I Epidemiologic Follow-up Study. *Journal of Clinical Epidemiology* 53(3):237–244.

Giovannucci E, Rimm EB, Stampfer MJ, Colditz GA, Ascherio A, Willett WC. 1994. Intake of fat, meat, and fiber in relation to risk of colon cancer in men. *Cancer Research* 54(9):2390–2397.

GISSI Study Investigators. 1999. Dietary supplementation with n-3 polyunsaturated fatty acids and vitamin E after myocardial infarction: Results of the GISSI-Prevenzione trial. Gruppo Italiano per lo Studio della Sopravvivenza nell'Infarto miocardico. *Lancet* 354(9177):447–455.

Goldbohm RA, van den Brandt PA, van 't Veer P, Brants HA, Dorant E, Sturmans F, Hermus RJ. 1994. A prospective cohort study on the relation between meat consumption and the risk of colon cancer. *Cancer Research* 54(3):718–723.

Gramenzi A, Gentile A, Fasoli M, Negri E, Parazzini F, La Vecchia C. 1990. Association between certain foods and risk of acute myocardial infarction in women. *British Medical Journal* 300(6727):771–773.

Grundt H, Nilsen DW, Hetland O, Aarsland T, Baksaas I, Grande T, Woie L. 1995. Improvement of serum lipids and blood pressure during intervention with n-3 fatty acids was not associated with changes in insulin levels in subjects with combined hyperlipidaemia. *Journal of Internal Medicine* 237(3):249–259.

Hanninen OO, Agren JJ, Laitinen MV, Jaaskelainen IO, Penttila IM. 1989. Dose-response relationships in blood lipids during moderate freshwater fish diet. *Annals of Medicine* 21(3):203–207.

Harper CR, Jacobson TA. 2005. Usefulness of omega-3 fatty acids and the prevention of coronary heart disease. *American Journal of Cardiology* 96(11):1521–1929.

He K, Rimm EB, Merchant A, Rosner BA, Stampfer MJ, Willett WC, Ascherio A. 2002. Fish consumption and risk of stroke in men. *Journal of the American Medical Association* 288(24):3130–3136.

He K, Song Y, Daviglus ML, Liu K, Van Horn L, Dyer AR, Goldbourt U, Greenland P. 2004a. Fish consumption and incidence of stroke: A meta-analysis of cohort studies. *Stroke* 35(7):1538–1542.

He K, Song Y, Daviglus ML, Liu K, Van Horn L, Dyer AR, Greenland P. 2004b. Accumulated evidence on fish consumption and coronary heart disease mortality: A meta-analysis of cohort studies. *Circulation* 109(22):2705–2711.

Holmes MD, Colditz GA, Hunter DJ, Hankinson SE, Rosner B, Speizer FE, Willett WC. 2003. Meat, fish and egg intake and risk of breast cancer. *International Journal of Cancer* 104(2):221–227.

Hooper L, Thompson RL, Harrison RA, Summerbell CD, Moore H, Worthington HV, Durrington PN, Ness AR, Capps NE, Davey Smith G, Riemersma RA, Ebrahim SB. 2005. Omega 3 fatty acids for prevention and treatment of cardiovascular disease. *Cochrane Database of Systematic Reviews* (4):CD003177.

Hooper L, Thompson RL, Harrison RA, Summerbell CD, Ness AR, Moore HJ, Worthington HV, Durrington PN, Higgins JPT, Capps NE, Riemersma RA, Ebrahim SBJ, Davey-Smith G. 2006. Risks and benefits of omega 3 fats for mortality, cardiovascular disease, and cancer: Systematic review. *British Medical Journal* 332(7544):752–760.

Hu FB, Bronner L, Willett WC, Stampfer MJ, Rexrode KM, Albert CM, Hunter D, Manson JE. 2002. Fish and omega-3 fatty acid intake and risk of coronary heart disease in women. *Journal of the Amercian Medical Association* 287(14):1815–1821.

Huang SL, Lin KC, Pan WH. 2001. Dietary factors associated with physician-diagnosed asthma and allergic rhinitis in teenagers: Analyses of the first Nutrition and Health Survey in Taiwan. *Clinical Exposures and Allergy* 31(2):259–264.

Iso H, Rexrode KM, Stampfer MJ, Manson JE, Colditz GA, Speizer FE, Hennekens CH, Willett WC. 2001. Intake of fish and omega-3 fatty acids and risk of stroke in women. *Journal of the American Medical Association* 285(3):304–312.

Iso H, Kobayashi M, Ishihara J, Sasaki S, Okada K, Kita Y, Kokubo Y, Tsugane S. 2006. Intake of fish and n3 fatty acids and risk of coronary heart disease among Japanese: The Japan Public Health Center-Based (JPHC) Study Cohort I. *Circulation* 113(2):195–202.

Jamrozik K, Broadhurst RJ, Anderson CS, Stewart-Wynne EG. 1994. The role of lifestyle factors in the etiology of stroke. A population-based case-control study in Perth, Western Australia. *Stroke* 25(1):51–59.

Kalmijn S, Feskens EJ, Launer LJ, Kromhout D. 1997a. Polyunsaturated fatty acids, antioxidants, and cognitive function in very old men. *American Journal of Epidemiology* 145(1):33–41.

Kalmijn S, Launer LJ, Ott A, Witteman JC, Hofman A, Breteler MM. 1997b. Dietary fat intake and the risk of incident dementia in the Rotterdam Study. *Annals of Neurology* 42(5):776–782.

Kato I, Akhmedkhanov A, Koenig K, Toniolo PG, Shore RE, Riboli E. 1997. Prospective study of diet and female colorectal cancer: The New York University Women's Health Study. *Nutrition and Cancer* 28(3):276–281.

Keli SO, Feskens EJM, Kromhout D. 1994. Fish consumption and risk of stroke: The Zutphen study. *Stroke* 25(2):328–332.

Kesavulu MM, Kameswararao B, Apparao CH, Kumar EG, Harinarayan CV. 2002. Effect of omega-3 fatty acids on lipid peroxidation and antioxidant enzyme status in type 2 diabetic patients. *Diabetes and Metabolism* 28(1):20–26.

Key TJ, Sharp GB, Appleby PN, Beral V, Goodman MT, Soda M, Mabuchi K. 1999. Soya foods and breast cancer risk: A prospective study in Hiroshima and Nagasaki, Japan. *British Journal of Cancer* 81(7):1248–1256.

Konig A, Bouzan C, Cohen JT, Connor WE, Kris-Etherton PM, Gray GM, Lawrence RS, Savitz DA, Teutsch SM. 2005. A quantitative analysis of fish consumption and coronary heart disease mortality. *American Journal of Preventive Medicine* 29(4):335–346.

Kromann N, Green A. 1980. Epidemiological studies in the Upernavik district, Greenland. Incidence of some chronic diseases 1950–1974. *Acta Medica Scandinavica* 208(5):401–406.

Kromhout D, Bosschieter EB, de Lezenne Coulander C. 1985. The inverse relation between fish consumption and 20-year mortality from coronary heart disease. *New England Journal of Medicine* 312(19):1205–1209.

Kromhout D, Feskens EJ, Bowles CH. 1995. The protective effect of a small amount of fish on coronary heart disease mortality in an elderly population. *International Journal of Epidemiology* 24(2):340–345.

Kvale G, Bjelke E, Gart JJ. 1983. Dietary habits and lung cancer risk. *International Journal of Cancer* 31(4):397–405.

Larsson SC, Kumlin M, Ingelman-Sundberg M, Wolk A. 2004. Dietary long-chain n-3 fatty acids for the prevention of cancer: A review of potential mechanisms. *American Journal of Clinical Nutrition* 79(6):935–945.

Le Marchand L, Kolonel LN, Wilkens LR, Myers BC, Hirohata T. 1994. Animal fat consumption and prostate cancer: A prospective study in Hawaii. *Epidemiology* 5(3):276–282.

Leaf A, Kang JX, Xiao Y-F, Billman GE. 2003. Clinical prevention of sudden cardiac death by n-3 polyunsaturated fatty acids and mechanism of prevention of arrhythmias by n-3 fish oils. *Circulation* 107(21):2646–2652.

Leaf A, Albert CM, Josephson M, Steinhaus, Kluger J, Kang JX, Cox B, Zhang H, Schoenfeld D. 2005. Prevention of fatal arrhythmias in high-risk subjects by fish oil n-3 fatty acid intake. *Circulation* 112(18):2762–2768.

Leng GC, Lee AJ, Fowkes FG, Jepson RG, Lowe GD, Skinner ER, Mowat BF. 1998. Randomized controlled trial of gamma-linolenic acid and eicosapentaenoic acid in peripheral arterial disease. *Clinical Nutrition* 17(6):265–271.

Lou J, Tizkalla SW, Vidal H. 1998. Moderate intake of n-3 fatty acids for 2 months has no detrimental effect on glucose metabolism and could ameliorate the lipid profile in type 2 diabetic men: Results of a controlled study. *Diabetes Care* 21(5):717–724.

MacLean CH, Newberry SJ, Mojica WA, Khanna P, Issa AM, Suttorp MJ, Lim YW, Traina SB, Hilton L, Garland R, Morton SC. 2006. Effects of omega-3 fatty acids on cancer risk: A systematic review. *Journal of the American Medical Association* 295(4):403–415.

Madsen T, Skou HA, Hansen VE, Fog L, Christensen JH, Toft E, Schmidt EB. 2001. C-reactive protein, dietary n-3 fatty acids, and the extent of coronary artery disease. *American Journal of Cardiology* 88(10):1139–1142.

Mann JI, Appleby PN, Key TJ, Thorogood M. 1997. Dietary determinants of ischaemic heart disease in health conscious individuals. *Heart* 78(5):450–455.

Marchioli R, Barzi F, Bomba E, Chieffo C, Di Gregorio D, Di Mascio R, Franzosi MG, Geraci E, Levantesi G, Maggioni AP, Mantini L, Marfisi RM, Mastrogiuseppe G, Mininni N, Nicolosi GL, Santini M, Schweiger C, Tavazzi L, Tognoni G, Tucci C, Valagussa F. 2002. Early protection against sudden death by n-3 polyunsaturated fatty acids after myocardial infarction: Time-course analysis of the results of the Gruppo Italiano per lo Studio della Sopravvivenza nell'Infarto Miocardico (GISSI)-Prevenzione. *Circulation* 105(16):1897–1903.

Marckmann P, Gronbaek M. 1999. Fish consumption and coronary heart disease mortality. A systematic review of prospective cohort studies. *European Journal of Clinical Nutrition* 53(8):585–590.

Martinez-Gonzalez MA, Fernandez-Jarne E, Serrano-Martinez M, Marti A, Martinez JA, Martin-Moreno JM. 2002. Mediterranean diet and reduction in the risk of a first acute myocardial infarction: An operational healthy dietary score. *European Journal of Nutrition* 41(4):153–160.

Mills PK, Beeson WL, Phillips RL, Fraser GE. 1989. Cohort study of diet, lifestyle, and prostate cancer in Adventist men. *Cancer* 64(3):598–604.

Mori TA, Vandongen R, Beilin LJ, Burke V, Morris J, Ritchie J.1994. Effects of varying dietary fat, fish and fish oils on blood lipids in a randomized controlled trial in men at risk of heart disease. *American Journal of Clinical Nutrition* 59(5):1060–1068.

Mori TA, Bao DQ, Burke V. 1999. Dietary fish as a major component of a weight-loss diet: Effect on serum lipids, glucose, and insulin metabolism in overweight hypertensive subjects. *American Journal of Clinical Nutrition* 70(5):817–825.

Morris MC, Manson JE, Rosner B, Buring JE, Willett WC, Hennekens CH. 1995. Fish consumption and cardiovascular disease in the physicians' health study: A prospective study. *American Journal of Epidemiology* 142(2):166–175.

Morris MC, Evans DA, Bienias JL, Tangney CC, Bennett DA, Wilson RS, Aggarwal N, Schneider J. 2003. Consumption of fish and n-3 fatty acids and risk of incident Alzheimer disease. *Archives of Neurology* 60(7):940–946.

Mozaffarian D, Lemaitre RN, Kuller LH, Burke GL, Tracy RP, Siscovick DS, Cardiovascular Health Study team. 2003. Cardiac benefits of fish consumption may depend on the type of fish meal consumed: The Cardiovascular Health Study. *Circulation* 107(10):1372–1377.

Mozaffarian D, Psaty BM, Rimm EB, Lemaitre RN, Burke GL, Lyles MF, Lefkowitz D, Siscovick DS. 2004. Fish intake and risk of incident atrial fibrillation. *Circulation* 110(4):368–373.

Mozaffarian D, Longstreth WT Jr, Lemaitre RN, Manolio TA, Kuller LH, Burke GL, Siscovick DS. 2005. Fish consumption and stroke risk in elderly individuals: The cardiovascular health study. *Archives of Internal Medicine* 165(2):200–206. Erratum in: *Archives of Internal Medicine* 165(6):683.

Nagata C, Takatsuka N, Shimizu H. 2002. Soy and fish oil intake and mortality in a Japanese community. *American Journal of Epidemiology* 156(9):824–831.

Ness AR, Whitley E, Burr ML, Elwood PC, Smith GD, Ebrahim S. 1999. The long-term effect of advice to eat more fish on blood pressure in men with coronary disease: Results from the Diet and Reinfarction Trial. *Journal of Human Hypertension* 13(11):729–733.

Ness AR, Hughes J, Elwood PC, Whitley E, Smith GD, Burr ML. 2002. The long-term effect of dietary advice in men with coronary disease: Follow-up of the Diet and Reinfarction trial (DART). *European Journal of Clinical Nutrition* 56(6):512–518.

Ngoan LT, Mizoue T, Fujino Y, Tokui N, Yoshimura T. 2002. Dietary factors and stomach cancer mortality. *British Journal of Cancer* 87(1):37–42.

Nilsen DW, Albrektsen G, Landmark K, Moen S, Aarsland T, Woie L. 2001. Effects of a high-dose concentrate of n-3 fatty acids or corn oil introduced early after an acute myocardial infarction on serum triacylglycerol and HDL cholesterol. *American Journal of Clinical Nutrition* 74(1):50–56.

Norat T, Bingham S, Ferrari P, Slimani N, Jenab M, Mazuir M, Overvad K, Olsen A, Tjonneland A, Clavel F, Boutron-Ruault MC, Kesse E, Boeing H, Bergmann MM, Nieters A, Linseisen J, Trichopoulou A, Trichopoulos D, Tountas Y, Berrino F, Palli D, Panico S, Tumino R, Vineis P, Bueno-de-Mesquita HB, Peeters PH, Engeset D, Lund E, Skeie G, Ardanaz E, Gonzalez C, Navarro C, Quiros JR, Sanchez MJ, Berglund G, Mattisson I, Hallmans G, Palmqvist R, Day NE, Khaw KT, Key TJ, San Joaquin M, Hemon B, Saracci R, Kaaks R, Riboli E. 2005. Meat, fish, and colorectal cancer risk: The European Prospective Investigation into cancer and nutrition. *Journal of the National Cancer Institute* 97(12):906–916.

Oomen CM, Feskens EJ, Rasanen L, Fidanza F, Nissinen AM, Menotti A, Kok FJ, Kromhout D. 2000. Fish consumption and coronary heart disease mortality in Finland, Italy, and The Netherlands. *American Journal of Epidemiology* 151(10):999–1006.

Orencia AJ, Daviglus ML, Dyer AR, Shekelle RB, Stamler J. 1996. Fish consumption and stroke in men. 30-year findings of the Chicago Western Electric Study. *Stroke* 27(2):204–209.

Osler M, Andreasen AH, Hoidrup S. 2003. No inverse association between fish consumption and risk of death from all-causes, and incidence of coronary heart disease in middle-aged, Danish adults. *Journal of Clinical Epidemiology* 56(3):274–279.

Ozasa K, Watanabe Y, Ito Y, Suzuki K, Tamakoshi A, Seki N, Nishino Y, Kondo T, Wakai K, Ando M, Ohno Y. 2001. Dietary habits and risk of lung cancer death in a large-scale cohort study (JACC Study) in Japan by sex and smoking habit. *Japanese Journal of Cancer Research* 92(12):1259–1269.

Pan SY, Ugnat AM, Mao Y, Wen SW, Johnson KC. 2004. A case-control study of diet and the risk of ovarian cancer. *Cancer Epidemiology, Biomarkers, & Prevention* 13(9):1521–1527.

Petridou E, Koussouri M, Toupadaki N, Youroukos S, Papavassiliou A, Pantelakis S, Olsen J, Trichopoulos D. 1998. Diet during pregnancy and the risk of cerebral palsy. *British Journal of Nutrition* 79(5):407–412.

Raitt MH, Connor WE, Morris C, Kron J, Halperin B, Chugh SS, McClelland J, Cook J, MacMurdy K, Swenson R, Connor SL, Gerhard G, Kraemer DF, Oseran D, Marchant C, Calhoun D, Shnider R, McAnulty J. 2005. Fish oil supplementation and risk of ventricular tachycardia and ventricular fibrillation in patients with implantable defibrillators: A randomized controlled trial. *Journal of the American Medical Association* 293(23):2884–2891.

Rodriguez BL, Sharp DS, Abbott RD, Burchfiel CM, Masaki K, Chyou PH, Huang B, Yano K, Curb JD. 1996. Fish intake may limit the increase in risk of coronary heart disease morbidity and mortality among heavy smokers. The Honolulu Heart Program. *Circulation* 94(5):952–956.

Sacks FM, Stone PH, Gibson CM, Silverman DI, Rosner B, Pasternak RC. 1995. Controlled trial of fish oil for regression of human coronary atherosclerosis. HARP Research Group. *Journal of the American College of Cardiology* 25(7):1492–1498.

Salonen JT, Seppanen K, Nyyssonen K, Korpela H, Kauhanen J, Kantola M, Tuomilehto J, Esterbauer H, Tatzber F, Salonen R. 1995. Intake of mercury from fish, lipid peroxidation, and the risk of myocardial infarction and coronary, cardiovascular, and any death in eastern Finnish men. *Circulation* 91(3):645–655.

Sasazuki S. 2001. Case-control study of nonfatal myocardial infarction in relation to selected foods in Japanese men and women. *Japanese Circulation Journal* 65(3):200–206.

Sauvaget C, Nagano J, Allen N, Grant EJ, Beral V. 2003. Intake of animal products and stroke mortality in the Hiroshima/Nagasaki Life Span Study. *International Journal of Epidemiology* 32(4):536–543.

Schaefer EJ, Lichtenstein AH, Lamon-Fava S. 1996. Effects of National Cholesterol Education Program Step 2 diets relatively high or relatively low in fish derived fatty acids on plasma lipoproteins in middle aged and elderly subjects. *American Journal of Clinical Nutrition* 63(2):234–241.

Singh RB, Niaz MA, Sharma JP, Kumar R, Rastogi V, Moshiri M. 1997. Randomized, double-blind, placebo-controlled trial of fish oil and mustard oil in patients with suspected acute myocardial infarction: The Indian experiment of infarct survival—4. *Cardiovascular Drugs Therapy* 11(3):485–491.

Sirtori CR, Crepaldi G, Manzato E, Mancini M, Rivellese A, Paoletti R, Pazzucconi F, Pamparana F, Stragliotto E. 1998. One-year treatment with ethyl esters of n-3 fatty acids in patients with hypertriglyceridemia and glucose tolerance: Reduced triglyceride, total cholesterol and increased HDL-C without glycemic alterations. *Atherosclerosis* 137(2):419–427.

Siscovick DS, Raghunathan TE, King I, Weinmann S, Wicklund KG, Albright J, Bovbjerg V, Arbogast P, Smith H, Kushi LH, Cobb LA, Copass MK, Psaty BM, Lemaitre R, Retzlaff B, Childs M, Knopp RH. 1995. Dietary intake and cell membrane levels of long-chain n-3 polyunsaturated fatty acids and the risk of primary cardiac arrest. *Journal of the American Medical Association* 274(17):1363–1367.

Skerrett PJ, Hennekens CH. 2003. Consumption of fish and fish oils and decreased risk of stroke. *Preventive Cardiology* 6(1):38–41.

Stolzenberg-Solomon RZ, Pietinen P, Taylor PR, Virtamo J, Albanes D. 2002. Prospective study of diet and pancreatic cancer in male smokers. *American Journal of Epidemiology* 155(9):783–792.

Stripp C, Overvad K, Christensen J, Thomsen BL, Olsen A, Moller S, Tjonneland A. 2003. Fish intake is positively associated with breast cancer incidence rate. *Journal of Nutrition* 133(11):3664–3669.

Takezaki T, Inoue M, Kataoka H, Ikeda S, Yoshida M, Ohashi Y, Tajima K, Tominaga S. 2003. Diet and lung cancer risk from a 14-year population-based prospective study in Japan: With special reference to fish consumption. *Nutrition and Cancer* 45(2):160–167.

Tavani A, Pelucchi C, Negri E, Bertuzzi M, La Vecchia C. 2001. n-3 polyunsaturated fatty acids, fish, and nonfatal acute myocardial infarction. *Circulation* 104(19):2269–2272.

Terry P, Lichtenstein P, Feychting M, Ahlbom A, Wolk A. 2001. Fatty fish consumption and risk of prostate cancer. *Lancet* 357(9270):1764–1766.

Terry PD, Rohan TE, Wolk A. 2003. Intakes of fish and marine fatty acids and the risks of cancers of the breast and prostate and of other hormone-related cancers: A review of the epidemiologic evidence. *American Journal of Clinical Nutrition* 77(3):532–543.

Troisi RJ, Willett WC, Weiss ST. 1995. A prospective study of diet and adult-onset asthma. *American Journal of Respiratory Critical Care* 151(5):1401–1408.

Vandongen R, Mori TA, Burke V, Beilin LJ, Morris J, Ritchie J. 1993. Effects on blood pressure of omega 3 fats in subjects at increased risk of cardiovascular disease. *Hypertension* 22(3):371–379.

Vatten LJ, Solvoll K, Loken EB. 1990. Frequency of meat and fish intake and risk of breast cancer in a prospective study of 14,500 Norwegian women. *International Journal of Cancer* 46(1):12–15.

Veierod MB, Laake P, Thelle DS. 1997. Dietary fat intake and risk of lung cancer: A prospective study of 51,452 Norwegian men and women. *European Journal of Cancer Prevention* 6(6):540–549.

Vericel E, Calzada C, Chapuy P, Lagarde M. 1999. The influence of low intake of n-3 fatty acids on platelets in elderly people. *Atherosclerosis* 147(1):187–192.

Whelton SP, He J, Whelton PK, Muntner P. 2004. Meta-analysis of observational studies on fish intake and coronary heart disease. *American Journal of Cardiology* 93(9):1119–1123.

Willett WC, Stampfer MJ, Colditz GA, Rosner BA, Speizer FE. 1990. Relation of meat, fat, and fiber intake to the risk of colon cancer in a prospective study among women. *New England Journal of Medicine* 323(24):1664–1672.

Yuan JM, Ross RK, Gao YT, Yu MC. 2001. Fish and shellfish consumption in relation to death from myocardial infarction among men in Shanghai, China. *American Journal of Epidemiology* 154(9):809–816.

Zhang J, Sasaki S, Amano K, Kesteloot H. 1999. Fish consumption and mortality from all causes, ischemic heart disease, and stroke: An ecological study. *Preventive Medicine* 28(5):520–529.

Zhang SM, Willett WC, Hernan MA, Olek MJ, Ascherio A. 2000. Dietary fat in relation to risk of multiple sclerosis among two large cohorts of women. *American Journal of Epidemiology* 152(11):1056–1064.

Recommendations for Seafood and EPA/DHAConsumption

TABLE B-3 Recommendations for Seafood and EPA/DHA Consumption

Organization	Audience	Purpose of Recommendtion
American Heart Association	Healthy adults (without documented coronary heart disease)	Reduce cardiovascular disease by dietary and lifestyle facts among the general population
American Heart Association	People with documented heart disease	Secondary prevention
American Heart Association	People with elevated triglycerides	Lower triglycerides
Dietary Guidelines Advisory Committee	Unspecified	Provide sound and current dietary guidelines to consumers
MyPyramid	Americans	Help Americans make healthy food choices, given their sex, age, and activity level
National Cholesterol Education Program, National Heart, Lung, and Blood Institute	People with high LDL-cholesterol/those adopting therapeutic lifestyle changes (TLC)	Healthy lifestyle recommendation for a healthy heart
American Diabetes Association	Unspecified	Lower risk of diabetes, and protect your heart and blood vessels
World Health Organization	Unspecified	To protect against coronary heart disease and ischaemic stroke
European Society of Cardiology	General population	To offer advice on food choices to compose a diet associated with the lowest risk of cardiovascular disease
United Kingdom Scientific Advisory Committee on Nutrition	General population and pregnant women	To reduce risk of cardiovascular disease
European Food Safety Authority	Unspecified	Reach daily intake for LC n-3 PUFA recommended for potential benefits to health
National Heart Foundation of Australia	People with coronary heart disease	Preventing cardiovascular events

Recommendations

Type of Fish/Seafood	Serving size	# of Servings
All fish, particularly fatty fish (salmon, albacore tuna, mackerel, lake trout, herring, and sardines)	3 ounces cooked (or 4 ounces raw)	Two per week
EPA+DHA per day, preferably from fatty fish; supplements can be considered with physician consultation	1 gram EPA+DHA	One per day
EPA+DHA per day as a capsule with physician consultation	2-4 grams EPA+DHA	One per day
Fish, especially salmon, trout, white (albacore or bluefin) tuna, mackerel, or other fish that are high in EPA and DHA	4 ounces	Two per week
Fish rich in omega-3 fatty acids, such as salmon, trout, and herring	Not specified	More often
Fish, type unspecified	≤5 ounces	One per day
Fish	Not specified	2–3 per week
Fish, type unspecified	Equivalent to 200–500 mg of EPA+DHA	1–2 per week
Fish, particularly oily fish	Not specified	Consumption encouraged
Fish	Not specified	Two per week, one of which should be oil fish (≈450 mg/day of LCPUFA)
Fish, especially fatty fish	130 grams	1–2 per week
Fish, preferably oily fish	Unspecified	At least 2 per week

FDA and EPA Safety Levels in Regulations and Guidance

TABLE B-4 FDA and US EPA Safety Levels in Regulations and Guidance

Product	Level	Reference
Ready-to-eat fishery products (minimal cooking by consumer)	Enterotoxigenic *Escherichia coli* (ETEC)—1×10^3 ETEC/gram, LT or ST positive.	Compliance Program 7303.842
Ready-to-eat fishery products (minimal cooking by consumer)	*Listeria monocytogenes*—presence of organism.	Compliance Program 7303.842
All fish	*Salmonella* species—presence of organism.	Sec 555.300 Compliance Policy Guide
All fish	1. *Staphylococcus aureus*—positive for staphylococcal enterotoxin, or 2. *Staphylococcus aureus* level is equal to or greater than 10^4/gram (MPN).	Compliance Program 7303.842
Ready-to-eat fishery products (minimal cooking by consumer)	*Vibrio cholerae*—presence of toxigenic 01 or non-01.	Compliance Program 7303.842
Ready-to-eat fishery products (minimal cooking by consumer)	*Vibrio parahaemolyticus*—levels equal to or greater than 1×10^4/gram (Kanagawa positive or negative).	Compliance Program 7303.842
Ready-to-eat fishery products (minimal cooking by consumer)	*Vibrio vulnificus*—presence of pathogenic organism.	Compliance Program 7303.842
All fish	*Clostridium botulinum*— 1. Presence of viable spores or vegetative cells in products that will support their growth, or 2. Presence of toxin.	Compliance Program 7303.842
Clams and oysters, fresh or frozen—imports	Microbiological— 1. *E. coli*—MPN of 230/100 grams (average of subs or 3 or more of 5 subs); 2. APC—500,000/gram (average of subs or 3 or more of 5 subs).	Sec 560.600 Compliance Policy Guide

continued

TABLE B-4 Continued

Product	Level	Reference
Clams, oysters, and mussels, fresh or frozen—domestic	Microbiological— 1. *E. coli* or fecal coliform—1 or more of 5 subs exceeding MPN of 330/100 grams or 2 or more exceeding 230/100 grams; 2. APC—1 or more of 5 subs exceeding 1,500,000/gram or 2 or more exceeding 500,000/gram.	Compliance Program 7303.842
Salt-cured, air-dried uneviscerated fish	Not permitted in commerce (Note: small fish exemption).	Sec 540.650 Compliance Policy Guide
Tuna, mahi mahi, and related fish	Histamine—500 ppm based on toxicity. 50 ppm defect action level, because histamine is generally not uniformly distributed in a decomposed fish. Therefore, 50 ppm is found in one section, there is the possibility that other units may exceed 500 ppm.	Sec 540.525 Compliance Policy Guide
All fish	Polychlorinated Biphenyls (PCBs)—2 ppm (edible portion).[a]	21 CFR 109.30
Fin fish and shellfish	Aldrin and dieldrin—0.3 ppm (edible portion).	Sec 575.100 Compliance Policy Guide
Frog legs	Benzene hexachloride—0.3 ppm (edible portion).	Sec 575.100 Compliance Policy Guide
All fish	Chlordane—0.3 ppm (edible portion).	Sec 575.100 Compliance Policy Guide
All fish	Chlordecone—0.4 ppm crabmeat and 0.3 ppm in other fish (edible portion).	Sec 575.100 Compliance Policy Guide
All fish	DDT, TDE, and DDE—5 ppm (edible portion).	Sec 575.100 Compliance Policy Guide
All fish	Heptachlor and heptachlor epoxide—0.3 ppm (edible portion).	Sec 575.100 Compliance Policy Guide
All fish	Mirex—0.1 ppm (edible portion).	Sec 575.100 Compliance Policy Guide
All fish	Diquat—0.1 ppm.[a]	40 CFR 180.226

continued

TABLE B-4 Continued

Product	Level	Reference
Fin fish and crayfish	Fluridone—0.5 ppm.[a]	40 CFR 180.420
Fin fish	Glyphosate—0.25 ppm.[a]	40 CFR 180.364
Shellfish	Glyphosate—3 ppm.[a]	40 CFR 180.364
Fin fish	Simazine—12 ppm.[a]	40 CFR 180.213a
All fish	2,4-D—1 ppm.[a]	40 CFR 180.142
Salmonids, catfish, and lobster	Oxytetracycline—2 ppm.	21 CFR 556.500
All fish	Sulfamerazine—no residue permitted.	21 CFR 556.660
Salmonids and catfish	Sulfadimethoxine/ormetoprim combination—0.1 ppm.	21 CFR 556.640
All fish	Unsanctioned drugs[b]—no residue permitted.	Sec 615.200 Compliance Policy Guide
Crustacea	Toxic elements: 76 ppm arsenic; 3 ppm cadmium; 12 ppm chromium; 1.5 ppm lead; 70 ppm nickel.	FDA Guidance Documents
Clams, oysters, and mussels	Toxic elements: 86 ppm arsenic; 4 ppm cadmium; 13 ppm chromium; 1.7 ppm lead; 80 ppm nickel.	FDA Guidance Documents
All fish	Methyl mercury—1 ppm.[c]	Sec 540.600 Compliance Policy Guide
All fish	Paralytic shellfish poison—0.8 ppm (80 µg/100 g) saxitoxin equivalent.	Sec 540.250 Compliance Policy Guide, and Compliance Program 7303.842
Clams, mussels and oysters, fresh, frozen or canned	Neurotoxic shellfish poison—0.8 ppm (20 mouse units/100 grams) brevetoxin-2 equivalent.	National Shellfish Sanitation Program Manual of Operations
All fish	Amnesic shellfish poison—20 ppm domoic acid, except in the viscera of dungeness crab, where 30 ppm is permitted.	Compliance Program 7303.842
All fish	Hard or sharp foreign object—generally 0.3 (7 mm) to 1.0 (25 mm) in length.	Sec 555.425 Compliance Policy Guide

[a]These values are tolerances;

[b]Sanctioned drugs are approved drugs and drugs used under an INAD;

[c]The term "fish" refers to fresh or saltwater fin fish, crustaceans, other forms of aquatic animal life other than birds or mammals, and all mollusks, as defined in 21 CFR 123.3(d) (FDA, 2005c).

SOURCE: CFSAN, 2001.

C

Tables and Scenarios

BOX C-1
A Case Scenario—The Pregnant Woman[a]

Pregnant women are advised of the potential advantage to their fetuses of EPA/DHA and other nutrients that seafood contains, as well as the potential consequences of exposure to toxicants (both microbiological and environmental). How do pregnant women balance these issues?

A woman establishes her food choices early in life and continues this pattern as she matures (*trajectory*). Pregnancy is a major transition in a woman's life. If this is her first pregnancy, the woman may rely on her family, her partner, medical professionals, and other authorities to provide information upon which to base her food choices (reflecting *cultural influences* and *linked lives*). If she has been pregnant before, she can base her decisions on her previous experience. If new information has been released since her last pregnancy (e.g., a seafood advisory), she may be unaware of the emerging issues (*contextual influences* and *timing in lives*) or she could consider them irrelevant to her own situation. Prior to making her food choices, she may make conscious decisions regarding which foods to eat or to avoid (*adaptive strategies*). For example, a woman who has eaten shrimp as her primary seafood choice throughout her life might consider choosing salmon during her pregnancy. If she was raised on local fish in Wyoming but moved to Michigan at the start of her pregnancy, she might cease to eat any fish (local or otherwise) in response to fish advisories.

---

[a]Italicized words reflect key concepts of the Life Course Perspective (Wethington, 2005; Devine, 2005).

TABLE C-1 Selected Theoretical Models Describing Health Behavior, Food Choice, and Behavior Change

Theory	Brief Description
Health Belief Model (Rosenstock, 1974)	Assumes individuals will protect their health if they think they are susceptible to the threat, believe that if they change behaviors they can reduce the threat (with benefits outweighing barriers), and that they are able to make the change.
Life Course Perspective (Wethington, 2005)	Key concepts: • trajectories (stable patterns of behavior over time); • transitions (changes in social responsibilities and roles); • turning points (major life events); • cultural and contextual influences (environmental events that shape and constrain change and adaptation); • timing in lives (interaction between the timing of the event and the age/stage of the life course); • linked lives (dependence of one person on another); and • adaptive strategies (conscious decisions)
Optimistic Bias (Shepard, 1999) (Weinstein, 1987)	Underestimation of the risk to oneself relative to others.
PEN-3 (Airhihenbuwa, 1995)	Consists of three interrelated and interdependent dimensions of health: health education diagnosis (identification of the target audience); education diagnosis of health behavior (exploration of target audience's supporting factors and beliefs); and cultural appropriateness of the health behavior (both positive and negative).
Transtheoretical Model (Stages of Change) (Prochaska, 1995) (Prochaska and Vellicer, 1997) (Weinstein et al., 1998)	Integrates a variety of theories (transtheoretical) to both describe progression of changes and to explain associated behaviors necessary to achieve change. Stages include: • *Precontemplation* (time when an individual is not considering or not aware that change is needed); • *Contemplation* (time when an individual is aware of a problem and is considering action to resolve it); • *Preparation* (time when an individual commits to taking action); • *Action* (time when effort is noted); • *Maintenance* (time when a person tries to stabilize the change); • *Termination* (time when no temptation to revert back to old behavior).

TABLE C-2 Processes of Change

Processes	Description
Thinking and Feeling Processes Occurring in *Precontemplation, Contemplation, Preparation, and Maintenance*	
Consciousness raising	Increases information, feedback and understanding about self and problem
Dramatic relief	Expresses and experiences feelings about one's problems and solutions
Self-reevaluation	Assesses one's feelings about oneself with respect to problem
Self-liberation	Consciously chooses and commits to act; believes in ability to change
Social liberation	Increases available alternatives for non-problem societal behaviors
Environmental reevaluation	Assesses how one's problems affect physical condition and social environment
Doing and Reinforcing Processes Occurring in *Preparation, Action, and Maintenance*	
Helping relationships	Is open and trusting about one's problems with someone who cares
Reinforcement management	Rewards self for making changes
Interpersonal systems control	
Counter-conditioning	Substitutes alternatives for problem behavior
Stimulus control	Avoids stimuli that produce problem behavior

SOURCE: Adapted from the *Journal of the American Dietetic Association,* 102(Supplement 3), Sigman-Grant, Strategies for counseling adolescents, S32–S39, Copyright (2002), with permission from the American Dietetic Association.

BOX C-2
A Family Seafood Selection Scenario

Description of Family Members

Tom: father; 57 years old; his father died of a heart attack at 56 years old

Nan: mother; 55 years old; no family history of cardiovascular disease

Dave: son; 32 years old; healthy, but his BMI is 28

Sharon: daughter; 25 years old; married to Jim and is 2 months pregnant with her first child

Cindy: cousin; 28 years old; lives in Alaska and is visiting Sharon

Context of their lives

Tom, Nan, Dave, Sharon, and Jim live near a lake in the Midwest. They are recreational fishers but tend to catch and release. They usually purchase seafood from the local supermarket.

The family is very health-conscious, and every member goes for yearly check-ups. During Tom's last visit to his cardiologist, the nurse gave him a pamphlet that encouraged him to eat two servings per week of fish high in omega-3 fatty acids.

Nan's gynecologist confirmed that she is in menopause, encouraged her to continue her healthy lifestyle, and suggested she might want to go to the MyPyramid.gov website to get a personalized diet plan using the new Food Guidance System. Since Tom's father died from a heart attack at a young age, Nan has tried to choose lean meat for dinner, including a weekly serving of lean seafood (primarily shrimp). She chooses shrimp because of local advisories warning against eating fatty fish, due to their DLC content. When she goes to her market, she is unable to tell where the fish came from, so she figured shrimp would be the safest.

Dave relies on fast foods. His primary seafood selection, which is a fried fish sandwich, is eaten at least three times a week. Dave was told by his general practitioner to lose weight and he suggested eating lean poultry, meat, and fish.

Sharon and Jim became more thoughtful about their eating patterns when Sharon's pregnancy was confirmed. Before this time, they rarely ate seafood except for canned white tuna which they used occasionally for luncheon sandwiches. On Sharon's first visit to her obstetrician, she told Sharon to increase her intake of DHA and EPA but then Sharon was given a pamphlet that warned her against eating certain fish because they contain methylmercury. Sharon left the office very confused.

Cindy lives in Alaska with her husband's family, who are Inuit. Cindy has acclimated to her new lifestyle with her husband and family. She now eats their traditional diet, including marine seafood. She is planning to get pregnant and is excited to learn what to expect from Sharon.

D

Open Session and Workshop Agendas

Nutrient Relationships in Seafood:
Selections to Balance Benefits and Risks

Institute of Medicine
Food and Nutrition Board

National Academy of Sciences
2100 C Street, N.W.
Washington, D.C.

Tuesday, February 1, 2005

Agenda for Open Session

1:00 p.m.   Welcome, Introductions, and Purpose of the Public Session
Malden Nesheim, Committee Chair

Presentations from the Sponsoring Agency:

1:10   US Department of Commerce, National Oceanic and Atmospheric Administration, National Marine Fisheries Service
E. Spencer Garret, Director, National Seafood Inspection Laboratory

2:10   US Department of Health and Human Services, Food and Drug Administration
David W. K. Acheson, Chief Medical Officer and Director, Office of Food Safety, Defense and Outreach

2:40   US Environmental Protection Agency
            *Denise Keehner, Director, Standards and Health Protection
                Division, Office of Water*

3:10   Break

3:30   Open Discussion

4:00   Adjourn

Nutrient Relationships in Seafood:
Selections to Balance Benefits and Risks

**National Academy of Sciences (NAS) Building
Auditorium
2101 Constitution Avenue, N.W.
Washington, D.C.**

Monday, April 11, 2005

Preliminary Agenda

8:30 a.m.   Welcome and Purpose of the Workshop
            *Ann Yaktine, Study Director, Food and Nutrition Board,
                IOM
            Malden Nesheim, Chair, Committee on Nutrient
                Relationships in Seafood*

8:45   *Seafood as a Dietary Component*

            Implications of Fatty Acids from Seafood in Chronic
                Disease and Health
            *Lawrence Appel, Johns Hopkins Bloomberg School of
                Public Health*

            Contributions of Seafood to the American Diet
            *Jennifer Weber, Office of Disease Prevention and Health
                Promotion, US Department of Health and Human
                Services*

            Recommendations for Use of Traditional Foods in Alaska
            *Jim Berner, Alaska Native Tribal Consortium
            John Middaugh, Alaska Division of Public Health*

10:00   Panel Questions

10:15   Break

10:30   *Dietary Practices and Vulnerable Populations*

              Traditional Diets in Native Populations
              Don Kashevarof, Alaska Native Tribal Health Consortium

              Communicating Nutrition Messages to Arctic Communities
              Eric Loring, Inuit Tapiriit Kanatami

              The Economic Impact of Fish Consumption Advisories
              Jay Shimshack, Tufts University

11:45   Panel Questions

Noon   Break for Lunch

1:00 p.m.   *Nutrient Benefits from Seafood*

              Population Studies on Health Benefits Associated with
                Seafood
              Joseph Hibbeln, National Institutes of Health

              Selenium Modulation of Toxicants in Seafood
              Nicholas Ralston, University of North Dakota

              Dietary Fatty Acids and Immune System Function
              Philip Calder, University of Southampton

2:15   Panel Questions

2:30   Break

2:45   *Mechanisms of Methylmercury Impact on Neurological*
                Outcomes
              Laurie Chan, McGill University

              Risk Relationships and Seafood Consumption

              Benefits and Risks of Seafood Selections
              Deborah Rice, Maine Bureau of Health

              Assessing Health Risks Associated with Seafood
                Contaminants
              Louise Ryan, Harvard University

3:45   Panel Questions

4:00   *Seafood Conservation and Sustainability*
              Mark Hixon, Oregon State University

4:20   *Interested individuals and organizations are invited to pres-*
            ent their views during this part of the open session. To
            be considered for a 3-minute presentation, please provide
            topic and contact information to Sandra Amamoo-Kakra
            no later than March 28, 2005, by fax (202) 334-2316, or
            by e-mail (samamook@nas.edu).

4:45   Adjourn

E

Committee Member Biographical Sketches

Malden C. Nesheim, Ph.D. (*Chair*), is Provost Emeritus and Professor of Nutrition Emeritus at Cornell. His previous positions have included Director of the Division of Nutritional Sciences and Vice President for the Planning and Budgeting Program at Cornell University. He has also served as Chair of the Board of Trustees of the Pan American Health and Education Foundation, President of the American Institute of Nutrition, Chair of the National Institutes of Health Nutrition Study Section, and Chair of the National Nutrition Consortium. He also chaired the 1990 US Department of Agriculture/Department of Health and Human Services Dietary Guidelines Advisory Committee and has served as an advisor to the Office of Science and Technology Policy. He is a fellow of the American Society for Nutritional Sciences and of the American Academy of Arts and Sciences. Dr. Nesheim is the recipient of numerous awards including the Conrad A. Elvehjem Award for Distinguished Service to the Public through the Science of Nutrition. His research interests are in human nutrition, nutritional requirements, dietary recommendations, and nutrition policy.

David C. Bellinger, Ph.D., is Professor of Neurology at the Harvard Medical School and Professor in the Department of Environmental Health at the Harvard School of Public Health. He also directs an interdisciplinary postdoctoral training program in Neurodevelopmental Toxicology at the Harvard School of Public Health. Dr. Bellinger has served on the National Research Council's Committee on Evaluation of Children's Health, the Committee on the Toxicological Effects of Mercury, the Committee on Measuring Lead Exposure in Critical Populations, and the Committee on Toxicology Subcommittee on Submarine Escape Action Levels. He has also served on the FAO/WHO Joint Expert Committee on Food Additives and Contaminants. He was a member of the Federal Advisory Committee of the National Children's Study to examine the effects of environmental influences on the health and development of children. Dr. Bellinger's research interests include early insults to the developing nervous system, exogenous chemical exposures, and endogenous metabolic insults related to serious medical conditions. Much of his research has focused on the neurodevelopmental effects of children's exposures to metals, including lead, mercury, arsenic, and manganese.

Ann Bostrom, Ph.D., is Associate Professor at the School of Public Policy, Georgia Institute of Technology. She is also Associate Dean for Research in the Ivan Allen College, the liberal arts college at Georgia Tech. Dr. Bostrom's research and expertise are in risk perception and communication. Her research focuses on mental models of hazardous processes, including the perception, communication, and management of global environmental change. Dr. Bostrom is currently a member of the US EPA Science Advisory Board Committee on Valuing the Protection of Ecosystems and Ecoservices, and has served on committees for the National Research Council and the Transportation Research Board. In 1997, Dr. Bostrom was awarded the Chauncey Starr Award for a young risk analyst from the Society for Risk Analysis. From 1999–2001, Dr. Bostrom directed the Decision, Risk and Management Science Program at the National Science Foundation. She has previously served on the National Research Council Committee on Optimizing the Characterization and Transportation of Transuranic Waste Destined for the Waste Isolation Pilot Plant, the Committee for the Study of a Motor Vehicle Rollover Rating System, and the Committee for a Study of Consumer Automotive Safety Information.

Susan E. Carlson, Ph.D., is the Midwest Dairy Council Professor of Nutrition at the University of Kansas Medical Center (Kansas City) in the Schools of Allied Health (Dietetics and Nutrition), Medicine (Pediatrics) and Nursing; and Clinical Professor of Obstetrics and Gynecology at the University of Missouri–Kansas City (Kansas City). Her research interests include the nutritional role of long-chain polyunsaturated fatty acids in pregnancy outcome and infant development. In 2002, she was made an honorary member of the American Dietetic Association for her pioneering work in proposing and testing the theory that dietary docosahexaenoic acid (DHA), a component of human milk, is important for the developing human central nervous system. Dr. Carlson is an author on numerous peer-reviewed articles and textbook chapters. She is a charter member of the International Society for the Study of Fatty Acids and Lipids (ISSFAL) and has been an organizer for two international conferences on the role of long-chain polyunsaturated fatty acids for maternal and infant health. She is also a member of the American Society for Nutrition, American Society for Nutritional Sciences, the American Pediatric Society, and the American Oil Chemists Society. Dr. Carlson reviews widely for journals devoted to publishing research in pediatrics, lipids, and nutrition.

Julie A. Caswell, Ph.D., is Professor and Chairperson in the Department of Resource Economics and Adjunct Professor of Food Science at the University of Massachusetts–Amherst. She served on the Institute of Medicine's Committee on the Implications of Dioxin in the Food Supply. Her research interests include the operation of domestic and international food systems, analyzing food system efficiency, and evaluating government policy as it affects systems operation and performance, in particular the economics of food quality, safety, and nutrition. Her edited book publications include *Economics of Food Safety, Valuing Food Safety and Nutrition*, and *Global Food Trade and Consumer Demand for Quality*. Dr. Caswell has provided her expertise to the UN Food and Agriculture Organization and the Organization for Economic Cooperation and Development on food safety issues. She is a member of the Food Safety Research Consortium. From 1989–2002 she chaired the Regional Research Project NE-165, an international group of over 100 economists who analyzed the operation and performance of the food system. She has also held numerous senior positions with the American Agricultural Economics Association and the Northeastern Agricultural and Resource Economics Association.

Claude Earl Fox, M.D., M.P.H., is Professor in the Department of Epidemiology at the University of Miami and was previously a Professor of Population and Family Health Sciences in the Johns Hopkins Bloomberg School of Public Health. Dr. Fox is also former Director of the Johns Hopkins Urban Health Institute in Baltimore. Prior to this, Dr. Fox was Administrator of the Health Resources and Services Administration of the US Department of Health and Human Services. His research focuses on population and family health and urban health. Dr. Fox served as the co-chair for the Institute of Medicine's Committee on Review of the Use of Scientific Criteria and Performance Standards for Safe Food. He has published widely on family and health issues and improving the nation's health. Dr. Fox is a recipient of the John Atkinson Farroll Prize for Outstanding Contributions to Preventive Medicine and Public Health; the Gay and Lesbian Medical Association Leadership Award; the Special Recognition Award from the National Rural Health Association; the Association of State and Territorial Health Officials Leadership Award; the National Hispanic Medical Association Leadership Award; and others, and he is a member of the Delta Omega Honorary Public Health Society.

Jennifer Hillard is a volunteer with the Consumer Interest Alliance of Canada. From 1996–2002, she served as National Vice President of Issues and Policy at the Consumer Association of Canada (CAC). She has produced informational booklets in collaboration with the CAC and the Food Biotechnology Communications network. Ms. Hillard also served on the National Research Council/Institute of Medicine's Committee on Identifying and Assessing Unintended Effects of Genetically Engineered Foods on Human Health. She has written many health and safety articles for publications designed for low-literacy consumers.

Susan M. Krebs-Smith, Ph.D., M.P.H., is Chief of the Risk Factor Monitoring and Methods Branch of the Division of Cancer Control and Population Sciences of the National Cancer Institute. She oversees a program of research on the surveillance of risk factors related to cancer—including diet, physical activity, weight status, tobacco use, sun exposure, genetics, and family history; methodological issues to improve the assessment of those factors; and issues related to guidance and food policy. In a previous position at US Department of Agriculture, Dr. Krebs-Smith was a member of the team that developed and tested food guidance recommendations that were subsequently adopted in the *Dietary Guidelines for Americans* and the original Food Guide Pyramid. More recently, she was a member of the drafting committee for the 2005 *Dietary Guidelines.* Her contributions in the area of dietary assessment methodology have focused on reported food intake differences between low energy reporters (LER) and non-LERs, on developing methods to assess dietary patterns, and on estimating usual dietary intake. Dr. Krebs-Smith is a member of the International Advisory Committee, Sixth International Conference on Dietary Assessment Methods, and has served on the editorial boards for both the *Journal of the American Dietetic Association* and the *Journal of Nutrition Education,* and on the Governing Council of the American Public Health Association.

Stanley T. Omaye, Ph.D., is Professor in the Department of Nutrition at the University of Nevada–Reno. Dr. Omaye served as Chief of the Applied Nutrition Branch and as research chemist for the Biochemistry Division, Department of Nutrition at Letterman Army Institute of Research, San Francisco, CA. He also served the US Department of Agriculture as project leader and research chemist at the Western Human Nutrition Center, San Francisco, and project leader and research nutritionist at the Western Regional Research Center, Berkeley. Dr. Omaye is a member of the American College of Nutrition, the Western Pharmacology Society, the American College of Toxicology, the Society of Toxicology, the American Society for Nutritional Sciences, the American Society for Pharmacology and Experimental Therapeutics, and the Institute of Food Technologists. He is author or coauthor of more than 160 publications and serves on the editorial boards of *Toxicology, Society of Experimental Biology and Medicine,* and *Nutritional and Environmental Medicine.* Dr. Omaye is a certified nutrition specialist and a Fellow of the Academy of Toxicological Sciences and of the American College of Nutrition. Dr. Omaye's research efforts are directed at air pollutants, food toxins, selected phytochemicals, tobacco smoke, and aging.

Jose M. Ordovas, Ph.D., is Senior Scientist and Director of the Nutrition and Genomics Laboratory, Jean Mayer USDA Human Nutrition Research Center on Aging at Tufts University. Dr. Ordovas' major research interests focus on the genetic factors predisposing to cardiovascular disease and their interaction with the environment and behavioral factors with special emphasis on diet, particularly omega-3 and -6 fatty acids. He has participated in the Framingham Heart Study for nearly 20 years and is carrying out multiple cross-cultural studies to determine cardiovascular risk in different populations around the world, including Asian Pacific and Mediterranean populations. He has written numerous reviews and edited several books on diet and coronary heart disease, diet and genetics, and the role of omega-3 fatty acids on lipoproteins and atherosclerosis. Dr. Ordovas serves on numerous editorial boards and is active with several American Heart Association and National Institutes of Health committees, including the National Heart, Lung, and Blood Institute Program Projects Parent Committee. Throughout his career, Dr. Ordovas has contributed his expertise to various global organizations. He has served as Nutrition Expert for the American Soybean Association, consulting for Mexico and Central America; was named Expert Consultant to the Singapore Ministry of Health; and is the recipient of the Francisco Grande Memorial Lecture for Excellence in Nutrition.

W. Steven Otwell, Ph.D., is a Professor in the Food Science and Human Nutrition Department of the University of Florida's Institute of Food and Agriculture Sciences. Dr. Otwell is recipient of the Institute of Food Technology's Myron Solberg Award for Excellence and Leadership. Dr. Otwell is the national director of the Seafood Hazard Analysis and Critical Control Points Alliance to help seafood processors and inspectors comply with federal food safety regulations. In 1997, he received Vice President Gore's National Performance Review Award for leadership of the nationwide seafood safety training program. His research focus is assuring quality, safety, and developments for the seafood industry and general public welfare.

Madeleine Sigman-Grant, Ph.D., R.D., is Professor and Area Specialist at the University of Nevada Cooperative Extension. Dr. Sigman-Grant is nationally known for her work in maternal and early childhood health and nutrition. She received an Early Extension Career Award in 1992 from Epsilon Sigma Phi, a Cooperative Extension honorary fraternity. She served as a member of the Food Advisory Committee for the Food and Drug Administration and is currently a member of the American Academy of Pediatrics panel revising Bright Futures. She is a member of the Society for Nutrition Education, the American Society of Nutrition, the American Dietetic Association and the International Society for Research in Human Milk and Lactation.

Nicolas Stettler, M.D., MSCE, is Assistant Professor of Pediatrics and Epidemiology at the Children's Hospital of Philadelphia and Senior Scholar at the Center for Clinical Epidemiology and Biostatistics at the University of Pennsylvania School of Medicine. Dr. Stettler is a pediatrician with specialty certification by the American Board of Physician Nutrition Specialists. He is a Fellow of the American Heart Association, the American Academy of Pediatrics, a member of the World Heart Federation, the International Epidemiology Association, and the European and American Societies for Pediatric Research. Dr. Stettler's research interest is in the epidemiology and prevention of obesity and related cardiovascular risk factors in childhood with special emphasis on a life course approach to the development of obesity and related complications.

FNB Liaison

Susan A. Ferenc, D.V.M., Ph.D., is the President of the Chemical Producers and Distributors Association in Alexandria, Virginia. Prior to this position, she served as the Executive Vice President for Scientific and Regulatory Affairs and Chief Science Officer at the Food Products Association, Washington, D.C. Previous experience includes serving as Principal and Senior Consultant, SAF*RISK LC, Madison, Wisconsin; and as Vice President, Scientific and Regulatory Policy, Grocery Manufacturers Association (GMA); Senior Scientist, ILSI Risk Science Institute; and Risk Science Specialist, US Department of Agriculture Office of Risk Assessment and Cost-Benefit Analysis, in Washington, D.C. She also has extensive experience in international field research, having coordinated projects in South America, Africa, and the Caribbean. Areas of expertise include food safety and risk assessment, international program coordination, agricultural policy analysis, food and resource economics, and veterinary medicine and parasitology. Dr. Ferenc belongs to a number of professional societies and has coordinated, chaired, or presented at numerous US and international working groups, expert consultations, and conferences dealing with food safety/risk analysis, etc. She has also published reports, abstracts, books, and presentations dealing with related topics.

Index